THE A-TO-Z GUIDE TO
ELDER C

362.609 Kan
Kandel, Joseph
A to z guide to elder care /
$19.95   ocn314017698

5
8
06/25/2009

WITHDRAWN

Joseph Kandel, M.D.
and
Christine Adamec

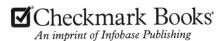

☑ Checkmark Books*
An imprint of Infobase Publishing

The A-to-Z Guide to Elder Care

Copyright © 2009 by Christine Adamec

All rights reserved. No part of this book may be reproduced or utilized in any form or by any means, electronic or mechanical, including photocopying, recording, or by any information storage or retrieval systems, without permission in writing from the publisher. For information contact:

Checkmark Books
An imprint of Infobase Publishing, Inc.
132 West 31st Street
New York NY 10001

ISBN-13: 978-0-8160-7910-0
ISBN-10: 0-8160-7910-2

The Library of Congress has cataloged the hardcover edition of this work as follows:

Kandel, Joseph.
The encyclopedia of elder care / Joseph Kandel and Christine Adamec.
        p. ; cm. — (Facts On File library of health and living)
Includes bibliographical references and index.
ISBN-13: 978-0-8160-7216-3 (alk. paper)
ISBN-10: 0-8160-7216-7 (alk. paper)
1. Older people—Care—United States—Encyclopedias. 2. Older people—Care—Canada—Encyclopedias.
3. Older people—Medical care—United States—Encyclopedias. 4. Older people—Medical care—Canada—
Encyclopedias. 5. Caregivers—United States—Encyclopedias. 6. Caregivers—Canada—Encyclopedias.
7. Geriatrics—United States—Encyclopedias. 8. Geriatrics—Canada—Encyclopedias.
I. Adamec, Christine A., 1949– II. Title.
HV1461.K34 2009
362.60973′03—dc22   2008018297

Checkmark Books are available at special discounts when purchased in bulk quantities for businesses, associations, institutions, or sales promotions. Please call our Special Sales Department in New York at (212) 967-8800 or (800) 322-8755.

You can find Facts On File on the World Wide Web at http://www.factsonfile.com

Text and cover design by Cathy Rincon

Printed in the United States of America

Bang Hermitage 10 9 8 7 6 5 4 3 2 1

This book is printed on acid-free paper.

This book is dedicated to my wife, Merrylee,
for her continued support, love, caring, and patience.
Her insight, wit, and wisdom make this and
every other project so worthwhile.

Always,
Joseph Kandel

❧

I dedicate this book to my husband, John Adamec, who is always
supportive and immensely helpful to me in all my endeavors.
I also thank my daughter, Jane, and my young grandson, Tyler,
for their patience and support.

—Christine Adamec

CONTENTS

FOREWORD

Increasing numbers of people in the United States and Canada, as well as in countries throughout the world, are living significantly longer lives than ever before, and, for the most part, this is a very good thing. However, at the same time, it is also important to acknowledge that older people, and especially the very old who are age 85 and older, often have serious physical, mental, and emotional health problems and other needs that cannot or should not be ignored by others.

As people attain the age at which most people regard them as elderly (age 65 and older), they frequently need the care and attention of others, such as their doctors and family members. Sometimes those other individuals are their own very busy middle-aged adult children who are struggling with managing their careers, caring for their children (and sometimes even their grandchildren), paying their mortgages and other bills, and coping with their own health problems. Often these adult children are exhausted by their current struggles to somehow balance the time and money needed to manage their multiple and complex responsibilities. It is also true that sometimes these "adult children" are actually age 65 and older themselves, and they are elderly retirees struggling to help their elderly parents who may be 85 years old or older.

Yet when the person who is in need is an elderly parent or another aged relative, many people try their best to marshal the emotional, physical, and financial strength and resources that are necessary to help the older person. This is true whether the tasks involve sorting out the elderly person's financial resources and bills, driving the older person to the doctor or dentist, or helping the elderly person understand specifically what the doctor has recommended as treatment for their ailments. Sometimes helping an elderly parent or relative involves accomplishing all of these tasks and many more.

Other tasks may involve helping the older person locate a new place to live that fulfills his or her needs, whether that be independent living, assisted living, a nursing home, or, sometimes, the home of the relative is the choice. In other cases, the elderly person chooses to stay in his or her own home, with backup help such as home health care or delivered meals, and with relatives or others periodically checking to make sure that he or she is really all right.

Many older people suffer from neurological and psychiatric problems, ranging from depression and anxiety disorders to Alzheimer's disease and other very debilitating forms of dementia. Others struggle with Parkinson's disease or the aftereffects of a major and devastating stroke. It can be extremely difficult for the older person as well as for his or her family members and others to deal with the major and ongoing health needs of elderly people with such profound problems.

Another key issue and concern with elder care is that some elderly people who live alone (and women are more likely than men to live alone) begin to neglect their health, through what is sometimes called "self-neglect." They fail to eat sufficiently, may stop paying their bills, and may begin to hoard many pets or disparate items, such as magazines or trinkets. A once neat and clean person living in a formerly tidy house may become disheveled and dirty because he or she forgets to bathe or is afraid of falling down in the tub. He or she may also become malnourished and forget to eat or cannot prepare meals. Their pets may become sickly looking, and old animal feces may be found throughout the house because the older person did not remember to take the dog out or clean the cat's litter box. These are warning signs to their family members and others that something is really wrong and that hard choices will have to be made. Understandably the older person may not appreciate these actions at all, seeing them instead as a personal attack and a cruel act. Very few people wish to go to a nursing home, no matter how ill they are. This can be a very painful emotional position for family members who are sincerely trying to help the older person.

Many older people suffer from serious illnesses that can cause emotional distress and confusion, such as cancer, heart disease, and kidney disease or failure. They may need to undergo frightening laboratory tests and may also be confused by their doctors' medical jargon and directions and complex medication dosage instructions that would be difficult for even a much younger person to comprehend. Often they rely upon their adult children or other family members, not only for moral support but also as interpreters for the medical information provided by busy doctors and nurses.

As medical knowledge continues to advance, many new diseases and disorders have been discovered in recent years, and many are discussed in this book. For example, sarcopenia, or the loss of skeletal muscle mass, is a serious problem in the elderly and affects up to 40 percent of those older than age 85. This loss leads to an increased risk of falling down as well as difficulties in managing day-to-day activities as simple as getting up from a chair. A variety of drugs and hormones have been tested and developed in an attempt to halt this loss, but so far only resistance/strength training has been proven to improve the condition significantly.

There are also very important but difficult end-of-life issues for caregivers to consider in relation to aging parents and older relatives. For example,

if an older person does not have a living will and refuses to create one, others may have to make lifesaving decisions for him or her if the elderly person needs heroic medical measures to stay alive. Again, adult children or other relatives usually make these choices.

Making these decisions is extremely difficult and it is also fraught with emotion for family members. If no one (such as a "health-care agent" or "health-care proxy") has been specifically designated in writing to make such decisions, adult siblings may worry about whether they should let Dad, unconscious and on a respirator, die. Or should they keep urging the doctors to try heroic measures because maybe that is what Dad would have wanted? These are difficult questions for any person to deal with.

For this reason *The A-to-Z Guide to Elder Care* includes an entry on talking with elderly parents about difficult issues, as well as entries on cremation, death, funerals, living wills, and other issues that are unpleasant to think about but which are important to consider before a serious health crisis or death occurs.

The A-to-Z Guide to Elder Care offers a comprehensive overview of medical, psychological, emotional, legal, and other issues that surround providing for the needs of many individuals age 65 and older in the United States and Canada. Some entries also concentrate on the caregivers themselves, such as entries on coping with compassion fatigue or even dealing with sibling rivalry issues when one sister wants Mom to take one course of action and a brother or another sister is strongly opposed.

In many cases some siblings and other relatives are in complete denial about the true capabilities of their parents, and as a result, they refuse to acknowledge that the older person may have (or does have) Alzheimer's disease or another form of dementia. At the same time, in many cases, other siblings or relatives are fully aware of their parent's abilities and limitations. For example, some family members may think that everything is just fine, while other family members are acutely aware that their relative has advanced dementia and needs help. These two mindsets may collide in a painful manner involving arguments and accusations. The relative who thinks that Dad should stay at home believes that she is acting in his best interest, while another relative realizes that Dad has advanced Alzheimer's and wants him to relocate to a nursing home where he will be safe. She is also convinced that she has her father's best interest at heart. Only by acknowledging the reality of the situation can an adult child or other relative truly help the elderly person.

In addition, sometimes the adult child or relative neglects his or her own health or personal needs to provide care and assistance to the older person, leading to development of what some call compassion fatigue and others call burnout. This basically means that the caregiver gives up and may behave in what seems to others like a very cold manner. If the caregiver becomes ill, then care can no longer be provided or can only be provided on a limited basis. Thus, it is important for caregivers to take into account their own health and personal needs.

We hope that *The A-to-Z Guide to Elder Care* will provide a good starting place for readers and that it may also be a resource to return to again and again for those who need information and understanding about the complexity of elder care as well as difficult end-of-life issues.

—Joseph Kandel, M.D.

INTRODUCTION

If you're worried about the current or future health, housing, or financial status of an elderly parent, spouse, or relative, then you are definitely not alone. As people in the United States and Canada (and worldwide) live increasingly longer lives, there are also many more aging relatives who need some looking after. Most people ages 65 and older have at least one serious health condition, according to the U.S. Census Bureau and other sources, and about 50 percent of them have two or more serious medical problems. Sometimes older people can monitor their own health conditions, but other times they need assistance from others.

In many cases, those "others" are their adult children, grandchildren, or other relatives, whether they directly help the older person with transportation, bill paying, personal care, or all of the above, or whether they find home-care professionals or other experts to take on jobs once handled by the older person. Providing help to an aging relative is a responsibility assumed from love, but it can also be a very daunting one, especially if the older person has or is developing one of the various forms of dementia or is physically disabled or both. In addition, working with relatives who are now struggling, when you still fondly remember them as healthy and alert people, can be emotionally painful and difficult for the most well-adjusted person.

The Increasing Population of Older People

Older people represent a much larger proportion of our society than ever before. For example, in 1900, people 65 to 74 years old represented only about 3 percent of the total population in the United States. By 2000 this percentage had more than doubled to 6.5 percent. Looking at the bigger picture of *all* older people, in 2006, people 65 and older made of 12.5 percent of the population, or a total of 37,424,750 people. By 2030, when all the baby boomers (born 1946–1964) will all be 65 and older, older people will represent 20 percent of all Americans. There were also 84,331 estimated centenarians (people who are age 100 or older) living in the United States as of 2007 (the latest information available as of this writing), more than double the 37,306 centenarians living in 1990.

A key reason for this radically improved longevity is the amazing breakthroughs in the treatment of very serious health problems that were certain killers throughout most of the 20th century, such as cancer, heart disease, and diabetes. Of course people still die from these diseases and others, since death itself has not been conquered. But physicians now carefully monitor most people with serious diseases, and they can also find and treat many diseases before they become severe or fatal. Ironically, however, this also means that a significant portion of the elderly population is older and sicker than ever before.

Who Are the Elderly in the United States?

According to the Census Bureau, in 2006, more than half of the elderly lived in nine states, including California, Florida, New York, Texas, Pennsylvania,

Illinois, Ohio, Michigan, and New Jersey. Florida had the highest percent of elderly individuals compared with individuals of all ages in the state (16.8 percent), followed by West Virginia (15.3 percent). The states with the lowest percentages of elderly people in 2006 were Alaska (6.8 percent) and Utah (8.8 percent). See Table 1 to find your state.

Some counties in the United States have a large percentage of older people, according to the Census Bureau; for example, McIntosh County, North Dakota, has the largest proportion of older people in the United States, a whopping 35 percent. Some Florida areas have more than 30 percent older people, such as the Clearwater–St. Petersburg–Tampa area.

TABLE 1: U.S. POPULATION AND PERCENT AGES 65 YEARS AND OLDER, BY STATE, 2006 (POPULATION DATA ARE IN THOUSANDS, ROUNDED OFF; THUS, 299,398 MEANS ABOUT 299,398,000 PEOPLE IN THE UNITED STATES, AND 4,599 IN ALABAMA MEANS 4,599,000 TOTAL PEOPLE IN ALABAMA.)

Numbers	Total Population	Percent 65 Years and Older
U.S. Total (50 States + D.C.)	299,398	12.5
Alabama	4,599	13.4
Alaska	670	6.8
Arizona	6,166	12.8
Arkansas	2,811	13.9
California	36,458	10.8
Colorado	4,753	10.0
Connecticut	3,505	13.4
Delaware	853	13.4
District of Columbia	582	12.3
Florida	18,090	16.8
Georgia	9,364	9.8
Hawaii	1,285	14.0
Idaho	1,466	11.5
Illinois	12,382	12.0
Indiana	6,314	12.4
Iowa	2,982	14.6
Kansas	2,764	12.9
Kentucky	4,206	12.8
Louisiana	4,288	12.2
Maine	1,322	14.6
Maryland	5,616	11.6
Massachusetts	6,437	13.3
Michigan	10,096	12.5
Minnesota	5,167	12.1
Mississippi	2,911	12.4
Missouri	5,843	13.3
Montana	945	13.8
Nebraska	1,768	13.3
Nevada	2,496	11.1
New Hampshire	1,315	12.4
New Jersey	8,725	12.9
New Mexico	1,955	12.4
New York	19,306	13.1
North Carolina	8,857	12.2
North Dakota	636	14.6
Ohio	11,478	13.4
Oklahoma	3,579	13.2
Oregon	3,701	12.9
Pennsylvania	12,441	15.2
Rhode Island	1,068	13.9
South Carolina	4,321	12.8
South Dakota	782	14.2
Tennessee	6,039	12.7
Texas	23,508	9.9
Utah	2,550	8.8
Vermont	624	13.3
Virginia	7,643	11.6
Washington	6,396	11.5
West Virginia	1,818	15.3
Wisconsin	5,557	13.0
Wyoming	515	12.2

Source: Adapted from *Resident Population by Age and State: 2006*. Washington, D.C.: U.S. Census Bureau.

Racial Makeup and Health Risks among Older Americans

In 2005 most older people in the United States were white, and about 19 percent of the elderly were minority members, including 8.3 percent who were African-American, 6.2 percent who were Hispanic, 3 percent who were Asian or Pacific Islander, and less than 1 percent who were American Indian or Native Alaskan. Table 2 shows a comparison of older people in 2000–2003 in terms of different ages, genders, and race/ethnicities, as well as the incidence of specific major diseases and disorders,

TABLE 2. NUMBER AND PERCENTAGE OF ADULTS AGES 65 AND OLDER BY SELECTED HEALTH STATUS, CONDITION OR IMPAIRMENT, AND OTHER CHARACTERISTICS, AVERAGE ANNUAL, 2000–2003

Selected Characteristic	Population (in thousands)	Fair or Poor Health	Hypertension	Heart Disease	Diabetes	Hearing Impairment	Vision Impairment	Lost All Natural Teeth
Age								
65 and over	33,219	26.0	50.1	31.1	15.9	38.5	17.4	27.6
65–74	17,876	22.9	47.9	26.7	17.0	31.4	13.9	24.0
75–84	12,075	28.5	53.2	35.6	15.5	43.9	19.1	29.5
85 +	3,268	33.6	50.5	38.5	11.0	58.0	30.3	40.2
Sex								
Men	14,147	26.4	46.7	36.3	18.1	47.5	16.0	26.2
Women	19,072	25.7	52.6	27.2	14.2	31.9	18.5	28.6
Race and Hispanic Origin								
White, not Hispanic	27,529	23.5	48.5	32.4	14.4	41.0	17.0	26.7
Black, not Hispanic	2,685	41.1	66.9	25.8	24.2	24.4	20.5	35.4
Asian, not Hispanic	649	25.7	53.5	24.6	14.6	34.0	15.2	24.3
Hispanic	2,015	39.6	46.9	21.5	23.5	24.5	19.1	28.7
Poverty Status								
Poor	2,479	42.5	56.2	32.7	20.4	36.8	24.7	44.6
Near poor	6,083	33.8	55.2	33.5	18.4	40.6	22.4	38.2
Not poor	12,791	19.7	48.6	31.2	14.8	40.0	15.7	20.9

Source: Adapted from Charlotte A. Schoenborn, Jackline L. Vickerie, and Eva Powell-Griner. "Health Characteristics of Adults 55 Years of Age and Over: United States, 2000–2003." In *Advance Data from Vital and Health Statistics* 370 (April 11, 2006): 14–15.

such as hypertension, heart disease, diabetes, and hearing and vision loss.

Diseases are not equal opportunity offenders, and some races are hit harder by them than others. For example, elderly blacks in 2003 had the highest rate of hypertension compared with other races (66.9 percent), followed by elderly Asians (53.5 percent). For example, as can be seen in Table 2, elderly blacks also had the highest rate of diabetes (24.2 percent), followed closely by Hispanics (23.5 percent). In addition, blacks were the most likely to have lost all their natural teeth by age 65 and older (35.4 percent), followed by Hispanics (28.7 percent).

In considering the issue of poor or fair health, African Americans age 65 and older in the United States had the greatest risk for poor or fair health (41.1 percent), followed by Hispanics (39.6 percent) and Asians (24.7 percent). In contrast, whites had the lowest rate of fair or poor health, at 23.5 percent.

Older white people had some higher rates of disease than other races; for example, elderly whites had the highest rates of hearing impairment (41 percent), followed by Asians (34 percent). Whites also had the highest rate of heart disease (32.4 percent), followed by blacks (25.8 percent).

Gender Disparities

In the United States, as well as in other countries, females are much more likely to live to advanced ages than are males, and, consequently, the percentage of the female population increases with age. Older men are much more likely to be married than older women; for example, among men ages 65–74, 78 percent are married, compared to 57 percent of women in the same age group.

Many older women are widows living alone, whether in their own homes or apartments or in assisted-living facilities. A minority of older females reside in nursing homes. According to the U.S. Census Bureau, in 2007 more than twice as many women age 65 and older lived alone (39 percent) compared with older men who lived alone (19 percent). It is not that older women necessarily *want* to live alone, but rather that they have often outlived their spouses or partners. For example, data in 2006 from the Census Bureau showed that 42.4 percent of women ages 65 and older were widowed, compared to only 13.1 percent of older men.

Elderly women are more likely to be physically disabled than older men, suffering from such non-fatal problems as back pain, fractures, osteoporosis, osteoarthritis, and depression than men, according to the *American Journal of Public Health*. In this survey of 1,348 men and women with an average age of 79, the researchers found that women were more likely to need assistance from others and to report activity limitations, largely because of their disabilities. The one area in which older men reported needing more help than older women was in dressing and grooming themselves. But women had more trouble than men in the areas of arising, eating, walking, hygiene, reaching items, performing errands, and gripping items.

The researchers also found that men were heavier smokers and drinkers than the women.

Military Veterans

Some elderly people are older military veterans living in the United States, primarily from World War II and the Korean War, with some veterans from the Vietnam War, and there were 400,000 male veterans over age 85 in 2000. (About 95 percent of older veterans are male.) The number of veterans ages 65 and older is expected to increase to nearly 1.2 million by 2010, with the aging of Vietnam War veterans. Many older veterans receive services from the Veterans Health Administration (VHA): in 2006, about 2.4 million veterans ages 65 and older received assistance from the VHA. Another 1.1 million veterans were enrolled to receive VHA services, although they did not use them in 2006.

Elders Have Increasingly Impaired Abilities

As most people who live with and/or love an older person know, with aging also comes an increased risk of the older person experiencing major dif-ficulties performing many everyday tasks, such as managing money, performing routine household chores, preparing food, and even just getting in and out of a chair or bed. As you can imagine, individuals who are age 80 and older have the greatest risk for having trouble performing these everyday tasks.

According to the National Center for Health Statistics, about 6 percent of people ages 60 to 69 in 1999–2002 had trouble managing their own money. This increased to 10 percent for those 70 to 79, and more than doubled again to 24 percent for those 80 and older. Table 3 provides data on the percentage of older adults who struggle with certain everyday tasks (or cannot perform them at all), such as preparing meals or getting dressed.

You may be providing your elderly relative with assistance in managing basic finances, which is a common problem. Sometimes family members are shocked when they find a sheaf of unpaid bills at a parent's house, because Mom was always a real stickler for paying bills on time.

Another area of concern is that even if your parent or other relative has never been a subject of a scam before, many elderly people are at high risk for being cheated, even of their life savings, by criminals who find that they are easy prey. Scam artists can be very aggressive and persistent. If they appear at the older person's door, wanting to perform roof repair because they are "in the neighborhood," they often act very friendly to obtain the trust of the older person so they can then "move in for the kill," financially speaking. Money is paid, and the roof isn't repaired—or a very shoddy job is performed. To avoid this problem, it is a good idea to warn elderly people that you cannot judge a salesperson by appearance, and even people who seem very nice can be very bad people.

Increasing numbers of older people are learning to use the Internet, wanting to see what all the fuss is about. They are very vulnerable to spam and scams and may need repeated warnings to NOT give their bank account numbers to people sending them "warnings" that their account is in danger. (It is in danger, but from the person trying to scam the older person.)

TABLE 3. PERCENTAGE OF ADULTS, AGE 60 AND OLDER, HAVING ANY DIFFICULTY PERFORMING SELECTED FUNCTIONAL ACTIVITIES OR WHO WERE UNABLE TO PERFORM THESE ACTIVITIES, BY AGE, 1999–2002

Functional Activities	60–69 years old		70–79 years old		80 and older	
	Sample Size	Percentage	Sample Size	Percentage	Sample Size	Percentage
Managing money	1,555	8	1,180	10	956	24
Walking for a quarter of a mile	1,418	21	1,070	30	831	49
Walking up 10 steps without resting	1,421	18	1,066	26	825	41
Stooping, crouching, or kneeling	1,556	42	1,183	52	963	66
Lifting or carrying something as heavy as 10 pounds	1,555	22	1,180	28	958	46
Doing chores around the house	1,555	20	1,180	28	960	44
Preparing one's own meals	1,554	8	1,179	12	961	27
Walking between rooms on the same floor	1,557	7	1,183	11	962	24
Standing up from armless chair	1,556	17	1,183	26	962	45
Getting in and out of bed	1,557	14	1,183	15	963	28
Holding a fork, cutting food, or drinking from a glass	1,557	3	1,183	6	963	11
Dressing oneself	1,557	10	1,182	13	963	24
Standing or being on one's feet for about two hours	1,544	32	1,171	43	952	63
Sitting for about two hours	1,556	20	1,180	22	961	21
Reaching up over one's head	1,567	16	1,181	15	962	26
Using one's fingers to grasp or hold small objects	1,557	12	1,182	17	962	25
Going out to do things like shopping, movies, or sporting events	1,556	15	1,180	21	961	39
Participating in social activities	1,552	13	1,179	16	961	34
Doing things to relax at home or for leisure	1,556	5	1,181	5	961	14

Source: R. Bethene Ervin. "Prevalence of Functional Limitations among Adults 60 Years of Age and Over: United States, 1999–2002." *Advance Data from Vital and Health Statistics* 375 (August 23, 2006): 5.

Alzheimer's Disease and Other Forms of Dementia

One of the biggest areas of concern when it comes to older people is Alzheimer's disease. Will your parent get it? Even worse, if your parent develops Alzheimer's, does this mean that *you* will inevitably get it too? The answer to the first question is that, by the time most individuals reach age 85, the National Institute on Aging reports that an estimated half of these people either have or may be developing Alzheimer's disease or another form of dementia. The answer to the second question is that the most hereditary form of Alzheimer's is the early-onset form, and the type that is associated with aging is apparently much less likely to be inherited.

However, researchers have found an increased risk for late-onset Alzheimer's disease on the apolipoprotein E (APOE) gene on chromosome 19. There are three common alleles, and APOE allele 4 apparently increases the risk for Alzheimer's disease. People inherit one APOE allele from each parent, and having one or two copies of allele 4 increases the risk for getting Alzheimer's. But even people who inherit two copies of allele 4 may not develop Alzheimer's disease, while some people who inherit no copies of allele 4 *do* develop Alzheimer's. So even if you could have your blood tested for its alleles (you cannot), you still could not know whether you were at risk for getting Alzheimer's.

In contrast, the Alzheimer's Disease Education & Referral Center (ADEAR) of the National Institute on Aging reports that it is largely early-onset Alzheimer's that runs in families, primarily caused by genetic mutations to chromosomes 1, 14, or 21. This is the form of Alzheimer's that starts before age 65, and it represents less than 5 percent of all cases of Alzheimer's disease.

Adult children and others with a relative who has Alzheimer's disease, and who worry that losing their car keys once in a while or forgetting someone's name means they have symptoms of Alzheimer's, should stop worrying. Forgetting where you put the car keys or forgetting the name of your neighbor of many years, Mrs. Magillicuddy, are not signs of Alzheimer's. However, if you forget what car keys are for (to start the car) or if that lady who has been your neighbor seems like a total stranger, these could be signs of Alzheimer's. Of course, only a physician can diagnose Alzheimer's disease.

Although your fears should be at least somewhat calmed, it's still true that your aging relative (or you) may develop Alzheimer's or another form of dementia. (The major and obscure forms of dementia are described in this book.) Scientists have found medications to slow the progression of Alzheimer's disease or control behavioral symptoms or both, such as donepezil (Aricept), galantamine (Razadyne), memantine (Namenda), and rivastigmine (Exelon). But what is needed is some way to prevent or significantly delay the onset of dementia, whatever the cause.

In 2008, preliminary studies indicated that a major breakthrough in treating Alzheimer's disease might be available in the future, if early favorable results prove effective in larger populations. Small studies conducted by principal investigator Edward Tobinick, director of the Institute for Neurological Research in Los Angeles, revealed that etanercept (Enbrel) injected in the spine improved the cognitive abilities of some individuals with Alzheimer's disease. For example, within two

hours of being injected with the drug, an 81-year-old man with Alzheimer's disease who previously could not identify nine of 10 everyday objects *was* able to identify the objects. He also appeared much less agitated than he was prior to the treatment. Dr. Tobinick also reported similar successes with a small number of other patients with Alzheimer's disease.

Discovered by accident (as are many scientific discoveries) when the doctor was treating patients with spinal pain, etanercept may represent an effective treatment for Alzheimer's disease, although further and larger studies are needed. Note that it is not a cure for the disease, but it may represent a breakthrough treatment.

Other Psychiatric Issues

Alzheimer's and other forms of dementia are generally considered neurological disorders. But many older people also have psychiatric problems such as depression and anxiety disorders. About 17 percent of older women reported depressive symptoms in 2004, compared to 11 percent of older men. (Among younger individuals, women are also more likely to be depressed than men.) The rate of depression is higher among people ages 85 and older (19 percent) than among people 65–74 (13 percent).

Depression   Some people think depression is a normal part of aging but it is not; however, it is often unrecognized and untreated, according to the National Institute of Mental Health (NIMH).

Even if an older person was never clinically depressed before, the death of a spouse or other family members, as well as distress from chronic illness and chronic pain, the inability to drive oneself around anymore and the necessity of having to rely upon others for transportation, and other age-related problems can lead to a depressive state. It can also lead to a state of anxiety.

Yet many older people are fearful of psychiatrists, seeing them as people who treat the severely mentally ill, such as people with schizophrenia. In fact, most psychiatrists treat the "worried well," who have problems such as depression and anxiety. Many primary care doctors are willing and able to treat depression and anxiety, so it is not necessary for the older person to see a psychiatrist. However, the older person may still be fearful of telling his or her "regular" doctor about extreme feelings of sadness, thinking that maybe the doctor will think he or she is insane or weak. As a result, depression is often undertreated in the elderly.

Depression can cause over- or undereating, sleep problems (constant sleeping or insomnia, as well as frequent wakenings and nightmares), and also worsened pain from chronic conditions, such as headaches, stomachaches, and so forth, that do not improve with treatment. Fatigue is common, as is a decreased level of energy. In addition, the depressed person may no longer take any interest in the activities that formerly interested him. Depression may also be present with serious physical illnesses such as cancer, stroke, diabetes, and Parkinson's disease, and it can make the symptoms of these diseases worse. Treatment with medications and therapy can improve both the depression and symptoms of the other disease.

Antidepressants are very effective at treating depression, and loneliness can also be alleviated through arranging for visits with the older person and outings to the park and other places.

There are a variety of types of antidepressants, including tricyclic antidepressants, which have been used for many years. Tricyclics can cause drowsiness and constipation, among other side effects. More recent antidepressants include selective serotonin reuptake inhibitors (SSRIs) such as fluoxetine (Prozac) or serotonin norepinephrine reuptake inhibitors (SNRIs) such as duloxetine (Cymbalta). SSRIs and SNRIs can cause insomnia and agitation.

Depression and Suicide Thoughts of suicide may become frequent and the person may also have inappropriate feelings of guilt. If depression is untreated, the older person is at risk for suicide. People 65 and older have a higher rate of suicide than younger people, or 14.3 for every 100,000 people compared to a rate of 11 per 100,000 for the general population. Elderly white males ages 85 and older have the greatest risk for suicide, according to the National Institute of Mental

Health (NIMH), with a rate of 49.8 suicide deaths per 100,000 people in this age group.

Older whites have the highest rate of suicide compared to Asians, Hispanics, and blacks, or 15.8 per 100,000. The rate for Asian and Pacific Islanders who died by suicide in 2004 was 10.6 per 100,000. The rate was 7.9 per 100,000 for Hispanics and 5.0 per 100,000 for non-Hispanic blacks.

People who are depressed and alone are the most at risk for suicidal thoughts and for carrying out their plans for suicide. Family members should remove guns, knives, and other items around the house that the older person could use to harm himself. The last thing a suicidal person needs is to be armed or have access to weapons.

Anxiety Disorders An estimated 11 percent of older persons suffer from anxiety disorders, particularly generalized anxiety disorder, which is a chronic and severe form of constantly worrying. Psychiatrist Gary Kennedy says that anxiety disorder symptoms in older people are like those seen in younger people, with the exception that older people with obsessive-compulsive disorder (OCD) are more likely to worry about having sinned. OCD refers to a disorder in which the person has recurrent thoughts and often a compulsion to perform frequent acts, such as constant hand washing or counting things.

Older people with anxiety disorders may startle easily and have trouble falling asleep. They may also have physical symptoms linked to their anxiety, such as indigestion or trouble swallowing. Anxiety disorders can be treated with medication and therapy.

Alcohol Disorders Sometimes alcohol misuse is linked with depression and anxiety in older adults. Faced with loneliness and chronic illness, older people may turn to alcohol for relief, and about a third of elderly alcoholics are late-onset drinkers according to researchers, first starting their drinking between the ages of 40 to 50 or older. However for some older people, particularly women, the onset of alcohol abuse occurs in their senior years. Of course alcohol is a bad choice because it is itself a depressant and can bring little relief from emotional pain. It is also true that many drugs interact with alcohol, often to an unsafe level.

Elderly drinkers are more receptive to therapy for this problem than younger drinkers, although many times alcohol abuse and alcoholism are not detected in elderly individuals. Doctors may forget to ask about the use of alcohol in older people, or older people themselves may withhold information about their drinking habits out of shame or embarrassment. Sometimes alcoholic behaviors are mistakenly attributed to normal aging.

In a study of over 1,000 elderly individuals published in the *International Journal of Geriatric Psychiatry* in 2008, the researchers found that men were more likely to abuse alcohol and that alcohol misuse was associated with depressive symptoms and poor functional status, as with people who have difficulty performing regular daily activities.

According to an article in *Advances in Psychiatric Treatment* in 2006, widowed or divorced older men are more likely to drink heavily (and to smoke) than elderly men who are married. (Interestingly, older married women had higher levels of alcohol consumption than those who were widowed or divorced—perhaps because they are under pressure by providing care to their elderly spouses.)

Alcohol abuse and alcoholism increase the risk of many health problems in older people, such as hypertension, stroke, and coronary heart disease. It is also a key factor in falls, which often lead to hospitalization and disability and even death. Older individuals who abuse alcohol also have greater problems with osteoporosis as well as with many liver problems, such as cirrhosis of the liver and liver cancer. An estimated 80 percent of older people take medications on a regular basis and many of them take alcohol with their medicines, leading to a risk for drug interaction.

According to Karim Dar, a psychiatrist specializing in substance abuse, the following are possible signs and symptoms of alcohol misuse in elderly people:

- depression
- anxiety
- blackouts
- disorientation
- falls and bruises
- incontinence
- an increased tolerance to alcohol
- memory loss
- poor nutrition
- poor hygiene
- an unusual response to medication

Some indicators that an older person needs help with a drinking problem, according to the National Institute on Aging, are the following behaviors:

- gulping down drinks
- drinking to calm nerves, forget worries, or reduce depression
- frequently drinking more than one drink a day
- lying about or trying to hide drinking
- hurting oneself or another person while drinking
- feeling irritable, resentful, or unreasonable when not drinking
- having medical, social, or financial problems caused by drinking

Making Healthy Choices

Even with the best medications and treatments, if elderly patients forget or refuse to take their medicine or to follow their doctors' recommendations (and no one is watching to make sure they are taking their medicine), they increase the risk of negative consequences from their illnesses. For example, doctors urge all people to quit smoking. This becomes particularly important for the older person, who may develop lung cancer, emphysema, chronic obstructive pulmonary disease (COPD), and many other serious diseases from smoking. (Older people who think it is too late to stop smoking are wrong: The lungs usually begin recovering very rapidly if no disease has yet set in, despite the person's age.)

Taking medicines as ordered can also be very hard for elderly individuals. Many older people cannot understand or comply with a complicated—or sometimes even a simple—drug regimen. They need others to tell them when to take their medicine and to make sure they don't take substances that could interact with their medicine. For example, if the older person is taking a blood thinner such as warfarin (Coumadin), he or she should avoid herbal remedies such as Gingko biloba that also thin the blood and potentially could lead to hemorrhage. Many older people do not even tell their doctors that they are taking herbal remedies (because they forget to tell the doctor or it just does not seem that important to mention it). So if the patient develops a bad reaction because of an interaction between a medication and an alternative remedy, often the patient, family members, and the doctor are all shocked. Yet it is simple to avoid blindsiding the doctor, by giving him or her all the information needed.

Difficult Family Issues

Providing advice, care, and assistance to older relatives can be cumbersome and uncomfortable, especially when those relatives are one's parents. Many older people are very resistant to relinquishing their former roles of authority and they see no reason why they should listen to their children, even when their children are doctors, lawyers, financial experts, or other successful people in their own right. In addition, natural pride and sometimes paranoia may come into play and older people may not wish to reveal anything about their financial or medical information, preferring to think that they are still in charge—although it may be clear to many others that their health is declining and they urgently need help.

It is also true that even when there are obvious signs of a parent's mental or physical deterioration, many adult children prefer to table any consideration of it, hoping that things will get better. They may also deny altogether that there *is* problem, basically because they do not *want* there to be a problem. Denial is a common response to difficult issues; unfortunately, it can be harmful to the elderly person who is consequently not protected from his or her own failings.

Sometimes family members disagree about what should be done with Mom or Dad, and one sibling may wish Mom to go in a nursing home while another insists that she is perfectly fine staying at home. Major battles may ensue and old rivalries from childhood may rear their heads. The important point, however, is for everyone to do his best to face the reality of the problem and attempt to work together.

Where Elderly People Live

Many people assume that most elderly people live in nursing homes, and this is not true. Instead, only about nine people in 1,000 ages 65–74 lived in a nursing home in 2004. This rate increased with age, and it was 36 people per 100,000 for those who were ages 75–84 in 2004, increasing further to 139 per 1,000 for those ages 85 and older.

The concept of assisted-living facilities was developed in the late 20th century in the United States and is a very popular one among older people who can afford it. This term describes a place, usually an apartment-style unit, which offers a lower level of care than a nursing home but a higher level of care than independent living. Assisted-living facilities vary dramatically in the services they offer their residents. The care in an assisted-living facility may be as minimal as having a call button in the resident's apartment in case of emergency and a few other amenities, or it may include a nurse or physician in residence, a dining hall that provides three meals per day, and numerous activities. Most people would much prefer to live in an assisted-living facility than in a nursing home.

State regulations on assisted-living facilities also vary drastically. In contrast, state governments and the federal government have very strict rules and regulations for nursing homes. It is also true that assisted living is very expensive and in most cases, it is not covered by Medicare. (In some few circumstances in some states, Medicaid will pay for assisted living.) As a result, most people cannot afford assisted living.

A minority of older people live in nursing homes, with especially high percentages in Kentucky, Tennessee, Alabama, and Mississippi. In contrast,

TABLE 4. POPULATION AGE 65 AND OLDER RESIDING IN A NURSING HOME BY REGIONS AND STATES, 1990 AND 2000

Region and State	1990	2000	Percentage Change
United States	1,590,763	1,557,800	-2.1
Northeast	**362,058**	**373,921**	**+3.3**
New England	109,403	110,156	0.7
Middle Atlantic	252,655	263,765	4.4
Midwest	**490,434**	**459,116**	**-6.4**
East North Central	309,247	293,245	-5.2
West North Central	181,187	165,871	-8.5
South	**498,340**	**520,512**	**4.4**
South Atlantic	240,760	253,818	5.4
East South Central	92,447	100,835	9.1
West South Central	165,133	165,859	0.4
West	**239,931**	**204,251**	**-14.9**
Mountain	58,954	59,275	0.5
Pacific	180,977	144,976	-19.9
New England	**109,403**	**110,156**	**0.7**
Maine	9,194	8,618	-6.3
New Hampshire	7,741	8,917	15.2
Vermont	4,399	3,796	-13.7
Massachusetts	50,852	50,962	0.2
Rhode Island	50,852	50,962	0.2
Connecticut	27,683	29,189	5.4
Middle Atlantic	**252,655**	**263,765**	**4.4**
New York	111,901	111,156	-0.7
New Jersey	42,883	46,773	9.1
Pennsylvania	97,871	105,836	8.1
East North Central	**309,247**	**293,245**	**-5.2**
Ohio	84,081	83,854	-0.3
Indiana	45,375	44,402	-2.1
Illinois	82,422	80,765	-2.0
Michigan	51,605	46,025	-10.8
Wisconsin	45,764	38,199	-16.5
West North Central	**181,187**	**165,871**	**-8.5**
Minnesota	43,475	37,542	-13.6
Iowa	33,429	31,399	-6.1
Missouri	46,844	44,198	-5.6
North Dakota	7,459	6,749	-9.5
South Dakota	8,278	7,253	-12.4
Nebraska	17,698	15,093	-14.7
Kansas	24,004	23,637	-1.5
South Atlantic	**240,760**	**253,818**	**5.4**
Delaware	4,330	4,405	1.7
Maryland	24,663	23,843	-3.3
District of Columbia	5,336	3,447	-35.4
Virginia	32,947	35,154	6.7
West Virginia	11,080	10,492	-5.3
North Carolina	40,260	44,837	11.4
South Carolina	16,009	19,080	19.2
Georgia	32,645	31,289	-4.2
Florida	73,490	81,271	10.6
Eastern South Central	**92,447**	**100,835**	**9.1**
Kentucky	24,436	26,198	7.2
Tennessee	31,678	33,584	6.0
Alabama	21,965	24,318	10.7
Mississippi	14,368	16,735	16.4
Western South Central	**165,133**	**165,859**	**0.4**
Arkansas	19,117	19,135	0.1
Louisiana	27,934	27,034	-3.2
Oklahoma	26,140	24,785	-5.2
Texas	91,942	94,954	3.2
Mountain	**58,954**	**59,275**	**0.5**
Montana	7,128	5,959	-16.4
Idaho	5,798	5,275	-9.0
Wyoming	2,441	2,588	6.0
Colorado	16,696	16,708	0.1
New Mexico	5,645	6,240	10.5
Arizona	12,743	12,163	-4.6
Utah	5,441	6,006	10.4
Nevada	3,062	4,336	41.6
Pacific	**180,977**	**133,976**	**-19.9**
Washington	29,735	20,887	-29.8
Oregon	16,076	13,010	-19.1
California	131,358	107,802	-17.9
Alaska	1,039	660	-36.5
Hawaii	2,769	2,617	-5.5

Source: Adapted from Charlotte A. Schoenborn, Jackline L. Vickerie, and Eva Powell-Griner. "Health Characteristics of Adults 55 Years of Age and Over: United States, 2000–2003." *Advance Data from Vital and Health Statistics* 370 (April 11, 2006): 163–164.

there was a decrease of 19.9 percent in nursing-home residents in the Pacific region (Washington, Oregon, California, Alaska, and Hawaii). It is unknown what drove these changes.

Global Aging

Many other countries have a rapidly aging population; for example, 20.4 percent of the population of Japan is made up of people ages 65 and older, compared to 12.5 percent in the United States. People in these countries face many of the same problems as Americans do, with providing help and assistance to their aging relatives while managing their own active lives. A key reason for this global increase in the elderly is an overall increased life expectancy that is largely driven by improved medical technology and medications and advances in infection control. The shift will be from infectious and parasitic diseases worldwide to chronic diseases such as cancer, diabetes, and heart disease.

In contrast, a few less-developed countries have seen population declines. In some countries in Africa, for example, the life expectancy fell from 60 years in 1996 to 43 years in 2006, largely because of large numbers of the population who were afflicted with the human immunodeficiency virus (HIV) and acquired immunodeficiency syndrome (AIDS).

See Table 5 for data on countries in which at least 10 percent of their population are ages 65 and older.

TABLE 5: POPULATION OF COUNTRIES OR AREAS WITH AT LEAST 10 PERCENT OF THEIR POPULATION AGES 65 AND OLDER, 2006

	Population (number in thousands)		Percent
Country or Area	Total	65 and Older	Percent 65 and Older
Japan	127,515	25,954	20.4
Italy	58,134	11,450	19.7
Germany	82,422	16,018	19.4
Greece	10,688	2,027	19.0
Spain	40,398	7,170	17.7
Sweden	9,017	1,588	17.6
Belgium	10,379	1,809	17.4
Bulgaria	7,385	1,279	17.3
Estonia	1,324	228	17.2
Portugal	10,606	1,822	17.2
Austria	8,193	1,401	17.1
Croatia	4,495	754	16.8
Georgia	4,661	768	16.5
Latvia	2,275	373	16.4
Ukraine	46,620	7,628	16.4
Finland	5,231	846	16.2
France	63,329	19,238	16.2
United Kingdom	60,609	9,564	15.8
Slovenia	2,010	315	15.7
Switzerland	7,524	1,171	15.6
Lithuania	3,586	554	15.5
Denmark	5,451	828	15.2
Hungary	9,981	1,518	15.2
Serbia	10,140	1,544	15.2
Belarus	9,766	1,462	15.0
Norway	4,611	683	14.8
Romania	22,304	3,275	14.7
Luxembourg	474	69	14.6

(Table continues)

(Table continued)

Population (number in thousands)		Percent	
Country or Area	Total	65 and Older	Percent 65 and Older
Czech Republic	10,235	1,481	14.5
Bosnia and Herzegovina	4,499	647	14.4
Netherlands	16,491	2,349	14.2
Russia	142,069	20,196	14.2
Malta	400	55	13.7
Montenegro	692	95	13.7
Canada	33,099	4,407	13.3
Poland	38,537	5,128	13.3
Uruguay	3,443	454	13.2
Australia	20,264	2,649	13.1
Hong Kong	6,940	890	12.8
Puerto Rico	3,928	504	12.8
United States	298,444	37,196	12.5
Slovakia	5,439	653	12.0
New Zealand	4,076	481	11.8
Iceland	299	35	11.7
Cyprus	784	91	11.6
Ireland	4,062	470	11.6
Virgin Islands (U.S.)	109	12	11.2
Armenia	2,976	332	11.1
Macedonia	2,051	225	11.0
Moldova	4,334	465	10.7
Argentina	39,922	4,244	10.6
Cuba	11,362	1,181	10.4
Taiwan	22,782	2,279	10.0

Source: Federal Interagency Forum on Aging-Related Statistics. *Older Americans 2008: Key Indicators of Well-Being*. Washington, D.C.: March 2008, 75.

End-of-Life Issues

We are all human and will eventually die. We know that this is a fact. But knowing it in general as a vague concept does not make it easy to face death in a loved one, and issues related to death are especially difficult to consider when it is your aging parent or other beloved relative, no matter how old the person is. For this reason, decisions about measures taken to prolong life at its end are difficult to make. Whether elderly relatives wish crash carts to be summoned in an attempt to prolong their lives, or breathing tubes inserted to manage their breathing when their failing lungs can no longer handle the task, or whether other devices and machinery are used, are all very difficult issues to think about and discuss.

If the older person creates an advance directive or a living will, he or she can stipulate whether extreme measures should be taken in the event that medical decisions must be made when he or she is incapable of making them (because of unconsciousness or the inability to communicate). Another option is for the older person to name a health-care agent, also known as a health-care proxy, to make medical decisions on his or her behalf if he or she is incapable of making them.

If such an individual is not named as a health-care agent or proxy, and if supporting legal documents are not created, then the decision about what to do in a crisis is left to the next of kin. It can be a wrenching decision to choose between letting your father die and watching him continue to suffer as machines perform basic functions for him.

Sometimes critically important organs fail, such as the kidneys, and it is left up to the elderly person or his or her family members (if the elderly person cannot make decisions) as to whether dialysis should occur. When the kidney fails, if dialysis does *not* occur, the person will die. Family members must balance their desire for their parent or other beloved relative to live, in spite of the pain he or she may be suffering, along with the prognosis for recovery.

At an extremely emotional point in their lives, such decisions are tremendously difficult. Thus, if these decisions have been previously planned, although the grief and pain are still present when death is imminent, the survivors are spared frantically trying to figure out what Mom or Aunt Lucy would have wanted.

The dying person may be placed in a hospice. This does not mean that death is imminent, although it does mean that the person is very ill and the illness cannot be resolved.

Personal End-of-Life Issues

When an older person is dying, it is important to see that his pain-relief needs are met. According to the National Institute of Aging in its publication *End of Life: Helping with Comfort and Care*, there should be no concern about drug abuse or dependence at the end of a person's life. Instead, it is more important to manage overwhelming pain. If the pain is not controlled, the doctor should be asked to arrange a consultation with a pain management specialist. Some people worry that giving morphine could hasten death, but most experts think this is unlikely, particularly when the dosage is carefully monitored.

It can also be important to provide other basic comforts, such as giving ice chips or swabbing lips with lip balm. A damp cloth over the eyes can alleviate dryness of the eyes. People who are dying may feel cold or hot and may be unable to tell anyone how they feel. If the person seems to be pushing away blankets, this may indicate that he or she feels too warm, and in that case, blankets should be removed. A cool cloth could be placed on the person's forehead.

Physical contact can make the dying person feel better. Warming your hands under water or rubbing them together before holding the person's hands gently can help.

There are also emotional issues that may be of concern to the dying person. Telling the person how much he or she has meant to you can be of major importance. Sharing memories, even if the dying person cannot speak, may be meaningful. Even if the person is unconscious, he or she may benefit from such acts.

The dying person may also be worried about a spouse, a pet, or other issues. He or she can be reassured that Fluffy the cat will be cared for or that other issues important to the dying person will be managed.

Caring for Your Needs

Do not forget about your own needs. Sometimes in caring for an elderly parent or other relative, people can become physically fatigued and emotionally overwhelmed. Everyone needs a break, and it is not bad to take one. It is also true that when a very sick relative dies, especially one who has been suffering or who has required extensive care, sometimes your initial reaction might be relief, followed by major guilt. Experts say that it is natural to be relieved that a burden has been lifted and this does not mean that you are a bad child or relative.

Let other people comfort you. In fact, before your loved one dies, make sure you take regular breaks from caregiving, to avoid *compassion fatigue*, a condition of feeling overwhelmed from caregiving. Do not dwell on your youthful indiscretions or ways you may have raised your parent's blood pressure by your actions when you were a teenager. Instead, pat yourself on the back emotionally for doing a good job in caring for your loved one and doing the best that you could in his or her final days.

Further Reading

American Hospital Association and First Consulting Group. "When I'm 64: How Boomers Will Change Health Care." Chicago, Ill.: American Hospital Association, 2007.

Cassels, Caroline. "Anti-TNF-alpha Therapy Produces Rapid Improvement in Alzheimer's Disease." *Medscape Medical News* (January 15, 2008). Available online. URL: www.medscape.com/viewartical/568812. Accessed February 28, 2008.

Dar, Karim. "Alcohol Use Disorders in Elderly People: Fact or Fiction?" *Advances in Psychiatric Treatment* 12, no. 3 (May 2006):173–181.

Ervin, R. Bethene. "Prevalence of Functional Limitations among Adults 60 Years of Age and Over: United States, 1999–2002." *Advance Data from Vital and Health Statistics* 375 (August 23, 2006).

Federal Interagency Forum on Aging-Related Statistics. *Older Americans 2008: Key Indicators of Well-Being.* Washington, D.C.: U.S. Government Printing Office, March 2008.

He, Wan, Manisha Sengupta, Victoria A. Velkoff, and Kimberly A. DeBarros. *65+ in the United States: 2005.* Washington, D.C.: U.S. Census Bureau, December 2005.

Kennedy, Gary J. *Geriatric Mental Health Care: A Treatment Guide for Health Professionals.* New York: Guilford Press, 2000.

Murtagh, Kirsen Naumann, and Helen B. Hubert. "Gender Differences in Physical Disability among an Elderly Cohort." *American Journal of Public Health* 94, no. 8 (2004): 1,406–1,411.

National Institute of Mental Health. "Women and Depression: Discovering Hope." Bethesda, Md.: 2008.

National Institute on Aging. *End of Life: Helping with Comfort and Care.* Bethesda, Md.: National Institutes of Health, January 2008.

———. "Why Population Aging Matters: A Global Perspective." Washington, D.C.: U.S. Department of State, 2007.

Schoenborn, Charlotte A., Jackline L. Vickerie, and Eva Powell-Griner. "Health Characteristics of Adults 55 Years of Age and Over: United States, 2000–2003." *Advance Data from Vital and Health Statistics* 370 (April 11, 2006).

St. John, Philip D., Patrick R. Montgomery, and Suzanne L. Tyas. "Alcohol Misuse, Gender and Depressive Symptoms in Community-Dwelling Seniors." *International Journal of Geriatric Psychiatry* (forthcoming).

abuse The unlawful and immoral maltreatment of an older person, whether the maltreatment is physical abuse, sexual abuse, emotional abuse, neglect, or another category of maltreatment. Some studies have indicated that for every reported case of the abuse of an older person, there are an estimated five abuse cases that have *not* been reported. In 2004, adult protective services agencies nationwide received more than 600,000 reports of older individuals who needed protection from others and sometimes who needed protection from themselves, as in self-neglect. (See NEGLECT/SELF-NEGLECT.)

The first known medical report of the abuse of an older person was made in 1975, and at that time it was also called "granny battering."

Each state in the United States has an office of adult protective services to investigate the abuse or neglect of adults, although states vary widely in how they define the abuse of adults as well as in how vigorously they prosecute the perpetrators of abuse against older people and other adults. There is no controlling federal authority for elder abuse and no federal statutes as there are with child-abuse cases.

Some older people are repeatedly abused, but even one incident of abuse can be traumatizing to the elderly person according to authors Carmel Bitondo Dyer, Marie-Therese Connolly, and Patricia McFeeley in *Elder Mistreatment: Abuse, Neglect, and Exploitation in an Aging America.* In their chapter on the clinical and medical forensics of elder abuse and neglect, the authors say that even *one* incident of victimization can be potentially harmful and even fatal for an older person:

> A single act of victimization can "tip over" an otherwise productive, self-sufficient older person's life. In other words, because older victims usually have fewer support systems and reserves—physi-

cal, psychological, and economic—the impact of abuse and neglect is magnified, and a single incident of mistreatment is more likely to trigger a downward spiral leading to loss of independence, serious complicating illness, and even death.

An additional issue is that often older people who have been abused or neglected do not wish (or even will refuse) to testify against their family members who have abused them, out of a misguided sense of loyalty, or of love, or for practical reasons; for example, they may fear what could happen to them if the perpetrator goes to jail, since they cannot live on their own and there may be no others with whom they can live. Thus, living *without* the abusive person may be perceived as worse than living *with* him or her.

Some may reason that the family member is usually nice to them when he or she is not intoxicated or on drugs, which is when abusive incidents occur. Others fear perceived stigmatization from others or they fear that the abuser will retaliate against them for telling others about the abuse or neglect. They may even feel embarrassed.

Often older people are victimized more readily than younger people for several reasons. The elderly are more physically vulnerable because they have less physical strength as well as a risk for multiple illnesses or disabilities, such as ARTHRITIS, CANCER, DIABETES, and HYPERTENSION. Also, many older people take one or more medications, which may affect their mental alertness (such as sedating drugs). (Note that it is an ageist assumption to assume that all older people are mentally incompetent, which is not true. See AGEISM.)

Elderly individuals may also be far more trusting than younger individuals, and thus, they are also more open to financial abuse involving schemes that are designed to cheat them of their savings.

Each state has its own laws on the specific types of actions that constitute maltreatment of elderly individuals. The National Center on Elder Abuse performs regular analyses of state laws on the maltreatment of older persons. A summary of the most recent statutes as well as other helpful information is available at: http://www.ncea.aoa.gov/NCEA-root/Main_Site/Find_Help/State_Resources.aspx.

Ageism and Abuse

Some authors attribute part of the reason for failing to identify abuse and neglect in elderly individuals to a problem of ageism that physicians and other health professionals may exhibit. In her chapter in *Elder Mistreatment: Abuse, Neglect, and Exploitation in an Aging America*, Patricia A. Bomba writes,

> Ageism refers to a tendency to dismiss many abnormal abuse processes as normal aging. Similarly, signs and symptoms of elder abuse may be written off as inevitable, or ascribed to other diseases. Fractures can be attributed to osteoporosis. Side effects of polypharmacy may be missed and ascribed to old age. Depression and pain may be underreported by the patient, unrecognized by the health care professional and undertreated by the physician.

Categories of Abuse and Neglect

Abuse generally refers to the suffering of physical and/or sexual harm or emotional abuse, while in contrast, *neglect* refers to the withholding of the items that are needed to sustain life, such as food, shelter, or medical care. Thus, abuse includes the *commission* of harmful acts, while neglect generally refers to acts of *omission*.

According to the Administration on Aging, neglect refers to the failure of a caretaker to provide goods or services that are necessary to avoid physical harm, mental anguish, or mental illness, including such acts as the denial of food or health-related services. Neglect also includes abandonment. In some states, if an individual fails to provide for his or her *own* self-care, this self-neglect is considered to be a form of neglect. Some studies indicate that self-neglect may be far more common than most people realize.

There are also subcategories of abuse and neglect; for example, according to the Administration on Aging, physical abuse is the willful infliction of physical pain or injury, such as slapping, bruising, or restraining the older person.

In her chapter on an overview of elder abuse in *Elder Abuse and Mistreatment: Policy, Practice, and Research*, social worker Lisa Nerenberg defined physical abuse as "intentionally or recklessly causing bodily injury, pain or impairment. Examples include striking, pushing, burning, and strangling elders, and using physical or chemical restraints." (Chemical restraints may include drugs or alcohol used to sedate the older person for the convenience of others.)

Sexual abuse may range from sexual touching to rape, depending on the particular state law. Nerenberg defined sexual abuse as "non-consensual sexual contact of any kind with an older person. It includes rape; molestation; lewd or lascivious conduct; coercion through force, trickery or threats; or sexual contact with any person who lacks sufficient decision-making capacity to give consent."

In her chapter in *Elder Abuse and Mistreatment: Policy, Practice, and Research*, Bomba says that finding bloody, torn, or stained underclothes may indicate that sexual abuse has occurred, as may bruises around the breasts, inner thighs, or genitals. Other signs of sexual abuse are unexplained sexually transmitted diseases or genital infections, unexplained vaginal or anal bleeding, and difficulty sitting or walking with no evidence of a musculoskeletal disease.

Emotional abuse (also known as psychological abuse) refers to emotional harm, such as the harm that can be suffered when the older person is constantly screamed at, denigrated, or threatened by another person. However, the definition of this category of abuse (if it exists in the state) varies considerably. According to the Administration on Aging, psychological abuse is the infliction of mental or emotional anguish, such as humiliating, intimidating, or threatening the elderly person.

Some states have a category of maltreatment called financial exploitation that encompasses the financial abuse or exploitation of elders, such as when their savings or other financial assets are used fraudulently or against the best interests of the older person. Such actions may be taken by a caregiver or by another person who has been placed in a position of trust, such as an attorney. According to the Administration on Aging, financial or material exploitation is the use of the resources of the older person without that person's consent and for someone else's benefit.

Evidence of Abuse

Sometimes abuse or neglect is obvious, as when there are clearly visible bite marks on the older person's skin, or there are rope, gunshot, or knife wounds, but in many cases, there are not obvious indications of abuse or neglect.

In their chapter on forensic evidence of abuse, Dyer and colleagues describe some types of injuries that are more likely to be from abuse than the result of normal aging. For example, bruises that are located on the palms or on the soles of the feet may indicate that abuse has occurred, since these areas are usually not injured accidentally to the extent of causing bruising. In addition, the authors say that most nonaccidental bruising occurs in the areas of the face, neck, the abdomen, buttocks, and the chest wall.

According to experts, fractures in the trunk, head, or spine—a problem that many elders face because of falls—are more likely to be caused by assaults than by falls. Falls, in contrast, often cause fractures of limbs, sprains, strains, and musculoskeletal injuries.

Malnutrition is a marker of neglect, according to the authors, particularly if the elderly person resides in an institution. In most cases, the malnutrition results because the older person is actually unable to feed him or herself and there are insufficient staff members available to feed the person.

Misuse of medication is another example of neglect or abuse. Dyer et al. write, "Abusive or neglectful caregivers may withhold necessary drugs, use the elders' drugs themselves, or overdose patients to keep them quiet and manageable."

If the older person is sexually abused, there is an increased risk of contracting a new sexually transmitted disease as well as lesions in the genital area. Dyer et al. report, "Behavioral signs indicating potential sexual abuse may include withdrawal, fear, depression, anger, insomnia, increased interest in sexual matters, or increased sexual or aggressive behavior."

Other examples of signs of abuse and neglect are included in Table 1; for example, signs of emotional abuse may include emotional upset or agitation, extreme withdrawal and lack of communication or the individual's nonresponsiveness, as well as unusual behavior that is usually attributed to dementia, such as sucking, biting, and rocking (and which may be caused by dementia but could also be a result of emotional abuse) or an older person's report of being verbally or emotionally mistreated.

Some individuals abandon elderly persons at hospitals, nursing homes, or other institutions, without making proper provisions for them. They may also abandon the older person at a mall or another public location.

Elderly Victims of Abuse and Neglect and Their Perpetrators

According to studies by the National Center on Elder Abuse, most elderly victims of maltreatment are white females, while most perpetrators of abuse against older people are also white females. In general, studies indicate that family members are more frequent abusers of elderly individuals than are nonfamily members. Spouses may also be the abusers, particularly elderly male spouses. (See SUICIDE for a discussion of homicide/suicide, which, when it occurs, is nearly always perpetrated by an elderly man.)

Some cases of abuse or neglect are unintentional, because the caregiver is unaware of the true needs of the older person. In some cases, elderly individuals actively seek to hide problems and needs, as well as their own failings, such as the inability to provide for themselves. Other cases of abuse are tied to an underlying stress as well as a lack of understanding or training about what the older person needs or should realistically be expected to be able to do.

In addition, many abusive and neglectful caregivers are also substance abusers, and their drug or alcohol use contributes to the overall problem. They are most likely to either abuse or neglect the older person when they are under the influence of alcohol or drugs.

Spouse/Partner Abuse Spouse or partner abuse refers to the physical, emotional, or sexual mistreatment that is perpetrated by one spouse or partner on another. Older men are much more likely to be spousal or partner abusers committing physical or sexual abuse than are older women, although women may perpetrate emotional abuse. In addition, in a case of suicide/homicide among older people, it is nearly always an elderly man who murders his wife or partner before killing himself, instead of an elderly woman who initiates the aggression.

Assisting an Older Person Who Is Abused or Neglected

If the elderly person is in imminent danger of abuse, the police or 911 should be called immediately to intercede. Alternatively, if it is likely but not certain that the person has been abused or neglected, each state has a hotline at a state adult protective services agency for reporting and investigation of abuse. (See Appendix IV for state hotline contact numbers to report maltreatment.)

Elder Abuse May Be Increasing

The incidences of maltreatment of the elderly may be increasing. The National Center on Elder Abuse published a report in 2006 that analyzed adult protective services reports. According to this report, entitled *The 2004 Survey of State Adult Protective Services: Abuse of Vulnerable Adults 18 Years of Age and Older,* 565,747 reports of elder and vulnerable adult abuse nationally were received in 2004, nearly a 20 percent increase from the data gathered in a 2000 survey. Those who were age 80 and older represented the largest category of abuse victims (30.9 percent), followed by those ages 70 to 79 (26.4 percent) and those ages 60 to 69 (15.1 percent). Nearly two-thirds of the victims age 18 and older were female.

See also AGEISM; BRUISING; COMPASSION FATIGUE; CRIMES AGAINST THE ELDERLY; FRAILTY; INAPPROPRI-

TABLE 1. SIGNS AND SYMPTOMS OF ELDER ABUSE	
Physical Abuse	• Bruises, black eyes, welts, lacerations, and rope marks
	• Bone fractures, broken bones, and skull fractures
	• Open wounds, cuts, punctures, untreated injuries in various stages of healing
	• Sprains, dislocations, and internal injuries/bleeding
	• Broken eyeglasses or frames, physical signs of being subjected to punishment, and signs of being restrained
	• Laboratory findings of medication overdose or underutilization of prescribed drugs
	• An elder's report of being hit, slapped, kicked, or mistreated
	• An elder's sudden change in behavior
	• A caregiver's refusal to allow visitors to see an older person alone
Sexual Abuse	• Bruises around the breasts or genital area
	• Unexplained venereal disease or genital infections
	• Unexplained vaginal or anal bleeding
	• Torn, stained, or bloody underclothing
	• An elder's report of being sexually assaulted or raped
Emotional/Psychological Abuse	• Emotional upset or agitation
	• Extreme withdrawal and lack of communication or nonresponsiveness
	• Unusual behavior usually attributed to dementia (such as sucking, biting, and rocking)
	• An elder's report of being verbally or emotionally mistreated
Neglect	• Dehydration, malnutrition, untreated bed sores, and poor personal hygiene
	• Unattended or untreated health problems
	• Hazardous or unsafe living condition/arrangements (such as improper wiring, no heat, or no running water)
	• Unsanitary and unclean living conditions (such as dirt, fleas, lice on person; soiled bedding; fecal/urine smell; inadequate clothing)
	• An elder's report of being mistreated

Abandonment	• Desertion of an elder at a hospital, nursing facility, or other similar institution
	• The desertion of an older person at a shopping center or other public location
	• An elder's own report of being abandoned
Financial or Material Exploitation	• Sudden changes in a bank account or banking practice, including an unexplained withdrawal of large sums of money by a person accompanying the elder
	• The inclusion of additional names on an elder's bank signature card
	• Unauthorized withdrawal of the elder's funds using the elder's ATM card
	• Abrupt changes in a will or in other financial documents
	• Substandard care being provided or bills unpaid despite the availability of adequate financial resources
	• Discovery of an elder's signature being forged for financial transactions for the titles of his/her possessions
	• Sudden appearance of previously uninvolved relatives claiming their rights to an elder's affairs and possessions
	• Unexplained sudden transfer of assets to a family member or someone outside the family
	• The provision of unnecessary services
	• An elder's report of financial exploitation
Self-Neglect	• Dehydration, malnutrition, untreated or improperly attended medication conditions, and poor personal hygiene
	• Hazardous or unsafe living conditions (for example, improper wiring, no indoor plumbing, no heat, no running water)
	• Unsanitary or unclean living quarters (for example, animal/insect infestation, no functioning toilet, fecal/urine smell)
	• Inappropriate and/or inadequate clothing, lack of necessary medical aids (such as eyeglasses, hearing aids, dentures)
	• Grossly inadequate housing or homelessness

Source: Adapted from the National Center on Elder Abuse, Administration on Aging, "Major Types of Elder Abuse." Available online. URL: http://www.ncea.aoa.gov/ncearoot/Main_Site/FAQ/Basics/Types_Of_Abuse.aspx. Accessed March 26, 2008.

ATE PRESCRIPTIONS FOR THE ELDERLY; LEARNED HELP-LESSNESS; NEGLECT/SELF-NEGLECT; SUBSTANCE ABUSE AND DEPENDENCE; SUICIDE.

Bomba, Patricia A. In *Elder Mistreatment: Abuse, Neglect, and Exploitation in an Aging America*. Washington, D.C.: National Academies Press, 2003, pp. 110–111.

Bonnie, Richard J., and Robert B. Wallace, eds. *Elder Mistreatment: Abuse, Neglect, and Exploitation in an Aging America*. Washington, D.C.: National Academies Press, 2003.

Brogden, Mike, and Preeti Nijhar. *Crime, Abuse and the Elderly*. Portland, Ore.: Willan Publishing, 2000.

Dyer, Carmel Bitondo, Marie-Therese Connolly, and Patricia McFeeley. "The Clinical and Medical Forensics of Elder Abuse and Neglect," in *Elder Mistreatment: Abuse, Neglect, and Exploitation in an Aging America*. Washington, D.C.: National Academies Press, 2003, pp. 339–381.

Mellor, M. Joanna, and Patricia Brownell, eds. *Elder Abuse and Mistreatment: Policy, Practice, and Research*. New York: The Haworth Press, 2006.

National Center on Elder Abuse, Administration on Aging, "Major Types of Elder Abuse." Available online. URL: http://www.ncea.aoa.gov/ncearoot/Main_Site/FAQ/Basics/Types_Of_Abuse.aspx. Accessed March 26, 2008.

Teaster, Pamela B., et al. *The 2004 Survey of State Adult Protective Services: Abuse of Vulnerable Adults 18 Years of Age and Older*. Washington, D.C.: National Center on Elder Abuse. March 2007.

accessibility to facilities Enabling the ease of use of public or private facilities for people who are age 65 or older and/or those who are physically disabled. For example, people who use wheelchairs should have access to ramps or elevators in most public buildings, parking lots, and shopping centers. Some facilities provide escalators, but these may be too difficult for disabled people to manage because they move too fast or are difficult to get on and off of.

The AMERICANS WITH DISABILITIES ACT requires that both public and private establishments provide reasonably accessible accommodations to disabled individuals; for example, restaurants must provide bathroom stalls that can accommodate a person using a wheelchair and have grab bars for disabled people who may be unsteady on their feet.

In addition, parking spots must be made available close to the entrance of stores and other types of buildings for those people who carry special stickers or car tags indicating that they are disabled. It is unlawful for others who are not disabled to park in these handicapped zones.

These stickers or special tag markings are usually provided by the state department of motor vehicles, the state department of aging, or another state agency, often after receiving a letter describing such a need from the disabled person's physician. These stickers or other indicators may also be made available for temporary use on some occasions, such as when someone is recovering from an injury or illness (such as recovering from a hip FRACTURE or knee replacement or back surgery). The stickers can also be made available on a longer basis for more chronic conditions such as a STROKE or PARKINSON'S DISEASE.

See ACTIVITIES OF DAILY LIVING; ASSISTED-LIVING FACILITY; DISABILITY; DRIVING.

accidental injuries Minor to major injuries that occur as a result of an accident, rather than occurring from a disease or disorder or from the abuse or neglect perpetrated by others. (See ABUSE; NEGLECT.) Such accidental injuries may be caused by a car crash, FALLS, or many other means; however, falls are the most common cause of accidental injuries.

Accidental injuries are more commonly seen among older people than other age groups because of the increased risk for poor vision, less flexible limbs, reduced mobility, and other issues related to aging. Many accidental injuries may result in FRACTURES of the hips and other bones, especially among those older people who have weakened bones due to OSTEOPOROSIS, VITAMIN AND MINERAL DEFICIENCIES/EXCESSES, and other medical problems.

Individuals with ALZHEIMER'S DISEASE or other forms of DEMENTIA have an increased risk for accidental injuries compared to most elderly individuals without dementia.

House Fires

According to a study reported in 2001 in the *New England Journal of Medicine*, based on more than 7,000 fires and 223 injuries and deaths in the Dallas, Texas, area, the fatality rate due to house fires was the highest among people age 65 and older and also among children younger than age 10. A lack of a smoke detector in the home was another major factor in injuries and deaths from house fires.

Car Crashes

According to the U.S. Census Bureau, the population age 65 and older had the second highest death rate from car crashes in 2000. (The highest rate was among those ages 15 to 24.) Death rates among men increased considerably with advancing age.

There were also racial differences among the older people; for example, American Indians or Alaska Natives had the highest death rates for both men and women (46.7 per 100,000 people for men and 22.9 per 100,000 for women), while African-American and Hispanic women had the lowest death rates (10.5 per 100,000 for African-American women and 12.0 per 100,000 for Hispanic women).

See also ACCESSIBILITY TO FACILITIES; ADVERSE DRUG EVENT; ASSISTIVE DEVICES; DEATH; DISASTER, NATURAL; DRIVING; ELDERIZING A HOME; EMERGENCY DEPARTMENT CARE; FRAILTY; HEALTH CARE AGENT/PROXY; NARCOTICS.

Istre, Gregory R., M.D., et al. "Deaths and Injuries from House Fires." *New England Journal of Medicine* 344, no. 24 (June 25, 2001): 1911–1916.

activities of daily living Basic activities that most healthy people can accomplish for themselves, such as dressing, eating, bathing, toileting, taking medications, and using the telephone. With increasing disability or disease, these activities become more difficult or impossible for individuals to manage on their own. As a result, individuals who cannot handle some or all of these activities must depend on others for assistance.

Some individuals who need assistance with their activities of daily living choose to live in an ASSISTED-LIVING FACILITY, while others require assistance that can only be obtained from the staff of a NURSING HOME. Others rely upon the assistance of a personal aide or home health attendant who comes to their home and provides the needed help. Some people live with other family members who provide the assistance that they need.

Some people refuse or do not know how to obtain help from others, such as when they have difficulty obtaining food or feeding themselves, and in the worst case, they can develop malnutrition or even die from insufficient nutrition. Others do not realize that they need help, such as individuals with ALZHEIMER'S DISEASE, DEMENTIA, ALCOHOLISM, or other serious health or medical problems, and they must depend on their family members and others to help them to realize that their basic functioning has severely declined and that help is urgently needed. Sometimes the help must be imposed, as when the older person does not have the cognitive ability to recognize that help is needed.

Some older people know that they need some help with daily activities, and they may have an idea where they could obtain such help, but they refuse to ask for help out of pride or embarrassment. Some older people neglect their own health and nutrition and can die as a result.

With increasing age comes an increasing difficulty in performing everyday activities, and according to the Centers for Disease Control and Prevention (CDC), of those aged 70 to 74, 47.4 percent of women and 45.5 percent of men need assistance with daily activities. This figure increases further to 53.4 percent of men and 60.7 percent of women age 75 to 79. Of those who are age 80 and older, 68.2 percent of men and 76.7 percent of women need help with their daily activities.

Some older individuals have difficulty with *instrumental activities of daily living.* These are activities that are not necessary to survive, yet which are important to most people such as the ability to drive a car, write checks, and balance a checkbook.

Some individuals facing difficulties in accomplishing their basic activities of daily living as well as with performing instrumental activities of daily living decide to move to assisted-living facilities, which provide meal services and often routinely check on residents. Other individuals move in with their family members and receive the needed help from them. If the individual has severe difficulties performing activities of daily living, he or she may require nursing home care.

In general, older women have a higher rate of activity limitations than older men. According to the CDC, 70.5 percent of older women have one or more activity limitations compared with 57.7 percent of older men. (See Table 1.) These limitations

TABLE 1. ACTIVITY LIMITATIONS AMONG PEOPLE AGE 65 AND OLDER, BY SEX: 1998		
Activity Limitations	**Men**	**Women**
Total (one or more limitations)	57.7	70.5
Very difficult/unable to walk a quarter of mile (about 3 city blocks)	16.8	28.3
Very difficult/unable to stand on one's feet for two hours	16.0	27.4
Very difficult/unable to climb 10 steps without resting	11.9	21.8
Very difficult/unable to sit for two hours	3.8	5.8
Very difficult/unable to reach over one's head	5.5	8.3
Very difficult/unable to use one's fingers to grasp or handle small objects	3.2	4.9
Very difficult/unable to lift/carry something as heavy as 10 pounds (such as a full bag of groceries)	7.4	19.1
Very difficult/unable to push/pull large objects (such as a living room chair)	13.1	27.9

Source: He, Wan, Manisha Sengupta, Victoria A. Velkoff, and Kimberly A. DeBarros. *65+ in the United States: 2005.* Washington, D.C.: U.S. Census Bureau, December 2005, p. 60.

range from walking a few blocks to standing for several hours to using fingers to grasp an object.

See also ACCESSIBILITY TO FACILITIES; AMERICANS WITH DISABILITIES ACT; ASSISTIVE DEVICES/ASSISTED TECHNOLOGY; BATHING AND CLEANLINESS; DISABILITIES; EXERCISE; FAMILY AND MEDICAL LEAVE ACT; FRAILTY; HOME HEALTH/HOME CARE; MENTAL COMPETENCY; NURSING HOMES; NUTRITION; VITAMIN AND MINERAL DEFICIENCIES/EXCESSES.

He, Wan, Manisha Sengupta, Victoria A. Velkoff, and Kimberly A. DeBarros. *65+ in the United States: 2005.* Washington, D.C.: U.S. Census Bureau, December 2005.

adaptive devices   See ASSISTIVE DEVICES/ASSISTED TECHNOLOGY.

adult children/children of aging parents   Men and women age 18 and older in relation to their elderly parents, who are age 65 and older. In most cases, the adult children of aging parents are age 30 and older, and in many cases, they are BABY BOOMERS, born between 1946 and 1964. However, sometimes the adult children are seniors themselves, and they may be providing care and assistance to their parents who are age 85 and older. This can be a considerable psychological burden for the adult children, who may have their own serious health problems, such as ARTHRITIS, CANCER, DIABETES, HYPERTENSION, and KIDNEY DISEASE.

Some adult children find themselves torn between balancing how they spend most of their nonwork time (and often making calls from work as well) caring for their aging parents and caring for their own children (such as adolescents) who are still living at home. Some experts have referred to these adults as the sandwich generation, because they are people who may feel trapped between the differing and sometimes equally intense demands and needs of two sets of generations.

In addition, some adult children who provide care and assistance for their aging parents also care for one or more grandchildren, who may have been abandoned or taken away from their parents by the state because of child abuse or neglect caused by drug abuse or other issues. This situation can lead to a great deal of stress on the adult child. Sometimes he or she must choose between providing what an elderly parent needs versus providing what a child needs, and such difficult conflicts can lead to chronic health problems and a lack of sleep.

It is also true that adult children who are siblings do not always agree on the best course of action for their parents. They may find themselves reenacting their childhood roles; for example, as the big brother who always decided what is best versus the younger sister, when in fact, the younger sister, who is now a competent adult, may be far better equipped to help the older parent. In addition, other sibling issues may arise out of a concern for financial issues (such as who can best help the aging parent financially or who will inherit the parent's money), as well as psychological issues, such as feelings of guilt.

See also ADULT DAY CENTERS; COMPASSION FATIGUE; DEATH, FEAR OF; FAMILY AND MEDICAL LEAVE ACT; FAMILY CAREGIVERS; HEALTH CARE AGENT/PROXY; LEARNED HELPLESSNESS; LIVING WILL; LONG-DISTANCE CARE; SIBLING RIVALRY AND CONFLICT; TALKING TO ELDERLY PARENTS ABOUT DIFFICULT ISSUES; TRANSPORTATION.

adult day centers   Facilities that provide day care to elderly individuals who cannot be safely left home alone because of health reasons or mental confusion, usually so that their family members with whom they live can work during the daytime. Individuals in adult day care centers receive social, recreational, and health-related services.

There are an estimated 3,500 adult day centers in the United States. Most are operated on a non-profit basis, according to the National Adult Day Services Association in Washington, D.C. Most day center participants are women in their 70s and older. Costs vary and most facilities are not covered by insurance, although financial assistance may be provided through state programs. The Eldercare Locator, available at (800) 677-1116 or http://www.eldercare.gov, can help individuals find adult day centers in their areas.

Adults Have Different Needs Than Children in Day Care

Adult day centers are not synonymous with child-care centers because the needs of older adults are different than those of infants and children. For example, many elderly adults need a variety of medications on a daily basis, as well as monitoring for diseases they may have, such as DIABETES and HYPERTENSION.

In contrast, although some children in day care require daily medications and medical monitoring, most do not. Another difference between children and elderly adults is that older adults with ALZHEIMER'S DISEASE or other forms of DEMENTIA may become agitated and distressed, requiring the specialized care of individuals who are experienced in dealing with older adults.

Older adults attending day centers may also require special diets, which is a relatively uncommon need among children. However, rarely, centers offer services to both older adults and children, providing an opportunity for both groups to interact.

Adult day centers may also provide a variety of services that would not usually be provided in child care, including physical therapy, MEDICATION MANAGEMENT, health screening, and even medical care. They may also provide personal care (bathing, shampooing) and assistance with ACTIVITIES OF DAILY LIVING. Most facilities are open during daytime hours during the week, although some day centers are also open during evenings or weekends. They may be located in hospitals, churches, schools, nursing homes, SENIOR CENTERS, and in other facilities.

Deciding If Adult Day Services Are Needed

Family caregivers considering adult day services for a loved one should ask themselves the following questions:

- Am I worried about my loved one's safety at home alone?
- Am I worried that my loved one is unhappy or bored sitting at home all day?
- Am I worried about my loved one's health?

- Do I want help to be able to keep my loved one at home as long as possible?
- Does my loved one seem depressed and have no one to talk to?

If the answer is "Yes" to any of these questions, adult day services can benefit both the caregiver and the loved one.

Identifying an Adult Day Center

In locating an adult day center, the following facility considerations should be taken into account:

- Where is the facility located?
- Is transportation to the facility available? Is there an extra charge for transportation?
- How long has the facility been in business?
- What is the ratio of staff to residents and the level of the skill/certification of the staff members?
- What are the days and hours of operation of the facility?
- Has the state health department received any significant complaints about the facility to date?
- What is the cost of care? Does the individual have to attend at least 2 days a week or some other minimum period of time?
- Does the facility accept individuals who have the following circumstances?
  - incontinence
  - in wheelchairs
  - memory loss
  - difficulty speaking
  - individuals who wander about (as with those with Alzheimer's disease or other forms of dementia)
  - special dietary constraints
  - behavioral problems
  - individuals who have catheters (urine drainage tubes)
- What activities are provided?
  - Are there individual and group activities?
  - Are the activities stimulating for the individual, such as exercise, crafts, music, etc.?

- Are individuals with dementia separated from the other participants?
- Are the meals well balanced and enjoyable?
- Is the facility clean, odorless, and pleasant?

See also ABUSE; ACCESSIBILITY TO FACILITIES; AMERICANS WITH DISABILITIES ACT; ASSISTED-LIVING FACILITIES; ASSISTIVE DEVICES/ASSISTED TECHNOLOGY; BABY BOOMERS; HOME HEALTH; NEGLECT; NURSING HOMES; OMBUDSMEN.

Administration on Aging. *Adult Day Services: How Can They Help You?* U.S. Department of Health and Human Services, November 4, 2004. Available online. URL: http://www.aoa.gov/press/nfc_month/2004/fact_sheets/Fact%20Sheet%20-%20Adult%20Day%20Services.pdf. Accessed February 13, 2008.

advance directive   See LIVING WILL.

adverse drug event   The negative consequence(s) of taking a medication, which may range from mild discomfort to death. Some doctors may be overly fearful of adverse drug events; some experts believe that some older people are undertreated (particularly for their pain) because of physicians' fears that medications could lead to an adverse event, such as a STROKE or a HEART ATTACK or even addiction to certain drugs. In such cases, patients fail to gain benefits from drugs because of excessive fear among doctors.

Because so many older people are likely to be taking more than one and sometimes many medications, their risk for an adverse drug event is heightened. In addition, many patients have multiple physicians and often receive prescriptions and take medications ordered by one or more doctors without the other physicians' knowledge. (This is not recommended. At every office visit, patients should advise every doctor about all drugs, prescribed, over-the-counter, and herbs or supplements that they take.)

It has also been scientifically established that older peoples' bodies often react differently than younger individuals' bodies to the same dose of medication. Also, in most cases, medications have not been tested on individuals older than age 65 prior to the pharmaceutical company receiving approval for the medication to be sold. Rates of metabolism, degrees of body fat (which acts as a storage reservoir for many medications), and levels of liver or kidney function are just a few reasons for erratic responses to some medicines in the senior population. For example, a dose of digoxin that is considered a normal dose for the average person who is younger than age 65 can sometimes induce a cardiac arrhythmia in an older person.

The older person may also have symptoms such as nausea, vomiting, confusion, and other side effects to drugs when these side effects to the same drugs are rarely seen in younger people. One key reason for this is that older people's hearts are generally not as healthy as younger individuals'.

According to Doctor Rosanne M. Leipzig in her 2001 article for *Geriatrics,* sometimes adverse events that are caused by drugs are mistaken by doctors for aging-related problems, such as incontinence or even DEMENTIA or confusion. Leipzig says that risk factors for an adverse drug reaction in an older person who is taking many drugs (POLYPHARMACY) should be considered, as should the dosage of the drug.

Some Drugs Are Inappropriate for Older People

Leipzig advises against prescribing certain drugs to people age 65 and older; for example, she recommends against prescribing the ANTIDEPRESSANT amitriptyline (Elavil), the sedative/anti-anxiety drug diazepam (Valium), the muscle relaxant cyclobenzaprine (Flexeril), and some nonsteroidal anti-inflammatory drugs (NSAIDs). In addition, indomethacin (Indocin) is among other drugs that Leipzig feels are either inappropriate or dangerous for many older people.

There is a list of inappropriate drugs for older people commonly referred to as the Beers' criteria that doctors and medical professionals use when considering drugs to avoid with people age 65 and older. It was originally developed by Dr. Mark H. Beers, the lead researcher on a 1991 study of drugs that were inappropriate or dangerous for nursing home patients. It was updated in 1997 and was most recently updated in 2003. (See INAPPROPRIATE PRESCRIPTIONS FOR THE ELDERLY.)

Leipzig recommends choosing another drug in the same class; for example, rather than ordering amitriptyline for the older person with DEPRESSION, she recommends prescribing nortriptyline (Pamelor) because it is more readily tolerated by older people and has fewer side effects.

Many doctors do not realize that it is important to take the age of their older patients into account when determining both *which* drug to use and the *dosage* to prescribe, and instead they often prescribe the same dosage of medication that they would order for a middle-aged or younger person. In a review of studies on medications prescribed for older people, reported in a 2000 issue of *The Annals of Pharmacotherapy,* the researchers found that about 14 to 24 percent of the patients that were studied had been prescribed medications that were not recommended for older people. It is important for older people and/or their family members to discuss all drug choices and their unique side effects with the senior adult's physician.

The researchers also found that the most commonly prescribed medications inappropriate for older people included amitriptyline (Elavil), propoxyphene (Darvon), and diazepam (Valium). Women older than age 80 and patients on MEDICAID were the most likely to be prescribed inappropriate medications. Patients in NURSING HOMES were also more likely than non-nursing home patients to be prescribed drugs inappropriate for older people. Making sure that the medicine prescribed, and not a generic substitution, is actually the one the patient is taking is another key issue.

Chronic Pain and Adverse Drug Events

Many older people take painkillers for the chronic pain of ARTHRITIS and other chronic illnesses. As a result, it is important for physicians to check that these drugs are not likely to interact with other medications that the patient takes; for example, that the painkiller will not cause excessive sedation or other ill effects.

Note that even common over-the-counter drugs such as acetaminophen (Tylenol) can cause liver damage over the long term. Aspirin is another drug that people often take for granted, but it can cause gastrointestinal bleeding, rashes, and even shock. Nonsteroidal anti-inflammatory drugs (NSAIDs)

are often prescribed for chronic pain, but frequent use may lead to ulcer disease. If the patient also consumes alcohol, the risk for gastrointestinal bleeding is increased. These anti-inflammatory drugs may also have an adverse impact on kidney function.

See also CHRONIC PAIN; DRUG ABUSE; HEALTH CARE AGENT/PROXY; MEDICATION COMPLIANCE; MEDICATION INTERACTIONS; MEDICATION MANAGEMENT; NARCOTICS; PAINKILLING MEDICATIONS; PRESCRIPTION DRUG ABUSE/MISUSE; SUBSTANCE ABUSE AND DEPENDENCE.

Feinberg, Steven D., M.D. "Prescribing Analgesics: How to Improve Function and Avoid Toxicity When Treating Chronic Pain." *Geriatrics* 55, no. 12 (2000): 44–62.
Leipzig, Rosanne M., M.D. "Prescribing Keys to Maximizing Benefit While Avoiding Adverse Drug Effects." *Geriatrics* 56, no. 2 (2001): 30–34.

African Americans Black Americans in the United States. In 2005, 8.3 percent of people age 65 and older were African American. In 2004, almost 50 percent of all elderly blacks lived in eight states, including New York, California, Florida, Texas, Georgia, Illinois, North Carolina, and Virginia.

In 2004, more than half of all older African-American males in the United States (56 percent) lived with their spouses, 13 percent lived with other relatives, 5 percent lived with nonrelatives, and 27 percent lived alone. Among African-American older women, 24 percent lived with their spouses, 33 percent lived with other relatives, 2 percent lived with nonrelatives, and 41 percent lived alone.

The poverty rate for elderly African Americans was 24 percent in 2004, greater than twice the amount for all older individuals (10.1 percent).

Most older African Americans have at least one chronic health problem, and many have more than one chronic disease or disorder. Older blacks have higher rates of HYPERTENSION, ARTHRITIS, and DIABETES than older people of all other races and ethnicities. In contrast, blacks have a lower rate of all types of heart disease and CANCER. (See Table 1.)

Older African Americans also have a lower risk than other races for developing some disorders, such as OSTEOPOROSIS and HEARING DISORDERS. They also have a significantly lower rate of dying

TABLE 1. PERCENTAGE OF OLDER BLACK AMERICANS WITH SPECIFIC CONDITIONS COMPARED WITH ALL OLDER AMERICANS, 2002–2003

Condition	Percentage of Older Blacks with the Condition	Percentage of All Older Americans with the Condition
Hypertension	68	51
Diagnosed arthritis	53	48
All types of heart disease	25	31
Diabetes	25	16
Cancer	11	21

Source: Data adapted from Administration on Aging. *A Statistical Profile of Black Older Americans Aged 65+.* U.S. Department of Health and Human Services, February 2006.

from FALLS than those of other races and ethnicities. Some studies of African Americans in facilities for military veterans show that African Americans have a significantly lower rate for mood disorders than veterans who are white or HISPANIC, but they have a significantly higher rate of being diagnosed with a psychotic disorder. (See VETERAN BENEFITS.)

See also ASIAN AMERICANS; CAUCASIANS; HISPANICS; NATIVE AMERICANS.

Administration on Aging. *A Statistical Profile of Black Older Americans Aged 65+.* U.S. Department of Health and Human Services, February 2006.

ageism The stereotyping of individuals based solely on their older age, and which usually centers on individuals age 65 and older, often concentrating on the perceived or presumed inabilities or infirmities that are assumed to be linked to their age. For example, some people mistakenly assume that all or most elderly people are or inevitably will become mentally incompetent or disabled.

Robert Butler, a psychiatrist to whom the term *ageism* is generally attributed, says,

> Underlying ageism is the awesome dread and fear of growing older, and therefore, the desire to distance ourselves from older persons who are a proxy portrait of our future selves. We see the young dreading aging and the old envying youth. Ageism not only reduces the status of older people but of all people.

Language That Demeans Older People

Older people may be infantilized by others, and terms such as old boys or old girls, young man, young lady, old coot, old codger, geezer, in their second childhood, and many other words and phrases are used to either pointedly or subtly deride older individuals.

Negative words and phrases were once used by many people to demean some racial and ethnic groups, but most people consider these usages to be unacceptable now. It is hoped that people will eventually realize that ageist terms are also inappropriate.

Ageist Physicians

Sometimes physicians have ageist attitudes, such as assuming that older people are "supposed" to be sicker than younger people when they become ill and labeling the causes of nearly all illnesses that older people have as "old age." Of course, many diseases and disorders are more prominent with aging, but it is the disease that causes the problem, not the person's chronological age.

Some patients are even ageist themselves. Frequently the patient will self-diagnose, saying, "I guess I am just getting old" when it comes to a medical problem. Often the doctor must remind patients that the opposite limb or joint is every bit as old as the one that is causing the problem.

Some doctors have their own pejorative acronyms and negative terms and phrases for older people in the hospital, such as GOMER (get out of my emergency room) or bed blocker (referring to very disabled and hospitalized elderly patients who are waiting to be transferred to nursing homes).

If older people are viewed as inevitably helpless and hopeless, or they are seen as useless individuals in society despite their individual circumstances and their personal past or present contributions, then older individuals may eventually and even unintentionally assume these negative roles in a form of LEARNED HELPLESSNESS. As reported by the International Longevity Center in their report *Ageism in America*, another consequence of ageism is that sometimes it can cause older people to be overmedicated:

> Drug interactions and diseases associated with a variety of other factors having nothing to do with

aging per se can cause dementia and delirium. Nonetheless, older women and men continue to be overmedicated because they have been stereotyped as being "set in their ways and unable to change their behavior," and cognitive impairment caused by drug interactions goes untreated.

Often, an overriding perception of the basic lifestyles of older people colors how people age 65 and older are viewed by younger individuals. For example, the ageist stereotypical perception is of the older person who sits in a rocking chair, complaining about many physical ailments. Although it is true that many older people do have physical ailments, it is also true that many can obtain relief from their pain and disabilities when seen and treated by caring physicians.

Measuring Ageism

Geriatric researchers have developed a tool to measure ageist attitudes. Some ageist events are such items as "a doctor or a nurse assumed ailments caused by age," "called an insulting name," "assumed I could not hear well," and "ignored or not taken seriously."

According to Erdman Palmore in his report on his ageism survey in a 2001 issue of *The Gerontologist*, the most commonly occurring form of ageism (reported by 58 percent of respondents) was "I was told a joke that pokes fun at old people." Individuals who think that this type of joke is all in good fun could perhaps reflect if they would feel the same way if someone told a joke that poked fun at their personal attributes, such as being short, fat, and so forth.

Palmore found that those with a high school education or less reported experiencing more incidents of ageism than college graduates, although the reason for this is unknown.

See also ABUSE; ADULT CHILDREN/CHILDREN OF AGING PARENTS; FRAILTY; NEGLECT.

International Longevity Center. *Ageism in America.* New York: International Longevity Center, 2006.
Palmore, Erdman. "The Ageism Survey: First Findings." *The Gerontologist* 41, note 5 (2001): 572–575.

age-related macular degeneration (AMD) Age-related macular degeneration is an eye disorder that destroys the central vision, and it can lead to blindness if it is untreated. AMD is the most common cause of blindness in individuals age 60 years and older, and thus, it is very important to diagnose this disease as soon as possible so that it can be treated. The macula is the part of the eye that enables individuals to view fine details. It lies in the center of the retina, which is the light-sensitive tissue at the back of the eye.

Symptoms and Diagnostic Path

There are two forms of age-related macular degeneration: the wet and dry forms. The majority of people with AMD have the dry form. These disorders are best diagnosed by an ophthalmologist, a medical doctor who specializes in eye diseases, rather than an optometrist.

With wet AMD, abnormal blood vessels behind the retina start to grow under the macula. Wet AMD can cause severe damage quickly. A key symptom is that straight lines appear wavy to the individual. There are no stages in wet AMD as with dry AMD. With dry AMD, the light-sensitive cells in the macula deteriorate and the person may see a blurred spot in the center of the vision. Slightly blurred vision is the most common symptom of wet AMD. The person may also have trouble with recognizing faces. Yellow deposits (drusen) may occur under the retina. The drusen can be identified in an ophthalmology examination.

Physicians test for AMD with a visual acuity test and a dilated eye examination. In addition, an instrument that measures the pressure inside the eye is also used. If the physician suspects AMD is present, he or she may order a fluorescein angiogram. A special dye is injected in the arm with this test and pictures are taken as the dye passes through the blood vessels of the retina. This test identifies leaky blood vessels.

Treatment Options and Outlook

AMD is treated with laser surgery, photodynamic therapy, and injections into the eye. These are not cures, and the disease may continue to progress. The laser surgery destroys the leaking blood vessels with a high-energy beam; however, sometimes this procedure also destroys adjacent healthy tissue.

In photodynamic therapy, a medication called verteporfin is injected into the arm, and it moves to the new blood vessels of the eye. A light is then shined into the eye for 90 seconds, and this light activates the verteporfin to destroy new blood vessels and also slow the rate of vision decline. This procedure does *not* destroy healthy tissue around the eye blood vessels. The person who has photodynamic therapy must avoid direct sunlight or even bright indoor light for five days after the treatment.

Injections into the eye can be given to treat wet AMD. There are high levels of a special growth factor that is present in the eyes of those with wet AMD, and drug treatment blocks the effects of the growth factor.

With dry AMD, high doses of a special formulation of ANTIOXIDANTS (such as vitamin C, vitamin E, and beta-carotene) and zinc can reduce the risk of further damage, based on research by the Age-Related Eye Disease Study (AREDS) of the National Eye Institute in 2001.

Risk Factors and Preventive Measures

Age is the primary risk factor for AMD; for example, people who are middle-aged have about a 2 percent risk of developing AMD, but the risk increases to 30 percent for those age 75 and older. Other risk factors for AMD are SMOKING, OBESITY, and a family history of AMD. Women have a greater risk for AMD than men. The severity of the disease also varies by race; for example, whites are more likely to go blind from AMD than blacks with the disorder. In addition, people who have had AMD in one eye are at risk to develop the disease in the other eye.

Preventive measures include quitting smoking and losing weight. Maintenance of normal blood pressure also decreases the risk of AMD.

See also BLINDNESS/SEVERE VISION IMPAIRMENT; EYE DISEASES, SERIOUS; GENDER DIFFERENCES.

Prevent Blindness America and the National Eye Institute. *Vision Problems in the U.S.: Prevalence of Adult Vision Impairment and Age-Related Eye Disease in America, 2002.* Available online. URL: http://www.nei.nih.gov/eyedata. Accessed February 13, 2008.

aggression, physical Acts of violence, which may become a problem among nursing home resi-

dents with ALZHEIMER'S DISEASE or other forms of DEMENTIA. Physical aggression is a major problem for nursing home residents and staffs, who can be injured when residents become violent. (Sometimes individuals with dementia who remain in the home can also become physically violent.)

In one study of more than 100,000 nursing home residents, as reported in 2006 in the *Archives of Internal Medicine*, 7,120 of all the residents (6.9 percent) in nursing homes in California, New York, Ohio, Pennsylvania, and Texas had been physically aggressive with those around them during a one-week period. The aggressive residents were physically aggressive at least once (hitting, scratching, or shoving) to the staff or other residents. Extrapolating to all nursing home residents, this translates to about 7 percent of all nursing home residents in the United States who have exhibited incidents of physical aggression each week.

The average age of the nursing home study subjects was 84. The researchers found that physical aggression was significantly associated with DEPRESSION, DELUSIONS, HALLUCINATIONS, and even CONSTIPATION. The factor that was the *most* correlated to physical aggression was depression.

The researchers also found that about 11 percent of the nursing home residents were verbally aggressive and, as with physical aggression, their behavior was linked to depression, delusions, and hallucinations. (However, constipation did not correlate with verbal aggression as it did with physical aggression.) The researchers recommended that treatment of the factors that were associated with physical and verbal aggression could theoretically change the behavior of the aggressive residents; for example, if depression was treated, physical and verbal aggression might then decrease, and so on.

See also ABUSE; COGNITIVE IMPAIRMENT; CONFUSION; IRRITABILITY; MANIA; NURSING HOMES; RAGE; SUICIDE.

Leonard, Ralph, M.D., et al. "Potentially Modifiable Resident Characteristics That Are Associated with Physical or Verbal Aggression among Nursing Home Residents with Dementia." *Archives of Internal Medicine* 166 (June 26, 2006): 1,295–1,300.

aging in place   Refers to older individuals who are able to remain in their homes or apartments despite the increased impairments due to their aging. Such individuals may receive HOME CARE that enables them to remain at home, and they may also receive delivered meals and other services. They may also receive assistance from COMPANIONS, live-in help, or relatives who may move in with them.

A key problem is that many elderly individuals insist on remaining in their homes even when they urgently need to live in a facility with a higher level of care, such as with another person or even in a NURSING HOME. There may also be a problem with transportation if they remain in their homes, such as when older people can no longer drive and bus service may be difficult to obtain or even nonexistent.

Many older people prefer to live in their own homes as long as possible, and they actively avoid moving to a nursing home if they become medically fragile. Some people can "age in place" in an ASSISTED-LIVING FACILITY, where both meals and emergency assistance are provided to older or disabled individuals. However, MEDICARE does not cover the cost of assisted living. In some few cases, MEDICAID covers the cost of assisted living for low-income seniors if the state has received a Medicaid waiver, but this option is generally only available in limited cases.

See also FRAILTY; HOUSING/LIVING ARRANGEMENTS; INDEPENDENT LIVING; LEARNED HELPLESSNESS; TALKING TO ELDERLY PARENTS ABOUT DIFFICULT ISSUES.

agoraphobia   See ANXIETY AND ANXIETY DISORDERS.

alcohol   A substance that is made from grains, fruits, or vegetables that includes an intoxicating ingredient called ethyl alcohol. In considering the ethyl alcohol content of different forms of alcohol,

TABLE 1. COMMONLY USED MEDICINES (BOTH PRESCRIPTION AND OVER-THE-COUNTER) THAT INTERACT WITH ALCOHOL

Symptoms/Disorders	Medication (Brand Name)	Medication (Generic Name)	Some Possible Reactions with Alcohol
Allergies/colds/flu	Alavert	Loratadine	Drowsiness, dizziness, increased risk for overdose
	Allegra, Allegra-D	Fexofenadin	
	Benadryl		
	Clarinex	Diphenhydramine	
	Claritin	Desloratadine	
	Claritin-D	Loratadine	
	Dimetapp Cold & Allergy		
	Sudafed Sinus & Allergy	Brompheniramine	
	Triaminic Cold & Allergy	Chlorpheniramine	
	Tylenol Allergy Sinus	Chlorpheniramine	
	Tylenol Cold & Flu	Chlorpheniramine	
Angina (chest pain), coronary heart disease	Isordil	Isosorbide	Rapid heartbeat, sudden changes in blood pressure, dizziness, fainting
		Nitroglycerin	
Anxiety, epilepsy	Ativan	Lorazepam	Drowsiness, dizziness, increased risk for overdose, slowed or difficulty breathing, impaired motor control, unusual behavior, and memory problems
	Klonopin	Clonazepam	
	Librium	Chlordiazepoxide	
	Paxil	Paroxetine	
	Valium	Diazepam	
	Xanax	Alprazolam	
	Herbal preparations (Kava Kava)		Liver damage, drowsiness
Arthritis	Celebrex	Celecoxib	Ulcers, stomach bleeding, liver problems
	Naprosyn	Naproxen	
	Voltaren	Diclofenac	

(Table continues)

(Table continued)

Symptoms/Disorders	Medication (Brand Name)	Medication (Generic Name)	Some Possible Reactions with Alcohol
Blood clots	Coumadin	Warfarin	Occasional drinking may lead to internal bleeding; heavier drinking also may cause bleeding or may have the opposite effect, resulting in possible blood clots, strokes, or heart attacks
Cough	Delsym Robitussin Cough Robitussin DAC	Dextromethorphan Pseudoephedrine, Guaifenesin and codeine	Drowsiness, dizziness, increased risk for overdose
Depression	Anafranil Celexa Desyrel Effexor Elavil Lexapro Luvox Norpramin Paxil Prozac Serzone Wellbutrin Zoloft Herbal preparations (St. John's Wort)	Clomipramine Citalopram Trazodone Venlafzine Amitryptyline Escitalopram Fluvoxamine Desipramine Paroxetine Fluoxetine Netazodone Bupropion Sertraline	Drowsiness, dizziness, increased risk for overdose, increased feelings of depression
Diabetes	Glucophage Micronase Orinase	Metformin Glyburide Tolbutamine	Abnormally low blood sugar levels, flushing reaction (nausea, vomiting, headache, rapid heartbeat sudden changes in blood pressure)
Enlarged prostate	Cardura Flomax Hytrin Minipress	Doxazosin Tamsulosin Terazosin Prazosin	Dizziness, light-headedness, fainting
Heartburn, indigestion, sour stomach	Axid Reglan Tagamet Zantac	Nizatidine Metoclopramide Cimetidine Ranitidine	Rapid heartbeat, sudden changes in blood pressure (metoclopramide), increased alcohol effect
High blood pressure	Accupril Caprozide Cardura Catapres Cozaar Hytrin Lopressor HCT Lotensin Minipress Vaseretic	Quinapril Hydrochlorothiazide Doxazosin Clonidine Losartan Terazosin Hydrochlorthizide Benzapril Prazosin Enalapril	Dizziness, fainting, drowsiness, heart problems such as changes in the heart's regular heartbeat (arrhythmia)

Symptoms/Disorders	Medication (Brand Name)	Medication (Generic Name)	Some Possible Reactions with Alcohol
High cholesterol	Advicor	Lovastatin and Niacin	Liver damage (all medications), increased flushing and itching (niacin), increased stomach bleeding (pravastatin and aspirin)
		Lovastatin	
	Altocor	Rosuvastatin	
	Crestor	Atorvastatin	
	Lipitor	Lovastatin	
	Mevacor	Niacin	
	Niaspain	Pravastatin	
	Pravachol	Pravastatin and Aspirin	
	Pravigard	Ezetimibe and	
	Vytorin	Simvastatin	
		Simvastatin	
	Zocor		
Infections	Acrodantin	Nitrofurantoin	Fast heartbeat, sudden changes in blood pressure, stomach pain, upset stomach, vomiting, headache, flushing or redness of the face, liver damage (isoniazid, ketokonazole)
	Flagyl	Metronidazole	
	Grisactin	Griseofulvin	
	Nizoral	Ketokonazole	
	Nydrazid	Isoniazid	
	Seromycin	Cycloserine	
	Tindamax	Tinidazole	
Muscle pain	Flexeril	Cyclobezaprine	Drowsiness, dizziness, increased risk of seizures, increased risk for overdose, slowed or difficult breathing, impaired motor control, unusual behavior, memory problems
	Soma	Carisoprodol	
Nausea, motion sickness	Antivert	Meclizine	Drowsiness, dizziness, increased risk for overdose
	Atarax	Hydroxyzine	
	Dramamine	Dimenhydrinate	
	Phenergan	Promethazine	
Pain (such as headache, muscle ache, minor arthritis pain), fever, inflammation	Advil	Ibuprofen	Stomach upset, bleeding and ulcers, liver damage (acetaminophen), rapid heartbeat
	Aleve	Naproxen	
	Excedrin	Aspirin and Acetaminophen	
	Motrin	Ibuprofen	
	Tylenol	Acetaminophen	
Seizures	Dilantin	Phenytoin	Drowsiness, dizziness, increased risk for seizures
	Klonopin	Clonazepam	
		Pheonbarbital	
Severe pain from injury, postsurgical care, oral surgery, migraines	Davorcet-N	Propoxyphene	Drowsiness, dizziness, increased risk for overdose, slowed or difficult breathing, impaired motor control, unusual behavior, memory problems
	Demerol	Meperedine	
	Fiorinal with codeine	Butalbital and codeine	
	Percocet	Oxycodone	
	Vicodin	Hydrocodone	

(Table continues)

(Table continued)

Symptoms/Disorders	Medication (Brand Name)	Medication (Generic Name)	Some Possible Reactions with Alcohol
Sleep problems	Ambien	Zolpidem	Drowsiness, sleepiness, dizziness, slowed or difficulty breathing, impaired motor control, unusual behavior, memory problems
	Lunesta	Escopiclone	
	Prosom	Estazolam	
	Restoril	Temazepam	
	Sominex	Diphenhydramine	
	Unison	Doxylamine	
	Herbal preparations (chamomile, valerian, lavender)		Increased drowsiness

Source: Adapted from National Institute on Alcohol Abuse and Alcoholism. *Harmful Interactions: Mixing Alcohol with Medicines.* NIH Publication No. 03-5329, National Institutes of Health, 2007.

12 ounces of beer is equivalent to 5 ounces of wine or 1.5 ounces of 80-proof distilled spirits. In some cases, alcohol is measured by *proof,* and an alcoholic beverage that is 80 proof is 40 percent alcohol. In general, aging slows down the older person's ability to metabolize alcohol and thus the alcohol remains in the system longer than it does in a younger person. As a result, lower amounts of alcohol can cause intoxication and ill effects in the older person.

Regular Drinkers and Binge Drinkers

According to the National Center for Health Statistics in their annual publication on health data, in 2004, 38 percent of older individuals ages 65 to 74 in the United States were regular drinkers and 16.4 percent were infrequent drinkers. About 6 percent were binge drinkers (consuming five or more drinks on at least one day in the past year) in 2004, the latest data available.

Alcohol consumption can cause sedation, dizziness, and even unconsciousness, depending on how much alcohol is consumed. It is also known to irritate, inflame, and depress the nervous system. Many medications interact with alcohol, and older people have a greater risk than others of suffering a bad outcome, such as a fall, a car crash, liver damage, impaired breathing, and many other reactions. See Table 1 for possible reactions of many drugs with alcohol.

Some people become dependent on alcohol, which is also referred to as ALCOHOLISM. Some older individuals who have not previously abused alcohol become alcoholic in their senior years due to loneliness, anxiety, or DEPRESSION.

Potential Effects of Alcohol

As seen in Table 1, many common medications can cause serious reactions when combined with alcohol, including over-the-counter drugs such as cold and allergy medications, as well as prescription medications, such as those taken for angina, hypertension, arthritis, and so forth. As a result, older people taking medications should talk to their doctor about whether it is safe to consume any alcohol—even a small amount—while they are taking medication.

See also ADVERSE DRUG EVENT; BINGE DRINKING; DRIVING; DRUG ABUSE; GENDER DIFFERENCES; PRESCRIPTION DRUG ABUSE/MISUSE; SUBSTANCE ABUSE AND DEPENDENCE.

National Center for Health Statistics. *Health, United States, 2006 with Chartbook on Trends in the Health of Americans.* National Institutes of Health. Hyattsville, Md.: 2006.

National Institute on Alcohol Abuse and Alcoholism. *Harmful Interactions: Mixing Alcohol with Medicines.* NIH Publication No. 03-5329, National Institutes of Health, 2007.

alcoholism   Addiction to ALCOHOL. Alcoholism is also known as *alcohol dependence,* and it is a form of substance abuse/dependence. Severe long-term alcoholism can lead to a thiamine deficiency and a DEMENTIA-like disorder that is known as WERNICKE-KORSAKOFF SYNDROME. Alcoholism causes many other serious health problems, including gastrointestinal disorders, liver cirrhosis, and some forms of cancer. Alcohol is the most common drug of abuse among individuals age 65 and older, according to the Substance Abuse and Mental Health Services Administration (SAMHSA). (See DRUG ABUSE.)

In 2005, alcohol was the primary substance of abuse among the majority (75.9 percent) individuals age 65 and older who were admitted for treatment of substance abuse. Most (76 percent) were male.

In moderation, alcohol (such as wine) can benefit some individuals by lowering blood pressure; however, excessive amounts of alcohol are very damaging to the body. The National Institute on Alcohol Abuse and Alcoholism recommends that people age 65 and older who choose to drink should markedly limit their alcohol consumption to no more than one drink per day.

The person who is an alcoholic is dependent on alcohol and has developed a tolerance to it such that he or she needs greater quantities than the nonalcoholic in order to achieve the same level of intoxication. Alcoholism is a major problem in the United States among all ages, and older people are at risk for alcohol dependence, particularly older men. Many elderly alcoholics have been heavy drinkers for years, but some elderly people only start their excessive drinking (or even drinking at all) when they are older because they are lonely, sick, depressed, or have other problems that concern or frighten them, such as financial problems or other issues.

According to the National Center for Health Statistics, about 45 percent of adults age 65 and older drank alcohol in 2004, and of those who were heavy drinkers, there was a greater percentage of males (53 percent) than females (37 percent). In addition, about 6 percent of adults ages 65 to 74 in 2004 who were current drinkers drank five or more drinks on at least one day in the past year. (This level of drinking is problematic, and it also indicates the presence of BINGE DRINKING and/or alcoholism.)

In 2005, there were 11,300 adults in the United States over age 65 who were admitted to treatment for some form of substance abuse. Alcohol was the abused substance in the majority of cases, according to the Substance Abuse and Mental Health Services Administration, and it represented 75.9 percent of all admissions. Most older adults (about 72 percent) who were admitted for treatment were white males. (The next most abused substances were opiates, representing the primary substance in 10.5 percent of all admissions.)

Symptoms and Diagnostic Path

According to the National Institute on Alcohol Abuse and Alcoholism (NIAAA), alcoholism is present when individuals have three or more of the following indicators:

- a tolerance to alcohol (more alcohol is needed to achieve the same level of intoxication than in the past)
- withdrawal symptoms (if alcohol is *not* consumed, physical symptoms such as nausea, sweating, and shakiness occur)
- use of the substance in a larger quantity than was intended by the individual
- the persistent desire to cut down or to control the use of alcohol
- a significant amount of time is spent on obtaining, using, or recovering from alcohol use
- drinking that occurs in order for the person to avoid the symptoms of withdrawal
- neglect of an individual's normal social, occupational, or recreational tasks (among older people, these indications may be mistakenly perceived by others as normal aging)
- continued use of alcohol despite the physical and psychological problems of the user

Treatment Options and Outlook

Some older individuals are treated for their alcoholism on an outpatient basis, while others receive treatment in a rehabilitative facility. Some studies have shown that older adults with alcoholism have the highest level of treatment success of all age groups, despite a generally worse physical health status. Studies have also shown that older patients in treatment often have more social support and a lower rate of psychological problems than individuals of other age groups. This may play a significant role in their greater levels of success with treatment for alcoholism.

However, many older people with alcoholism refuse to acknowledge that they have a problem and/or they refuse treatment. In addition, some family members may believe that it would be embarrassing, cumbersome, expensive, or even pointless to send an elderly person to a rehabilitative facility. Another problem is that most facilities that treat alcoholism are not designed for the treatment of older individuals and thus, they cannot provide for their medical needs.

Sometimes medications to treat alcoholism may be given to the older alcoholic, although care must be used. The primary medications that are used to treat alcoholism are acamprosate (Campral), naltrexone (ReVia), or disulfiram (Antabuse). Because disulfiram causes copious vomiting even when very minute quantities of alcohol are consumed by accident (as with cooking sherry or wine that is present in food), many physicians are very hesitant to prescribe this drug to patients over age 65.

It is also true that older people taking disulfiram may have difficulty understanding that they must completely avoid all over-the-counter medications that contain any alcohol, such as Nyquil or generic cold medicines with alcohol, as well as even minute amounts of alcohol in food. In addition, disulfiram is dangerous for older adults because the alcohol-disulfiram reaction may cause hypotension or tachycardia (rapid heartbeat). Naltrexone appears to be well tolerated in some small studies of older individuals with alcoholism; however, further studies are needed.

BENZODIAZEPINES are another category of medication that may be used to help alcoholics who are suffering from the symptoms of withdrawal; however, some benzodiazepines are not recommended for the treatment of older people, as these medications may have harmful side effects in older people. They are sedating drugs and can increase the risk of falls among older people.

Behavioral therapy is also used effectively to treat alcoholism in patients of all ages. In addition, many patients benefit from attending meetings of self-help groups, such as Alcoholics Anonymous.

Risk Factors and Preventive Measures

There are genetic predispositions to alcoholism, and in many cases, the elderly alcoholic person had a mother and/or a father with alcoholism. However, some children of alcoholics never drink, and it is also true that some children of nondrinking parents do become alcoholics.

In some cases, older individuals apparently develop alcoholism because of serious problems that they face, such as the death of a loved one, severe pain from an illness, family problems, or other issues. Sometimes alcoholism does not appear until the person is elderly.

Women who were not alcoholics in the past are more likely to become alcoholics at a late age than men. According to Frederick C. Blow and Kristen Lawton Barry in their article for *Alcohol Research & Health,* older women who formerly did not abuse alcohol have a greater risk of turning to alcohol than older men because they are more likely to outlive their spouses and be faced with losses that may cause depression and loneliness. For example, widowed women may feel shut out from couples with whom they formerly associated, and they may feel like the "odd woman out."

In most cases, men begin their heavy drinking in early adulthood or even before then, such as in adolescence or childhood. Individuals who are depressed may turn to alcohol for psychological relief; however, alcohol is a depressant and it cannot provide permanent or substantial emotional improvements.

The best preventive measure against alcoholism is to avoid drinking altogether, because alcohol can contribute to many health problems of the liver, kidneys, heart, and other organs, and alcohol abuse and alcoholism exacerbate the risk.

See also ACCIDENTAL INJURIES; AGGRESSION, PHYSICAL; ALCOHOL; ANEMIA; DRIVING; FALLS; GENDER DIFFERENCES; NARCOTICS; PRESCRIPTION DRUG ABUSE/MISUSE; SUBSTANCE ABUSE AND DEPENDENCE.

Blow, Frederick C., and Kristen Lawton Barry. "Use and Misuse of Alcohol Among Older Women." *Alcohol Research & Health* 26, no. 4 (2002): 308–315.

Gwinnell, Esther, and Christine Adamec. *The Encyclopedia of Addictions and Addictive Behaviors.* New York: Facts On File, 2005.

———. *The Encyclopedia of Drug Abuse.* New York: Facts On File, Inc., 2008.

Substance Abuse and Mental Health Services Administration. "Adults Aged 65 or Older in Substance Abuse

Treatment: 2005." May 31, 2007. Available online. URL: http//oas.samhsa.gov/2k7/older/TX/olderTX.htm. Accessed October 12, 2007.

alternative/complementary medicine (CAM)
See COMPLEMENTARY/ALTERNATIVE MEDICINE.

Alzheimer's disease/dementia A degenerative brain disease and the most common form of DEMENTIA. This disease was first discovered by Dr. Alois Alzheimer in 1906 after an autopsy on a female patient, Auguste D., who had suffered from an early onset of the disease. Dr. Alzheimer discovered that the brain cells in the cerebral cortex of Auguste D. were very different from normal brain cells. The cerebral cortex is the region of the brain that manages memory and reasoning. Dr. Alzheimer also found tangles of a plaque substance in the brain, a substance that is not seen in a normal brain.

Alzheimer's disease (AD) is also known as *senile dementia of the Alzheimer's type*. This form of dementia causes deteriorating brain function, and it is nearly always devastating for the individual in the early stages (who has sufficient awareness to know that he or she will get worse) as well as for family members, who must often face the fact that their relative will eventually not recognize them at all. The average patient with Alzheimer's disease lives from eight to 10 years after they are diagnosed, although the disease may last as long as 20 years in some patients.

In some cases, other diseases may mimic the symptoms of early Alzheimer's disease, such as the presence of DEPRESSION, thyroid disease, brain tumors, chemical imbalances or deficiencies, or blood vessel disease in the brain. As a result, other illnesses should be ruled out first through laboratory tests and careful diagnosis before Alzheimer's disease is diagnosed. In addition, another form of dementia may be present, which may need treatment that is different from the recommended treatment for Alzheimer's disease.

An estimated 4.5 to 5 million people in the United States have Alzheimer's disease. According to the Alzheimer's Association, someone in the United States develops Alzheimer's disease every 72 seconds.

The onset of Alzheimer's disease usually occurs after age 60, and the risk for the disease increases with age. There is also an early-onset form of the disease, although most people with Alzheimer's disease have the form with the later onset. An estimated 5 percent of men and women ages 65 to 74 have Alzheimer's disease and nearly half of all individuals age 85 and older may have the disease according to the National Institute on Aging.

Of course, the converse is also true; an estimated 95 percent of men and women ages 65 to 74 do *not* have Alzheimer's disease, and about half of all individuals 85 years old and older do not have it either. This fact is often forgotten in ageist assumptions that all or most older people have Alzheimer's disease. (See AGEISM.)

There are many different theories as to the cause of Alzheimer's disease. According to the Alzheimer's Disease & Education (ADEAR) Center, a service of the National Institute on Aging, the genetic risk for Alzheimer's disease lies largely with the early-onset (before age 65 years) form of the disease. An ADEAR expert says that the early-onset form of Alzheimer's disease is often caused by genetic mutations on chromosomes 1, 14, and 21. However, this is a *risk* and not a certainty, contrary to the fears of many relative caregivers of individuals with Alzheimer's disease who wonder if their brain is a ticking time bomb ready to develop Alzheimer's disease at some future point.

There are no obvious inheritance patterns, as of this writing, with the late-onset form of Alzheimer's disease, and this form encompasses more than 95 percent of all cases. There are, however, genetic risk factors with late-onset Alzheimer's, but only one gene, apolipoprotein E, that is found on chromosome 19, has been identified as a risk factor to date.

Symptoms and Diagnostic Path
The symptoms of Alzheimer's disease may be subtle and go unnoticed in the very early stages; however, the disease progressively worsens. Neurologists are the best-qualified specialists to diagnose and treat Alzheimer's disease, although many

general practitioners also treat individuals who are still in an early stage of the disorder.

In the early stages of Alzheimer's disease (sometimes referred to as *mild* AD) the person may experience one or more of the following symptoms:

- personality changes, such as AGITATION, depression, and anxiety
- frequent and unexplained mood swings
- difficulties with thinking and reasoning
- temporary CONFUSION while outside his or her house or neighborhood
- difficulty performing tasks that the person could perform in the past, such as writing checks or making minor repairs

In the next stage, or the *moderate* stage of Alzheimer's, the disease is easier for the doctor to diagnose because the symptoms are significantly more obvious and prominent. They may include the following symptoms and signs:

- an inability to perform personal tasks that could be performed in the past, such as bathing or toileting
- loss of good personal hygiene (such as wearing the same dirty clothes, day after day)
- aggressive or combative behavior, which is problematic to the family and to others the person with Alzheimer's disease deals with
- difficulty with speech and with responses that require more than a one- or two-word answer

In the late stage of Alzheimer's disease (sometimes referred to as *severe* AD), the person may exhibit the following symptoms and signs:

- total incontinence of both the bowels and bladder, requiring the use of adult diapers
- rages that occur for no apparent reason, as well as other mood changes
- aphasia (difficulty speaking to others or understanding the words that are spoken by others)
- extreme paranoia or suspiciousness

- speech that is slow or impossible to understand
- trouble with simple tasks that the individual could perform in the past, such as tying shoes or dressing oneself

Treatment Options and Outlook

Medications may be prescribed to delay the progression of the symptoms, although there are no medications available to date that can permanently halt or cure Alzheimer's disease. As of this writing, there are five medications that are approved for the treatment of early Alzheimer's disease, and there is also one medication that is approved to treat individuals who have been diagnosed as in the moderate to severe stage of the disease. (See Table 1 for a description of the four most commonly used medications.)

In 2008 preliminary studies indicated that in a major breakthrough, etanercept, a medication that is approved for treating RHEUMATOID ARTHRITIS, may also be effective in treating Alzheimer's disease, if early preliminary results prove effective in further large-scale clinical studies. Very small studies with about 15 subjects, conducted by principal investigator Edward Tobinick, director of the Institute for Neurological Research in Los Angeles, revealed that etanercept (Enbrel, Amgen) injected in the spine significantly improved the cognitive abilities of some individuals with Alzheimer's disease. For example, within two hours of being injected with the drug in his spine, an 81-year-old man with Alzheimer's disease who was unable identify nine of 10 everyday objects *was* able to identify the objects. He was also less agitated than prior to treatment. (Agitation is a major problem among many individuals with Alzheimer's disease.)

Etanercept does not cure Alzheimer's disease, but it may represent a breakthrough treatment. It is the first major hope that researchers have identified in years.

Risk Factors and Preventive Measures

Individuals whose parents or siblings now have Alzheimer's disease or whose deceased parents or siblings had Alzheimer's disease have an increased risk for the disease, although they may not develop it. As mentioned earlier, the primary genetic risk is with early-onset Alzheimer's disease. Past studies

TABLE 1. MEDICATIONS PRESCRIBED FOR PATIENTS WITH ALZHEIMER'S DISEASE

Drug Name and Action	Drug Type and Treatment	Manufacturer's Recommended Dosage	Common Side Effects	Possible Drug Interactions
Namenda (memantine) Blocks the toxic effects associated with excess glutamate and regulates glutamate activation	N-methyl D-aspartate (NMDA) antagonist prescribed to treat symptoms of moderate to severe AD	• 5 mg once a day, available in tablet form • Increase to 10 mg/day (5 mg twice a day), 15 mg/day (5 mg and 10 mg as separate doses), and 20 mg/day (10 mg twice a day) at minimum of one week intervals if well-tolerated	Dizziness, headache, constipation, confusion	Other NMDA antagonist medications, including amantadine (an antiviral used to treat the flu), dextromethorphan (prescribed to treat coughs due to cold or flu), and ketamine (sometimes used as an anesthetic) have not been systematically evaluated and should be used with caution in combination with this medication.*
Razadyne (galantamine, formerly known as Reminyl) Prevents the breakdown of acetylcholine and stimulates nicotine receptors to release more acetylcholine in the brain	Cholinesterase inhibitor prescribed to treat symptoms of mild to moderate AD	• 4 mg twice a day (8 mg/day), available in tablet or capsule form • Increase by 8 mg/day after 4 weeks to 8 mg, twice a day (16 mg/day), if well-tolerated • After another 4 weeks, increase to 12 mg, twice a day (25 mg/day) if well-tolerated	Nausea, vomiting, diarrhea, weight loss	Some antidepressants such as paroxetine, amitriptyline, fluoxetine, fluvoxamine, and other drugs with anticholinergic action may cause retention of excess Reminyl in the body, leading to complications. NSAIDs should be used with caution in combination with this medication.*
Exelon (rivastigmine) Prevents the breakdown of acetylcholine and butyrycholine (a brain chemical similar to acetylcholine) in the brain	Cholinesterase inhibitor prescribed to treat symptoms of mild to moderate AD	• 1.5 mg, twice a day (3 mg/day), available in capsule and liquid form • Increase by 3 mg/day every 2 weeks to 6 mg, twice a day (12 mg/day) if well-tolerated	Nausea, vomiting, weight loss, upset stomach, muscle weakness	None observed in laboratory studies. NSAIDs should be used with caution in combination with this medication.*
Aricept (donepezil) Prevents the breakdown of acetylcholine in the brain	Cholinesterase inhibitor prescribed to treat symptoms of mild to moderate and moderate to severe AD	• 5 mg once a day, available in tablet form. • Increase after 4–8 weeks to 10 mg, once a day if well-tolerated	Nausea, diarrhea, vomiting	None observed in laboratory studies. NSAID should be used with caution in combination with this medication.*
Cognex (tacrine) Prevents the breakdown of acetylcholine in the brain (Note: Cognex is still available but is no longer actively marketed by the manufacturer)	Cholinesterase inhibitor prescribed to treat symptoms of mild to moderate AD	• 10 mg, four times a day (40 mg/day), in capsule form • Increase by 40 mg/day every 4 weeks to 40 mg, four times a day (160 mg/day), if liver enzyme functions remain normal and if well-tolerated	Nausea, diarrhea, possible liver damage	NSAIDs should be used with caution in combination with this medication.*

*Note: Use of cholinesterase inhibitors can increase the risk of stomach ulcers, and because prolonged use of nonsteroidal anti-inflammatory drugs (NSAIDs) such as aspirin or ibuprofen can also cause stomach ulcers, NSAIDs should be used with caution in combination with these medications.
Source: Adapted, modified, and derived from Alzheimer's Disease Education and Referral Center. "Alzheimer's Disease Medications: Fact Sheet." Bethesda, Md.: National Institutes of Health, November 2006. Available online. URL: http://www.nia.nih.gov/Alzheimers/Publications/medicationsfs.htm. Accessed July 15, 2007.

have indicated the following risks for adult children and identical twins:

- 11 percent if neither parent has Alzheimer's
- 36 percent if one parent has the disease
- 54 percent if both parents have the disease
- 40–50 percent if an identical twin has Alzheimer's disease

Alzheimer's disease cannot be prevented, although the deterioration can be somewhat delayed through the use of medication. Stimulation through encouraging the individual to use the mind through doing even simple crossword puzzles or other forms of mental challenges are also often a good idea.

Caregiving Suggestions

Caregiving for a relative with Alzheimer's can become extremely stressful and cumbersome, particularly as the disease progresses and the mental deterioration of the individual increases. The National Institute on Aging offers suggestions for caregiving for individuals with Alzheimer's disease in their *Caregiver's Guide,* published in 2007. Other suggestions are offered in *Home Safety for People with Alzheimer's Disease,* published by the National Institute on Aging in 2007.

Some suggestions for more successful communication include

- minimizing distractions and noise, such as the television and radio, to enable the individual with Alzheimer's to focus on what you are saying
- choosing simple words and short sentences to communicate and speaking in a calm and gentle voice
- calling the individual by name and making sure that you have his or her attention before continuing
- giving the person enough time to respond and not interrupting
- gently providing the word that he or she appears to be looking for if the person struggles to communicate an idea or thought
- framing instructions and questions in a positive manner

- having the discussion in a familiar setting if possible

Some suggestions for bathing the person with Alzheimer's disease include

- planning the bath or shower for the time of day when the individual is usually the most agreeable and trying to develop a routine
- understanding that bathing can be frightening and uncomfortable for some people who have Alzheimer's disease, so be patient, gentle, and calm
- testing the water temperature before the person enters the bath or shower to make sure it is not too hot or cold
- using a handheld showerhead, shower bench, or shower chair and grab bars and nonskid bath mats
- never leaving the person alone in the shower or bath, where he or she may become injured
- using a sponge bath for days between showers and baths
- telling the person what you are going to do, step by step, as you bathe him or her, and allowing the person to do as much as possible

Some suggestions for dressing the person with Alzheimer's disease include

- having the person get dressed at the same time each day so it will become part of a daily routine
- encouraging the person to dress himself or herself as much as possible and allowing extra time
- allowing the person to choose from a limited selection of outfits
- choosing clothing that is easy to take on and off, such as pants with elastic waists or clothes with Velcro closures, to avoid struggling with buttons and zippers
- arranging the clothes in the order in which they are to be put on to minimize confusion

Some suggestions for helping people with Alzheimer's with eating include

- giving the person food choices but limiting the number of choices
- serving small portions throughout the day and having healthy snacks and finger foods available (be aware of the risk of the person overeating while in the early stages of dementia)
- using dishes that encourage independence, such as a bowl instead of a plate or eating utensils with large handles, and using straws or cups with lids to make drinking easier
- making mealtimes calm and limiting noise
- realizing that as the disease progresses, the risk for choking increases

Some suggestions for dealing with sleep problems include

- limiting daytime napping so that the individual will need to sleep at night, while making sure that the individual gets sufficient rest
- scheduling more physically demanding tasks for earlier in the day (bathing may be best in the morning, while large family meals may be best around noon)
- restricting access to caffeine in the evening
- using night-lights in the hallway, bedroom, and bathroom so that the darkness will not be disorienting

As the illness worsens, the person with Alzheimer's disease may experience hallucinations (seeing, hearing, smelling, tasting, or feeling something that is not there) or delusions (false beliefs that are strongly held).
Some suggestions for dealing with hallucinations and delusions include

- not arguing with the person about what he or she hears or sees. Try instead to respond to the person about the feelings expressed (such as fear or anxiety). Do not, however, say that you also see or hear the hallucinations.
- distracting the person to perform another activity, such as going for a walk or even just leaving the room.
- turning off the television when violent programs are shown. The person with Alzheimer's may

have trouble distinguishing television programming from real life.
- ensuring that the person is safe and has no access to any items that can harm anyone (guns should be removed and placed in a location where the individual cannot access them)

Because many people with Alzheimer's disease have a problem with WANDERING from their homes, the following suggestions may help:

- Be sure that the person has some form of identification or wears a medical bracelet. Consider enrolling the person in the Alzheimer's Association Safe Return program if such a program is available in your area (contact the Alzheimer's Association at [800] 272-3900 or http://www.alz.org). Tell neighbors that the individual has a tendency to wander so they can notify you or another person when it happens.
- Keep a recent photograph or videotape of the person with Alzheimer's to show police if the individual becomes lost.
- Keep the doors locked. Consider using a keyed deadbolt or an additional lock that is high or low on the door.
- Put away anything that could cause danger to the individual, both inside and outside the house.

Suggestions for improving home safety for the person with Alzheimer's disease include

- installing secure locks on all outside doors and windows and removing bathroom door locks to prevent the person from locking himself or herself in the bathroom
- installing smoke alarms near all bedrooms and place carbon monoxide detectors in appropriate places and check the batteries frequently
- hiding a spare key outside in case the person with Alzheimer's locks you out of the house
- using childproof plugs on unused outlets
- making sure there are light switches at both the top and bottom of stairs
- locking up all medications

- locking up alcohol because drinking increases confusion
- keeping plastic bags out of reach
- locking up all power tools and machinery
- removing all poisonous plants
- keeping fish tanks out of reach because the combination of water, glass, and electrical pumps could harm the person
- using a monitoring device (such as one used for infants) to alert you to noises indicating a need for help
- placing locks on exit doors either high or low rather than in the direct line of sight
- placing signs such as STOP, DO NOT ENTER, or CLOSED in strategic areas around the home
- If the person should no longer drive, ask his or her doctor to write DO NOT DRIVE on a prescription pad. Show this to the person with Alzheimer's disease. In addition, ask the doctor to write to the Department of Motor Vehicles at the state capitol to tell them the person should no longer drive. (State laws on removing driving privileges vary greatly from state to state.) Consider having a mechanic install a kill switch or alarm system that disengages the fuel line and prevents the car from starting at all.
- placing red tape around radiators, floor vents, and other heating devices to deter the person from standing on or touching a hot grid
- using childproof latches on cabinets where cleaning supplies are kept
- making the house clutter free to decrease the risk for falls
- installing an automatic shut-off switch on the stove in order to prevent burns or a fire

See also ACTIVITIES OF DAILY LIVING; ADULT CHILDREN/CHILDREN OF AGING PARENTS; AGGRESSION, PHYSICAL; COGNITIVE IMPAIRMENT; COMPASSION FATIGUE; DELUSIONS; DEMENTIA; ELDERIZING A HOME; END-OF-LIFE ISSUES; FAMILY AND MEDICAL LEAVE ACT; FAMILY CAREGIVERS; HALLUCINATIONS; HEALTH CARE AGENT/PROXY; IRRITABILITY; LEARNED HELPLESSNESS; MEMORY IMPAIRMENT; NURSING HOMES; RAGE; SUNDOWNING; TOILETING; TRANSPORTATION.

Alzheimer's Disease Education and Referral Center. "Alzheimer's Disease Medications: Fact Sheet." Bethesda, Md.: National Institutes of Health, November 2006. Available online. URL: http://www.nia.nih.gov/Alzheimers/Publications/medicationsfs.htm. Accessed July 15, 2007.

Cassels, Caroline. "Anti-TNF-alpha Therapy Produces Rapid Improvement in Alzheimer's Disease." *Medscape Medical News,* January 15, 2008. Available online. URL: http://www.medscape.com/home. Accessed February 28, 2008.

National Institute on Aging. *Alzheimer's Disease Fact Sheet.* Hyattsville, Md.: National Institutes of Health. July 2006. Available Online. URL: http://www.nia.nih.gov/alzheimer's/publications/adfact.htm. Accessed February 13, 2008.

———. *Caregiver Guide: Tips for Caregivers of People with Alzheimer's Disease.* Hyattsville, Md.: National Institutes of Health. (Undated.) Available online. URL: http://www.nia.nih.gov/Alzheimers/Publications/caregiverguide.htm. Accessed July 10, 2007.

———. *Home Safety for People with Alzheimer's Disease.* Hyattsville, Md.: National Institutes of Health. Available online. URL: http://www.nia.nih.gov/Alzheimers/Publications/homesafety.htm. Accessed July 30, 2007.

Americans with Disabilities Act A federal law that was first enacted in 1990 and which prohibits discrimination in areas that are used by individuals with disabilities, such as public places (city hall, public libraries, etc.), restaurants and cafeterias, medical clinics and hospitals, libraries, and many other locations. The law requires that toilets, sinks, alarms, ramps, drinking fountains, stairs, parking areas, and elevators be accessible to the disabled. As a result of the Americans with Disabilities Act, individuals who are disabled find such areas far easier to navigate than in past years.

See also ACCESSIBILITY TO FACILITIES; DISABILITY; FAMILY AND MEDICAL LEAVE ACT.

Department of Justice. "Nondiscrimination on the Basis of Disability by Public Accommodations and in Commercial Facilities: Excerpt from 28 CFR Part 36: ADA Standards for Accessible Design." Washington, D.C.: Code of Federal Regulations. Available online. URL: http://www.usdoj.gov/crt/ada/stdspdf.htm. Accessed November 23, 2007.

amyotrophic lateral sclerosis (ALS) Also known as Lou Gehrig's disease and named after the baseball player who was first identified with this degenerative disease. It is a progressive disease of the spinal cord and the brain motor neurons that control movement, and as a result, eventually walking, eating, speaking, and even breathing will become very difficult or impossible for the individual and aids such as a breathing ventilator become necessary. About 30,000 people in the United States have ALS. Most patients die within three to six years from the onset of their symptoms, but some live for many years, particularly if they choose to be maintained on a ventilator.

Symptoms and Diagnostic Path

According to the National Institute of Neurological Diseases and Stroke, the symptoms of ALS are often subtle in the early stages and may include cramping and stiff muscles, muscle weakness of a leg or an arm, slurred speech or difficulty with chewing and swallowing. The individual may also have severe difficulty with breathing. These symptoms worsen into obvious weakness.

Sometimes only one leg may be affected and patients experience weakness when walking or tripping or stumbling. They may have difficulty writing a note or buttoning a shirt. The weakness and muscle atrophy eventually spread to the rest of the body, and patients develop difficulty speaking, walking, and even swallowing. Brief muscle twitches can be observed under the skin.

ALS is diagnosed based on the signs and symptoms that the doctor observes. Tests are used to rule out other diseases, such as electromyography (EMG), a test to measure electrical activity in the muscles. Computerized tomography (CT) scans or magnetic resonance imaging (MRI) scans can help physicians with the diagnosis. Laboratory tests of blood and urine will also be ordered to rule out other diseases. In some cases, infectious diseases such as the human immunodeficiency virus (HIV) have symptoms that can mimic ALS symptoms.

Treatment Options and Outlook

There is no cure for this disease. The drug riluzole (Rilutek) is the only medication approved by the U.S. Food and Drug Administration (FDA) for the treatment of ALS, and it may prolong the patient's survival for several months. Other types of drugs such as antidepressants may be prescribed because often patients with ALS suffer from depression. In addition, medications are given to treat symptoms, such as pain, cramping, and muscle spasms. Supportive therapies may be provided, such as physical therapy, speech therapy, and occupational therapy. Patients may use computer-assisted communication devices to communicate with others when they can no longer speak. A ventilator may become needed if the patient can no longer breathe on his or her own.

The prognosis for ALS is poor as of this writing, because the disease causes progressive deterioration and no known treatments can break the cycle. According to the National Institute of Neurological Disorders and Stroke, most people with ALS die from respiratory failure, usually within three to five years of the onset of symptoms.

Risk Factors and Preventive Measures

A small percentage (less than 10 percent) of ALS is caused by an inherited predisposition.

Men have a greater risk for ALS than women. Most individuals stricken with ALS are diagnosed between ages 40 and 60. There are no known preventive measures.

See also DEMENTIA.

National Institute of Neurological Disorders and Stroke. "Amyotrophic Lateral Sclerosis Fact Sheet." Updated February 2008. Available online. URL: http://www.ninds.nih.gov/disorders/amyotrophiclateralsclerosis/detail_amyotrophiclateralscleros is.htm. Accessed February 13, 2008.

Zeller, John L., M.D., Cassio Lynn, and Richard M. Glass, M.D. "Amyotrophic Lateral Sclerosis." *Journal of the American Medical Association* 298, no. 2 (July 11, 2007): 248.

anemia A blood disease in which there is an insufficient number of red blood cells and a deficiency of either the hematocrit or hemoglobin blood levels. *Hematocrit* refers to the percentage of red blood cells in a blood test, while *hemoglobin* refers to a substance that carries oxygen in the blood throughout the body.

Anemia may be a short-term problem that responds to treatment or it can become a long-term disorder that is difficult to diagnose and treat. Many older people suffer from some form of anemia, often caused by deficiencies of vitamin B_{12} or iron, gastrointestinal bleeding, or resulting from chronic diseases. In addition, sometimes the treatments for other diseases can cause anemia, such as chemotherapy or radiation therapy given to treat CANCER. An estimated 61 percent of individuals age 65 and older have some form of anemia, according to the National Anemia Action Council, and the risk is particularly high for men.

There are three primary types of anemia, including iron deficiency anemia, Vitamin B_{12} deficiency anemia (also known as pernicious anemia), and the anemia that occurs as a result of some chronic diseases, which is also known as anemia of chronic disease. According to Doctors Weiss and Goodnough in their article on anemia for the *New England Journal of Medicine* in 2005, the anemia of chronic disease is the second most common form of anemia after iron deficiency anemia.

Iron deficiency anemia may be caused by the heavy use of nonsteroidal anti-inflammatory medications (NSAIDs), which may lead to gastrointestinal blood loss. Individuals with ARTHRITIS are often prescribed NSAIDs to relieve pain and inflammation, and thus their blood should be checked periodically for the possible presence of iron deficiency anemia. Poor NUTRITION may also lead to iron deficiency anemia in older individuals, who may neglect eating a balanced diet because of DEPRESSION, their inability to prepare meals, or another problem. If the individual has an iron deficiency anemia, iron supplements should be administered while the underlying cause for the anemia is being determined.

When anemia of chronic disease is present, it is often associated with the following diseases:

- cancer
- INFECTIONS, including bacterial, viral, parasitic, or fungal infections
- autoimmune disorders such as systemic lupus erythematosus, inflammatory bowel disease, or RHEUMATOID ARTHRITIS
- chronic kidney disease

According to Weiss and Goodnough, the key difference between iron deficiency anemia and the anemia of chronic disease is that iron deficiency anemia is caused by iron deficiency *only*, whereas many possible factors can cause anemia of chronic disease.

When the cause of the anemia is determined and the problem is treated, the anemia should improve.

Vitamin B_{12} anemia is common among older adults and according to the Office of Dietary Supplements of the National Institutes of Health, up to 30 percent of adults 50 years old and older may have *atrophic gastritis,* a condition in which there is an increased growth of intestinal bacteria and an inability to absorb vitamin B_{12} from food; however, individuals *are* able to absorb synthetic Vitamin B_{12} from dietary supplements or fortified foods. As a result, they should take Vitamin B_{12} supplements as well as enhance their diet with foods rich in Vitamin B_{12}. If B_{12} levels still do not rise, then often these individuals will require injections of B_{12} on a routine basis.

There are a variety of common medications that may interact with the absorption of Vitamin B_{12}, and one such example is metformin (Glucophage, Glucophage XL), a drug that is used to treat DIABETES. In addition, some drugs that are taken to treat gastroesophageal reflux disease (GERD) or for a peptic ULCER may decrease the individual's vitamin B_{12} levels. (See Table 1). Older individuals who are taking these drugs should check with their doctors to see if they may be deficient in vitamin B_{12}. Chronic alcohol use may also block the absorption of Vitamin B_{12}.

Symptoms and Diagnostic Path

Symptoms of anemia may sometimes be mistakenly attributed to "old age." In addition, anemia should also be considered a possibility if the older person has cancer, hepatitis, OSTEOARTHRITIS, rheumatoid arthritis, or tuberculosis, because of the treatments associated with those diseases. If older individuals exhibit any of the following symptoms or signs, their blood should be tested for anemia:

TABLE 1. IMPORTANT VITAMIN B$_{12}$ DRUG INTERACTIONS THAT MAY LEAD TO ANEMIA

Drug Class and Drugs	Potential Interaction
Proton pump inhibitors (PPIs) are used to treat gastroesophageal reflux disease (GERD) and peptic ulcer disease. Examples of PPIs are omeprazole (Prilosec) and lansoprazole (Prevacid).	PPI medications can interfere with vitamin B$_{12}$ absorption from food by slowing the release of hydrochloric acid into the stomach. This is a concern because acid is needed to release vitamin B$_{12}$ from food prior to absorption. So far, however, there is no evidence that these medications promote vitamin B$_{12}$ deficiency, even after long use.
Histamine 2 (H2) receptor antagonists are used to treat peptic ulcer disease. Examples are Tagamet, Pepsid, and Zantac.	H2 receptor antagonists can interfere with vitamin B$_{12}$ absorption from food by slowing the release of hydrochloric acid into the stomach. This is a concern because acid is needed to release vitamin B$_{12}$ from food prior to absorption. So far, however, there is no evidence that these medications promote vitamin B$_{12}$ deficiency, even after long-term use.
Metformin is a drug used to treat diabetes.	Metformin may interfere with calcium metabolism. This may indirectly reduce vitamin B$_{12}$ absorption because vitamin B$_{12}$ absorption requires calcium. Surveys suggest that from 10 to 30 percent of patients taking Metformin have evidence of reduced vitamin B$_{12}$ absorption.

Source: Office of Dietary Supplements. "Vitamin B$_{12}$." Dietary Supplement Fact Sheet, 2006. Available online. URL: http://ods.od.nih.gov/factsheets/VitaminB12_pf.asp. Accessed August 22, 2007.

- weakness
- worsening dizziness
- frequent infections
- HEADACHE
- rapid heartbeat
- pale skin
- cold hands and feet
- CONFUSION
- impaired balance
- chest pain
- fatigue

Some of the symptoms of anemia are symptoms that are also commonly seen in the elderly, such as cold hands and feet, fatigue, and so forth. As a result, physicians often may mistakenly assume that the individual's symptoms are related to aging rather than to anemia or another disease or disorder. However, regular laboratory tests should avoid this problem of misdiagnosis.

If anemia is suspected, in many cases, the primary laboratory test that is needed is a complete blood count (CBC), which is a common laboratory test to measure red and white blood cells.

Treatment Options and Outlook

Iron supplements are prescribed if the individual has iron deficiency anemia. If the patient is deficient in vitamin B$_{12}$, then B$_{12}$ supplements are given. However, the patient should be monitored by their physician if the anemia stems from chronic disease. Some patients are given erythropoietin to treat their anemia, but as of this writing, this treatment is controversial. Many forms of anemia are readily treatable, while some cases are more difficult and require further and sometimes intensive investigation and analysis by the physician before any real improvement is seen. The patient may also need to consult with a hematologist, an expert in blood diseases.

Risk Factors and Preventive Measures

Older individuals who are losing weight unintentionally may be at risk for anemia. Individuals with kidney disease are also at risk for anemia, as well as those who are undergoing kidney DIALYSIS. In addition, patients who are receiving chemotherapy for cancer may be at risk for the development of anemia, and when the chemotherapy ends, the anemia may resolve itself.

See also COLONOSCOPY; NEGLECT; VITAMIN AND MINERAL DEFICIENCIES/EXCESSES.

Office of Dietary Supplements. "Vitamin B12." Dietary Supplement Fact Sheet, 2006. Available online. URL:

http://ods.od.nih.gov/factsheets/VitaminB12_pf.asp. Accessed August 22, 2007.

Weiss, Guenter, M.D., and Lawrence T. Goodnough, M.D. "Anemia of Chronic Disease." *New England Journal of Medicine* 352, no. 10 (March 10, 2005): 1,011–1,023.

antidepressants Medications that are used to treat a clinical DEPRESSION. Antidepressants should be used carefully with older individuals because elderly people often need a lower dose than individuals of other ages to sustain a clinical improvement.

Elderly individuals may experience depression for many different reasons, such as the loss of a spouse, increased health problems, the fear of death or disease, chronic pain, and even the complete loss of independence. Some individuals who rely heavily on alcohol or who are alcoholics have an underlying problem with depression. Antidepressants may provide significant relief to depressed individuals for a short term or for a longer period.

Osteoporosis Risk with Some Antidepressants

A study published in 2007 in the *Archives of Internal Medicine* indicated that antidepressants that are in the selective serotonin reuptake inhibitor (SSRI) category may affect bone density negatively in older women. This finding was based on studies of older individuals who were taking such drugs and who had about a 6 percent lower bone density in the spine and about a 4 percent lower bone density in the hip than among same-aged individuals who were *not* taking SSRIs.

Those individuals who were taking tricyclic antidepressants for their depression were not similarly affected. As a result of this information, older people with OSTEOPOROSIS who are depressed should use caution before taking an SSRI. (There are several other categories of antidepressants, such as monoamine oxidase inhibitors and atypical antidepressants that do not seem to contribute to lower bone density.) However, individuals who are already taking an SSRI antidepressant should *not* immediately stop taking the SSRI drug but instead should first consult with their physicians. (Sometimes abruptly halting a medication that has been taken for some time can cause other problems, and it may be necessary to taper off the medication.) They should also exercise, and they may need to take calcium and vitamin D supplements if their physicians recommend them. Screening with bone density examinations may be appropriate for individuals on long-term SSRI drug therapy.

Categories of Antidepressants

There are several categories of antidepressants, including tricyclic antidepressants, selective serotonin reuptake inhibitors (SSRIs), and serotonin norepinephrine inhibitors (SNRIs). There are also atypical antidepressants, such as bupropion (Wellbutrin and Wellbutrin XL). Some physicians continue to prescribe monoamine oxidase (MAO) inhibitors, although because of the very strict dietary restrictions that are required for patients taking this category of drugs, MAO inhibitors are chosen far less frequently than the other types of antidepressants.

Because many older people take an array of medications, it is important for the physician to consider whether a particular type of antidepressant could cause a medication interaction. For example, if the patient is already taking medications that are sedating, an antidepressant that is sedating could cause excessive sleepiness in some patients.

Tricyclic antidepressants have been available for many years, and they are effective in treating many people with depression. They are also sometimes used to treat patients with chronic pain. Their primary side effects are sedation and weight gain. They may affect vision and alertness, and in males, there may be difficulty with starting to urinate. Some examples of tricyclics are amitriptyline (Elavil), imipramine (Tofranil), and desipramine (Norpramin).

SSRIs are prescribed by many physicians, and they are often effective in treating depression. Some SSRIs, such as fluoxetine (Prozac) may inhibit sexual response (such as inhibiting ejaculation in men and lubrication and orgasm in women). If the individual is still sexually active, this makes the drug undesirable. However, there are many different SSRIs to choose from, and few affect sexual desire.

Some newer antidepressants inhibit the reuptake (reabsorption) of both serotonin and norepinephrine, two key brain chemicals. Examples of these SNRIs are duloxetine (Cymbalta) and venlafaxine (Effexor). Some studies have shown that duloxetine is also effective in inhibiting pain. Since pain from arthritis, diabetic nerve damage, and many other diseases and disorders is very common among older individuals, this drug may be prescribed by some physicians for depressed patients who also have chronic pain, since it may improve both conditions.

Some antidepressants do not fit within the tricyclic, SSRI, or SNRI category. The best example of the atypical antidepressant is bupropion (Wellbutrin, Wellbutrin XL). It is not clear how this drug works, but it does bring relief from depression for many people.

Monoamine oxidase (MAO) inhibitor antidepressants are rarely used anymore because they require strict adherence to a low tyramine diet, and most doctors consider the diet too difficult for most patients to comply with. Tyramine is naturally produced in foods; it is not a food additive. Tyramine is found in numerous foods and drinks including bacon, sausage, bologna, figs, and raisins.

Patients taking an MAO inhibitor antidepressant must avoid all foods that have been aged, fermented, pickled, or smoked, and thus should avoid cheese, beer, wine, liver, pepperoni, and yogurt (as some examples). They should also avoid a high consumption of foods with caffeine or chocolate. In addition, they must also avoid taking any over-the-counter medications containing dextromethorphan (a cough suppressant) and should also avoid nasal medications and cold medications.

Some examples of MAO inhibitors are phenelzine (Nardil, Nardelzine), isocarboxazid (Marplan), tranylcypromine (Parnate), and selegiline (Eldepryl).

See also ADVERSE DRUG EVENT; AGGRESSION, PHYSICAL; ANXIETY AND ANXIETY DISORDERS; BENZODIAZEPINES; DEPRESSION; FRAILTY; GENDER DIFFERENCES; INAPPROPRIATE MEDICATIONS FOR THE ELDERLY; MEDICATION COMPLIANCE; NEGLECT/SELF-NEGLECT; SUICIDE; VITAMIN AND MINERAL DEFICIENCIES/EXCESSES.

Diem, Susan J., M.D., et al. "Use of Antidepressants and Rates of Hip Bone Loss in Older Women: The Study of Osteoporotic Fractures." *Archives of Internal Medicine* 167 (June 25, 2007): 1,240–1,245.

Stahl, Stephen M. *Essential Psychopharmacology: The Prescriber's Guide.* New York: Cambridge University Press, 2005.

antioxidants Substances such as vitamins and minerals that are added to foods or taken as supplements and that may protect the body against the negative effects of free radicals, which are molecules that are produced when the body breaks down food or environmental exposures, such as tobacco smoke from SMOKING. As a result, antioxidants may prevent the development of CANCER, HEART DISEASE, and other diseases. Cancer is a matter of great concern to many older individuals since it is the second leading cause of death after heart disease.

Some examples of antioxidants are beta-carotene; vitamins A, C, and E; lutein; lycopene; and selenium. Antioxidants are available in many foods, such as vegetables, fruits, grains, and some poultry, meat, and fish.

The tannin in red wine is considered to be an antioxidant by some experts; however, it is important to consider the risks of consuming excessive quantities of alcohol and to exercise moderation. Note that taking antioxidants is *never* a substitute for receiving treatment from a medical doctor when a patient has already been diagnosed with cancer.

See also COMPLEMENTARY/ALTERNATIVE MEDICINE; HYPERTENSION.

Butler, Robert N., et al. "Anti-Aging Medicine: Efficacy and Safety of Hormones and Antioxidants." *Geriatrics* 55, no. 7 (2000): 48.

anxiety and anxiety disorders Anxiety is a general feeling of distress that may accompany bad news, severe pain, or a variety of other experiences, such as the sudden death of a loved one. (See BEREAVEMENT.) In contrast, *anxiety disorders* refer to serious and chronic psychiatric illnesses that commonly occur among older people. An estimated 11 percent of older persons suffer from anxiety disorders, according to the Substance Abuse & Mental Health Technical Assistance Center.

Yet many older people actively resist the idea that they may have a psychiatric problem, often fearing that this may mean that they will be institutionalized. In contrast, most older people with anxiety disorders and other psychiatric problems can improve considerably with medications and psychotherapy, and they rarely need to be placed in an institution. (Individuals with advanced ALZHEIMER'S DISEASE or other forms of DEMENTIA may eventually need to be placed in an institution, but it will usually be a NURSING HOME rather than a psychiatric facility such as the state hospital.)

The primary types of anxiety disorders that older people suffer from are generalized anxiety disorder, post-traumatic stress disorder, panic disorder, and specific phobias. Some older individuals also suffer from obsessive-compulsive disorder. Others may have agoraphobia, a fear of being helpless in a situation, and a condition that is often manifested by people staying in their homes and shunning others.

Symptoms and Diagnostic Path

According to psychiatrist Gary Kennedy in his book *Geriatric Mental Health Care: A Treatment Guide for Health Professionals,* the symptoms of anxiety disorders that are evinced by older individuals are similar to those seen in younger people with the same diagnosis, with the exception that older people with obsessive-compulsive disorder are more likely to fear that they have sinned. Kennedy says of geriatric patients with anxiety disorders:

> Anxious persons are apprehensive and tense and have a sense of dread. They may be irritable, startle easily, feel restless or on edge, and find it difficult to fall asleep. As with depression, they have physical symptoms. They have difficulties with gastrointestinal function, including trouble swallowing, indigestion, excessive flatulence, and either too frequent or too few bowel movements. They may worry excessively about their health, their memory, their money, the safety of the neighborhood, and falling or being mugged while out of the house.

Treatment Options and Outlook

Anxiety disorders are highly treatable with medication and therapy. In general, it is best to see a psychiatrist, a physician who specializes in treating behavior disorders, for treatment of anxiety disorders, since most primary care doctors are not as knowledgeable about the disorders or the best medications to treat them. However, some older people may be fearful of seeing a psychiatrist, mistakenly assuming that they only treat the severely mentally ill.

They may conclude that if others think that they need to see a psychiatrist, others may believe that the older person is severely mentally ill; however, the elderly should be comforted by the fact that most psychiatrists treat people who are not psychotic and instead have emotional disorders that respond well to medication and therapy. Despite such information, however, some older people will refuse treatment unless it comes from their primary care physician.

Psychotherapy may also be effective in treating older individuals with anxiety disorders. Cognitive behavioral therapy (CBT), in which the individual is trained to challenge irrational or damaging thoughts, has been shown to be helpful in some older individuals. Lang and Stein write in their article on anxiety disorders in older people:

> A number of studies have found that relaxation training reduces overall anxiety in older persons who report anxiety symptoms. In case studies, CBT has been used successfully to treat anxiety disorder (including GAD [generalized anxiety disorder], panic disorder, specific phobia and OCD) in older patients. Results of controlled trials of cognitive-behavior therapy for GAD are promising.

Risk Factors and Preventive Measures

The elderly individual with an anxiety disorder often has suffered from the disorder before reaching the senior years, and the problem is often either a continuation or a worsening of past symptoms (which often went undiagnosed). However, in some cases, anxiety is an entirely new problem that appears in older individuals. Anxiety disorders often coexist with depression. Lang and Stein write in their article on anxiety in *Geriatrics,*

Anxiety is one of the most common psychiatric symptoms in older adults; yet it has been studied less than depression or dementia. As a result, the diagnosis and treatment of late-life anxiety are evolving and may be based more on a physician's clinical experience than on scientific evidence.

Types of Anxiety Disorders

Elderly people are susceptible to the same variety of anxiety disorders that affect the general populace.

Generalized Anxiety Disorder (GAD) Generalized anxiety disorder is an overwhelming and distressing form of anxiety/severe worry that pervades the individual's entire life and inhibits his or her level of happiness and success in all areas. The individual simply cannot stop worrying about the many terrible things that may occur, even when it is very unlikely that such things would actually happen. In most cases, they *know* that their fears are unwarranted, yet they worry anyway because they cannot stop themselves.

GAD is treated with medications such as BENZODIAZEPINES, as well as some antidepressants, and it is also treated with psychotherapy.

Post-traumatic Stress Disorder (PTSD) Post-traumatic stress disorder (PTSD) is an anxiety disorder that presents weeks, months, or even years after an extremely distressing or shocking event or series of events occur, such as an experience in wartime combat or a violent encounter with another person (such as a rape or another form of assault). The consequences of a severe natural DISASTER (such as Hurricane Katrina) or other extreme events may also result in the development of PTSD. Simpler courses of PTSD may result from minor and moderate injuries, such as those that occur after a motor vehicle accident.

The individual may experience flashbacks to the emotionally painful event that feel like they are reliving it. They may also feel emotionally overwhelmed and numbed and unable to participate in normal activities.

PTSD can be treated with therapy and medications for depression and anxiety, as needed. In one small study performed by the National Institute of Mental Health (NIMH), researchers found that the medication prazosin (Minipress), a drug for high blood pressure, helped to decrease the symptom severity of PTSD. (Prazosin should not be taken with ALCOHOL.) Propranolol (Inderal), a beta-blocker drug, is under study to see if it can reduce the stress of a traumatic event.

Panic Disorder Everyone feels nervous or even panicked at some times in his or her life, but the person with panic disorder has a chronic problem with panic. He or she has a frequent and desperate feeling that everything is out of control, and this emotion pervades and negatively affects all aspects of the individual's life. In some cases, the panic becomes so severe that he or she is unable to leave home because of an overwhelming fear and anxiety. This condition is also known as agoraphobia.

Obsessive-Compulsive Disorder (OCD) Obsessive-compulsive disorder (OCD) is characterized by repetitive actions (compulsions) that the individual usually knows are irrational, yet he or she feels helpless to stop them. Such actions may include constant checking (that the door is locked, the refrigerator is closed, and so on) or counting (such as counting the steps to the front door or any number of senseless things). Some individuals with OCD obsessively wash their hands over and over, seemingly unable to stop even when their hands are red and raw. Whatever the obsessive and compulsive behaviors are, they cause distress and unhappiness to the individual.

People with OCD also often have repeated thoughts (obsessions) that they cannot block despite every effort, including recurrent thoughts about germs, intruders, dirt, sexual acts, being extremely neat, and other recurring thoughts. The thoughts, as well as the rituals, often take at least an hour of their time each day.

These disorders may be treated with therapy and with antidepressants in various classes, such as clomipramine (Anafranil), which is a tricyclic antidepressant; fluvoxamine (Luvox), a selective serotonin reuptake inhibitor (SSRI); fluoxetine (Prozac), an SSRI; paroxetine (Paxil, Paxil CR), an SSRI; and sertraline (Zoloft), an SSRI. Sometimes antianxiety medications or beta-blockers are used to treat OCD.

Specific Phobias Many people report that they dislike or are afraid of snakes and spiders (a natural fear that most people are apparently born with), but individuals with specific phobias are extremely terrified of the thing(s) that they fear, and they may even fear leaving their home lest they should encounter the thing that they fear the most.

The phobic individual usually knows that the phobia is irrational (similarly as do most individuals who have OCD), yet the extreme fear persists despite this knowledge. Specific phobias can be treated with therapy, such as desensitization to the feared items, as well as with many other forms of therapy.

See also DEPRESSION; GENDER DIFFERENCES; INAPPROPRIATE PRESCRIPTIONS FOR THE ELDERLY; MEDICATION COMPLIANCE; SUBSTANCE ABUSE AND DEPENDENCE.

Kahn, Ada, Ronald Doctor, and Christine Adamec. *The Encyclopedia of Phobias, Fears, and Anxieties.* Third Edition. New York: Facts On File, 2008.

Kennedy, Gary. *Geriatric Mental Health Care: A Treatment Guide for Health Professionals.* New York: Guilford Press, 2000.

Lang, Ariel J., and Murry B. Stein, M.D. "Anxiety Disorders: How to Recognize and Treat the Medical Symptoms of Emotional Illness." *Geriatrics* 56, no. 5 (2001): 24–34.

National Institute of Mental Health. *When Unwanted Thoughts Take Over: Obsessive-Compulsive Disorder.* National Institutes of Health: Bethesda, Md., 2006.

Substance Abuse & Mental Health Technical Assistance Center. *Depression and Anxiety Prevention for Older Adults.* Washington, D.C.: U.S. Department of Health and Human Services. (Undated.)

appetite, chronic lack of A lack of appetite or a poor appetite lasting weeks or longer, and which causes a significant weight loss in the older person. A chronic lack of appetite may stem from a metabolic disorder (such as a thyroid disease), as well as from a serious illness such as ANEMIA or CANCER. It may also result from an emotional disorder such as DEPRESSION or ANXIETY or from another cause. A lack of appetite may stem from as simple a cause as a diminished sense of taste.

In some cases, prescribed medications may decrease the individual's appetite, as in the case of some disease-modifying antirheumatic drugs (DMARDs) that are used to treat RHEUMATOID ARTHRITIS.

A lack of appetite should be explored with the individual (and the family, if relevant) as well as with the individual's physician for possible causes. It should never be assumed that a person's appetite is poor simply or solely because he or she is an "old person." To make such an assumption would be ageist. (See AGEISM.)

If the lack of appetite problem becomes severe, the individual could develop malnutrition, requiring hospitalization.

See also BEREAVEMENT; FRAILTY; SARCOPENIA.

arteriosclerosis A general term that describes several conditions in which fatty substances accumulate on the walls of the arteries and cause a blockage. It is popularly known as "hardening of the arteries." The presence of arteriosclerosis leaves the individual with an increased risk for a HEART ATTACK or STROKE. Depending on where the blockage is located and how extensive it is, arteriosclerosis can be disabling or fatal. Older people have an increased risk for developing arteriosclerosis.

Coronary arteriosclerosis, also known as coronary artery disease (CAD), is the most common form of heart disease, and it is the leading cause of death in the United States for both men and women. With this form of arteriosclerosis, the arteries that supply blood to the heart become narrowed and hard because of a buildup of CHOLESTEROL and other substances.

As the buildup increases, the blood flow becomes insufficient, and if a blood clot forms and stops the blood supply to the heart altogether, this results in a heart attack. Coronary arteriosclerosis also weakens the heart muscle and can cause irregular heart rhythms (arrhythmias) and HEART FAILURE.

There is also a cerebral form of arteriosclerosis that occurs when the artery walls in the brain (or the blood vessels going to the brain) are too thick, which may lead to a blocked or sluggish blood flow to the brain and result in an ischemic stroke. Cerebral arteriosclerosis may also occur if a blood clot is caught within the artery. This may lead to bulges that are called *aneurysms*. If the bulge ruptures, the bleeding that occurs in the brain may lead to a hemorrhagic stroke, which can be fatal. Cerebral arteriosclerosis is also linked to DEMENTIA in the elderly, and in that case, it is caused by a series of small and symptom-free or minimally symptomatic strokes.

Peripheral arterial disease is an arteriosclerosis of the extremities, which first presents in the legs and the feet. The narrowing of the arteries may worsen to the point that the blood vessel is completely blocked. Calcium deposits in the walls of the arteries may be present, exacerbating the stiffness and narrowness. The individual may have leg pain, abnormalities in walking (also known as gait), cold feet or legs, and numbness of the legs or feet when not moving. Cramping in the legs with walking, which is quickly relieved by resting, is a classic sign of this type of blockage.

Symptoms and Diagnostic Path

In addition to taking a complete medical history and performing a medical examination, physicians may use any or all of several different techniques to diagnose arteriosclerosis. For example, the coronary arteriogram (angiogram) procedure involves injecting a contrast agent (dye) into the arteries and then taking X-rays to identify any narrowing of the arteries as well as any blockage or other irregularities in the path through which the blood passes on its way to the heart.

Doppler sonography uses a device known as a transducer to channel sound waves into a blood vessel in order to assess blood flow. If it is difficult or impossible to hear the sound of the blood moving, then the artery may be obstructed.

Radionuclide angiography (Multiple-Gated Acquisition; MUGA scan) uses radioactive tracers to determine if the heart wall moves and to measure the amount of blood each heartbeat expels while the patient is resting.

Myocardial effusion imaging (thallium scanning) may reveal some areas of the heart where the blood supply is inadequate. This test is performed after exercise or when the patient is resting.

If peripheral arterial disease is suspected, the doctor may order a blood pressure comparison that involves taking the blood pressure in both the arms and ankles for comparison and to determine whether the patient's circulation is impaired. A magnetic resonance angiogram (MRA) scan of the legs may be taken. In addition, angiography of the leg arteries may also be performed. If a blockage of the arteries going to the brain is suspected, then magnetic resonance angiography of those arteries may be helpful.

Treatment Options and Outlook

Coronary arteriosclerosis may be treated with coronary angioplasty, a procedure in which a special balloon is used to enlarge the affected artery and improve the blood flow to the heart. (The balloon is inserted surgically, and then it is subsequently inflated.) Angioplasty usually decreases the individual's chest pain, and it also minimizes the damage to the heart muscle that was caused by a heart attack. Often stents are placed in the vessels to keep them open.

An estimated one million angioplasties are performed each year in the United States, according to the National Heart, Lung, and Blood Institute of the National Institutes of Health. Coronary arteriosclerosis is also treated with medications, such as blood thinners.

Peripheral arterial disease is treated with blood thinners, pain relievers, and drugs to enlarge the affected arteries. In severe cases, surgery is required. Exercise is often recommended, even to the point of pain. Wearing properly fitting shoes is very important, as is attention to any injuries in the feet or legs.

Cerebral arteriosclerosis is treated with medications or, rarely, with surgery. Patients are usually advised to control any existing HYPERTENSION, stop SMOKING cigarettes, and reduce their CHOLESTEROL levels. All of these actions are necessary to reduce the risk for cerebral arteriosclerosis.

Risk Factors and Preventive Measures

The key risk factors for developing any form of arteriosclerosis are:

- smoking
- hypertension
- DIABETES
- OBESITY
- elevated CHOLESTEROL levels

Preventive measures involve countering any risk factors that can be controlled; for example, individuals who smoke should stop smoking immediately. Those with hypertension should seek to get their blood pressure under control as best they can. Individuals with diabetes should seek to maintain a tight control over their blood sugar. Obese individuals should lose weight. Performing these tasks will usually work to improve the person's overall cholesterol levels.

See also HEART DISEASE.

arthritis Includes a wide variety of debilitating and degenerative diseases that affect the joints. Many are commonly found in older people. The most frequently occurring form of arthritis in the United States is OSTEOARTHRITIS, followed in prevalence by RHEUMATOID ARTHRITIS. Other forms of arthritis are GOUT and lupus. (There are at least 100 different forms of arthritis, too numerous to list here.)

According to the Centers for Disease Control and Prevention (CDC), arthritis is the leading cause of DISABILITY in the United States. Arthritis affects about 17 million older people in the United States, or 50 percent of all adults age 65 and older. Some individuals suffer from two or more forms of arthritis; for example, they may have both osteoarthritis and rheumatoid arthritis, among many other possible arthritic combinations. Note that by 2030, it is expected that the number of all Americans with arthritis will increase from 46 million in 2007 to 67 million, and about 26 million of these individuals will be BABY BOOMERS with arthritis. (See JOINT REPLACEMENT.)

Older people age 65 and older are the most likely to report any level of joint pain as well as to report suffering from severe joint pain, and women are more likely to suffer from joint pain than men. For example, nearly half of all individuals age 65 and older reported any joint pain in 2003, while the percentage of any joint pain for all adults was 31.4 percent. In addition, 13.6 percent of older individuals reported suffering from severe joint pain, compared to 8.4 percent of all adults. (See Table 1.) Some individuals with severe joint pain will opt for joint replacement surgery.

Arthritis causes many older people to limit their activities; for example, the CDC reports that about 12 percent of those ages 65 to 74 years old are forced to limit their activities because of arthritis and other musculoskeletal conditions, and this percentage increases to about 19 percent for those individuals age 75 and older. In contrast, only about 2 percent of individuals ages 18 to 44 must limit their activities because of arthritis.

As the BABY BOOMERS (individuals who were born between the years 1946 and 1964) begin to age into their retirement years, the number of people with arthritis and other serious chronic diseases will increase dramatically.

Symptoms and Diagnostic Path

The symptoms and diagnosis of arthritis depend on the type of arthritis that is present, and treatment also varies with the specific type. Arthritis is strongly linked to DEPRESSION, probably because of the limitations it places on the individual's lifestyle as well as the pain it causes.

Treatment Options and Outlook

In general, individuals go to their physicians when they are suffering from the acute and chronic pain caused by their arthritis. They may need medications, physical therapy, injections, and other treatments, up to and including surgery. The treatment depends on the type of arthritis that is present.

TABLE 1. ADULTS 18 YEARS OF AGE AND OLDER REPORTING JOINT PAIN IN THE 30 DAYS PRIOR TO INTERVIEW, BY SEVERITY LEVEL, AGE, AND GENDER, BY PERCENTAGE, 2003

Characteristic	Any Joint Pain	Severe Joint Pain
Age		
18 and older	31.4	18.4
18–44	20.5	4.9
45–64	39.9	11.5
65 and older	49.9	13.6
Sex		
Men	28.5	6.5
Women	34.1	10.1

Source: Adapted from National Center for Health Statistics. *Health, United States, 2006 with Chartbook on Trends in the Health of Americans.* Hyattsville, Md.: National Institutes of Health, 2006, p. 118.

For example, massage therapy of the affected area would be inappropriate and painful for the person with gout but may be helpful for the individual with osteoarthritis. The medications that are used vary considerably as well. Some individuals improve with periodic injections of steroids. In general, the goal is to improve the pain and decrease the disability, as well as to prevent further deterioration when possible.

Most people with arthritis need to take some form of painkilling medication, including NARCOTICS.

Risk Factors and Preventive Measures

The risk for arthritis and other musculoskeletal conditions increases with age, according to the Centers for Disease Control and Prevention (CDC), and 117.8 people per 1,000 ages 65 to 74 years must limit their activities because of this problem. The rate increases to 193.1 per 1,000 for those who are age 75 and older.

The incidence of arthritis varies by gender and is weighted heavily toward females. According to CDC data published in an analysis in a 2007 issue of the *Journal of Women's Health,* women have a higher level of arthritis at every age group, as well as at every race and ethnicity. Among women of all ages, nearly a quarter of them (22.4 percent) say that arthritis or rheumatism is their main cause of disability, compared to 11 percent of all men.

The risk for arthritis increases for both genders with age but remains higher for women; for example, about 40 percent of men ages 65 to 74 years have been diagnosed with arthritis compared to about 50 percent of women in this age group. In addition, about 48 percent of men ages 75 to 84 years have arthritis compared to nearly 60 percent of women in this age group. Finally, about 45 percent of men age 85 and older have been diagnosed with arthritis compared to an estimated 60 percent of women in this age group.

Many people with arthritis are overweight or obese. According to the CDC, 66 percent of adults with arthritis are either overweight or obese compared with 53 percent of adults who are not overweight or obese and do *not* have arthritis. A weight loss of even as little as 11 pounds can dramatically reduce the risk of the development of knee osteoarthritis in women by 50 percent.

See also AMERICANS WITH DISABILITIES ACT; DISABILITY; FAMILY AND MEDICAL LEAVE ACT; GENDER DIFFERENCES; OBESITY.

He, Wan, Manisha Sengupta, Victoria A. Velkoff, and Kimberly A. DeBarros. *65+ in the United States: 2005.* Washington, D.C.: U.S. Census Bureau, December 2005.

Kandel, Joseph, M.D., and David Sudderth, M.D. *The Arthritis Solution.* Rocklin, Calif.: Prima Publishing, 1997.

National Center for Health Statistics. *Health, United States, 2006 with Chartbook on Trends in the Health of Americans.* Hyattsville, Md.: National Institutes of Health, 2006.

Theis, Kristina A., Charles G. Helmick, M.D., and Jennifer M. Hootman. "Arthritis Burden and Impact Are Greater Among U.S. Women Than Men: Intervention Opportunities." *Journal of Women's Health* 16, no. 4 (2007): 441–452.

Asian Americans Individuals of Asian or Pacific Islands ancestry or who were born in other countries and then moved to the United States. Asian Americans include such racial and ethnic groups as Chinese, Japanese, Asian Indians, Koreans, and people of Filipino genetic ancestry. Some people originated from the Pacific islands of Micronesia, Polynesia, and Melanesia. In 2005, 3.1 percent of all older people were of Asian or Pacific Islander ethnicity.

According to reports from the Centers for Disease Control and Prevention (CDC), Asian Americans age 65 and older in the United States have the lowest percentage of the races (including whites, blacks, Hispanics, and Asians) of reporting themselves to be in fair or poor health, which means that they regard themselves as having at least average health. (See Appendix VI.) This may be why Asian Americans are reportedly the least likely of the races and ethnicities to require home care.

In addition, Asian Americans have the lowest rate of vision impairment and of having lost all their natural teeth. However, they have the second highest rate (after African Americans) of HYPERTENSION, and the second highest rate (after Caucasians) of having HEARING DISORDERS. Asian Americans are the least likely of the races to be impoverished;

in 2005, they had the highest median income of $49,163. Of course, some individual Asian Americans are poor, while others may be very wealthy.

See also AFRICAN AMERICANS; CAUCASIANS; HISPANICS; NATIVE AMERICANS; POVERTY.

aspirin therapy The daily use of a baby aspirin as a preventive therapy against HEART ATTACK or STROKE, particularly among those who have previously experienced a heart attack or stroke. Aspirin therapy may also be used by individuals who are believed to be at risk for a heart attack or stroke, usually because they have HYPERTENSION, DIABETES, or another disorder that is linked to heart disease. However, before starting aspirin therapy (or any other medication regimen, including taking over-the-counter medications or supplements), the physician should be consulted to ensure that the therapy is needed and that it will not cause any MEDICATION INTERACTIONS with other drugs that the patient is taking, such as blood thinners.

Aspirin does have several side effects. For example, it can thin the blood and cause it to clot more slowly. In addition, according to the U.S. Food and Drug Administration (FDA), aspirin can also lead to KIDNEY FAILURE and some kinds of STROKES. The FDA recommends medical professionals consider the following factors before advising a person to start aspirin therapy:

- the individual's medical history as well as the medical history of other close family members
- the person's use of other prescribed and over-the-counter medications
- the use of dietary supplements and herbs
- possible side effects that the individual could experience

The doctor will also take into account the patient's current health, including uncontrolled hypertension, bleeding disorders, asthma, peptic ULCERS, KIDNEY DISEASE, or liver disease, all of which could make continued aspirin therapy a bad choice.

See also ADVERSE DRUG EVENT; ARTERIOSCLEROSIS; CARDIOVASCULAR DISEASE; HEART DISEASE.

assault See CRIMES AGAINST THE ELDERLY.

assets Items of value, such as cash, a home or other property, stocks, bonds, and certificates of deposit (CDs), as several key examples. When considering an individual's eligibility for some state programs, such as MEDICAID, the state considers the assets of the applicant, and if the total of these assets exceed a predetermined level, then the person is ineligible for benefits. In addition, if a person is initially eligible for a program such as Medicaid but that individual acquires assets (such as an inheritance or winning the lottery), these new assets usually then make them ineligible for programs such as Medicaid.

Some individuals try to shelter their assets through legal mechanisms such as a LIVING TRUST, which enable them to transfer assets during their lifetimes to a trust that includes the older person and one or more others, usually family members.

Some older adults who might otherwise choose either MARRIAGE or remarriage decide to remain single because of the negative impact on their finances should they get married. The assets of both individuals would be considered by the federal government if they were married, and if one of them needed to move into a NURSING HOME and then sought MEDICAID eligibility they would possibly be denied coverage. However, if they remain single, even if they reside with the other person, only the individual's assets will be considered in their eligibility for Medicaid. Some older adults also decide against remarriage because they fear that their adult children could lose some or all of their inheritance when they die.

See also ATTORNEYS; DURABLE POWER OF ATTORNEY; END-OF-LIFE ISSUES; ESTATE PLANNING; GUARDIANSHIP; LIVING WILL; POWER OF ATTORNEY; WILLS.

assistance program A program providing money, medication, or other benefits, generally to low-income individuals. MEDICAID is a state government assistance program that provides medical assistance to categories of individuals, including older people, with low incomes. The level of income an individual must have in order to qualify depends on state law. Supplemental Security Insurance (SSI) is another program. SSI provides monthly payments to those who are eligible, as well as Medicaid. In addition, Medicaid pays for medications needed by the older person. There is either no co-payment or a very low co-payment for adults who qualify for Medicaid, depending on state law.

There are a variety of other assistance programs, such as rental assistance programs and food stamps. Older individuals may qualify for a variety of assistance programs, based on the state. Contact the state aging office for further information. (See Appendix II.)

See also POVERTY.

assisted-living facility (ALF) Long-term housing for elderly individuals that also provides an array of services, such as meals, emergency call buttons, and may also include assistance with ACTIVITIES OF DAILY LIVING, such as eating, dressing, bathing, and so forth. There are an estimated 36,000 assisted-living facilities in the United States in which about 900,000 to one million people live, with as many as 50,000 people receiving financial support from MEDICAID. According to the National Center for Assisted Living, the average monthly fee for private units in 2006 was $2,627. However, this is about half the price of the fees charged by nursing homes. (Contrary to popular belief, many people pay for their own nursing home care. Medicaid does not cover nursing home care unless the individual's financial resources have been exhausted.)

There are many different names that are used for assisted living, including retirement community, senior housing complex, residential care, board and care, and personal care, among some of the more popular phrases. The phrase "assisted-living facility" also has very different meanings in different states and even within states. Anyone who is considering a move to a particular facility, for either themselves or a family member, should request a clear definition of what is included in the services that are provided by the assisted-living facility they are considering before making a commitment.

Assisted-living facilities may be comprised of one or many buildings, and they may be simple or very lavish. In most cases, residents live in apartmentlike housing, ranging from studio apartments to apartments with one to two bedrooms, and one to two bathrooms. The majority of people live in either a studio apartment or a one-bedroom apartment. They may also have an area for their washer and dryer, or they may use a common laundry room. The services usually also include meals, housekeeping, and transportation to the supermarket, doctor appointments, and so forth.

There is often a clubhouse or other area in which to socialize, and the facility may also offer a swimming pool and exercise facilities. Usually a dining facility is available, which may provide two or three meals per day for the residents.

Most assisted-living facilities provide residents with transportation to their doctor appointments, shopping, and to other activities that older individuals need. In addition, they also usually provide a wealth of social activities, from the traditional bingo games to access to many different clubs. Buses may take residents to movies, shows, and to a broad array of entertainment.

Many elderly individuals actively dislike the idea of living in NURSING HOMES, and whenever possible, they prefer to live in an assisted-living facility because it offers varying degrees of independence, depending on the needs of the individual, the facility, state laws, and other factors.

The assisted-living concept is becoming increasingly popular with the rapid aging of the elderly nationwide. According to the National Center for Assisted Living, the average community includes 58 units; however, some facilities are smaller or larger. About half of all assisted-living units are either studio or efficiency apartments, while 29 percent are one-bedroom units and 6 percent are two-bedroom units.

Many states offer information about assisted-living facilities on their Web site. For example, the Colorado Department of Public Health and Environment offers a consumer guide to selecting assisted living and offers topics with questions for consumers to ask. In Florida, the Florida Department of Elder Affairs offers information on assisted-living facilities on their Web site, as well as an option that allows consumers to search for a facility in their location and price range.

Demographics of Assisted-Living Residents

According to the National Center for Assisted Living in Washington, D.C., in 2006 the average age of residents was 85 years old and about 76 percent of residents were female. Many of the residents needed help accomplishing their activities of daily living, such as bathing and dressing. In addition most (91 percent) needed assistance with performing housework. (Many assisted-living facilities provide maid service.) Most residents stayed for an average of 27 months. Of those who left the facility, about 34 percent moved to a nursing home, 20 percent died, and the others moved to other locations.

Medicaid Vouchers for Assisted Living

As of this writing, 41 states in the United States provide vouchers to some elderly citizens, enabling them to live in assisted-living facilities, using either a Medicaid waiver or a state plan service (personal care or home health care). Only 20 states authorized Medicaid spending on assisted living in 1998. It is estimated that more than 10 percent, or about 120,000 people, receive Medicaid to pay for their assisted living.

Veterans and Assisted Living

In recent years, the Veterans Administration (VA) has begun placing some elderly veterans in assisted-living facilities. Most are elderly males, largely because most older military veterans are men. A report in a 2007 issue of the *Gerontologist* described the characteristics of the residents and providers in the VA assisted-living pilot program. This report was based on 743 residents placed over the period 2002 to 2004 in 58 adult family homes, 56 assisted-living facilities, and 46 residential-care facilities.

The pilot program for assisted living provided up to six months of assisted living, as well as living in adult family homes and residential-care facilities. According to this report, the basic services offered in assisted-living units included such items as regular nursing assessment and oversight, medication oversight, and social and recreational activities. The assisted-living units the residents lived in were apartments with private baths with either a kitchenette or a kitchen.

In the study, 410 residents (55 percent of the study subjects) were placed in assisted living, followed by 29 percent who were placed in residential-care facilities and 16 percent placed in adult family homes. The researchers found that nearly all of the subjects placed in any type of facility needed help with preparing meals, doing housework, and managing their medications.

The researchers also surveyed assisted-living facilities, and they found that these facilities were less likely to admit residents with such problems as needing skilled nursing care or having behavioral or psychological problems. For example, 66.5 percent of adult family homes said that they would admit residents needing skilled nursing care, but the rate was 42.3 percent for assisted living. With regard to behavioral or psychological problems, 39.8 percent of the adult family homes said they would admit such patients compared to 29.5 percent of assisted facilities. According to the researchers,

> These comparisons support our finding that the smallest facilities in our study, the adult family homes, enrolled residents who required greater levels of assistance with ADLs [activities of daily living], as they were dependent in an average of 2.5 of 6 ADLs compared to 1.6 for both assisted living and adult residential care facility residents. Adult family home residents also had the highest levels of skilled care need; had limited life expectancy; were homebound; needed physical, speech, or occupational therapies; and used wheelchairs.

In other words, the residents of the assisted-living facilities were in better physical and mental health that the residents of adult family homes.

Choosing an Assisted-Living Facility

According to the Administration on Aging, the following should be considered in a search for an assisted-living facility:

- Think ahead. What will the resident's future needs be and how will the facility meet those needs?
- Is the facility close to family and friends? Are there any shopping centers or other businesses nearby (within walking distance)?

- Do admission and retention policies exclude people with severe cognitive impairments or severe physical disabilities?
- Does the facility provide a written statement of its philosophy of care?
- Visit each facility more than once, sometimes unannounced.
- Visit at mealtime, sample the food, and observe the quality of the food and the service.
- Observe interactions among residents and staff as well as interactions among the residents.
- Check to see if the facility offers social, recreational, and spiritual activities.
- Talk to the residents.
- Learn about the type of training the staff receives and how frequently they receive training.
- Review state licensing reports about the facility.

Consider taking the following steps before signing a contract with an assisted-living facility:

- Contact your state's long-term care OMBUDSMAN to see if any complaints have been filed against the facility. In many states, the ombudsman checks on conditions at assisted-living facilities as well as at nursing homes.
- Contact the local Better Business Bureau to see if that agency has received any complaints about the assisted-living facility.
- If the assisted-living facility is associated with a nursing home, ask for information about it also.

See also AMERICANS WITH DISABILITIES ACT; ASSISTIVE DEVICES/ASSISTED TECHNOLOGY; DISABILITY; GENDER DIFFERENCES; HOME CARE; HOUSING/LIVING ARRANGEMENTS; INDEPENDENT LIVING.

Administration on Aging. *Assisted Living.* Washington, D.C.: Department of Health and Human Services, August 27, 2003.

Hedrick, Susan, et al. "Characteristics of Resident and Providers in the Assisted Living Pilot Program." *The Gerontologist* 47, no. 3 (2007): 365–377.

Mollica, Robert L. *Informing Consumers about Assisted Living: State Practices.* Washington, D.C.: National Academy for State Health Policy, June 2005.

assisted suicide   Causing or helping to cause the death of another person who has stated that he or she wishes to die. Assisted suicide is very controversial, and state laws vary considerably on this topic. Oregon and Washington are thus far the only states to allow physicians to assist patients to commit suicide.

Jack Kevorkian, a pathologist, is considered a pioneer of assisted suicide. Nicknamed "Dr. Death," he was convicted of murder and began serving a 10-to-20-year prison term in 1999. According to Kervorkian, he has helped 130 people commit suicide since 1990. He was released from jail in 2007 and has promised to provide no further assistance to anyone wishing to commit suicide.

Oregon Death with Dignity Act

In 1994, Oregon legalized physician-assisted suicide in its Oregon Death with Dignity Act. The act was immediately challenged in the courts, and in 2001 the U.S. Attorney General ruled that it was not lawful for doctors to use controlled substances to assist in a suicide. However, in 2006 the U.S. Supreme Court overruled the federal government in *Gonzales v. Oregon*, saying that doctors could not be prevented from prescribing scheduled drugs to assist patients in commiting suicide under Oregon law.

According to attorney Lawrence Gostin in his 2006 article on physician-assisted suicide in the *Journal of the American Medical Association*, doctors can assist patients with suicide in Oregon only under strict conditions:

> The physician must diagnose an incurable and irreversible disease that, within reasonable medical judgment, will cause death within 6 months. The law requires the attending physician to determine that the patient, who must be an Oregon resident, has made a voluntary request and that the patient's choice is informed; the physician must refer the patient to counseling if the patient may have a mental disorder or depression causing impaired judgment. A second "consulting" physician must examine the patient and review the medical records to confirm the attending physician's conclusions. The reviewing physicians must keep detailed medical records of the process leading to the prescription.

Arguments for and against Assisted Suicide

Some individuals support the concept of assisted suicide because they believe that individuals have the right to choose the time of their own death. They may also support the concept because the individual suffers from an incurable disease, such as advanced CANCER or from another severely painful or debilitating disease. Proponents of assisted suicide may point out that when pets become severely ill, pet owners may choose to end the pet's life to avoid further suffering for the animal. They believe humans should also be able to end their own lives if they wish to do so.

Those who oppose assisted suicide say that others may unduly influence an ill person or may even cause the death of an individual who wishes to die a natural death. Nefarious purposes may be related to the wish for an inheritance, the desire to cease caring for an aging parent or relative, or other reasons. They also fear that individuals who are clinically depressed may choose assisted suicide when treatment could actually resolve their depression.

It is likely that assisted suicide will continue to be a controversial topic with the aging of many Americans and their increased risk for major diseases.

See also DEATH; DEPRESSION; SUICIDE.

Gostin, Lawrence O., J.D., LLD. "Physician-Assisted Suicide: A Legitimate Medical Practice?" *Journal of the American Medical Association* 295, no. 16 (April 26, 2006): 1,941–1,943.

assistive devices/assistive technology Items that enable a person to perform daily activities, such as a cane or wheelchair. Assistive technology generally refers to devices that make life easier for the older person, such as an amplification device to make the sound louder on the telephone or the television for individuals with hearing impairments. These devices are also sometimes called ADAPTIVE DEVICES. According to the Administration on Aging, there are many different types of assistive devices, including

- walkers, which are assistive devices that are used by those with severe difficulty with walking unassisted or with mobility

- adaptive switches that may be voice-activated to adjust a variety of equipment, including air conditioners, computers, telephone answering machines, wheelchairs, and other equipment
- home modifications, such as ramps that allow wheelchair access
- mobility aids, such as a power wheelchair or a wheelchair lift to enable movement for those with mobility problems
- prosthetic equipment, such as an artificial limb for someone with an amputated arm or leg
- seating aids, such as modifications to chairs, wheelchairs, or motor scooters so that the individual can sit upright
- sensory enhancements, such as a telecaption decoder on a television set for the person with a hearing disorder
- aids that will enable a disabled person to more easily get into and out of their vehicle

According to the Administration on Aging, when trying to decide whether an assistive device is needed, individuals should ask the following questions:

- Does a more advanced device meet more than one of my needs?
- Does the manufacturer of the assistive technology have a preview policy that will let me try out a device and return it for credit if it does not work as expected?
- How are my needs likely to change over the next six months? How about over the next six years or longer?
- How up-to-date is this piece of assistive equipment? Is it likely to become obsolete in the immediate future?
- What, if any, types of assistive technology have I used in the past, and how did that equipment work?
- What type of assistive technology will give me the greatest personal independence?
- Will I always need help with this task? If so, can I adjust this device and continue to use it as my condition changes?

Paying for Assistive Devices

In general, Medicare Part B will pay for up to 80 percent of the cost of assistive technology if the items can be defined as durable medical equipment. To determine whether MEDICARE will pay for a particular item, individuals may call Medicare at (800) 633-4227 or go to the Web site http://www.medicare.gov.

In some cases, another program, MEDICAID, may pay for an assistive device for eligible individuals (such as very low-income older people). Military veterans may be able to receive payment for some assistive items from the Veterans Administration.

Use of Assistive Devices

In a study of the use of assistive devices among elderly individuals published in the *Journal of Applied Gerontology* in 2004, researchers studied 694 cognitively intact (without DEMENTIA) but physically frail elderly people ages 60 and older who lived at home. The researchers found that physical disability was the strongest predictor of the use of an assistive device, as was increased medication intake. (The more medicine that the older person took, the more likely he or she would need an assistive device.)

The researchers also found some demographic predictors of the use of assistive devices, including being Caucasian and living in the southern part of the United States, as well as living alone. In considering factors that *hindered* the use of assistive devices, DEPRESSION was a significant factor mitigating against the use of these devices. Based on this last finding, among older individuals who need yet still refuse to use assistive devices, the possibility of depression should be considered.

See also ACCESSIBILITY TO FACILITIES; ACTIVITIES OF DAILY LIVING; AMERICANS WITH DISABILITIES ACT; DISABILITY; FAMILY AND MEDICAL LEAVE ACT.

Tomita, Mackiko R., William C. Mann, Linda F. Fraas, and Kathleen M. Stanton. "Predictors of the Use of Assistive Devices That Address Physical Impairments Among Community-Based Frail Elders." *Journal of Applied Gerontology* 23, no. 2 (June 2004): 141–155.

attitudes toward elderly   See AGEISM.

attorneys   Individuals who are educationally qualified and licensed by their states to provide legal assistance. Older individuals may need attorneys to provide assistance with drawing up WILLS, as well as with LEGAL GUARDIANSHIPS and the preparation of other legal documents, such as a LIVING TRUST. If family members or others think their older relatives suffer from emotional incompetence (an inability to manage their own legal or financial affairs or all of their affairs), attorneys may represent the family in court. Conversely, attorneys may represent older individuals who are disputing with others about whether they are mentally incompetent.

Competent attorneys can save individuals a great deal of time, money, and emotional distress. However, incompetent attorneys can create financial ruin and emotional hardships for their clients.

See also DURABLE POWER OF ATTORNEY; END-OF-LIFE ISSUES; ESTATE PLANNING; HEALTH CARE AGENT/PROXY; LEGAL GUARDIANSHIP; LIVING WILL; MENTAL COMPETENCY; POWER OF ATTORNEY.

audiologist   See HEARING DISORDERS.

baby boomers The population bulge of individuals who were born in the United States between 1946 and 1964; an estimated 78 million people. The oldest baby boomers are attaining early retirement age as of this writing, and this surge of retirement will continue for nearly 20 years, with the leading edge of the surge becoming eligible for Medicare after 2010. There are also baby boomers in Canada, including individuals born between 1946 and 1965. (See CANADA.)

According to the American Hospital Association in their booklet *When I'm 64*, there are four major factors that will influence how baby boomers will affect the health-care system: (1) many of them will need more health care than any other generation; (2) the prevalence of chronic diseases, such as arthritis, diabetes, and other diseases and disorders, is increasing among baby boomers; (3) baby boomers have different needs and expectations than past generations—in general, they may be a more demanding population than past generations; and (4) baby boomers have more medical facilities and technology available to them than have ever been available and many will wish to take advantage of these facilities and new technology.

Some experts question whether the federal government system of Social Security and MEDICARE in the United States will be able to successfully accommodate the sharply increased demand for retirement benefits from this very large group of people. Others worry about managing the physical and mental health problems of this group, with the potential for numerous baby boomers with such diseases as ALZHEIMER'S DISEASE and other forms of DEMENTIA, as well as the many chronic diseases common in older people. They speculate about how society will be able to pay for and cope with large numbers of individuals with these disorders.

It is also true that many baby boomers age 50 and older who are not yet elderly have already been diagnosed with many chronic conditions, such as OBESITY, DIABETES, ARTHRITIS, and HYPERTENSION, and they have also been diagnosed with these conditions to a significantly greater extent than individuals in this age group in the past. Some experts fear that the baby boomers will ultimately require considerably more care than their parents currently require, not only because there are so many of them but also because they are considerably less healthy than their parents were at their age.

Some conditions, such as obesity, exacerbate the risk for diabetes and hypertension and also may make arthritic pain more severe as the body struggles to support the greater weight of the obese person. Baby boomers have a high rate of obesity, as well as related health problems. These medical problems are worsened by increasing age, so that when the baby boomers themselves *are* elderly, their health-care needs may well be considerable, as experts in the early 21st century currently fear.

According to some studies, such as the one by Soldo et al., baby boomers who were born between 1948 and 1953 were reportedly less healthy in 2006 than people of the same age in the mid-1990s. In addition, the baby boomers reported more chronic health problems, more pain, more drinking, and more psychiatric problems. They also had more problems with walking, climbing stairs, getting up from a chair, and performing other normal daily tasks than were reported by previous pre-retirees when they were the same age. These are all ominous signs for these future retirees, as well as for those who must provide the funds to pay for their Social Security and Medicare benefits.

Richard W. Johnson and his colleagues looked at the likely outcomes of DISABILITY and disease with aging baby boomers, and they found that between the years 2020 and 2040, the disability rates for older individuals would likely increase to about 28 percent. According to the authors,

> Because the overall size of the older population will expand rapidly, the number of frail older Americans will soar in coming decades. Between 2000 and 2040, the numbers of older adults with disabilities will more than double, increasing from about 10 million to about 21 million. The number of older Americans with severe disabilities will increase by more than 3 million, to about 6 million adults.

This rapid growth will significantly increase the burden on the younger and smaller-sized population.

The authors project that the frail older population will be primarily non-Hispanic white (67.1 percent) and female (61.5 percent). The mean age of this older population will be 79.8 years.

The Sandwich Generation

In many cases in the early 21st century, baby boomers find themselves providing care for their aging parents who are in their eighties and nineties, and some may also provide care for their own adolescent children or even their grandchildren of all ages from infants to teenagers. Thus, these baby boomers are also known as the sandwich generation. Caring for both older and younger generations may take its own health toll on the baby boomers in terms of their physical and emotional health. Baby boomers who are pre-retirees will hopefully recognize this problem and exercise more and eat more nutritiously, as well as eating less calorie-laden foods.

See also ADULT CHILDREN/CHILDREN OF AGING PARENTS; AMERICANS WITH DISABILITIES ACT; ASSETS; CANCER; COMPASSION FATIGUE; END-OF-LIFE ISSUES; FAMILY AND MEDICAL LEAVE ACT; FAMILY CAREGIVERS; SIBLING RIVALRY AND CONFLICT; TALKING TO ELDERLY PARENTS ABOUT DIFFICULT ISSUES.

American Hospital Association. *When I'm 64: How Boomers Will Change Health Care.* Chicago, Ill.: American Hospital Association, 2007.

Johnson, Richard W., Desmond Tooney, and Joshua M. Wiener. *Meeting the Long-Term Care Needs of the Baby Boomers: How Changing Families Will Affect Paid Helpers and Institutions.* Washington, D.C.: The Urban Institute, 2007.

Soldo, B. J., et al. *Cross-Cohort Differences in Health on the Verge of Retirement.* Cambridge, Mass.: National Bureau of Economic Research, 2007.

back pain Moderate to severe discomfort that occurs in the spinal column or the general back area. Back pain is very common among older individuals, and the risk for back pain increases with aging.

Back pain may be caused by trauma to the back caused by many different reasons, such as an injury or a car crash. It may also be caused by many chronic diseases, such as CANCER, OSTEOARTHRITIS, RHEUMATOID ARTHRITIS, ruptured discs, KIDNEY DISEASE, INFECTIONS, or spasms in the muscles of the back. Many older individuals suffer from chronic back pain. In many cases of back pain, the problem goes away on its own; however, in many instances, the pain persists and becomes chronic pain.

Extremely severe back pain may be caused by kidney stones or other kidney disease. Other causes of back pain are infections, such as bladder or kidney infections or infection of the prostate gland in a man. Rarely, there may be an infection in the bones of the spine (the vertebrae). However, in many cases, the specific cause of back pain cannot be determined.

People of all ages can develop back pain, but according to the Centers for Disease Control and Prevention (CDC), low back pain causes a greater percentage of people ages 65 and older to limit their activities. (See Table 1.) For example, older individuals have more than three times the risk of those 18 to 44 years old of having to limit their activities because of their low back pain (52.9 percent versus 14.8 percent for those ages 18 to 44).

Symptoms and Diagnostic Path

Back pain may occur in any part of the spine, from the cervical spine (neck area) to the thoracic spine (the vertebrae below the neck area), and the

TABLE 1. HEALTH STATUS MEASURES AMONG ADULTS 18 YEARS OF AGE AND OLDER WITH LOW BACK PAIN, BY AGE: UNITED STATES, 2004

Health Status Measure and Age	Percent
Limitation of activity caused by chronic conditions	
18 years and older	28.1
18–44	14.8
45–64	32.4
65 and older	52.9

Source: Adapted from National Center for Health Statistics. *Health, United States, 2006 with Chartbook on Trends in the Health of Americans.* Hyattsville, Md.: National Institutes of Health, 2006, p. 124.

lumbar spine, where most individuals with back problems experience their pain, particularly in the lower lumbar spine. Some neck pain is referred to the head and experienced as headache, particularly the cervicogenic headache. (See HEADACHE.)

To diagnose the cause of back pain, physicians take a complete medical history and perform a physical examination to check for where the pain is the most severe. In many cases, diagnostic tests such as a computerized tomography (CT) scan are ordered. Alternatively (or in addition to the CT scan), magnetic resonance imaging (MRI) scan or ultrasound may be ordered to help the physician with diagnosis. Laboratory tests such as the complete blood count (CBC) can rule out infection or ANEMIA. An erythrocyte sedimentation blood test can check for rheumatoid arthritis, lupus, and other autoimmune diseases. A urinalysis and/or culture can check for infection of the kidneys or bladder.

A physical examination of the back is essential, because the doctor needs to know exactly where it hurts the patient, how much it hurts, and whether the pain extends into the legs or elsewhere. (Pain extending from the low back into one or both legs is called sciatica.) The doctor will evaluate various movements by the patient, such as having him or her bend sideways, forward, and backward, as the physician reviews how difficult these particular movements are. The doctor may also check the patient's gait to see if he or she can walk normally. These are just a few of the many tests used when diagnosing back pain.

Treatment Options and Outlook

Depending on the cause and intensity of the back pain, treatment may include applying heat or ice to the painful area, limited bed rest, and painkillers, sometimes including NARCOTICS. Other drugs that may be helpful are the muscle relaxant cyclobenzaprine (Flexeril) or dextromethorphan (a medication that is commonly used for cough but which is also helpful in pain control).

Sometimes antiseizure drugs such as carbamazepine (Tegretol), topiramate (Topamax), gabapentin (Neurontin), lamotrigine (Lamictal), or pregabalin (Lyrica) may help control an individual's chronic back pain. However, the physician should first verify that the medication is considered appropriate for an elderly person. (See ADVERSE DRUG EVENT; INAPPROPRIATE PRESCRIPTIONS FOR THE ELDERLY.)

If the back pain becomes severe, back surgery is recommended in some cases. There are many different types of back surgery depending on the type of problem that the patient is experiencing, whether it is degenerative disc disease, a herniated disc, or another type of back problem. Often doctors will first try injections in the spine (epidural or facet blocks) in the hope of the patient avoiding spine surgery.

Lifestyle changes are often recommended to the patient with chronic back pain, such as instituting an exercise program as soon as the pain becomes tolerable. Doctors may also use transcutaneous electrical nerve stimulation (TENS), ultrasound, and related therapies. Aquatic exercise is often very helpful because it is low impact and puts less stress on already sore muscles and enables many patients to move around more easily.

Risk Factors and Preventive Measures

Individuals who have had back pain in the past have an increased risk for suffering from back pain again. If the pain stems from arthritis, often the individual's parents and other relatives also had back pain from arthritis. Exercise and weight loss often may alleviate much (or even all) of the back pain, because less weight and a better level of fitness will decrease the overall strain on the body.

See also AMERICANS WITH DISABILITIES ACT; ARTHRITIS; CHRONIC PAIN; FAMILY AND MEDICAL LEAVE

ACT; RHEUMATOID ARTHRITIS; SARCOPENIA; SUBSTANCE ABUSE AND DEPENDENCE.

Kandel, Joseph, M.D., and David B. Sudderth, M.D. *Back Pain—What Works! A Complete Guide to Back Problems.* New York: Prima Publishing, 1996.

bathing and cleanliness Some older individuals, including those who were meticulously clean in the past, may begin to bathe infrequently as they get older. This may be due to ALZHEIMER'S DISEASE or another form of DEMENTIA. It may also be true that the older person is less physically coordinated than in the past and, as a result, is fearful of falling down in the bathtub or shower. One solution to this problem is to provide grab bars to hold onto or a seat to sit on in case the individual becomes fatigued or dizzy. These adaptations can be made in a private home.

The older person also may be fearful of bathing because it seems too complicated. Stella Mora Henry, a registered nurse, writes, "Simply adjusting the hot and cold water controls in the shower can get confusing. It may also be difficult for older people to maintain their balance as they step in and out of the bathtub."

Another problem may be that the individual feels too weak, ill, or fatigued to take a bath or shower. Some older people may be suffering from DEPRESSION, and they may think that there is no point to bathing anymore. In any case in which the person is clearly chronically dirty or has a diminished interest in bathing regularly, the cause of this behavior should be investigated and resolved.

If the older person frequently wears dirty and stained clothing, this should be investigated as well. The person may no longer be able to launder his or her clothes or possibly his or her vision is extremely poor and he or she does not realize the clothes are dirty, or they may have forgotten to change their clothes because of a memory impairment. Once the cause for the dirty clothing is determined, other individuals can assist the older person in finding a solution.

See also ACTIVITIES OF DAILY LIVING; BEDSORES; HOME HEALTH/HOME CARE; NEGLECT/SELF-NEGLECT.

Mora Henry, Stella, R.N., with Ann Convery. *The Eldercare Handbook: Difficult Choices, Compassionate Solutions.* New York: Collins, 2006.

bedsores Pressure sores that occur as a result of a patient lying in bed for a long time and not moving about. The pressure causes reduced blood flow and may eventually result in an open wound. Bedsores are also known as pressure ulcers or decubitus ulcers. These sores result from a breakdown of the skin when a patient stays in one position for too long and may occur because the individual is unable to leave the bed because of severe illness or he or she is confined to a wheelchair. People with generally fragile skin are also at risk. In people with light skin, a pressure sore may cause the skin to turn red or dark purple. In people with dark skin, the skin becomes even darker than usual.

Symptoms and Diagnostic Path

The bedsore initially appears as reddened skin but then forms a blister. If untreated, the blister becomes an open sore and eventually a crater. Bedsores can appear anywhere on the body but are most likely to appear where bones are close to the skin, such as the ankles, hips, heels, elbows, shoulders, back, and the back of the head.

There are four stages of a bedsore. In Stage I, the skin is red and when it is pressed, it does not turn white, indicating that a bedsore is forming. In Stage II, the skin develops blisters or an open sore forms. The skin around the sore may become irritated and red. In Stage III, the skin has a craterlike appearance, and there is damage to the body below the skin. In Stage IV, the damage is so deep that the muscle and bone are harmed and the tendons and joints may also be harmed.

Bedsores can become infected, and the infection can then spread to the rest of the body. One indicator of an infected bedsore is when the skin near the sore is swollen and warm. Other indicators are when there is a bad odor from the sore itself or the area around the sore is tender and red. Weakness and fever are also signs that the infection may have spread to the bloodstream or elsewhere.

The physician diagnoses the pressure sore based on a visual examination and determines the severity and the stage of the sore.

Treatment Options and Outlook

Treatment depends on the stage of the bedsore and is also determined by the physician. In general, the bedsore is cleaned with salt water to remove the dead tissue (also called *debridement*), and then the damaged area is covered with a dressing that is specially made to treat bedsores.

Pressure must be relieved from the area, using pillows, sheepskin, or special foam cushions that the patient lies against. The sheets may be lightly powdered to reduce friction against the skin. There are special Medicare-approved beds that can help to reduce and eliminate bedsores if the problem is recurrent or chronic. If the patient has a problem with nutrition, as often happens, this issue should be resolved.

The patient or others should *not* massage the area of the pressure sore because this could cause further damage. Round or donut-shaped cushions are not recommended for patients with bedsores because they would further reduce blood flow to the area and could cause complications.

Risk Factors and Preventive Measures

In addition to being bedridden or using a wheelchair, there are other risk factors contributing to the development of bedsores including

- urinary incontinence
- fecal incontinence
- malnourishment
- DIABETES
- ARTERIOSCLEROSIS
- an inability to move about without assistance, such as may occur after a brain or spinal injury
- ALZHEIMER'S DISEASE
- older age

Patients at risk for bedsores should check their bodies daily (or have others check for them) for the presence of such sores. They should also change their position at least every two hours, eat a nutritious diet, keep the skin dry and clean, and use items that will reduce the pressure.

See also BATHING AND CLEANLINESS; HOME HEALTH/ HOME CARE; HOSPITALIZATION; INFECTIONS; NEGLECT.

Beers criteria See INAPPROPRIATE PRESCRIPTIONS FOR THE ELDERLY.

benzodiazepines Medications that are prescribed for the treatment of anxiety disorders. (See ANXIETY AND ANXIETY DISORDERS.) Some benzodiazepines are also prescribed as a sleep remedy to treat insomnia and other SLEEP DISORDERS since most benzodiazepines are sedating. Note that many older individuals may already be taking other medications that are significantly sedating, and thus this effect should be considered by the physician in determining whether a benzodiazepine should be prescribed, as well as in determining the type of benzodiazepine and the dosage. Also, these medications may take a long time to be metabolized (removed from the body), so their effects may last long after the medication has been taken.

Some examples of benzodiazepines are diazepam (Valium), clonazepam (Klonopin), and lorazepam (Ativan). Benzodiazepines can be habit-forming, and for this reason, they are controlled by the federal government. Some people abuse and misuse benzodiazepines, although they are not commonly abused by older people. Benzodiazepines should never be offered to a friend or another person. This is not only illegal but could also cause serious side effects to the other person and even death.

See also ADVERSE DRUG EVENT; ANTIDEPRESSANTS; CHRONIC PAIN; DEPRESSION; DRUG ABUSE; INAPPROPRIATE PRESCRIPTIONS FOR THE ELDERLY; MEDICATION COMPLIANCE; PRESCRIPTION DRUG ABUSE/MISUSE; SUBSTANCE ABUSE AND DEPENDENCE.

Stahl, Stephen M. *Essential Psychopharmacology: The Prescriber's Guide.* New York: Cambridge University Press, 2005.

bereavement Deep feelings of grief and sadness that are suffered by an individual who is emotionally distressed because someone close to him or her has died, such as a husband or wife, a close friend, or even an adult child. Bereavement is a more common and frequent problem for older individuals because they are more likely to lose their spouses, siblings, and friends to death than are younger individuals. However, although it is more common, it is not an easy experience for the older person, who may be grieving the loss of nearly all (and sometimes all) the people that he or she loved.

The bereaved person may develop DEPRESSION or ANXIETY DISORDERS. Some bereaved individuals develop a problem with late-onset ALCOHOLISM. Although it is not common, when it does occur, it is more likely to be a problem among older women than older men.

See also CREMATION; DEATH; DEATH, FEAR OF; END-OF-LIFE ISSUES; FUNERAL; SLEEP DISORDERS.

bill paying, problems with Older individuals may have mild or severe difficulty with paying their bills because of serious mental and cognitive illnesses such as ALZHEIMER'S DISEASE or another form of DEMENTIA or because of physical illnesses that prevent them from attending to their routine financial affairs. As a result, although there may be sufficient income, bills are not paid, and threatening letters to shut off the utilities or other services that will affect the individual's credit are ignored and may even be left unopened.

Sometimes adult children who are visiting their parents are shocked to discover a sheaf of unpaid bills and threatening letters that have been completely ignored by their parents who had always been very conscientious about paying bills in the past. In most cases, if the situation is explained to creditors and the bills are paid, such a situation can be resolved. However, the adult children or others may have to take over managing the older person's financial affairs.

Taking over responsibility for managing the bills can cause considerable stress between the parent and adult child as well as between other siblings and relatives. The parent may be angry or distressed at the loss of financial independence and even suspicious of the motives of the adult child. The adult child may be angry and distressed that his or her altruistic motives are challenged.

See also COGNITIVE IMPAIRMENT; CONFUSION; LEGAL GUARDIANSHIP; TALKING TO ELDERLY PARENTS ABOUT DIFFICULT ISSUES.

binge drinking Drinking five or more alcoholic drinks on the same occasion, either at the same time or within a few hours of each other on at least one day in the past 30 days. *Heavy use of alcohol,* a different category, is defined as drinking five or more drinks on the same occasion in each of five or more days in the past 30 days.

Binge drinking is less of a problem among older people than among other age groups. According to the Substance Abuse and Mental Health Services Administration, in 2006, 7.6 percent of individuals age 65 and older had a problem with binge drinking. This is a serious problem, because many older people take medications, and excessive alcohol can cause severe MEDICATION INTERACTIONS. The rate of heavy drinking was lower than binge drinking among older adults, or 1.6 percent in 2006.

Another problem is that some people drive while intoxicated. According to the Substance Abuse and Mental Health Services Administration, an estimated 1.7 percent of individuals ages 65 and older drove while intoxicated in 2006. (The highest rate for driving while intoxicated occurred among individuals ages 21 to 25 years old, or 27.3 percent of that age group.) Older people who get into car crashes are more likely to be harmed or killed than individuals in other age groups because of their more fragile bones and other health problems.

Males in all age groups are more likely to be binge drinkers than females, and binge drinking is more common among American Indians and Alaska Natives, followed by whites.

See also ADVERSE DRUG EVENT; ALCOHOL; ALCOHOLISM; DRUG ABUSE; GENDER DIFFERENCES; MEMORY IMPAIRMENT; SUBSTANCE ABUSE AND DEPENDENCE.

Substance Abuse and Mental Health Services Administration. *Results from the 2006 National Survey on Drug Use and Health: National Findings.* Rockville, Md.: Office of Applied Studies, 2007.

Binswanger's disease Also called subcortical vascular dementia (or simply vascular dementia) or subcortical arteriosclerotic encephalopathy, Binswanger's disease is caused by microscopic damage to the deep white layers of the brain, which is caused by the thickening and hardening of the arteries that supply the subcortical areas of the brain. (See ARTERIOSCLEROSIS.) This disease was named after Swiss psychiatrist Otto Binswanger (1852–1929), who described a new clinical diagnosis that he called "encephalitis subcorticalis chronica progressive" in 1894. The illness was named after Binswanger in 1902 by Dr. Alzheimer (for whom ALZHEIMER'S DISEASE was named).

Symptoms and Diagnostic Path

Binswanger's disease can start when a person is in their 40s, and it becomes progressively worse as the person ages. Slowness of action, known as psychomotor slowness, is the key feature of this disease. Individuals with Binswanger's often have an unsteady gait, and they may suffer from frequent FALLS.

Other common symptoms are forgetfulness (which is usually a less severe form of forgetfulness than found with Alzheimer's disease), changes in speech, and personality changes; for example, according to Bonelli and Cummings in their article in *Neurologist* in 2008, the individual with any form of subcortical dementia may develop apathy or DEPRESSION.

Individuals with Binswanger's disease are much less likely to have sleep disturbances than patients with Alzheimer's disease. In one study in *Current Alzheimer's Research,* about 35 percent of the subjects with Alzheimer's disease had sleep disturbances compared to 3.6 percent of the subjects with vascular dementia. The subjects with Binswanger's were also less likely to have appetite changes than the subjects with Alzheimer's disease.

If Binswanger's disease is suspected, brain imaging will reveal its characteristic lesions and confirm its presence.

Treatment Options and Outlook

There is no treatment for Binswanger's disease, other than treatment for the accompanying emotional disorders, such as depression and anxiety. Atypical antipsychotic drugs such as risperidone (Risperdal) and olanzapine (Zyprexa) may help with agitation. Careful management of any existing HYPERTENSION and/or DIABETES can help to slow the progressive deterioration of the disease.

Risk Factors and Preventive Measures

Individuals with hypertension and/or diabetes have an increased risk for developing Binswanger's disease. Increased age increases the risk for this disease. There are no known preventive measures to stop the disease from developing, but its further progression can be slowed with exercising, eating a healthy diet, and avoiding SMOKING.

See also DEMENTIA.

Bonelli, R. M., and J. L. Cummings. "Frontal-Subcortical Dementias." *Neurologist* 14, no. 2 (March 2008): 100–107.

Fernández-Martinez, M., et al. "Prevalence of Neuropsychiatric Symptoms in Alzheimer's Disease and Vascular Dementia." *Current Alzheimer's Research* 5, no. 1 (February 2008): 61–69.

Hoff, Paul, M.D. "Images in Psychiatry: Otto Binswanger (1852–1929)." *American Journal of Psychiatry* 159, no. 4 (April 2002): 538.

Olsen, Cynthia G., M.D., and Mark E. Clasen, M.D. "Senile Dementia of the Binswanger's Type." *American Family Physician* (December 1998). Available online. URL: http://www.aafp.org/afp981200ap/olsen.html. Downloaded March 28, 2008.

blindness/severe vision impairment Inability or extreme difficulty in seeing. Blindness or severe vision impairment may be caused by serious EYE DISEASES that are untreated (or treated too late), such as CATARACTS, GLAUCOMA, or AGE-RELATED MACULAR DEGENERATION. Diabetic retinopathy may also cause blindness if individuals with diabetes are unable or unwilling to tightly control their blood sugar levels. Another common cause of vision loss is STROKE.

Symptoms and Diagnostic Path

The symptoms for eye diseases such as cataracts, glaucoma, and age-related macular degeneration vary with each disorder. There are also behavioral signs of severely deteriorating vision or blindness. According to authors Alberta L. Orr and Priscilla Rogers in their book *Aging and Vision Loss: A Handbook for Families,* indicators of possible vision loss in an older person may include the following behaviors:

- going up and down stairs with extreme caution
- constantly bumping into things
- discontinuing reading or watching television
- having trouble getting food on a fork
- pouring liquids over the top of a cup
- no longer reading the mail or newspapers
- reaching out for objects uncertainly

If the person may be blind or have severely bad eyesight, the advice of a doctor should be sought. In the case of very bad eyesight, an eye care professional should be consulted to see if any actions can be taken to improve or reverse the condition, such as eye surgery.

Treatment Options and Outlook

Some people who are blind wish to learn Braille (a tactile language for the blind), while others do not. In addition, some wish to use trained guide dogs, while others do not.

There are many products for people who are visually impaired, and a blind or severely sight-impaired person will often appreciate learning about these products. For example, there are talking watches, clocks, scales, and thermometers. It is possible for many people with "caller ID" on their telephones to purchase a talking phone that says aloud the phone number of the person who is calling. Blind people may appreciate books on tape or disks.

If the individual is already blind, he or she will need to take adaptive measures, with the help of family members and others. For example, clutter in the home should be reduced and small area rugs that could be tripped over should be eliminated. The older person may need to use a long white cane to help him or her locate hazards (although many older people are resistant to this idea). About 109,000 people in the United States use canes to move about according to the American Foundation for the Blind.

People who become blind may develop a loss of their sense of self-worth or may be embarrassed because they can no longer perform tasks such as paying bills or cleaning the house. It is important to tell such individuals that they are still important to others who care about them. It should be noted that it is usually extremely difficult for a formerly sighted person to lose his or her vision. The person may feel that he or she has lost independence, the enjoyment of seeing family and friends, and the ability to perform tasks that were easily performed in the past. The person may suffer from DEPRESSION or anxiety, and psychological counseling is often recommended. However, older people are often resistant to receiving therapy, seeing it as a weakness or as only for someone who is severely mentally ill.

According to Orr and Rogers, individuals who live with the blind or severely visually impaired person should take the following actions:

- Install smoke detectors, fire extinguishers, and carbon monoxide detectors.
- Remember to close doors and drawers so that the sight-impaired person will not risk walking into them.
- Mark the hot water setting in the tub with tactile identification. Also, make sure the hot-water setting is at a safe level.
- Do not walk away from the person without telling him or her that you are leaving.
- Do not worry about using words such as "see" or "look" and being very politically correct. The person with the vision impairment will usually not be offended.
- Give specific directions, such as, "Your chair is to the right of you, about three feet ahead."
- Avoid moving furniture without telling the individual.
- If the older person has a stain on clothing, let him or her know privately.

Risk Factors and Preventive Measures

Blindness may also be caused by long-term DIABETES, and individuals with diabetes have an increased risk for blindness caused by diabetic retinopathy. The risk for blindness or severe vision impairment increases with aging, and the risk is especially marked after age 75.

In as many as half of all cases, blindness can be prevented altogether by annual eye examinations with an ophthalmologist, a physician who specializes in treating the eyes, or an optometrist, a health-care professional who treats the eyes, who will check for serious eye diseases. According to Prevent Blindness America, individuals age 65 and older should have a comprehensive eye examination with dilated pupils at least once every one to two years.

Older African Americans have a greater risk for blindness than individuals of other races and ethnicities.

See also AMERICANS WITH DISABILITIES ACT; EYE DISEASES, SERIOUS; FAMILY AND MEDICAL LEAVE ACT; GLAUCOMA; HEARING DISORDERS.

Orr, Alberta L., and Priscilla Rogers. *Aging and Vision Loss: A Handbook for Families.* New York: American Foundation for the Blind, 2006.

blood pressure monitoring Periodically taking the blood pressure of an individual. This is particularly important in those individuals with severe HYPERTENSION (high blood pressure) as well as those with HYPOTENSION (low blood pressure). Monitoring the blood pressure can help individuals considerably by providing important information to give to their doctors, particularly if their blood pressure is very high or low.

Blood pressure monitoring is also important for physicians to help them determine whether prescribed medications are effective and if dosages need to be changed. Sometimes blood pressure changes indicate the presence of an underlying illness, such as an infection. Individuals with blood pressure problems should take their own blood pressure each day so that they can identify whether their blood pressure drops too low or climbs too high, and if so, contact their physician.

When the blood pressure is taken, two numbers are important, including the systolic pressure (the number on the top, as in 120/80, when the systolic pressure is 120) and the number on the bottom, or the diastolic pressure (which is 80, in this example). The systolic pressure measures the pressure when the heart is beating, and the diastolic pressure measures the pressure when the heart relaxes.

See also ARTERIOSCLEROSIS; CARDIOVASCULAR DISEASE; FRAILTY; HEART DISEASE.

breast cancer Most cases of breast cancer occur in women, and women age 60 and older have the greatest risk for this form of cancer. According to the American Cancer Society, there were an estimated 180,510 new cases of breast cancer diagnosed in 2007, including 178,480 women and 2,030 men. Breast cancer is the most frequently diagnosed form of cancer in women. An estimated 40,910 people died of breast cancer in 2007, including 40,460 women and 450 men.

Mammograms help to identify many cases of breast cancer. The Centers for Disease Control and Prevention (CDC) has set a goal that 70 percent of women age 40 and older will have a mammogram by 2010, and 47 states have already met this goal. In considering the states with the worst and best rates of number of older women who have mammograms, only 66.3 percent of women obtain mammograms in Mississippi (the worst state), while 84.8 percent of women obtain mammograms in Rhode Island (the best state).

Symptoms and Diagnostic Path

Some common symptoms of breast cancer are

- a lump or thickening in or near the breast or in the underarm area
- a change in how the breast or nipple looks (a change in the size or shape of the breast, such as a nipple turned inward into the breast; or a change in the skin of the breast, such as the areola or nipple may be scaly, red, or swollen, and it has ridges or pitting that is similar to the skin of an orange)
- the presence of a nipple discharge of fluid

When the tumor is localized to the breast, the disease can be treated, and many women will lead normal life spans after receiving treatment. However, if the tumor has spread to other parts of the body, such as to the bones, this type of cancer is usually not curable as of this writing.

If a lump is identified as a result of the mammogram, the physician will usually order more screening tests such as X-rays and/or an ultrasound to confirm the diagnosis. A biopsy (the removal of tissue that includes the cancer cells for analysis) will be taken. A biopsy for breast cancer is usually performed by a fine-needle aspiration, a core biopsy, or a surgical biopsy.

With the fine-needle aspiration procedure, a very thin needle is used to remove fluid from a breast lump. The pathologist will then examine the fluid and check for the presence of any cancer cells. With a core biopsy, the doctor will use a thick needle to remove breast tissue, and this tissue is checked by the pathologist for cancer cells. With a surgical biopsy, the doctor removes a sample of the abnormal area, and the pathologist evaluates the tissue for cancer cells.

Sometimes doctors also order special laboratory tests, such as the hormone receptor test or the human epidermal growth factor receptor-2 (HER2) test, which provide further information about the breast tissue.

Treatment Options and Outlook

Treatment of breast cancer depends on how advanced the cancer is and how far it has spread within the body. In the best case, when the cancer is not advanced and it is confined to the breast, a lumpectomy may be performed. In some cases, however, the entire breast and surrounding tissues must be removed as well.

Surgery, radiation therapy, hormone therapy, and chemotherapy are the primary treatment choices for breast cancer. Often a combination of treatments is used, such as both surgery and radiation.

Before treatment begins, the patient should ask the doctor the following questions:

- What did the hormone receptor test show? What did other lab tests show?
- Do any lymph nodes show signs of cancer?
- What is the stage of the disease? Has the cancer spread?
- What is the goal of treatment? What are my treatment choices? Which do you recommend for me? Why?
- What are the expected benefits of each kind of treatment?
- What are the risks and possible side effects of each treatment? How can side effects be managed? What can I do to prepare for treatment?

- Will I need to stay in the hospital? If so, for how long?
- How will treatment affect my normal activities?
- If I were your parent, what treatment would you recommend?
- Would a clinical trial be appropriate for me?

If surgery is to be performed, the patient may have breast-sparing surgery or may have a mastectomy, an operation to remove as much of the breast as possible.

Before having surgery for breast cancer, the patient should ask the following questions:

- What kinds of surgery can I consider? Is breast-sparing surgery an option for me? Which operation do you recommend for me? Why?
- Will my lymph nodes be removed? How many? Why?
- How will I feel after the operation? Will I have to stay in the hospital?
- Will I need to learn how to take care of myself or my incision when I get home?
- Where will the scars be? What will they look like?
- Will I have to do special exercises to help regain motion and strength in my arm and shoulder? Will a physical therapist or nurse show me how to do the exercises?
- Is there someone I can talk with who has had the same surgery I'll be having?

Radiation is another treatment option for breast cancer. Doctors use both external radiation from a large machine and implanted radiation that stays in place for several days. Before having radiation therapy, the patient should ask the doctor the following questions:

- How will radiation be given?
- When will treatment start? When will it end? How often will I have treatments?
- How will I feel during treatment? Will I be able to drive myself to and from treatment?
- How will we know the treatment is working?

- What can I do to take care of myself before, during, and after treatment?
- Will treatment affect my skin?
- How will my chest look afterward?
- What is the chance that the cancer will come back in my breast?
- How often will I need checkups?

Chemotherapy may be the treatment used to kill cancer cells. Chemotherapy may cause hair loss, nausea and vomiting, diarrhea, and mouth sores. Biological therapy may also be given to help the immune system fight the cancer. Trastuzumab (Herceptin) is one form of biological therapy. However, it may cause heart damage that could lead to heart failure.

Risk Factors and Preventive Measures

Most studies show that white women have the greatest risk for a breast cancer diagnosis. However, African-American women who develop breast cancer have a worse prognosis than white women and also a higher mortality rate than women of other races, which may be related to the more advanced level of the tumors that they develop. In addition, they may receive the cancer diagnosis at a later stage of the disease. Most cases of breast cancer occur in women age 60 and older, and it rarely occurs before menopause.

Other risk factors for female breast cancer include

- women who experienced menopause after age 55
- women who never had children
- women who are overweight or obese after menopause
- women who have had breast cancer previously
- women whose mother, sister, or daughter had breast cancer
- women who took diethylstilbestrol (DES), a drug given to some pregnant women from 1940 to 1971 to prevent morning sickness
- women who have had radiation therapy to the chest before age 30, such as women who have been treated with radiation for Hodgkin's lymphoma

Some studies have also shown that ALCOHOLISM increases the risk for breast cancer in both men and women.

See also CANCER.

bruising Black and blue marks on the skin. Older people are often more likely to have broken capillaries and to bruise more easily than younger individuals, and when an individual has many bruises, physicians may attribute the cause to sensitive skin and bones. Sometimes medications can cause more frequent bruising, such as warfarin (Coumadin), a blood thinner. However, in some cases, the appearance of excessive bruising may be a sign that the older individual is suffering from ABUSE at the hands of caregivers or others. Frequent bruising with no apparent cause should be questioned by a physician and family members.

See also NEGLECT/SELF-NEGLECT.

Canada There is an increasingly large elderly population in Canada, and according to Health Canada, in 2001, one in eight Canadians was age 65 or older. By 2026, one in five Canadians will be age 65 or older. This is largely due to Canada's own baby boomers, born between 1946 and 1965. The most rapidly growing part of the elderly population are the oldest Canadians. In 2001, there were 430,000 Canadians age 85, more than twice as many people in this age group as in 1981.

As in the United States, women represent the majority of elderly people, or about 56 percent of all seniors and 70 percent of those age 85 and older.

According to Health Canada, one in four seniors in Canada was born outside the country but most moved to Canada when they were children or young adults.

Chronic Health Problems

More than 80 percent of seniors in Canada report suffering from a chronic health problem such as HEART DISEASE, CANCER, STROKE, respiratory disease, or chronic liver disease. However, the most common chronic health problems are ARTHRITIS, HYPERTENSION, BACK PAIN, CATARACTS, and DIABETES. In addition, among Canadians ages 65 to 74, 25 percent were obese in 2004. Among Canadians age 75 and older, 24 percent were obese. Women age 75 and older were more likely to be obese than men; 27 percent of females in this group were obese compared with 19 percent of males of the same age range.

Falls and Accidental Injuries

Accidental injuries are also a problem for Canadian seniors, and in 1997, seniors who were age 85 and older had a 70 percent higher risk than those ages 65 to 74 of suffering from a serious injury according to the Public Health Agency of Canada in its "Report on Seniors' Falls in Canada." In most cases, the injuries were caused by FALLS.

Older women have a greater risk of falling than older men, and the older the person is, the higher is the risk that they will fall and be injured. For example, 22.3 percent of those ages 65 to 69 were injured in a fall in 2003 in Canada, but this rate increased to 28 percent for those age 80 and older. In considering gender and age, an estimated 39,000 Canadian women age 80 and older were injured in a fall in 2003 compared with 11,000 men.

The largest percentage of those who were injured in a fall (44 percent) slipped, tripped, or stumbled on any surface. The next largest percentage (26 percent) were injured going up or down the stairs. Twenty percent of the subjects were injured in cold weather injuries, such as skating, skiing, snowboarding, or simply slipping, tripping, or stumbling on ice or snow.

Of the areas of the body that were injured, the largest percentage (37 percent) of individuals injured their hip, thigh, knee, lower leg, ankle, or foot. The next largest area of injury (17 percent) was an injury that occurred to the wrist or hand, followed by injuries to the upper or lower spine (14 percent).

The site of the fall was also noted in the report, and almost half (47 percent) of the falls took place inside or around the person's home. Twenty-one percent of the falls that led to hospitalizations occurred to residents of institutions.

Division of Aging and Seniors, Health Canada. *Canada's Aging Population.* Ottawa, Ontario: Minister of Public Works and Government Services, Canada, 2002.

———. *Report on Seniors' Falls in Canada.* Ottawa, Ontario: Minister of Public Works and Government Services, Canada, 2005.

Tjepkema, Michael. *Measured Obesity: Adult Obesity in Canada: Measured Height and Weight.* Ottawa, Canada: Analytical Studies and Reports.

cancer Malignant tumor. An estimated 77 percent of all cancers are diagnosed in people age 55 and older. Among adults age 65 and older, all forms of cancer together represent about 22 percent of deaths from all causes of death among older people, according to the Centers for Disease Control and Prevention (CDC).

According to the American Cancer Society, in 2007 there were 10.5 million people living in the United States with a history of cancer. In addition, in 2007 there were 1,444,920 new cases of cancer diagnosed, and 559,650 people died of cancer, including 289,550 men and 270,100 women.

Cancer is the second most common form of death in the United States, after heart disease. However, many forms of cancer can be treated and even cured if the cancer has not already metastasized (spread) to the adjacent or distant organs or to the bones. This is true for older individuals as well as for younger people.

The five-year survival rate for all forms of cancer during the period 1996 to 2002 was 66 percent, up from 51 percent from 1975 to 1977, although survival rates vary considerably based on the type of cancer and its stage at the time of the diagnosis.

Among older individuals, men over age 75 have the highest rates of cancer, about 28 percent, according to the CDC. Women ages 65 to 74 and women age 85 and older have significantly lower rates of cancer than men experience, or about 17 percent. In considering all people in the United States older than age 65, about 24 percent of men have been diagnosed with some type of cancer compared to 18 percent of older women.

Older people are at risk for many forms of cancer, including lung, prostate, colon, or BREAST CANCER as well as SKIN CANCER. The leading cause of cancer death among people age 65 and older in the United States is LUNG CANCER, which is often linked to many years of smoking cigarettes. Among women of all ages in the United States, the risk of death from lung cancer is 20 times greater for those who smoke two or more packs of cigarettes per day than is the risk among nonsmokers.

Physicians with specialized training treat different types of cancer; for example, a pulmonologist, a physician who specializes in treating the lungs, treats lung cancer, while a urologist treats PROSTATE CANCER, and a gastroenterologist, a physician who specializes in treating digestive diseases, treats STOMACH CANCER. However, many people with cancer also need treatment from an oncologist, a doctor who is a specialist in treating cancer, such as a radiation oncologist.

In most cases, cancer is confirmed by a biopsy of the area where the cancer is suspected, unless this is ill advised because it is clearly evident that cancer is present or the biopsy could be dangerous for the patient or very difficult to perform, as with PANCREATIC CANCER.

In many forms of cancer, the disease is treated with surgery and/or radiation. Sometimes chemotherapy is used. Some cancers use specialized forms of therapy; for example, THYROID CANCER may be treated with radioactive iodine or thyroid hormone.

As mentioned, lung cancer is the most prominent form of cancer among older people, and it is nearly always caused by smoking. Note that older people who smoke and who have not yet been diagnosed with cancer should *not* tell themselves that it is too late to stop smoking because of their age. Ending the smoking habit may mean that lung cancer does not ever develop.

Lung cancer occurs in two primary forms: non-small cell lung cancer and small cell lung cancer, but the majority of cases of lung cancer are non-small cell lung cancers, a slower spreading type of lung cancer. Some symptoms include a cough that gets worse over time and frequent infections with bronchitis or pneumonia.

Depending on the level of advancement of the cancer and many other factors, the doctor may recommend surgery, radiation therapy, or chemotherapy, or may recommend several different types of therapies.

According to the American Cancer Society, black males have the highest rate of developing lung cancer, but white women have a greater rate than black women of developing lung cancer.

When considering gender only, after lung cancer, prostate cancer is the next most frequently occurring form of cancer among older men, and breast cancer is the next most common form of cancer among older women.

The majority of prostate cancer cases are diagnosed in men older than age 65. The diagnosis of prostate cancer is very frightening, but many men can be treated and the problem resolved. With prostate cancer, there may be no symptoms or symptoms may include frequent urination and pain during urination, as well as a weak urine flow. Prostate cancer is often diagnosed with a rectal examination, and the diagnosis is confirmed with a biopsy. Prostate cancer may be treated with surgery, radiation, chemotherapy or hormone therapy (or a combination of therapies), depending on the individual and what his doctor recommends.

Note that if a man's father or brother was diagnosed with prostate cancer, this means his risk for prostate cancer is elevated. Because African-American men have a greater risk for prostate cancer, they should be especially vigilant in having checkups for prostate cancer, although older men of any race are at risk for prostate cancer.

Among women, breast cancer is a frightening diagnosis, but it is also often treatable and should not be regarded as a death sentence as long as treatment occurs. Older women should have periodic mammograms as recommended by their physicians, because this screening test is a major means of identifying breast cancer. Some common symptoms of breast cancer are a lump in the breast or nearby and a change in how the nipple or breast looks. A GYNECOLOGIST treats breast cancer.

Surgery, radiation therapy, hormone therapy, and chemotherapy are the primary treatment options for breast cancer. A combination of treatments may also be used, such as both surgery and radiation. Having a mother or a sister with breast cancer increases the odds that a woman may develop breast cancer. African-American women have an especially high risk of death from breast cancer and should be sure to have mammograms on the schedule recommended by their physicians.

COLORECTAL CANCER is another common form of cancer occurring in older people, appearing at about the same level in men and women. Some common symptoms of colorectal cancer include a change in bowel habits, as well as an unintended weight loss, and a feeling of constant exhaustion. A gastroenterologist, a specialist in the digestive system, can determine whether colorectal cancer is present by examining the patient with a rectal examination and diagnosing or confirming the disease with a COLONOSCOPY.

The preparation medication taken before the colonoscopy can be unpleasant because it causes severe diarrhea in order to completely empty the bowel prior to the procedure. However, it is worth some temporary discomfort because this test can detect cancer and treatment can then begin.

Patients with colorectal cancer may be treated with surgery, radiation, or chemotherapy, or a combination of treatments, depending on the individual needs of the patient and the doctor's recommendation. Individuals whose parents, children, or siblings have had colorectal cancer have an increased risk for this disease. The highest rates of colorectal cancer occur among black men and black women.

Another cancer that may occur in older people is ORAL CANCER. People who have not been diagnosed with cancer (as well as people who *have* been diagnosed) and who smoke should stop smoking immediately, since smoking is a major cause of oral cancer. An oral and maxillofacial surgeon or an otolaryngologist may treat oral cancer.

Most oral cancers start on the tongue or the floor of the mouth. Some symptoms of oral cancer are bleeding inside the mouth or sores in the mouth that do not heal. Regular dental checks are important because often it is the dentist who detects possible cancer, and dental X-rays of the mouth can also show if cancer has spread to the jaw. The medical doctor may order an endoscopy, a procedure done by a gastroenterologist using local anesthesia, to check the person's lungs, windpipe, and throat.

The person with oral cancer may be treated with surgery or radiation therapy or a combination of both treatments. Chemotherapy may also be needed. The highest rates of oral cancer occur among black men and white women.

Stomach cancer is a problem for some older people, and there are usually no early warning symptoms. When symptoms do occur, they may include weight loss and nausea and vomiting. If stomach cancer could be a problem, the patient is usually referred to a gastroenterologist, an expert in digestive diseases. The doctor checks the abdomen for swelling and orders tests such as an upper gastrointestinal series and an endoscopy. Treatment may include surgery, radiation, or chemotherapy, or a combination of treatments.

Older men have a higher risk for stomach cancer than older women, and whites have the lowest risk of developing stomach cancer compared to other races and ethnicities. Smoking is a risk factor for stomach cancer. The highest rates of stomach cancer occur among black and Hispanic males and among Asian/Pacific Islander and Hispanic females.

Skin cancer is diagnosed in some older people, particularly those who have had extensive sun exposure, and this type of cancer is usually treatable. Basal cell cancer and squamous cell cancer are the most commonly occurring forms of skin cancer. Changes in the skin may indicate skin cancer but a dermatologist, a physician specialist in skin diseases and disorders, should be consulted for an expert opinion.

If the patient does have skin cancer, it may be treated with surgery, chemotherapy, or radiation treatment, or a combination of treatments. People with relatives who have had skin cancer have an increased risk for this form of cancer.

LIVER CANCER may develop in older people, and the risk for liver cancer increases with age. Often there are no symptoms but, as the cancer grows, symptoms may include weight loss, a bloated abdomen, and pain on the right side upper abdomen. Liver cancer may be treated by a hepatologist, an expert in liver disease.

The physician feels the abdomen to check the liver and surrounding organs for possible abnormalities and any abnormal fluid buildup. The skin and eyes are checked for jaundice, another sign of possible cancer.

Imaging tests such as a CT scan and ultrasound may be used. Liver cancer is difficult to control but surgery that removes part of the liver may improve the condition. Specialized treatment may be used, such as percutaneous ethanol injection, an injection of alcohol into the liver to destroy cancer cells. Chemotherapy may also be used.

Individuals with chronic hepatitis are at risk for liver cancer, as are those with cirrhosis of the liver. Men have double the risk of developing liver cancer than women. The rate for liver cancer is highest among Asian/Pacific Islander men and Hispanic men and among Asian/Pacific Islander women, American Indian/Alaska Native women and Hispanic women. (The rate is the same for the last two racial categories.)

Some older people develop KIDNEY CANCER. Symptoms may include a constant pain on the side, weight loss, and blood in the urine. The doctor will check for general health signs and for the presence of high blood pressure. She or he will also feel the patient's abdomen and side for any apparent tumors. Urine tests will check for blood and other indicators of disease.

The doctor, usually a nephrologist, a physician expert in kidney disease, may order an intravenous pyelogram (IVP), a test in which dye is injected into the arm and X-ray images are taken as the dye moves through the urinary tract. This test can help detect kidney cancer. The doctor may also order a computerized tomography (CT) scan or an ultrasound test. Treatment may include surgery, radiation therapy, or chemotherapy as well as specialized treatments to shrink the tumor before surgery.

Smokers have double the risk of developing kidney cancer compared to nonsmokers, and men are more likely to develop kidney cancer than women. High blood pressure (HYPERTENSION) increases the risk for kidney cancer. Individuals receiving long-term dialysis for kidney failure have an elevated risk for kidney cancer. The rate for kidney cancer is highest among American Indian/Alaskan Native males and black males and among American Indian/Alaskan Native females.

Pancreatic cancer is a distressing diagnosis for most people because it is often not detected until the individual is in the later stages of the disease, and it is often fatal. An estimated 4 percent of patients survive. Pancreatic cancer is the fourth leading cause of cancer death.

The most common sign of pancreatic cancer is jaundice, or yellowing of the skin and eyes. The individual may also have back pain or abdominal pain and may have had an unintended weight loss. Pancreatic cancer may be treated by a gastroenterologist, but the specialist should be experienced in treating this form of cancer since it is so difficult to treat.

The doctor usually orders tests such as computerized tomography (CT) scans, and the gastroenterologist may order other specialized tests.

Most patients with pancreatic cancer are elderly. People with DIABETES have an elevated risk for pancreatic cancer. The rate for pancreatic cancer is highest among black and white males and black and white females.

Thyroid cancer is another form of cancer that occurs among some older people, and it is much more common among older women than older men. Most thyroid cancers are papillary thyroid cancers, a slow-growing form of cancer. Symptoms often do not occur in early stages, but in the later stages, the individual may have a lump in the neck and have a hoarse voice and trouble breathing and swallowing.

An endocrinologist, an expert in endocrine diseases, may diagnose and treat thyroid cancer. A physical examination, an ultrasound, and a thyroid scan will help determine if thyroid cancer may be present and, if necessary, a biopsy will be taken to confirm the presence of cancer.

Treatment for thyroid cancer includes surgery and/or radiation. Other treatments, such as thyroid hormone treatment, chemotherapy, or radioactive iodine therapy, may also be used.

People with a family history of thyroid disease have an increased risk for thyroid cancer. Among men, the highest rates of thyroid cancer occur among whites, and among women, the highest rates also occur among whites, closely followed by American Indians/Pacific Islanders.

Coping with Fears of Cancer Returning

Many people who are treated for cancer have a deep and underlying fear that the cancer will come back, no matter what the doctor says. This fear is normal and common, but it can be dealt with. The National Cancer Institute recommends the following steps in its publication *Facing Forward: Life after Cancer Treatment*:

- Be informed. Learning about your cancer, understanding what you can do for your health now, and finding out about the services available to you can give you a greater sense of control. Some studies even suggest that people who are well informed about their illness and treatment are more likely to follow their treatment plans and recover from cancer more quickly than those who are not.

- Express your feelings of fear, anger, or sadness. People have found that when they express strong feelings like anger or sadness, they are better able to let go of them. Some sort out their feelings by talking to friends or family, other cancer survivors, or a counselor. Even if you prefer not to discuss your cancer with others, you can still sort out your feelings by thinking about them or writing them down.

- Look for the positive. Sometimes this means looking for the good even in a bad time or trying to be hopeful instead of thinking the worst. Try to use your energy to focus on wellness and what you can do now to stay as healthy as possible.

- Do not blame yourself for your cancer. Some people believe that they got cancer because of something they did or did not do. Remember, cancer can happen to anyone.

- You do not have to be upbeat all the time. Many people say they want to have the freedom to give in to their feelings sometimes. As one woman said, "When it gets really bad, I just tell my family I'm having a bad cancer day and go upstairs and crawl into bed."

- Exercise can help you relax. (See Appendix XIV.)

- Be as active as you can. Getting out of the house and doing something can help you focus on other things besides cancer and the worries it brings.

- Look at what you *can* control. Some people say that putting their lives in order helps them. Being involved in your health care, keeping your appointments, and making changes in your lifestyle are among the things you can control. Even setting a daily schedule can give you a sense of control, and while no one can control every thought, some say that they try not to dwell on the fearful ones.

Deaths from Cancer

Often the first thoughts that occur to most people when they or someone whom they love is diagnosed with cancer are thoughts of dying and death. However, the reality is that many people do recover from cancer with treatment. Despite this, there are many cancer deaths, particularly among older people. For example, according to data from the National Cancer Institute for 2004, of the deaths from breast cancer among people of all ages, 20.4 percent of the deaths occurred to people ages 65 to 74 and 23 percent of the deaths occurred to individuals ages 75 to 84.

In addition, 14.6 percent of the breast cancer deaths were among those age 85 and older. This means that the majority, or a total of 58 percent of all the deaths from breast cancer, occur among individuals age 65 and older. (See Table 1.) The percentage of deaths from prostate cancer is even higher.

In adding up the percentages of deaths from prostate cancer for the three age categories of older men, 91.9 percent of all the deaths from prostate cancer occurred to individuals age 65 and older. Cancer deaths are lower among older people for some types of cancer; for example, testicular cancer is generally a disease of a younger man. As a result, only 12.4 percent of all the deaths from testicular cancer occurred to men age 65 and older.

In considering all sites of cancer deaths, individuals ages 65 to 74 represented 26 percent of all deaths, while those ages 75 to 84 represented 30 percent. Individuals age 85 and older represented 14.2 percent of all cancer deaths at all sites of the body. As a result, 70.2 percent of all deaths from any form of cancer occurred to people age 65 and older.

See also ADVERSE DRUG EVENT; AMERICANS WITH DISABILITIES ACT; CHRONIC PAIN; DEATH; DEATH, FEAR OF; END-OF-LIFE ISSUES; FAMILY AND MEDICAL LEAVE ACT; FRAILTY; GENDER DIFFERENCES; HEALTH CARE AGENT/PROXY; LIVING WILL; NARCOTICS; OBESITY; SMOKING; WILLS.

TABLE 1. AGE DISTRIBUTION (PERCENTAGE) OF ALL DEATHS BY SITE, AGE 65 AND OLDER, ALL RACES, BOTH SEXES, 2000–2004*

Site	65–74	75–84	85+
All Sites	26.0	30.0	14.2
Oral Cavity & Pharynx:	24.7	22.3	11.0
Lip	17.6	32.1	24.7
Tongue	23.9	21.3	9.7
Salivary gland	22.4	28.7	18.2
Floor of mouth	27.9	17.8	8.5
Gum & other oral cavity	23.5	26.3	19.5
Nasopharynx	21.3	17.2	6.5
Tonsil	23.5	16.3	4.8
Oropharynx	26.0	20.9	8.5
Hypopharynx	30.1	20.3	5.7
Other oral cavity & pharynx	27.7	23.0	9.0
Digestive System:	25.1	30.2	16.3
Esophagus	28.9	26.4	9.2
Stomach	23.6	29.8	17.2
Small intestine	24.5	28.7	12.8
Colon & rectum	23.6	31.1	20.1
Anus, anal canal & anorecum	20.0	21.2	10.8
Liver and intrahepatic bile duct:	25.2	26.9	10.9
Liver	25.2	25.9	9.9
Intrahepatic bile duct	25.2	30.6	14.2
Gallbladder	26.0	33.5	16.3
Other biliary	23.4	34.7	22.8
Pancreas	26.8	31.5	14.5
Retroperitoneum	24.7	29.6	11.2
Peritoneum, omentum & mesentery	31.8	29.4	7.6
Other digestive system	22.2	31.9	24.3
Respiratory System:	32.0	30.1	8.7
Nose, nasal cavity & middle ear	22.1	25.3	13.3
Larynx	30.0	24.5	7.7
Lung & bronchus	32.1	30.3	8.7
Pleura	28.3	38.1	12.2
Trachea & other respiratory organs	23.7	25.8	10.2
Bones & Joints	13.9	18.5	11.1
Soft Tissue (including heart)	19.7	21.5	9.8
Skin (except basal & squamous):	21.4	24.3	14.1
Melanoma of the skin	21.6	23.1	10.7
Other non-epithelial skin	20.9	28.0	24.8
Breast (female)	20.4	23.0	14.6
Female Genital System:	23.7	26.8	13.1
Cervix uteri	15.3	13.7	7.1
Corpus uteri	28.9	29.6	14.6
Uterus, not otherwise specified	24.7	28.7	17.1

Site	65–74	75–84	85+
Ovary	25.0	28.8	12.2
Vagina	20.2	27.0	26.5
Vulva	17.4	34.3	29.6
Other female genital system	24.0	28.2	13.5
Male Genital System:	20.7	41.3	28.9
Prostate	20.8	41.8	29.3
Testis	5.5	4.6	2.3
Penis	25.4	25.1	12.0
Other male genital system	16.3	38.6	15.2
Urinary System:	24.3	32.7	18.7
Urinary bladder	22.6	37.1	24.7
Kidney & renal pelvis	26.0	27.9	12.4
Ureter	27.6	37.4	20.1
Other urinary system	22.7	37.4	20.3
Eye & Orbit	21.0	24.5	13.1
Brain & Nervous System	22.8	19.4	5.8
Endocrine System:	21.8	24.3	11.8
Thyroid	24.2	30.7	16.2
Other endocrine & thymus	18.1	14.5	5.0
Lymphoma:	23.3	32.6	15.8
Hodgkin lymphoma	16.9	19.8	8.3
Non-Hodgkin lymphoma	23.7	33.4	16.3
Myeloma	27.8	35.2	14.4
Leukemia:	22.5	31.6	17.2
Lymphocytic:	20.1	30.7	22.3
Acute lymphocytic	12.5	11.6	5.7
Chronic lymphocytic	22.6	36.4	27.4
Other lymphocytic	19.8	35.5	25.3
Myeloid & monocytic:	24.6	30.7	11.9
Acute myeloid	25.4	30.5	10.7
Chronic myeloid	20.6	27.1	15.0
Acute monocytic	20.7	35.6	18.9
Other myeloid & monocytic	24.6	39.6	18.3
Other:	21.3	34.5	21.2
Other acute	23.2	35.6	18.1
Aleikemic, subleuk, and not otherwise specified	19.9	33.7	23.7
Ill-defined and unspecified	24.5	31.2	16.9

*Chart does not include percentages of deaths for those younger than age 65, which make up the balance.

Source: Ries, L., et al. *SEER Cancer Statistics Review 1975–2004.* Bethesda, Md.: National Cancer Institute. Available online. URL: http://seer.cancer.gov/csr/1975_2004/. Downloaded July 29, 2007.

American Cancer Society. *Cancer Facts & Figures 2007.* Atlanta, Ga.: American Cancer Society, 2007.

Centers for Disease Control and Prevention. *Prostate Cancer Screening: A Decision Guide.* Available online. URL: http://www.cec./gov/cancer/prostate/prospdf/prosguide.pdf. Downloaded July 2, 2007.

He, Wan, Manisha Sengupta, Victoria A. Velkoff, and Kimberly A. DeBarros. *65+ in the United States: 2005.* Washington, D.C.: U.S. Census Bureau, December 2005.

Lange, Paul H., M.D., and Christine Adamec. *Prostate Cancer for Dummies.* New York: Wiley, 2003.

National Cancer Institute. *Facing Forward: Life After Cancer Treatment.* Bethesda, Md.: National Institutes of Health, September 2006.

———. *What You Need to Know About Breast Cancer.* Bethesda, Md.: National Institutes of Health, May 2005.

———. *What You Need to Know About Kidney Cancer.* Bethesda, Md.: National Institutes of Health, April 2003.

———. *What You Need to Know About Oral Cancer.* Bethesda, Md.: National Institutes of Health, June 2003.

———. *What You Need to Know About Stomach Cancer.* Bethesda, Md.: National Institutes of Health, August 2005.

———. *What You Need to Know About Thyroid Cancer.* Bethesda, Md.: National Institutes of Health, August 2007.

Ries, L., et al. *SEER Cancer Statistics Review 1975–2004.* Bethesda, Md.: National Cancer Institute. Available online. URL: http://seer.cancer.gov/csr/1975_2004/. Accessed July 29, 2007.

cardiologist   See HEART ATTACK; HEART DISEASE.

cardiopulmonary resuscitation (CPR)   Specialized training that instructs individuals in a method for reviving a person who has stopped breathing due to a HEART ATTACK, STROKE, drowning, choking, or another life-threatening event that has interrupted breathing. Alternate names for CPR are rescue breathing and chest compressions, adult; or resuscitation-cardiopulmonary, adult. According to the National Institutes of Health, CPR combines rescue breathing to provide oxygen to the individual's lungs with chest compressions to keep the person's blood circulating in the body. (If blood flow stops, brain damage or death can occur in minutes; for example, permanent brain damage starts within four minutes when the person is deprived of oxygen, and death can occur within four to six minutes later.)

CPR should not be performed on a person with normal breathing or movement, or who is coughing.

The rescuer should avoid seeking a pulse, according to Dr. Gordon A. Ewy in his article on CPR for *Circulation.* Instead, says Ewy, the individual should first be spoken to loudly. If an adult victim fails to respond, then the individual should be shaken to see if he or she is unconscious. Then breathing should be assessed for normal or abnormal breathing. (Abnormal breathing is no breathing or an intermittent gasping for breath.) The next step is to call 911. If the person on the scene knows how to do CPR, the dispatcher may instruct him or her to perform continuous-chest-compression or CPR. If the person on the scene does not know CPR, then often instructions will be provided on the phone.

Some rescuers are concerned that they may harm the patient and are fearful of performing CPR. Says Dr. Ewy, "Yes, you may break ribs, but the alternative is almost certainly death. The patient's medical history is not important; conditions such as a pacemaker or bypass surgery should not concern you as a bystander."

Ewy says that continuous-chest-compression CPR is the best method for a sudden and unexpected collapse, but conventional mouth-to-mouth breathing CPR is the best for patients experiencing respiratory arrest, as in the case of alcohol intoxication, a drug overdose, carbon monoxide poisoning, a severe asthma attack, choking, or drowning.

Individuals performing CPR should have a current state certification in the procedure. Special care should be taken with elderly individuals when possible, because they are more likely to suffer injuries from aggressive CPR; however, as mentioned, even an injury is a better option than death from the adverse event.

Survival rates from CPR are not uniformly reported; however, according to the American Heart Association, in cities such as Seattle, Washington, where many people have received CPR training and emergency response is rapid, the survival rate

for a person who has experienced cardiac arrest and received CPR is 30 percent. In contrast, in cities such as New York City, where few people have received CPR training and emergency response is longer, the survival rate is about 1 to 2 percent.

See also CARDIOVASCULAR DISEASE; HEART DISEASE; DEATH; DEATH, FEAR OF; EMERGENCY DEPARTMENT CARE; END-OF-LIFE ISSUES; FRAILTY; HEART FAILURE; LIVING WILL.

American Heart Association. "Cardiopulmonary Resuscitation (CPR) Statistics." Undated. Available online. URL: http://www.americanheart.org/presenter.jhtml?identifier=4483. Accessed February 20, 2008.

Ewy, Gordon A., M.D. "New Concepts of Cardiopulmonary Resuscitation for the Lay Public." *Circulation* 116 (2007): e566–e568. Available online. URL: http://circ.ahajournals.org/cgi/content/full/116/25/e566. Accessed February 20, 2008.

cardiovascular disease (CVD) Encompasses HEART DISEASE, HYPERTENSION, and STROKE. Cardiovascular disease is a leading cause of death, and it is a major health problem in the United States and worldwide. It is most common among the following individuals:

- smokers
- black males
- Mexican-American men and women
- individuals age 65 and older
- NATIVE AMERICANS
- those who are obese
- individuals with DIABETES

Symptoms and Diagnostic Path

Doctors diagnose CVD based on blood pressure readings, electrocardiograms, MAGNETIC RESONANCE IMAGING (MRI scans), stress tests, and various other means.

Treatment Options and Outlook

The treatment depends on the nature and the severity of the problem. EMERGENCY DEPARTMENT CARE is required in the case of a heart attack or stroke, usually followed by maintenance doses of medications, as well as recommended lifestyle changes, such as weight loss, better control of diabetes among diabetic individuals, and regular EXERCISE. In the case of hypertension, the goal is to lower the blood pressure. There is a broad array of medications used to treat hypertension, and individuals should contact their physicians to determine the right medicines for them. Some individuals need to take three or more different hypertension medications before they are able to control their hypertension.

Risk Factors and Preventive Measures

Smoking and high cholesterol levels are risk factors for hypertension. In addition, obesity increases the risk for high blood pressure.

Smokers must stop smoking immediately. Individuals with high blood CHOLESTEROL levels need to change their diets and often must also take cholesterol-lowering medications as well. Patients are also advised to watch their cholesterol levels and to lose weight if they are obese.

See also ARTERIOSCLEROSIS; BLOOD PRESSURE MONITORING; HEART ATTACK; HEART FAILURE.

caregivers Term usually used to denote family individuals who care for an ill member, although it is sometimes used to refer to private individuals who are paid to provide care in a nursing home or other environment. Many family caregivers are married middle-aged women who still have children in the home.

See also FAMILY CAREGIVERS.

Parks, Susan Mockus, M.D., and Karen D. Novielli, M.D. "A Practical Guide to Caring for Caregivers." *American Family Physician* 62 (2000): 2613–2620, 2621–2622.

caregiver stress It can be very stressful and distressing to provide frequent or constant care to an elderly loved one who is a parent or other relative. The caregiver may feel that he or she cannot ever leave the elderly person and thus has no independent life. The caregiver may develop ANXIETY or DEPRESSION, as well as a variety of physical symptoms such as HEADACHES, stomachaches, and other CHRONIC PAIN syndromes.

It is important for caregivers to acknowledge their stress symptoms to themselves and to work on means to alleviate them, such as taking time off from caregiving by seeking help from other family members, ADULT DAY CENTERS, or other individuals or groups who can provide respite assistance.

Some organizations provide respite care to caregivers of the elderly, although most people agree that respite care is hard to find and insufficient. For the caregiver who could take some time off but refuses to do so, it may help to point out that if the caregiver becomes ill from overwork and must be hospitalized, then he or she will no longer be able to assist the elderly person.

See also ADULT CHILDREN/CHILDREN OF AGING PARENTS; BABY BOOMERS; COMPASSION FATIGUE; FAMILY AND MEDICAL LEAVE ACT; IRRITABILITY; LONG-DISTANCE CARE; TALKING TO ELDERLY PARENTS ABOUT DIFFICULT ISSUES.

cataracts A cataract is an eye disease that causes an opaqueness of the lens of the eye, and it can cause blindness if it is not treated. More than half of all Americans age 80 and older have cataracts. The World Health Organization says that cataracts are the leading cause of blindness worldwide. People with DIABETES have an increased risk for developing cataracts compared to nondiabetics.

Symptoms and Diagnostic Path

In the early stages of cataracts, there may be slight clouding of vision, but as the disease progresses, it becomes increasingly difficult for the person to see through the cloudy film of the cataract. Some people in the early stages of cataracts may find sunlight more glaring than in the past, and they may have found the oncoming headlights of a car at night too bright or distorted. In addition, colors may seem duller than in the past.

An optometrist, a professional with specialized training in treating the eyes, or ophthalmologist, a physician specialist trained in treating the eyes and eye diseases, diagnoses cataracts using an eye chart as well as a dilated eye examination. The eye professional may also use tonometry, which is an instrument that measures internal eye pressure, after numbing drops are inserted into the eye. If surgery is required, the ophthalmologist can perform the procedure.

Treatment Options and Outlook

If surgery is performed, the cataract and the natural lens of the eye are removed and an artificial clear plastic lens is implanted. According to the National Institutes of Health, cataract surgery is one of the safest forms of surgery and 90 percent of those who have it experience better vision after this outpatient procedure. If a person has cataracts in both eyes, then the surgery is performed on one eye at a time, according to the National Eye Institute, and these surgeries are usually performed from four to eight weeks apart.

One of two types of cataract surgery may be used, including *phacoemulsification* or *extracapsular surgery*. If phacoemulsification is used, a tiny incision is made on the cornea's side (the cornea covers the front of the eye). Then a tiny probe is inserted that emits ultrasound waves that break up the lens, which is then removed by suction. The artificial lens, or intraocular lens (IOL), is then implanted to become a permanent part of the eye.

A less popular form of cataract surgery is called *extracapsular surgery*, in which the doctor makes a long incision on the side of the cornea and removes the cloudy lens as one piece. Any leftover pieces are suctioned out. As in phacoemulsification, the artificial lens is then implanted.

Whichever surgery is performed, the procedure takes less than an hour and there is no pain; in fact, many people remain awake and alert during the operation.

After the surgery, the vision may be blurred at first because the eye needs time to heal. Patients should ask their doctors when they can drive again.

Risk Factors and Preventive Measures

Some people have an increased risk for developing cataracts, according to the National Eye Institute; for example, people with diabetes have a greater risk than others, as do older people who are constantly out in the sun with little or no eye protection. Patients who have had cataracts can have recurrences and consequently should have regular eye examinations. They should also avoid excessive sun exposure. In addition, those who smoke should stop smoking to reduce the risk of developing or redeveloping cataracts. According to the NIH, some research indicates that good nutrition can reduce the risk of an age-related cataract, and researchers recommend eating fruit, leafy vegetables, and other foods that contain antioxidants. In addition, wearing a hat with a brim and sunglasses in bright sunlight may help to delay the development of a cataract.

See also EYE DISEASES, SERIOUS.

Prevent Blindness America and the National Eye Institute. *Vision Problems in the U.S.: Prevalence of Adult Vision Impairment and Age-Related Eye Disease in America.* 2002. Available online. URL: http://www.nei.nih.gov/eyedata. Accessed February 13, 2008.

Caucasians Individuals generally referred to as *white*, although their skin tone may vary from very light to medium to dark brown. In general, elderly white males have a greater risk than older individuals of other races for the development of some illnesses, such as HEART DISEASE. Caucasians also have the highest rate of hearing impairments. White women have a greater risk of dying from ALZHEIMER'S DISEASE than do women of other races. White women also have a higher risk than women of other races of developing OSTEOPOROSIS.

According to the Centers for Disease Control and Prevention (CDC), whites age 65 and older have the lowest rate of DIABETES when compared with blacks, Hispanics, Asians, and Native Americans.

See also AFRICAN AMERICANS; ASIAN AMERICANS; HISPANICS; NATIVE AMERICANS; RACIAL AND ETHNIC DIFFERENCES.

cemetery, choice of The choice of the cemetery where a loved one will be interred can be difficult sometimes. The family may wish to bury the remains (or *cremains,* in the case of a CREMATION) of the loved one in a cemetery at the location where the deceased person grew up or, alternatively, they may wish the burial to occur at a cemetery that is near certain family members. If the cemetery is distant from where the deceased died, the remains can be shipped by air to the location of the cemetery. This arrangement is made by the funeral home. The family may also choose for the burial to occur in a military cemetery, if the deceased was a veteran. In some cases, the family may wish to retain the cremated remains of the deceased in an urn or other special container that they maintain at home.

In some cases, some family members may wish to bury the loved one at a cemetery for military veterans, while other family members may disagree because the cemetery may be far away and hard to visit. Sometimes family members disagree on where the remains should be buried and arguments can become intense.

See also BEREAVEMENT; DEATH; DEATH, FEAR OF; END-OF-LIFE ISSUES; FUNERALS; TALKING TO ELDERLY PARENTS ABOUT DIFFICULT ISSUES.

centenarians Individuals who have lived to the age of 100 years or beyond. In the United States as of November 1, 2000, there were 68,000 people who were centenarians, according to the U.S. Census Bureau. There were 37,000 centenarians in 1990; thus, the number increased by about 84 percent in 10 years. In contrast, the population for individuals of all ages increased by about 11 percent during the same 10-year period. The global population of centenarians is also anticipated to be on the rise, with the global aging of citizens in many countries throughout the world.

In a Danish study of centenarians, reported in 2001, researchers found that only about half of the study subjects had Alzheimer's or another form of DEMENTIA. This largely disproves the generally accepted belief that nearly all very old people will develop some form of dementia.

See also ALZHEIMER'S DISEASE.

cervicogenic headaches The cervicogenic headache is a severe headache that is caused by referred pain in the neck, such as pain caused by ARTHRITIS in the upper spine, or by a pinched nerve, or by an array of other possible causes. It was first described in 1983 by Ottar Sjaastad

et al., and its diagnostic criteria was revised by Sjaastad in 1998. Often people with cervicogenic headaches are misdiagnosed with MIGRAINE or tension headaches.

Symptoms and Diagnostic Path
According to Doctors Kandel and Sudderth in their book *The Headache Cure,* the following are some key symptoms of cervicogenic headaches:

- tenderness when the doctor examines the neck
- minor neck pain that develops into severe head pain
- pain that increases when the person sits or lies down for several hours
- shoulder pain
- headache pain that occurs when pressure is applied to the neck

According to Kandel and Sudderth, many patients with cervicogenic headaches suffer from head pain that is so severe that they do not actually notice that they have neck pain until it is physically demonstrated to them by a physician who presses on the neck. However, the neck pain must be resolved in order to treat the head pain in this case, since it is the source of the problem.

Treatment Options and Outlook
Cervicogenic headaches can be treated with over-the-counter or prescribed nonsteroidal anti-inflammatory drugs (NSAIDs) and muscle relaxants such as carisprodol (Soma) or cyclobenzaprine (Flexeril). Some patients improve with low dosages of ANTIDEPRESSANTS, such as amitriptyline (Elavil) or Aventyl (nortriptyline). Others find relief with antiseizure drugs such as carbamazepine (Tegretol) or topiramate (Topamax).

Patients may also benefit from using over-the-counter ointments with lidocaine or capsaicin. Others benefit from using Lidoderm, a prescribed transdermal skin patch of lidocaine. Trigger injections or joint injections of steroids may provide temporary relief, as may nerve blocks. Botulinum toxin injections (Botox) may be quite helpful if there is a strong component of muscle spasm as the pain generator.

Massage therapy is often helpful in treating cervicogenic headaches, as is physical therapy and regular exercises of the neck and head.

Risk Factors and Preventive Measures

Individuals who remain sitting and working on computers for long periods of time are at risk for developing cervicogenic headaches. Sometimes bright light and/or noise can trigger this type of headache. Women have about twice the risk of suffering from cervicogenic headaches than men. FALLS increase the risk for cervicogenic headaches, and older people have an increased risk for falls compared to other age groups of adults. Some illnesses, such as osteoarthritis in the cervical spine (neck area) also increase the risk for cervicogenic headaches.

Frequent short breaks walking around and moving about can decrease the risk for these headaches. Individuals who often talk on their phones may have an increased risk for cervicogenic headaches, especially if they crane their necks to balance the phone between their head and shoulder. Women who carry large purses should remove unnecessary items that add weight (and potential pain), such as large amounts of coins. Large-breasted women should also use appropriate support, such as a sports bra, to alleviate stress on the neck.

See also HEADACHES.

Kandel, Joseph, M.D., and David Sudderth, M.D. *The Headache Cure: How to Uncover What's Really Causing Your Pain and Find Lasting Relief.* New York: McGraw-Hill, 2006.

cholesterol Refers to lipoproteins (fats) that are circulating in the bloodstream, including low-density lipoproteins (LDL), also known as "bad" cholesterol, and high-density lipoprotein (HDL), often referred to as "good" cholesterol. Elevated LDL levels increase the risk for HEART DISEASE, HEART ATTACK, and STROKE. Triglyceride levels are also linked to cholesterol levels, and individuals with high triglyceride levels may need to take medications and also make changes in their diet to bring those levels down.

According to the National Heart, Lung, and Blood Institute of the National Institutes of Health, the total desirable cholesterol level is less than 200 mg/deciliter (dL) of blood. In addition, the optimal LDL cholesterol level is less than 100 mg dL. (See Table 1.)

Effects on Cholesterol Levels

There are several factors that affect cholesterol levels, including some that can be changed and others that cannot. For example, diet is a key factor among those factors that can be changed. Reducing the amount of cholesterol and saturated fat in the diet will lower the cholesterol level. Another risk factor for raising cholesterol levels is OBESITY, and weight loss can improve the cholesterol count. The third key factor is the individual's level of activity, and regular exercise can lower LDL levels as well as help the individual lose weight.

Cigarette SMOKING is also a risk factor for high cholesterol, as is hypertension of 140/90 mm Hg or higher. Individuals can stop smoking. Hypertension can be controlled with medication and often with weight loss as well.

Among several risk factors that individuals cannot control are their age and gender. For example, as men and women age, their cholesterol levels generally rise. In general, women have a lower cholesterol level than men before the onset of menopause, but after menopause, the cholesterol levels of both men and women are about the same. Heredity is another risk factor for high cholesterol, and members of some families have

TABLE 1. RANGES OF CHOLESTEROL LEVELS AND DESIRABLE LEVELS

Total Cholesterol Level	Category
Less than 200 mg/dL	Desirable
200–239	Borderline high
240 mg/dL and above	High

LDL Cholesterol Level	LDL Cholesterol Category
Less than 100 mg/dL	Optimal
100–129 mg/dL	Near optimal/above optimal
130–159 mg/dL	Borderline high
160–189 mg/dL	High
190 mg/dL and above	Very high

Source: National Heart, Lung, and Blood Institute. *High Blood Cholesterol: What You Need to Know.* Washington, D.C.: National Institutes of Health, June 2005.

higher cholesterol levels than others. In addition, individuals with DIABETES have an increased risk for the development of high cholesterol levels.

Treating High Cholesterol

Some individuals can lower their cholesterol levels through diet and physical activity. Others may need to take cholesterol-lowering medications, along with changing their diet and level of physical activity.

See also ARTERIOSCLEROSIS; OBESITY.

chronic obstructive pulmonary disease (COPD)

A serious and incurable (although treatable) lung disease that causes a severe obstruction of a person's airflow and also is the cause of death for many older people in the United States and other countries. COPD is the fourth leading cause of death in the United States according to the Centers for Disease Control and Prevention (CDC). Chronic obstructive pulmonary disease is also known as chronic obstructive airway disease and chronic obstructive lung disease.

The disease occurs as a result of a combination of chronic bronchitis and EMPHYSEMA, although it can also result from emphysema alone. The primary cause of COPD is smoking, and 15 to 20 percent of long-term smokers develop COPD. As with asthma, the airways are hyperresponsive to stimuli and the illness can cause extreme and even life-threatening coughing and choking as the person attempts to catch a breath.

Symptoms and Diagnostic Path

Chronic coughing, wheezing, and frequent occurrences of shortness of breath are possible symptoms of COPD. The person with COPD is also more prone to developing colds and other infections. A pulmonologist, a physician who specializes in lung diseases, treats patients with COPD.

Doctors may order a chest X-ray to diagnose COPD, which will show an over-expanded lung. There are also breathing machines that can measure how effectively the lungs are working. During a physical examination, the doctor can see how hard the patient works at breathing. In addition, the patient may exhibit such signs as pursing the lips when exhaling.

Treatment Options and Outlook

When experiencing an attack of breathing difficulties, patients may use bronchodilators, which are inhaled medications. Sometimes the drug theophylline is used to treat COPD. Antibiotics are administered to fight infections. Steroid drugs may also be used for short periods of several weeks. For severe cases, steroids may be given intravenously. Some patients may need oxygen therapy, administered by special tubes (cannula) through the nose. Oxygen therapy can occur at home with home health-care workers providing assistance. In some severe cases, surgery may be required, such as a lung transplant. A lung reduction procedure may also be possible.

Anyone diagnosed with COPD who still smokes must stop SMOKING immediately to increase the odds of survival. Patients may also need antidepressants or smoking cessation products to stop smoking. Ending their smoking habit is the most important action that COPD patients can take and it should be emphasized. People who smoke but who do not have COPD should also stop smoking immediately to avoid the future development of COPD.

Risk Factors and Preventive Measures

Smoking is the cause of 90 percent of the cases of people who are diagnosed with COPD. Environmental exposure to chemicals can also cause or worsen COPD, and people who have worked in certain professions, such as mining, firefighting, and metalworking have a higher risk of developing COPD as well as many other diseases linked to smoking.

Triggers for COPD

There are a variety of triggers for the symptoms of COPD according to the Environmental Protection Agency (EPA), including air pollution, which may lead to the need for HOSPITALIZATION. In addition, there are also often pollutants found in the home, such as direct and secondhand tobacco smoke, animal dander, dust mites, mold, cockroaches, and pollen. Other items that may trigger a COPD attack are the combustion products of oil, gas, kerosene, and coal as well as building materials made of pressed wood products. In addition, household cleaning substances and pesticides with irritating odors may also trigger an attack.

According to the EPA, individuals with COPD (or asthma) should take the following actions to reduce the risk of breathing difficulties:

- stay away from tobacco smoke
- avoid smoke from wood-burning stoves
- reduce mold, dust mites, and cockroaches in the home
- keep pets out of sleeping areas
- check the furnace and heating units annually to make sure they are working properly
- fix water leaks promptly
- check the air quality index (AQI). To learn more, go to www.epa.gov/airnow

See also LUNG CANCER.

Environmental Protection Agency. *Fact Sheet: Age Healthier, Breathe Easier: Information for Older Adults and their Caregivers,* June 2007.

chronic pain Frequent or constant discomfort. Many older people suffer from chronic pain that is caused by ARTHRITIS, BACK PAIN, CANCER, DIABETES, HEADACHES, and other serious medical problems that cannot be cured but can be treated. In some cases, over-the-counter medications such as ibuprofen or acetaminophen (Tylenol) will provide sufficient pain relief to the individual with chronic pain. In other cases, stronger painkillers and even NARCOTICS may be needed to relieve the pain adequately.

Sometimes chronic pain becomes extremely severe, and some individuals with excessive pain levels rely on an implanted morphine pump to provide them with steady relief from their extreme pain. This may be true for patients who have had failed back surgery or who have cancer.

In a study of more than 7,000 older individuals with chronic pain, reported in a 2007 issue of the *Annals of Clinical Psychiatry,* the majority of elderly individuals suffered from chronic pain, and the six-month prevalence of chronic pain was evident in 76.2 percent of the subjects. In addition, chronic

pain was directly associated with disturbed sleep in some of the chronic conditions that were included in the study, such as headaches (49.7 percent), gastrointestinal pain (47.6 percent), chest pain (45.3 percent), joint pain (42.7 percent), and back pain (42.5 percent).

Some studies have shown that older people are often undertreated for their pain, or they are not treated at all for their pain, even when they suffer from the severe pain of cancer. Some physicians worry that the use of narcotics could cause the older person to develop an addiction to the drug. They may wait until the patient becomes frantic with pain before prescribing strong analgesics.

This is a mistake, because in general, pain should be treated *before* it reaches very high levels. In general, once the pain has peaked, it is more difficult to treat than when it is treated at a lower level.

It is also untrue (and it is an ageist assumption) that chronic pain is a normal state in an older person. (See AGEISM.) Although older people are more likely to experience chronic pain than younger people, treatment can usually alleviate or at least decrease the older person's pain; thus, chronic pain should not be accepted as a normal part of the aging process and one that simply must be endured. It is not true that older people are somehow *supposed* to suffer with pain, although there are still some physicians and older patients who apparently believe this to be true.

EXERCISE can sometimes help to relieve chronic pain, as may spiritual exercises, such as meditation and prayer. Weight loss can often improve chronic pain among those with problems with OBESITY.

Chronic pain is often significantly associated with SLEEP DISORDERS based on a study published in the *Annals of Clinical Psychiatry.* In this study, such chronic pain problems as headaches, gastrointestinal disorders, joint pain, and back pain were all significantly associated with a 30-day prevalence of disturbed sleep. Whites were more likely to be affected than individuals of other races, and disabled individuals were more likely to be affected than the nondisabled.

In this study, nearly half of the subjects with disturbed sleep reported having a problem with chronic headaches, and nearly 48 percent reported gastrointestinal pain. About 45 percent said they had chest pain and approximately 43 percent had joint pain, the same percentage found with respondents who reported disturbed sleep and back pain. According to the researchers, "Elderly subjects with a combination of disturbed sleep and chronic pain condition appear to be seriously handicapped and suffer role disability as demonstrated by the use of medical services, self-rated health and socioeconomic status."

The researchers found that the presence of psychiatric problems, the number of pain disorders, and the presence of headaches were key factors in predicting sleep disorders among those who were white. However, age was also somewhat of a protective factor, and the risk of a sleep disorder deceased with increasing age.

See also AMERICANS WITH DISABILITIES ACT; BACK PAIN; FAMILY AND MEDICAL LEAVE ACT; GENDER DIFFERENCES; HEART DISEASE; INAPPROPRIATE PRESCRIPTIONS FOR THE ELDERLY; IRRITABILITY; PAINKILLING MEDICATIONS; PRESCRIPTION DRUG ABUSE; SUBSTANCE ABUSE AND DEPENDENCE.

Blay, Sergio Luis, Sergio Baxter Andreoli, and Fabio Leite Gastal. "Chronic Painful Physical Conditions, Disturbed Sleep and Psychiatric Morbidity: Results from an Elderly Survey." *Annals of Clinical Psychiatry* 19, no. 3 (2007): 169–174.

cocoa/chocolate See HYPERTENSION.

cognitive impairment Difficulty in thinking that was not present in the individual in past years. The person may have ALZHEIMER'S DISEASE or another form of DEMENTIA or may be cognitively impaired due to chronic ALCOHOLISM.

In some cases, a vitamin deficiency, such as a deficiency of Vitamin B_{12}, may cause a cognitive impairment. In other cases, a medication or a MEDICATION INTERACTION may be impeding a person's thought processes. If the impairment results from a vitamin deficiency, it will often be resolved when the underlying vitamin deficiency is corrected. If a medication is causing the problem, changing the medication dose may improve the person's ability to think clearly.

It is very difficult for older people in the early stages of Alzheimer's disease or dementia to accept that their cognitive abilities will continue to decline markedly as they age. It is also extremely hard for family members to cope with this fact. Many individuals have said that seeing a parent or a loved one's mind deteriorate was much harder than observing an increase in their physical disabilities.

See also ADULT CHILDREN/CHILDREN OF AGING PARENTS; AGGRESSION, PHYSICAL; CONFUSION; DELUSIONS; FAMILY CAREGIVERS; HALLUCINATIONS; IRRITABILITY; MEMORY IMPAIRMENT; RAGE; VITAMIN AND MINERAL DEFICIENCIES/EXCESSES.

colonoscopy Procedure in which a colonoscope, a special instrument that is used to examine the colon, is inserted into the sedated person's colon by a gastroenterologist, a physician who specializes in treating digestive diseases. The colonoscopy is done for the purpose of checking for *polyps,* an extra piece of tissue that grows inside your body and which may be cancerous or precancerous, and for other digestive diseases and disorders, such as gastric or duodenal ulcers, irritable bowel syndrome, diverticulitis, and so forth.

Procedure

The patient's colon must be empty prior to the colonoscopy in order for the procedure to be thorough. The physician will provide the patient with instructions about preparing for the colonoscopy. These include taking medication that causes diarrhea and a complete cleaning out of the stool, so that the physician may more easily view the colon during the procedure. The patient fasts before the test, usually eating nothing after midnight, although the instructions may vary depending on the doctor, the scheduled time of the test, and so forth.

It is important that the doctor is aware well before the colonoscopy of any medications the patient takes on a regular basis (including aspirin, blood thinners, DIABETES medications, and vitamins that contain iron). In addition, it is important to inform the doctor about any diagnosed medical conditions that the patient has, including heart or lung disease. Also because the patient will be sedated for the procedure, it is important to make arrangements ahead of time for someone to drive him or her home after the colonoscopy.

In addition to a sedative, the patient may be given pain medication prior to the procedure. The doctor will insert a long, flexible, lighted tube into the rectum and guide it into the colon. The tube has a tiny camera that projects images onto a screen for the doctor to view as he or she examines the colon. Following the procedure the tube is carefully withdrawn.

The colonoscopy is a very valuable diagnostic tool for gastroenterologists. It is also a tool for treatment in some cases, as when polyps are identified in the procedure and they are then removed and biopsied to test for cancer. Finding the polyps early will often reduce the need for major surgery later.

The colonoscopy procedure generally takes 30 to 60 minutes to complete. Sometimes patients remain at the treatment location for one to two hours after the procedure to allow the sedative to wear off.

Risks and Complications

Most individuals find the preparation for the colonoscopy much more discomforting than the actual colonoscopy. There is usually no pain after the colonoscopy has been completed although some people experience mild and temporary gas or cramping.

It is important to notify your doctor if you experience severe abdominal pain, fever, bloody bowel movements, or dizziness or weakness after the procedure. A rare complication of the procedure is a puncture of the bowel or colon.

Outlook and Lifestyle Modifications

Most elderly individuals should have a colonoscopy every several years, depending on the advice of their gastroenterologist. If previous problems were detected in a colonoscopy, such as the presence of precancerous polyps or other digestive disorders, the procedure should be repeated more frequently.

Your physician will tell you if you need to stop taking any medications before or after the colonoscopy. Generally patients are fully recovered 24 hours after the procedure and can resume their normal activities.

See also CANCER.

National Digestive Diseases Information Clearinghouse (NDDIC). "Colonoscopy." Available online. URL: http://digestive.niddk.nih.gov/ddiseases/pubs/colonoscopy/#1. Accessed March 26, 2008.

colorectal cancer   Colorectal cancer is a common form of cancer, and the risk of developing colorectal cancer increases with age. According to the National Cancer Institute, there were an estimated 112,340 cases of colon cancer and 41,420 cases of rectal cancer in 2007. Men and women get colorectal cancer at about the same rate.

Colon cancer forms in the colon (the long part of the large intestine), and rectal cancer forms in the last inches of the large intestine before the anus. There were an estimated 52,180 deaths from both colon and rectal cancer together in 2007.

Symptoms and Diagnostic Path

A change in bowel habits may indicate colorectal cancer. Other symptoms that may be present may include

- a feeling that the bowel does not completely empty
- the presence of blood in the stool (sometimes blood is also found with hemorrhoids, thus blood in the stool does not inevitably indicate cancer)
- frequent gas pains or cramps or a bloated feeling
- unintended weight loss
- constant fatigue
- nausea and vomiting
- a change in routine bowel habits

A digital rectal examination, performed by a physician during a routine physical examination, may reveal abnormalities in the colon or rectum that require further testing. Many people are embarrassed by the digital rectal examination and may even try to avoid it altogether, but this simple test can be a lifesaver for many people.

There are three primary tools to check for the presence of colorectal cancer, including the fecal occult blood test (FOBT), which is a small stool sample that is analyzed for occult blood; the sigmoidoscopy and the COLONOSCOPY are the other two tests. The sigmoidoscopy and the colonoscopy are tools that check the colon from the inside, with the colonoscopy examining the entire colon. Most gastroenterologists, physicians who specialize in treating digestive diseases, prefer the colonoscopy to the sigmoidoscopy, because the colonoscopy is a considerably more comprehensive test. (Some doctors have said that using a sigmoidoscopy to detect cancer rather than a colonoscopy is like taking a mammogram of one breast.)

If any precancerous polyps are identified during the sigmoidoscopy or colonoscopy, the physician will remove them during the procedure and submit them to a pathologist for a biopsy and further analysis.

Other tests that may be performed include a chest X-ray to see if cancer has spread to the lungs, or a computerized tomography (CT) scan to see if cancer has spread to the liver, lungs, or other organs.

Treatment Options and Outlook

As with other forms of cancer, a biopsy of sample tissue is taken when colorectal cancer is suspected (which can be done during a colonoscopy), and the tissue is then examined by a pathologist. The pathologist determines whether cancer if present, and if so, how advanced the cancer is. Treatment for colorectal cancer may include surgery, radiation, or chemotherapy, and the choice of treatment depends on how advanced the tumor is and whether it has spread to other parts of the body.

According to the National Cancer Institute, patients with colorectal cancer should ask their physicians the following questions before treatment begins:

- What is the stage of my disease? Has the cancer spread?

- What are my treatment choices? Which do you suggest for me? Will I have more than one kind of treatment?

- What are the expected benefits of each kind of treatment?

- What are the risks and possible side effects of each treatment? How can the side effects be managed?

- What can I do to prepare for treatment?

- How will treatment affect my normal activities? Am I likely to have urinary problems? What about bowel problems, such as diarrhea or rectal bleeding? Will treatment affect my sex life?

- If I were your parent, what treatment would you recommend for me?

Risk Factors and Preventive Measures

Patients who have had colorectal cancer in the past are at risk for a recurrence. In addition, women with a history of breast cancer or cancer of the ovary or uterus have a slightly increased risk of developing colorectal cancer.

Individuals who now have polyps are at risk for colorectal cancer, as are those who have had polyps in the past. Removing polyps may reduce the risk of cancer.

Individuals age 50 years and older have a greater risk for a diagnosis with colorectal cancer than younger individuals, and according to the National Cancer Institute, the average age at diagnosis of colorectal cancer is 72.

A family history of colorectal cancer in the patient's parents, siblings, or children is another risk factor for colorectal cancer, particularly if the other relative had cancer at a younger age.

A change in some genes increases the risk for colorectal cancer, and if family members have hereditary nonpolyposis colon cancer (NHPCC), the common type of inherited colorectal cancer or familial adenomatous polyposis (FAP), a rare inherited disorder that causes hundreds of polyps to occur in the colon and rectum, then other family members can receive genetic testing to see if genetic changes have occurred in them that will make them at risk for the development of one of these diseases.

Ulcerative colitis (also known as Crohn's disease) is another risk factor for colorectal cancer. SMOKING may increase the risk of colorectal cancer.

See also CANCER.

companions Paid or unpaid individuals who are not family members but who provide care and assistance to those older individuals who need it.

Such individuals may play games with the older person, talk with them about current events, go for walks, and provide a variety of different services. Some aging organizations provide volunteer companions to older individuals. Many elderly individuals report that they look forward to the visits of their companions. Companions can play a vital role in filling the void of a departed loved one, or may even be a contact for out-of-town family members who can check in with the companion on the health and well-being of elderly individuals.

See also ACTIVITIES OF DAILY LIVING.

compassion fatigue Refers to the "burnout" that many professionals and FAMILY CAREGIVERS experience after attending very closely to the comprehensive and sometimes complex needs of others. When compassion fatigue becomes a problem, the person loses empathy and understanding for the ill person. Compassion fatigue may occur because the caregiver has ignored his or her own emotional and physical needs and, as a result, can be suffering from physical and emotional exhaustion.

Some family caregivers delay seeking needed medical treatment for themselves because they worry that it will take time away from an older person needing care. They may not have access to (or may not know about) ADULT DAY CENTERS that could provide respite care. They may also feel an intense sense of obligation to the person they are providing care for and believe that any other options for care should not be considered.

In some cases, the older person that is being cared for really needs the assistance that is provided in a nursing home, but the family caregiver is resistant to placing the relative in a nursing home because they are fearful that the older person will not receive adequate care or because they have promised the elderly person that they would never put him or her in a nursing home.

See also ADULT CHILDREN/CHILDREN OF AGING PARENTS; COGNITIVE IMPAIRMENT.

complementary/alternative medicine (CAM) Treatments and remedies that are outside the realm of mainstream medicine, including the use of dietary supplements, herbal products, homeopathic remedies, as well as procedures or practices such as meditation, acupuncture, and many other treatments or remedies. Complementary/alternative medicine is also known as alternative/complementary medicine.

A key misconception about alternative medicine that is shared by many people of all ages and walks of life is the apparently unfaltering belief that alternative medicines are inherently safe because they are "natural." The reality is that some herbs and supplements can be very dangerous and even fatal for some people.

Some individuals have died as a result of combining herbal remedies or vitamin supplements with their prescription medications. This risk is increased when the patient takes multiple drugs, as is the case for many elderly people. (See POLYPHARMACY; MEDICATION INTERACTIONS.) It is also true that physicians should specifically ask their patients about their use of alternative medicine and explain why this information is needed. Studies have shown that patients often forget or fail to tell their doctors about their use of alternative medicine.

Since alternative medicine such as herbal remedies or vitamin supplements can interact with prescription medications, it is extremely important for patients to report this use to their physicians. For example, coumadin (Warfarin) causes blood thinning, and if patients also take Vitamin E and/or gingko biloba, they could cause excessive blood thinning and even internal bleeding.

According to a survey of 1,559 people age 50 and older that was jointly released by the AARP and the National Center for Complementary and Alternative Medicine in 2007, more than half (54 percent) of survey respondents age 65 and older used a CAM practice or therapy. Most of the respondents (84 percent) age 65 and older reported also taking prescription medications and 25 percent said they took five or more prescriptions.

Information derived from the survey released in 2007 revealed that, of those age 65 and older who had used some form of CAM, 58 percent used the therapy or treatment for their overall wellness. About 38 percent used CAM to supplement the conventional medicine they used. However, few older people (15 percent) had discussed their use of CAM with their physician.

The most common reasons among people of all ages who had not discussed CAM with their doctors were that the doctor had never asked them about their use (42 percent), or they did not know that they should discuss it with their doctor (30 percent), or that there was not enough time during the office visit to discuss this issue (19 percent).

Of those respondents who *did* discuss their use of CAM with their doctors, 67 percent said that they had discussed the effectiveness of a particular CAM therapy with their physicians, and 64 percent said they had discussed what to use. In addition, 60 percent said that they had asked the doctor if CAM could interact with the other treatments or medications they received, and the same percentage had asked the doctor whether they should pursue a particular CAM therapy.

See also ANTIOXIDANTS; MEDICATION COMPLIANCE; PRESCRIPTION DRUG ABUSE; VITAMIN AND MINERAL DEFICIENCIES/EXCESSES.

AARP and the National Center for Complementary and Alternative Medicine. *Complementary and Alternative Medicine: What People 50 and Older Are Using and Discussing with Their Physicians.* Washington, D.C.: AARP, 2007. Available online. URL: http://www.aarp.org/research/health/prevention/cam_2007.html. Downloaded January 18, 2007.

conflicts, with adult children/physicians/others
Disagreements may arise when an elderly person's medical, financial, relocation, or other important decisions that need to be made conflict with what his or her adult children may believe is best for the older person. In addition, in some cases, older people may also act directly against the wishes of their physicians, attorneys, or other professionals who provide advice.

ADULT CHILDREN/CHILDREN OF AGING PARENTS and others may assume that because the elderly person refuses to follow the advice of others, this refusal means that the older person is mentally incompetent. However, although they may be correct in this assumption, the designation of mental incompetence can only be made in a court by a judge, based on testimony from physicians, mental health professionals, and others.

Some potential areas of conflict may include the choice for or against medical treatments and medications, choices about what items to spend money on, and even vacation choices. For example, the aging parent may choose to go on a vacation abroad when the adult child believes such a trip would be risky because of the parent's health. Sometimes older parents decide to remarry, to the consternation of their adult children. There are many potential areas of disagreement.

Sometimes other family members, such as siblings or even aunts, uncles, and cousins, may have their own opinions about what is best for the aging parent, and the dispute may become very heated. Assuming that the elderly parent is mentally competent, often it is best to let him or her make their own choices, even when they are not the choices the adult child or others approve of.

See also BABY BOOMERS; COGNITIVE IMPAIRMENT; COMPASSION FATIGUE; END-OF-LIFE ISSUES; LEARNED HELPLESSNESS; MARRIAGE/REMARRIAGE; SIBLING RIVALRY AND CONFLICT; TALKING TO ELDERLY PARENTS ABOUT DIFFICULT ISSUES.

confusion The uncertainty or the inability to understand what is going on or to analyze information that could be perceived by the average person or by the individual at previous points in time. Confusion is a common symptom of ALZHEIMER'S DISEASE as well as of many other forms of DEMENTIA.

Confusion may also result as a side effect of some medications, especially NARCOTICS such as morphine. Alternatively, confusion may result from some MEDICATION INTERACTIONS. In addition, some illnesses may lead to mental confusion, and if they are not diagnosed, their symptoms and signs may lead to a mistaken diagnosis of dementia, such as when a person has severe vitamin deficiencies or has some types of endocrine disorders, such as hypothyroidism.

The confusion of an older person with a cognitive impairment is one of the most difficult aspects of aging for family members to accept. Fear, ANXIETY, DEPRESSION, and rage may also accompany the older person's confusion. Alternatively, depression may present as confusion, making the diagnosis even more difficult.

See also AGGRESSION, PHYSICAL; COGNITIVE IMPAIRMENT; DELUSIONS; HALLUCINATIONS; IRRITABILITY; MEMORY IMPAIRMENT; RAGE; VITAMIN AND MINERAL DEFICIENCIES/EXCESSES.

congregate living   A form of senior housing that may provide housekeeping services as well as one or two meals per day but does not offer other services, such as transportation to physicians' appointments or supermarkets, medication oversight, and so forth. Each state has its own laws and terminology regarding senior housing, so the state office for elder care services should be consulted to determine the individual state laws and definitions of terminology. (See Appendix II.)

See also ASSISTED-LIVING FACILITY; CONTINUING CARE RETIREMENT CENTERS; HOUSING/LIVING ARRANGEMENTS; NURSING HOMES.

constipation   Difficulty and infrequency in having a bowel movement. Constipation is a common problem among many older people, although some experts say that too many older people worry excessively about having a bowel movement every day. Some people have a bowel movement twice a week, and others have one three or four times a week. In one study, researchers found that nursing home patients with DEMENTIA who were constipated were significantly more physically aggressive than other patients. This finding indicates that treating the constipation could help restore harmony. (See AGGRESSION, PHYSICAL.)

According to the National Institute on Aging, doctors often ask individuals who may be constipated the following questions:

- Do you often have a feeling of being blocked or not having fully emptied your bowel when you have a bowel movement?
- Are your stools often hard and lumpy?
- Do you often have a difficult time passing stools?

- Do you often have fewer than three bowel movements per week?

If the answer to one or more of these questions is "yes," then the individual may have a problem with constipation.

Constipation may be caused by insufficient exercise, lack of eating enough foods rich in fiber, such as vegetables, eating an overall poor diet, or relying on laxatives too often. Some foods, such as sweets or high-fat meats, can cause constipation. Another cause is the failure to drink enough water or other fluids.

Some medical problems can lead to constipation, such as DIABETES, STROKE, or irritable bowel syndrome.

Some medications can cause constipation, such as some antidepressants or antacids that have aluminum or calcium in them. In addition, antihistamines can cause constipation, as well as some drugs for HYPERTENSION or for PARKINSON'S DISEASE.

Treatments for constipation (if the doctor has ruled out a more serious illness), include

- eating more fresh fruits and vegetables and more whole grain breads and cereals
- adding small amounts of unprocessed bran ("miller's bran") to cereals, fruits, and baked goods
- drinking more fluids
- increasing the level of physical activity

See also EXERCISE; NUTRITION.

continuing care retirement centers   A retirement community that offers a broad range of housing based on the developing needs of elderly residents, from INDEPENDENT LIVING to assisted living to nursing home care, all in the same general "campus" arrangement. As a result, as the older individual's health declines, he or she can remain in the community but will begin to receive care that is commensurate with his or her increased needs.

Residents usually pay a large entry fee before they move into a continuing care retirement center, and they will also pay monthly fees that cover rent and services. State laws vary on how continuing care retirement centers are managed. Most people who live in such an arrangement are affluent.

See also ASSISTED-LIVING FACILITY; CONGREGATE LIVING; HOUSING/LIVING ARRANGEMENTS; NURSING HOMES.

coronary heart disease   See HEART ATTACK; HEART DISEASE.

cremation   The disposal of deceased human remains by burning the body at extremely high temperatures in a special oven so that only shards of the body are left. These human remains weigh from three to nine pounds, depending on the body weight of the deceased. (The remains, often called cremains, are also frequently referred to as ashes by the general public, but they do not actually physically resemble ashes.) Any pacemakers or similar electronic devices that remain in the deceased must be removed before the cremation process, because pacemakers can explode under extreme heat.

Cremation is increasingly popular in the United States as an option for the disposal of the remains of loved ones. It is significantly less costly than the fees for a funeral, such as the funeral fees for the embalming of the remains, the viewing of the body, the costs of the casket and the tombstone, and the multiple other fees that are usually charged by the funeral home.

Other reasons why individuals may choose cremation rather than burial in a cemetery is because cremation saves land, it may be considered a simpler process, and because it does not involve placing the body under the ground. (Some individuals have a fear or even a horror of an underground burial, which they may project onto others, such as deceased loved ones.)

In his article on cremation for *Generations*, Michael C. Kearl says that another reason for the growing appeal of cremation is a declining sense of connections with both ancestry and the place where one is from: "For a number of reasons, Americans' ties to place are dissolving as is their sense of connectedness to familial generations past.

Geographic mobility and continuously changing social landscapes have made quaint the idea of a cemetery plot populated with eight or nine generations of family members."

Another reason for the current increased popularity of cremation is that some religions have relaxed their past objections to cremation. In the past, some religious groups believed that a body had to be available in order for an afterlife to occur. Many mainstream religions no longer believe this to be true.

Some individuals bury the cremated remains of the deceased person while others keep the remains in an urn in a special place in their homes. Some cemeteries offer niches or special shelves where funeral urns are kept.

Who Chooses Cremation?

According to the Cremation Association of North America, a trade association for crematoriums in the United States and Canada, most individuals who were cremated in 2005 were white and Protestant, and the median age at the time of their deaths was 74. In considering the number of cremations as a percentage of all deaths in 2005, Hawaii ranked highest with 66.3 percent of deaths that were cremated, followed by Nevada (65 percent) and Washington (64 percent). In contrast, the states with the lowest percentage of deaths that were cremated in 2005 were Alabama (9.4 percent), followed by Mississippi (9.9 percent) and Tennessee (10.5 percent).

The Cremation Association of North America has reported that there were 1,971 crematories in operation in 2005 and 784,962 cremations occurred in the United States that year (an estimated one-third of all deaths in 2005). The Cremation Association of North America projects that by 2010, 39 percent of all deaths in the United States will be cremated, and by 2025, that figure will increase further to a majority of 57 percent.

Cremation is even more popular in CANADA, where the Cremation Association of North America reported that 56 percent of all deaths were cremated in 2004, the latest figures available as of this writing.

See also BEREAVEMENT; CEMETERY, CHOICE OF; DEATH; DEATH, FEAR OF; END-OF-LIFE ISSUES; FUNERALS.

Cassell, Dana K., Robert C. Salinas, M.D., and Peter A. S. Winn, M.D. *The Encyclopedia of Death and Dying.* New York: Facts On File, 2005.

Cremation Association of North America. *Final 2005 Statistics and Projections to the Year 2025, 2006 Preliminary Data.* Chicago, Ill.: Cremation Association of North America, September 4, 2007. Available online. URL: http://www.cremationsassociation.org/docs/CANA-Final06Prelim.pdf. Accessed September 7, 2007.

Kearl, Michael C. "Cremation: Desecration, Purification, or Convenience?" *Generations* 27, no. 11 (Summer 2004): 15–20.

Creutzfeldt-Jakob disease (CJD)   A very rare and fatal brain disorder, Creutzfeldt-Jakob disease usually has its onset at about age 60. According to the Centers for Disease Control and Prevention (CDC), "classic" CJD has been known to exist since the early 1920s. The CDC says that the median age at death for the person with CJD is 68 years.

There are three primary types of CJD, according to the National Institutes of Health, including sporadic CJD, which develops for no known reason and represents at least 85 percent of all cases. A second form, hereditary CJD, is caused by a genetic link, and five to 10 percent of all cases of CJD are inherited. A third form, acquired CJD, occurs after contact with infected tissue, often during a medical procedure. This form represents only about one percent of all cases of CJD.

CJD occurs in about one person for every million people worldwide, according to the National Institute of Neurological Disorders and Stroke. About 300 cases of CJD are identified each year in the United States.

Symptoms and Diagnostic Path

Initially CJD sufferers experience memory problems, behavioral changes, failing visual disturbances up to and including blindness, and decreased coordination. These symptoms escalate to dementia, coma, and then death. Patients with CJD also have personality changes and may have DEPRESSION and INSOMNIA. The mental and physical deterioration of CJD is more rapid than with other forms of dementia, such as Alzheimer's disease.

There are no diagnostic tests for CJD. Instead, doctors rule out treatable forms of dementia such as chronic meningitis or encephalitis (inflammation of the brain). A spinal tap may be used to rule out more common forms of dementia, and an electroencephalogram (EEG) may be used to record the brain pattern because there is a characteristically distinct brain wave pattern among those with CJD. A brain biopsy could definitely diagnose CJD, but it is very dangerous and thus generally contraindicated for patients.

Treatment Options and Outlook

There is no treatment for CJD; however, the symptoms can be treated; for example, narcotics can relieve pain if it occurs. Drugs such as clonazepam (Klonopin) can help alleviate muscle jerking. When the patient becomes confined to bed, it is important to change his or position frequently to help prevent BEDSORES. Many people with CJD die within a year.

Risk Factors and Preventive Measures

Because CJD is so rare, the risk of contracting this disease is very low.

Health workers and others who live or work with a person with CJD should take the following precautions:

- Wash hands before eating or drinking.
- Cover any cuts and abrasions with waterproof dressings.
- Wear surgical gloves when handling the patient's tissues or fluids or dressing the patient's wounds.
- Avoid cutting or sticking oneself with instruments contaminated by the patient's blood.
- Use face protection if there is a risk of splashed contaminated material such as blood or cerebrospinal fluid.
- Soak medical instruments that came into contact with the patient in undiluted chlorine bleach for at least an hour, then use a pressure cooker (autoclave) to sterilize them in distilled water for at least an hour at 132°–134°C.

See also DEMENTIA.

National Institute of Neurological Disorders and Stroke. "Creutzfeldt-Jakob Disease Fact Sheet." Available online. URL: http://www.ninds.nih.gov/disorders/djd/detail_djd.htm?css=print. Accessed April 4, 2008.

crimes against the elderly Includes violent and nonviolent crimes perpetrated against older individuals. Violent crimes against older individuals include such acts as murder or assault, as well as acts of physical and sexual ABUSE, including rape. Examples of nonviolent crimes include fraud, property theft, identity theft, and embezzlement, among the many different types of nonviolent crimes that are perpetrated against older individuals. For example, a common tactic is to tell the older person that he or she has won a prize, and then manipulate the person into buying products or providing personal information, such as their Social Security number or bank account numbers.

Home repair scams are also common, in which individuals go throughout neighborhoods offering to fix roofs or make other repairs and requiring a deposit. The work is either never done or it is very shoddy. According to the American Bar Association in *The American Bar Association Legal Guide for Americans Over 50,* some signs to watch out for are if the worker demands cash and refuses to take a check for payment or if workers are driving a truck with license tags from another state. If the worker pressures the older person for an immediate decision, this is another warning sign. (For a listing of state consumer protection offices, see Appendix XIII.)

Some older people may be more vulnerable to criminals than others because they may be more trusting, particularly in the case of a person who is a recent widow or widower. As a result, if someone calls them and says they are from the bank and need to know their bank account number, credit card number, Social Security number, or other confidential information, the older person may provide this information without challenging the caller. Then the criminal can steal money from the individual's bank account, charge items on his or her credit card, and even steal the older person's identity.

Common frauds against the elderly include the following types of scams (although there are many more than these few examples):

- The older person is sent a fictitious bill for items that he or she never received. Many older people believe that they must pay every bill they receive. They may also think that they *did* purchase the item for which they are being billed but simply forgot about it.

- The older person may be a victim of a "work-at-home" plan that offers extremely large profits if the person purchases a special kit. Few people make any money from using these kits.

- Young attractive people who are overtly friendly travel from door-to-door selling magazines to people in their homes. Often these young people do not represent publishers at all and fail to deliver any magazines after payment is made.

- Older people are sometimes offered sweepstakes prizes that are completely bogus.

- Older people are often encouraged to purchase insurance that he or she does not need, such as mechanical repair insurance on a car that is already under warranty with a dealer.

According to the National Institute on Aging, older individuals should take the following steps to be safer in their homes:

- Make sure that all locks, doors, and windows cannot be broken into easily and consider installing a good alarm system.

- Keep the doors and windows locked when you are at home and make sure they are locked before you leave your home.

- Check through the peephole before opening the door and always insist that all strangers show identification. Remember that you do not have to open your door if you feel uncomfortable.

- Ask the local police about marking valuables with an identification number so they are more easily recognized if they are stolen.

- Do not keep large amounts of cash in your home.

- Join a neighborhood watch program if one is available, and try to get to know your neighbors.

- Make a list of valuable items in your home and consider taking photographs of them. Keep the list and photographs in a safe place.

Suggestions from the National Institute on Aging to stay safe in public in one's car include the following:

- Avoid dark parking lots or alleys and always park in well-lit areas.
- Keep car doors locked at all times.
- Avoid rolling down the car window for strangers.
- Do not fight back if confronted by a robber; just hand over your cash or jewelry immediately without an argument.

Suggestions for financial safety for elderly individuals include the following:

- Have monthly pension checks sent by direct deposit to the bank rather than mailed to your home.
- Avoid carrying large amounts of cash.
- Avoid keeping credit cards and checkbook together.
- Check your monthly bank statement carefully.
- If you shop online, verify that the Web site has a "secure server" before entering your credit card information.

See also NEGLECT.

American Bar Association. *The American Bar Association Legal Guide for Americans Over 50.* New York: Random House Reference, 2006.

National Institute. "Staying Safe and Planning Ahead—Crime and Older People." Available online. URL: http://www.niapublications.org/pubs/PDFs/E_Section4-Staying%20Safe%20and%20Planning%20Ahead.pdf. Accessed April 3, 2008.

deafness Partial or total inability to hear. Many older people have hearing impairments but most have some hearing or can hear with the use of hearing aids. The deafness may have been caused by illnesses or by a deterioration of part of the ear. Some level of deafness is increasingly likely as a person ages. For example, according to the National Institute on Deafness and Other Communication Disorders, about a third of individuals older than 65 have some hearing loss and half of those ages 75 and older have a hearing loss.

Symptoms and Diagnostic Path

The individual with hearing loss may have trouble hearing high-pitched sounds, such as the voices of women and children. If he or she is completely deaf, they will hear nothing at all. A hearing assessment by an otolaryngologist (ear/nose/throat doctor) can verify if there is a partial or complete hearing loss.

Treatment Options and Outlook

If hearing loss is partial, then hearing aids are often helpful. If hearing loss is total, surgery such as a cochlear implant may help the individual regain hearing. A cochlear implant allows individuals who are deaf to understand speech and may allow them to use the telephone. A cochlear implant is a tiny electronic device that is surgically inserted under the skin behind the ear. It receives sounds that it transforms into electrical signals that are sent past the nonworking ear and into the brain.

It can be very difficult for a person who has had hearing all his or her life to become deaf, and as a result, the individual may develop depression and/ or anxiety, which should be treated.

Risk Factors and Preventive Measures

As mentioned, aging is a risk factor for hearing loss and deafness. In general, men have a greater risk for hearing loss than women. In addition, some medications, particularly some antibiotics, are "ototoxic," which means that they may be damaging to the ear and can impair hearing.

Ear infections may cause hearing loss and deafness, especially if they are untreated. Some ear diseases that cause deafness may be genetically linked.

See also HEARING DISORDERS; HEARING LOSS.

death Cessation of life and of all vital functions, including total and irreversible cessation of all cerebral functions, as well as cessation of the respiratory and circulatory systems and irreversible cessation of any perceptible heartbeat. According to *The Encyclopedia of Death and Dying,* indicators of death also include all cessation of the heart, any reflexes, and any electrical activity in the brain, as well as manifestation of rigor mortis (a stiffening of the body that occurs after death).

According to Cassell, Salinas, and Winn in *The Encyclopedia of Death and Dying,*

> In the past, it was customary to attribute non-accidental death to "natural causes," which were thought to bring about a termination of life as if by unavoidable destiny and with no particular cause specified. Since the early 1900s, however, death has no longer been thought to happen unavoidably without specific cause. Today, physicians who fill out death certificates usually must enter a specific disease or condition that caused the death.

Elderly people may die from many different diseases and disorders, particularly HEART DISEASE (the number-one killer in the United States) and CANCER (the number-two killer). They may also die from injuries that were incurred as a result of FALLS or other traumas.

According to the Census Bureau, of the 1.8 million deaths in people age 65 and older in 2000, the largest percentage (33 percent) were deaths that were caused by heart disease, followed by 22 percent of deaths caused by cancer and 8 percent caused by STROKE. Other common causes of death were chronic lower respiratory diseases, FLU/INFLUENZA and PNEUMONIA, ALZHEIMER'S DISEASE, DIABETES, and KIDNEY DISEASE. (See Table 1.)

Preparing for Death

Death can be extremely hard for those who survive, and it is often extremely difficult for an elderly person to cope with the loss of a spouse or other loved one. Sometimes the older person's normal BEREAVEMENT may markedly worsen into a clinical DEPRESSION that requires medical treatment with ANTIDEPRESSANTS and psychotherapy.

Common fears represent another issue; older individuals may fear that they have not accomplished important goals or taken care of loved ones adequately. To avert this fear, it is best for older individuals to prepare important legal documents ahead of time and when they are relatively healthy. For example, many older people die without having created a will, believing that only millionaires need to create a will or assuming that they can simply add their child's name to a bank account and he or she can withdraw the money.

Both assumptions are unrealistic. If the older person owns a house and/or a car, even if there are no other assets, it is best to create a will for how the assets should be managed. It is also best to investigate other options, such as a LIVING TRUST, in which the individual's assets pass to the designated child or children. (State laws on such matters vary greatly.)

It is a good idea, too, for the older person to create a LIVING WILL, which states the lifesaving means (if any) the older person wishes to be performed in the event of severe injury or illness. It is very difficult for adult children to know what their parent would want in such a situation, and they may become laden with guilt if they try to guess at the parent's wishes. They may also choose to prolong the parent's life when he or she is in severe pain, not knowing if this choice was what the parent would have wanted.

TALKING TO ELDERLY PARENTS ABOUT DIFFICULT ISSUES is not easy or pleasant, but it can alleviate the strain on an older person who is terminally ill and who may be worried about such issues. The older person may also have specific wishes with regards to whether he or she would be interested in HOSPICE care in the event of a terminal illness. In addition, he or she may have definite wishes regarding a FUNERAL and where he or she wishes to be buried or whether he or she would wish for cremation to occur after death.

See also ABUSE; ADVERSE DRUG EVENT; ASSISTED SUICIDE; CEMETERY, CHOICE OF; CREMATION; DEATH, FEAR OF; END-OF-LIFE ISSUES; NEGLECT; SUICIDE; WILLS.

TABLE 1. THE TOP 10 CAUSES OF DEATH FOR PEOPLE AGE 65 AND OLDER: 2000

Cause of Death	Number	Percentage
All causes	1,799,825	100.0
Heart disease	593,707	33.0
Malignant neoplasms (cancer)	392,366	21.8
Cerebrovascular (stroke)	148,045	8.2
Chronic lower respiratory disease	106,375	5.9
Pneumonia/influenza	58,557	3.3
Diabetes	52,414	2.9
Alzheimer's disease	48,993	2.7
Nephritis, nephrotic symptoms, and nephrosis	31,225	1.7
Accidents and adverse effects	31,051	1.7
Septicemia	24,786	1.4
All other causes of death	1,487,519	17.4

Source: He, Wan, Manisha Sengupta, Victoria A. Velkoff, and Kimberly A. DeBarros, *65+ in the United States: 2005*. Washington, D.C.: U.S. Census Bureau, December 2005, p. 42.

Cassell, Dana K., Robert C. Salinas, M.D., and Peter A. S. Winn, M.D. *The Encyclopedia of Death and Dying.* New York: Facts On File, 2005.

He, Wan, Manisha Sengupta, Victoria A. Velkoff, and Kimberly A. DeBarros. *65+ in the United States: 2005.* Washington, D.C.: U.S. Census Bureau, December 2005.

death, fear of Older people may be fearful of death, especially of a painful and/or a lingering death. In some cases, the fear of death leads to constructive actions. For example, some people create a LIVING WILL, a document that stipulates the medical lifesaving measures that they wish to have taken or not taken in the event that they are incapacitated or unconscious and cannot respond to questions about their treatment.

Some individuals may stipulate that they do not wish to be kept on life support if it is believed that they will have no chance of recovery. They may also stipulate that they do not wish for a breathing tube to be inserted if they have little or no chance of recovering from an illness. There are many different provisions that may be included in the living will, and they may ease the fears of the older person who feels that with the document, his or her wishes will be respected and followed.

Older individuals may also fail to make a living will and, consequently, their adult children or others, such as physicians, will have to make decisions about whether medical care should be continued if the adult becomes seriously ill and unconscious, taking into account what they believe the older person would have wanted and also affected by their own values and beliefs.

The fear of death may also lead to inaction and denial on the part of the older person, and it is one key reason why many older people refuse to take any financial and legal steps to ensure that their adult children and other heirs will not be burdened with difficult decisions at a very hard time (upon the severe illness or the death of their parent), such as how finances should be managed should their parents become incapable of managing them or how to help an aging parent afford to move into an ASSISTED-LIVING FACILITY or a NURSING HOME.

See also CEMETERY, CHOICE OF; CREMATION; DEATH; END-OF-LIFE ISSUES; FUNERAL; TALKING TO ELDERLY PARENTS ABOUT DIFFICULT ISSUES.

Cassell, Dana K., Robert C. Salinas, M.D., and Peter A. S. Winn, M.D. *The Encyclopedia of Death and Dying.* New York: Facts On File, 2005.

"death tax" Refers to the estate tax charged by federal and state governments in the United States upon the death of an individual whose estate exceeded a limit that was decreed by the state or federal government.

Some individuals believe that estate taxes are unfair because they are high and because they diminish the amount that the person can leave to family members. Others believe that the tax burden falls primarily on wealthy people, whose families can afford such a tax, and they also argue that these tax revenues are needed by society. It is clear that the vast majority of money from death tax comes from the wealthiest 2 percent of individuals.

Whether there is a lack of equity in this matter is and will continue to be a hotly discussed topic among those with the most to lose: owners of small and large family businesses, small-farm owners, entrepreneurs, and big-business owners. This is a political issue that will continue to be debated as the population ages.

See also ESTATE PLANNING.

decision making, difficulty with Making choices can be hard for some older people, particularly in the case of those whose spouse or partner has recently died, and thus they are in the midst of BEREAVEMENT. Even simple choices such as what to eat for dinner (or actually remembering to eat dinner) may seem to be overwhelming in the face of the loss of a spouse. In some cases, the spouse made most of the life choices for the bereaved person for many years, and it can be difficult for the person still living to learn to make decisions for himself or herself.

The confusion and the distress surrounding bereavement should not be confused with the chronic decision-making difficulty of the older person who has ALZHEIMER'S DISEASE or another form of DEMENTIA. In addition, major choices may also be hard to make for elderly individuals who suffer from chronic and undertreated pain stemming from a variety of diseases, such as BACK PAIN, CANCER, DIABETES, and so forth, primarily because they are so distracted by the pain.

Decision making can also be difficult for adult children if their parents have not made financial and legal decisions about their estates, where they wish to be buried, and so forth, and the children have to guess at what their parents would have wanted when they become ill or die. They may have difficulty finding the parents' wills and other legal documents that are needed by attorneys and the court system.

See also ADULT CHILDREN/CHILDREN OF AGING PARENTS; COGNITIVE IMPAIRMENT; CONFUSION; END-OF-LIFE ISSUES; MEMORY IMPAIRMENT; SIBLING RIVALRY AND CONFLICT; TALKING TO ELDERLY PARENTS ABOUT DIFFICULT ISSUES.

decubitus ulcers See BEDSORES; HOSPITALIZATION; NURSING HOMES.

delusions False beliefs, such as the belief that one is being persecuted when there is no evidence of such persecution. Delusions may be caused temporarily by medications that older people take (particularly NARCOTICS, such as morphine) or they may be a part of the overall symptomology of DEMENTIA or ALZHEIMER'S DISEASE. An example of a delusion is believing that the sky is purple rather than blue.

It can be frustrating dealing with a person who is delusional, but it may help to understand that the person truly believes the delusion is real. One means to cope with delusional behavior is for another individual to try to inculcate doubt; for example, if a person believes that Martians are landing in the backyard, the other individual can say that he or she sees nothing out of the ordinary.

See also AGGRESSION, PHYSICAL; COGNITIVE IMPAIRMENT; CONFUSION; HALLUCINATIONS; IRRITABILITY; MEMORY IMPAIRMENT; RAGE.

dementia A group of symptoms that is characterized by CONFUSION, memory loss, language difficulties, and, in many cases, eventually psychosis. Dementia is not a specific disease. Personality changes may also occur, and the formerly kindly man or woman may become aggressive and combative with dementia. HALLUCINATIONS (seeing or hearing things that are not there) and DELUSIONS (false beliefs, such as the delusion of persecution by others) may be present. These changes can be

frightening for the elderly person's family members, and an accurate medical diagnosis is important so that treatment can begin and plans for long-term care of the individual can be considered. Although some memory loss is common with aging, *serious* memory loss is not a normal function of aging.

The most common form of irreversible dementia is ALZHEIMER'S DISEASE, followed by vascular dementia (See BINSWANGER'S DISEASE). There are also some forms of reversible dementias, but the majority of dementias cannot be reversed as of this writing.

The risk for the development of dementia increases with age, although dementia is less common than often assumed by the general public. According to the Centers for Disease Control and Prevention (CDC), the risk of dementia is about 6 to 10 percent among individuals age 65 and older. However, in considering significantly older people, the prevalence of dementia increases to 30 percent or greater for those age 85 and older. Some studies have shown that dementia peaks at about 60 percent for those individuals age 94 and older. The National Institute of Neurological Disorders and Stroke estimates that about 6.8 million people in the United States had some form of dementia in 2008.

In general, the rates of dementia are higher for institutionalized adults than those who are not living in institutions, and some studies have shown that about half of all nursing home residents have dementia. This circumstance is likely because family members cannot deal with the symptoms of dementia and, as a result, they place the older person in an institution.

Most forms of dementia have a poor outcome; however, some activities, such as doing puzzles, reading, playing word games, and playing a musical instrument, have been associated with a decreased risk for cognitive impairment. In some studies, walking is associated with mental improvement among those with dementia.

Some dementias are reversible, such as those caused by vitamin deficiencies, thyroid disease, and hydrocephalus. However, according to the CDC only about 9 percent of all cases of dementia are reversible.

In addition to Alzheimer's disease, other causes of irreversible dementia include PICK'S DISEASE,

Binswanger's disease, DEMENTIA WITH LEWY BODIES (DLB), HUNTINGTON'S DISEASE, CREUTZFELDT-JAKOB DISEASE, MULTI-INFARCT DEMENTIA (MID), AMYO-TROPHIC LATERAL SCLEROSIS (Lou Gehrig's disease), and the dementia that is caused by late PARKIN-SON'S DISEASE.

Only a physician can determine which form of dementia is most likely present in a patient. Dementia is usually treated by a neurologist, a physician who specializes in diagnosing and treating brain diseases, or by a psychiatrist, a physician who specializes in treating maladaptive behavior.

When symptoms such as confusion, memory loss, and significant behavioral changes are present, an accurate diagnosis of the cause of the dementia begins with a thorough medical and neurological exam. Because the elderly individual is exhibiting signs of memory loss, it is important that someone accompany him or her to the medical exam to answer questions and provide details about the person's behavior.

The physician will want to know about when the symptoms such as memory loss and/or behavioral changes began, as well as the order in which they began. He or she will also ask how these changes are affecting the elderly individual's ability to function on a daily basis. The rate at which these changes have progressed is also quite important.

The physician will also need information regarding the elderly person's medical history as well as any medication the person takes. The medical history may help the physician recognize conditions that lead to a higher risk for a certain kind of dementia. In addition, providing an accurate list of the person's medications may allow the physician to identify medications that might be contributing to the elderly person's confusion or memory loss.

A neurological examination may also be necessary to accurately diagnose the cause of dementia. This exam tests the person's vision, reflexes, movement, and speech. In addition, the physician may request laboratory tests to check for vitamin deficiencies or infection that may be causing the person's confusion.

If necessary the physician may request brain-imaging tests such as a computerized tomography (CT) scan or magnetic resonance imaging (MRI) scan to look for changes in certain parts of the brain, or to find evidence of a stroke or brain tumor. Finally, the physician may request mental status testing to evaluate the person's memory, language, and judgment. These mental status tests are written tests and are sometimes also called cognitive tests or neuropsychological tests.

After the physician has analyzed the results of all of these tests and examinations, he or she may recommend observing the elderly individual for a period of time before confirming a diagnosis.

As the dementia progresses and the individual's symptoms worsen, an accurate diagnosis often becomes increasingly obvious, particularly if the individual has one of the more common forms of dementia, such as Alzheimer's disease or vascular dementia (Binswanger's disease).

As mentioned earlier, dementia itself is not a disease; it is caused by other disorders and/or conditions, and treatment, life-care decisions, and prognosis vary depending on the diagnosis.

Alzheimer's disease (AD) is the most common cause of dementia and is characterized by progressive deterioration of brain function. Alzheimer's generally manifests after age 60, and patients generally live eight to 10 years after a confirmed diagnosis. Alzheimer's can be particularly heartbreaking for both patients and family members because of their awareness that the patient's symptoms will eventually worsen to the point when he or she will no longer recognize family members.

Symptoms of Alzheimer's in the early stages (mild AD) include temporary disorientation, forgetfulness, mood swings, and personality changes (including depression and anxiety). These symptoms worsen as the disease progresses, and in the middle stage (moderate AD), patients often exhibit aggressive behavior as well as an inability to perform simple, everyday tasks such as bathing. In the final stages of Alzheimer's (severe AD), patients exhibit unprovoked rage, incontinence, difficulty speaking (aphasia), slowed speech, and extreme paranoia. Treatment for Alzheimer's includes medications that may slow the progression of the disease, but there is no known cure.

Pick's disease (also known as frontotemporal dementia) is a possible cause of dementia. It is caused by shrinking of parts of the brain and generally presents before age 75. Patients with

Pick's disease generally exhibit extreme (and often very inappropriate) behavioral changes as well as significant difficulty with language. Although there is no cure for Pick's disease, behavior modification and medication can sometimes control the person's undesirable behavior. Pick's disease progresses over a two- to 10-year time span and the person will require 24-hour supervision in the advanced stage.

Binswanger's disease (also known as vascular dementia) is caused by damage to the deep layers of the brain and is another possible cause of dementia. Binswanger's disease can present as early as age 40 and gets progressively worse over time. The principal symptom of Binswanger's disease is slowness of action, often accompanied by an unsteady gait, which can result in injuries from falls. Brain-imaging scans will reveal the lesions in the brain to confirm the diagnosis. Treatment for Binswanger's disease is confined to controlling the accompanying depression and anxiety; there is no cure for the disease itself. Individuals with hypertension and/or diabetes have an increased risk of Binswanger's disease.

Dementia with Lewy Bodies (DLB) represents 15 to 20 percent of all cases of dementia and is caused by excessive deposits of a protein, sometimes referred to as Lewy bodies, within the brain cells. Symptoms of DLB include excessive daytime drowsiness and other sleep disorders, confusion, hallucinations, and unusual movement. There is no cure for DLB, and the disease progresses over about eight years.

Amyotrophic Lateral Sclerosis (ALS), also known as Lou Gehrig's disease, is a progressive disease of the spinal cord and parts of the brain that control movement. Eventually patients with ALS have extreme difficulty walking, eating, speaking, and even breathing. Early symptoms of ALS may include cramping and weak muscles, slurred speech, and difficulty with chewing and swallowing. There is no cure for ALS, and patients generally die from respiratory failure.

Huntington's disease is a hereditary disease caused by the degeneration of nerve cells in the brain and generally begins around age 30 to 40. Symptoms of Huntington's disease include dementia, uncontrolled movements, and unusual facial expressions. In addi-

tion, individuals with Huntington's disease may be irritable and paranoid. Eventually they exhibit memory loss and personality changes. There is no treatment for Huntington's disease, but medications can help control symptoms. Individuals generally die within 20 years of diagnosis and, as a result, few elderly people have Huntington's disease.

Creutzfeldt-Jakob disease (CJD) is a rare, degenerative brain disease characterized by extreme confusion, extreme (and often inappropriate) behaviors, memory loss, vision problems, and decreased coordination. The classic forms of CJD are not related to mad cow disease (bovine spongiform encephalitis), and there is no known cause. There are no diagnostic tests for CJD, and patients usually die within a year.

Multi-infarct Dementia (MID) is caused by damaged brain tissue resulting from multiple strokes and is the third most likely cause of dementia in the elderly. Individuals are sometimes not even aware they have suffered these "silent" strokes. Strokes often are the result of hypertension, diabetes, high cholesterol, or heart disease. Symptoms of MID include extreme disorientation, short-term memory loss, and inappropriate laughing or crying. Treatment for MID is focused on preventing further strokes, and the prognosis for patients with MID is poor.

Parkinson's disease is a degenerative disease of the nervous system, the most common symptom of which is severe tremor and slowed movements. Parkinson's disease is sometimes a cause of dementia.

Patients with dementia may face other problems; for example, sometimes they are not given needed pain medication. According to Cotter in her 2007 article for the *American Journal of Managed Care*, patients with dementia who are in long-term care are less likely to receive pain medicine than other patients. Says Cotter,

> Patients with dementia are at particular risk for suboptimal pain management and are less likely to receive pain medication when prescribed on an as-needed basis, compared with other LTC [long-term care] patients. Yet, pain management in dementia is crucial not only because it improves quality of life, but [also] because unmanaged pain often gives rise to behavioral disturbances and inappropriate psychotropic use [psychiatric drugs].

Cotter says that patients with dementia are also more likely than others to suffer from malnutrition or dehydration because they have a diminished sense of taste and smell. In addition, they may not recognize their own symptoms of hunger and thirst, and they often need help with eating. Also, their medications may decrease their appetite or cause nausea. Caregivers need to consider these issues, and family members should not assume that if Mom or Dad is not eating, it is all right because he or she is simply not hungry.

Cotter, Valerie T. "The Burden of Dementia." *The American Journal of Managed Care* 13, no. 8 (2007): S193–S197.
National Institute of Neurological Disorders and Stroke. "Dementia: Hope through Research." Available online. URL: http://www.ninds.nih.gov/disorders/dementias/detail_dementia.htm. Downloaded March 28, 2008.

dementia with Lewy Bodies (DLB) Dementia with Lewy Bodies (DLB) is caused by excessive deposits of alpha-synuclein, a protein that forms inside the brain cells. These deposits are also sometimes referred to as *Lewy bodies.* Lewy bodies are also found in patients with Parkinson's disease and in some patients with Alzheimer's disease. According to the Centers for Disease Control and Prevention (CDC), DLB represents about 15 to 20 percent of all cases of dementia.

Symptoms and Diagnostic Path

Individuals with DLB exhibit confusion, daytime drowsiness (sleeping for two or more hours during the day), movement symptoms (such as shakiness, foot shuffling, and staring off into space), and visual HALLUCINATIONS. In about half the cases, individuals with DLB also have abnormal sleep patterns, such as rapid eye movement (REM) sleep disorder. With normal REM sleep, individuals do not move about or act out their dreams; however, with REM sleep disorder, individuals may actually act out their dreams violently, making their behavior dangerous to themselves and others.

Treatment Options and Outlook

According to the National Institute of Neurological Disorders and Stroke, there is no cure for DLB, and medications such as donepezil (Aricept) or rivastigmine (Exelon) are given to improve cognitive symptoms as well as psychiatric and motor symptoms. Antipsychotics are usually avoided because they could worsen motor symptoms. Some individuals may show some improvement with levodopa, a drug also used to treat Parkinson's disease.

Individuals with DLB will become increasingly disabled until they die, about eight years from the time of diagnosis.

Risk Factors and Preventive Measures

There are no known risk factors although, very rarely, familial cases have been reported. There are no preventive measures.

dentures Artificial teeth, also known as false teeth. Many older people lose their teeth due to periodontal disease (gum disease), cavities, and a variety of dental problems. However, it is not inevitable that all older people must invariably lose all their teeth, and some studies have shown that up to half of the elderly retain their own teeth. Yet many seniors do lose their teeth because of poor oral hygiene and their failure to obtain regular (or any) dental services. At least an annual visit to the dentist is a good idea for many older people. Some individuals are bedridden and cannot travel to a dentist's office, and transportation may need to be arranged.

According to the Centers for Disease Control and Prevention (CDC), AFRICAN AMERICANS age 65 and older are the most likely to lose all of their natural teeth in comparison to CAUCASIANS, ASIAN AMERICANS, and HISPANICS; for example, 35.4 percent of older blacks lose all their teeth. The next highest group of older people at risk for losing all their teeth is Hispanics (28.7 percent). See Appendix VI for a further age breakdown and more information on health issues by race and other characteristics.

When an older person obtains his or her dentures, it is very important to ensure that the dentures fit properly, because ill-fitting dentures may make it difficult or even impossible for the individual to eat, and in the worst case, this problem ultimately could lead to malnutrition. Dentures should be kept clean and brushed daily. During sleep, the dentures should be soaked in an appropriate cleaning liquid. Individuals who have partial dentures should care for their "partials" in the same proper way as those individuals with full dental replacements.

Sometimes dentures need some adjustment or repair, and these changes should only be made by the dentist or others that he or she recommends and *not* by the older person, spouse, or anyone else.

See also BATHING AND CLEANLINESS.

depression   Chronic sadness that may occur as a result of a distressing situation, such as a death of a spouse or other loved one. Depression may also occur independently from life events and even when an individual's life seems to be successful. According to the Substance Abuse & Mental Health Technical Assistance Center, an estimated 3 to 7 percent of older adults suffer from depression and a lower level of depressive symptoms may be present in 8 to 16 percent of adults living in the general community and up to 50 percent of those living in long-term facilities such as nursing homes.

The Substance Abuse and Mental Health Services Administration estimates that about 7 million people age 65 and older have a psychiatric illness (about 20 percent of the older population), such as depression, bipolar disorder, or schizophrenia. (Note that ALZHEIMER'S DISEASE and other forms of dementia are not generally considered psychiatric disorders but are considered neurological disorders.) Depression is also a risk factor in SUICIDE and attempted suicide. In general, older individuals are more successful at suicide than younger people.

Note that depression is also common among family caregivers, although one study indicated that providing information and assistance significantly decreased the rate of depression. (See FAMILY CAREGIVERS.)

Symptoms of depression may coexist with serious medical problems such as CANCER, DIABETES, heart disease, and PARKINSON'S DISEASE. Other factors that may lead to depression are being victimized by abuse, as well as the experience of social isolation, alcohol use and ALCOHOLISM, and widowhood or BEREAVEMENT.

Some other predictive factors of depression in older individuals include disability, past depression, and SLEEP DISORDERS. In addition, other predictive factors for depression may include:

- low or medium levels of physical activity
- having two or more chronic health problems
- having fewer than three close relatives or friends
- being somewhat satisfied or dissatisfied with friendships

Many individuals, including some physicians, believe that depression is a normal part of aging and thus should be accepted. (See AGEISM.) The reality is that when depression is present, it is often highly treatable among individuals of any age and, in most cases, should be treated.

In general, older women have a greater risk for clinically relevant depressive symptoms than older men; for example, according to the National Center for Health Statistics, 18 percent of women age 65 and older have depression compared to 11 percent of older men. However, older men are more likely to commit suicide than older women.

Symptoms and Diagnostic Path

Many people feel sad at different points in their lives, and depression is much more serious than a feeling of sadness. Instead, depression is a profound and hopeless feeling that can cause people to question the point of their existence or even actively wish to die. If older relatives are making statements that they (or others) would be better off if they were dead or talking about ways that they would choose to commit suicide, they are likely to be depressed and urgently need treatment. It should not be assumed that an older person would never actually carry out a suicide threat, because some will do so. Older people who are chronically depressed may present with some or all of the following symptoms:

- significant weight gain or loss without having tried to gain or lose weight
- loss of interest in activities formerly found pleasurable
- refusal to see family or friends
- initiates discussion about death or the wish for the release of death

- discusses the existence of a suicide plan
- changes in sleep patterns, either sleeping much more or much less than usual
- extreme fatigue or lack of energy, with no apparent cause
- expression of feelings of worthlessness, self-hate, or inappropriate guilt

Depression is diagnosed based on the patient's statements, behavior, and sometimes on the statements of others, such as caregivers. Physicians should rule out other causes of symptoms through laboratory tests, screening for such medical problems as low thyroid levels, anemia, or other medical problems that could present as depressive symptoms.

Treatment Options and Outlook

Psychotherapy may be very helpful for the older person. ANTIDEPRESSANTS are often prescribed by the primary care doctor or by a psychiatrist, a physician who treats maladaptive behaviors, to relieve the symptoms of depression. Some older individuals prefer to receive a prescription for antidepressants from their primary doctor, because they are apprehensive or fearful of psychiatrists or they may mistakenly believe that psychiatrists treat only psychotic patients.

There are several major classes of antidepressants used to treat depression, including tricyclic antidepressants, selective serotonin reuptake inhibitors (SSRIs), atypical antidepressants, and serotonin norepinephrine reuptake inhibitors (SNRIs). Some SNRIs, such as duloxetine (Cymbalta) may provide relief from chronic pain as well as depressive symptoms.

Risk Factors and Preventive Measures

Individuals who have been depressed in the past are at risk for developing depression again. In addition, when other family members are depressed, although the disease is not contagious in the same way as is an infection, sometimes others in the family may become depressed as well. Individuals who have suffered multiple losses in the past year or two have an increased risk for depression, such as the death of a loved one, the sale of a home that the individual lived in for many years, and other major life changes.

See also AGGRESSION, PHYSICAL; ANXIETY DISORDERS; ASSISTED SUICIDE; ASSISTIVE DEVICES/ASSISTED TECHNOLOGY; DIABETES; FRAILTY; GENDER DIFFERENCES; IRRITABILITY; SUICIDE.

Substance Abuse & Mental Health Technical Assistance Center. *Depression and Anxiety Prevention for Older Adults.* Washington, D.C.: U.S. Department of Health and Human Services.

dermatologist See CANCER; SKIN CANCER.

DEXA scan (dual-energy X-ray absorptiometry) See OSTEOPOROSIS.

diabetes Either the inability of the pancreas to produce any of the insulin (Type 1 diabetes) that is needed for digestion *or* the inability of the body to adequately use the insulin that is produced by the pancreas (Type 2 diabetes). According to the Centers for Disease Control and Prevention (CDC) in 2007, six in 10 older adults either had diabetes or they were at a very high risk for developing diabetes. An estimated 575,000 new cases of diabetes developed in people age 60 years and older in 2005. An endocrinologist is a medical doctor who is a specialist in the treatment of endocrine diseases and disorders, such as diabetes, thyroid disease, and other major medical problems that involve the endocrine glands. The physician can often help patients prevent their borderline elevated blood sugar levels from escalating into diabetes with the combination of counseling, medications, and exercise. Endocrinologists are often the group of physicians who diagnoses and treats calcium disorders, most notably OSTEOPOROSIS.

It is important to note that studies have demonstrated that even among well-functioning older adults who have maintained good control of their diabetes, the disease is linked to an increased risk for the development of the symptoms of DEPRESSION. In addition, diabetes can cause CARDIOVASCULAR DISEASE, KIDNEY FAILURE, BLINDNESS/SEVERE

VISION IMPAIRMENT, and many other severe health problems. For example, diabetes accounted for 44 percent of kidney failure cases in 2002, according to the CDC. More than 60 percent of nontraumatic limb amputations occurred to people with diabetes.

Patients with diabetes have from two to four times the risk of STROKE as those without diabetes. Diabetes is also the leading cause of kidney failure in the United States. In addition, diabetes causes many other medical problems, such as nervous system damage causing pain or impaired sensation in the hands or feet; for example about 30 percent of those age 40 and older with diabetes have impaired sensation. Adults with diabetes have a 100 to 200 percent increased risk of DISABILITY compared with those without diabetes.

The risk for death from PNEUMONIA or INFLUENZA is increased among those with diabetes. Individuals with diabetes also have an increased risk of blindness. Some research indicates that older individuals with diabetes have a greater risk for ALZHEIMER'S DISEASE than those without diabetes, although the reason for this is yet unknown. The tighter the glucose control that diabetic individuals can maintain of their blood sugar, the lower the risk for these and other medical problems.

Researchers studied older people who were newly diagnosed with diabetes and followed them up for 10 years. They found that the individuals with diabetes experienced high rates of complications that far exceeded the experiences of individuals without diabetes. For example, according to a study reported in 2007 in the *Archives of Internal Medicine*, newly diagnosed diabetics had a higher risk of cardiovascular disease, and 57.6 percent of the newly diagnosed diabetes patients had cardiovascular complications compared with 34.1 percent of the nondiabetic controls.

Diabetes requires frequent monitoring through blood testing and heeding the results of the blood test in determining dietary changes; for example, if the blood sugar is high, the individual must avoid products high in natural or artificial sugar. If the individual's blood sugar is low (as sometimes happens with individuals with diabetes), then an item high in sugar is needed. Individuals who must take insulin also use the results of their blood test to determine how frequently to self-inject the insulin,

unless they are on an automatic pump that generates insulin as needed.

Older people with diabetes must also self-monitor or have someone else monitor their blood sugar level. In some cases, the older person is too confused or otherwise impaired to manage the demands of the disease and may need to live with others who will test their blood, monitor their diet, and administer needed medication, or they may need to move to a NURSING HOME. Elderly people also have a greater risk for the development of other serious diseases and medical problems, such as coronary HEART DISEASE, HYPERTENSION, FRACTURES, and osteoporosis.

According to the U.S. Census Bureau, diabetes significantly limits the activity of adults and the activity limitation increases with age; for example, 38.4 of 1,000 people ages 65 to 74 limited their activities because of diabetes in 2000. This rate increased for individuals with diabetes age 75 and older, and for this group, 42.5 per 1,000 limited their activities.

Symptoms and Diagnostic Path

Nearly all individuals with Type 1 diabetes are diagnosed in childhood or adolescence, since the disease is very debilitating and the symptoms are obvious. However, most people with diabetes, about 90 percent, have Type 2 diabetes, which is often linked to OBESITY and is usually diagnosed in adulthood. Some individuals are diagnosed with insulin resistance, sometimes called prediabetes, which is a blood sugar rate that is higher than normal but is not high enough to be diagnosed as diabetes.

The most common symptoms of diabetes are

- constant thirst
- frequent urination
- itching of the skin
- frequent infections
- blurred vision
- frequent skin infections
- slow healing from cuts and bruises
- chronic fatigue
- unexplained weight loss
- very dry skin

Physicians diagnose diabetes by ordering laboratory tests of the blood sugar level, as well as by reviewing the patient's symptoms and medical history. They may check blood glucose levels with the fasting plasma glucose test, which measures the level of blood sugar after the individual fasts for eight hours. Blood glucose levels are checked within one hour, two hours, and then three hours later. A result greater than 126 mg/dl indicates the possibility of diabetes. If blood sugar levels are still high with a repeated test on another day, then diabetes is diagnosed. Other tests may also be given.

If patients with diabetes have emergency symptoms, they need to seek medical care immediately, either with their own physician or at a hospital emergency room. Examples of key emergency symptoms include

- The individual is unable to keep food or fluids down for more than six hours.
- The individual suddenly loses five pounds or more without seeking to lose weight.
- The individual's body temperature exceeds 101°F.
- The individual's blood glucose level is lower than 60 mg/dl or stays more than 300 mg/dl.
- The person has trouble breathing.
- The person cannot think clearly.

Treatment Options and Outlook

Individuals who are diagnosed with diabetes are trained to test their own blood sugar levels with a device that pricks the finger. They are also trained on what actions to take should the blood sugar level be too high or too low. For example, if the individual is hypoglycemic (low blood sugar), as occurs with some diabetics, he or she must bring up their blood sugar level with fruit or another item with sugar. If the blood sugar level is too high (which is far more common), then the individual must carefully watch consumption of items containing natural or artificial sugar.

Individuals with Type 1 diabetes must inject themselves with insulin, and they are expected to maintain a very tight control over their disease. Some patients with diabetes use an implanted insulin pump that releases insulin on a preprogrammed basis. The management of Type 1 diabetes is more difficult than Type 2 diabetes. However, sometimes people with Type 2 diabetes will also require insulin; for example, if they are severely injured and hospitalized, their blood sugar levels may go dangerously out of control unless they receive insulin.

Most people with Type 2 diabetes can manage their illness by daily blood testing and monitoring and by taking oral medications such as metformin (Glucophage) and other drugs; however, according to the CDC, metformin does not work as well in older people as it does in younger individuals.

Medicare provides coverage for glucose monitors, test strips, and lancets used to test blood sugar. It is also recommended that patients with diabetes eat regular meals every four to five hours; for example, three meals and one or two snacks can help maintain normal or close to normal blood sugar.

Older individuals with diabetes have an increased risk for many medical problems, including cardiovascular disease, kidney disease, hypertension, and so forth. Physical activity and exercise can decrease these risks for many individuals.

Risk Factors and Preventive Measures

The risk for the development of diabetes increases among some groups of older individuals. One risk factor is age. For example, according to the National Center for Health Statistics, the prevalence of diabetes was higher among those ages 65 to 74 (19.0 percent) but it is significantly lower among those age 75 and older (16.0 percent). About 21 percent of all people age 60 and older have diabetes.

In considering GENDER DIFFERENCES, older men have a higher risk for diabetes than women; for example, an estimated 20 percent of men age 65 and older have diabetes compared with 15 percent of older women.

Some racial and ethnic groups have a higher risk for diabetes; for example, blacks have a much greater risk for diabetes than whites. According to the CDC, based on 2005 statistics, non-Hispanic blacks of any age are about 1.8 times as likely to have diabetes compared to non-Hispanic whites. Hispanic Americans are about 1.7 times as likely to be diagnosed with diabetes as non-Hispanic whites. Native Americans and Alaska Natives have the highest risk for diabetes: 2.2 times the risk of non-Hispanic whites.

Individuals with a family history of diabetes have a greater risk for developing the disease themselves. OBESITY is also a risk factor for Type 2 diabetes. Physical inactivity is another risk factor. In addition, Type 2 diabetes is much more common among individuals over age 65 than it is among younger individuals. Diabetes is a greater problem for older NATIVE AMERICANS, AFRICAN AMERICANS, ASIAN AMERICANS, and HISPANICS than for CAUCASIANS. (See Appendix VI.)

See also AMERICANS WITH DISABILITIES ACT; CARDIOVASCULAR DISEASE; DEATH; DISABILITY; ENVIRONMENTAL HAZARDS; EYE DISEASES, SERIOUS; FAMILY AND MEDICAL LEAVE ACT; KIDNEY DISEASE; SARCOPENIA.

Bethel, M. Angelyn, et al. "Longitudinal Incidence and Prevalence of Adverse Outcomes of Diabetes Mellitus in Elderly Patients." *Archives of Internal Medicine* 167 (May 14, 2007): 921–927.

He, Wan, Manisha Sengupta, Victoria A. Velkoff, and Kimberly A. DeBarros. *65+ in the United States: 2005.* Washington, D.C.: U.S. Census Bureau, December 2005.

Miraldi, Cinzia, M.D., et al. "Diabetes Mellitus, Glycemic Control, and Incident Depressive Symptoms among 70–79 Year Old Persons: The Health, Aging, and Body Composition Study." *Archives of Internal Medicine* 167 (June 11, 2007): 1137–1144.

Moran, S. A., C. J. Caspersen, G. D. Thomas, D. R. Brown and The Diabetes and Aging Work Group (DAWG). *Reference Guide of Physical Activity Programs for Older Adults: A Resource for Planning Interventions.* Atlanta, Ga.: National Center for Chronic Disease Prevention and Health Promotion, Centers for Disease Control and Prevention, 2007.

National Diabetes Information Clearinghouse, "National Diabetes Statistics," November 2005. Available online. URL: http://diabetes.niddk.nih.gov/dm/pubs/statistics/index.htm. Downloaded February 14, 2008.

Petit, William A., Jr., and Christine Adamec. *The Encyclopedia of Diabetes.* New York: Facts On File, 2002.

Pompei, Peter. "Diabetes Mellitus in Later Life." *Generations* 30, no. 3 (Fall 2006): 39–44.

Schoenborn, Charlotte A., Jackline L. Vickerie, and Eva Powell-Griner. "Health Characteristics of Adults 55 Years of Age and Over: United States, 2000–2003." *Advance Data from Vital and Health Statistics,* no. 370. Hyattsville, Md.: National Center for Health Statistics, 2006.

dialysis The filtering of the blood by machine, as a result of KIDNEY FAILURE (end-stage renal disease or ESRD). (Dialysis can also be used to treat people who have ingested poisons or drugs and are at risk for acute kidney failure.) People with DIABETES have an increased risk for kidney failure, and when both diabetes and hypertension are present, the risk is further escalated. When the kidneys fail, the only recourse to sustaining the individual's life is to receive either kidney dialysis or a kidney transplant. Hemodialysis may be managed at a dialysis center while peritoneal dialysis can be provided at home. Most elderly people receive their dialysis in a dialysis center. Dialysis removes contaminants from the blood and maintains a normal level of electrolytes in the blood.

In some cases, the elderly person needing dialysis is unconscious and other family members, such as a spouse or adult children, must make the decision for or against dialysis, knowing that if they do not choose dialysis, the patient will die. This is a very difficult decision for any person to make about a loved one. It can help enormously if the older person had earlier prepared a LIVING WILL, stipulating the types of lifesaving measures that he or she would prefer if unable to make medical decisions at a later date.

Procedure

The two types of dialysis are *hemodialysis* and *peritoneal dialysis*. When patients have hemodialysis, they usually go to a dialysis center three times a week for three to four hours each time, and a machine filters their blood of impurities. (Some patients receive hemodialysis at home.) According to the National Institutes of Health, before each session of hemodialysis begins, the health-care provider checks the following in the patient:

- blood pressure
- breathing rate
- chest assessment
- examination of the access
- heart rate
- temperature
- body weight

A permanent access to the bloodstream (*arteriovenous fistula*) is created in the patient's body by joining an artery to a vein, which allows the vein to receive blood at a high pressure and also thickens the walls of the vein. This is the access point for the dialysis machine. However, a temporary access may also be created with dialysis catheters, which are generally used in emergency situations.

Simply put, the patient is connected to the machine at the access point, and the blood is diverted from the access point in the body to the dialysis machine. The blood flows into a solution called *dialysate,* where it is purified and chemical imbalances are corrected. Then the blood is returned back to the body. Each hemodialysis session lasts from three to four hours.

According to authors Dimkovic and Oreopoulos in their chapter on dialysis in *The Aging Kidney in Health and Disease,* most elderly individuals (about 81 percent) receive hemodialysis compared to 65 percent for their younger counterparts. These experts say that hemodialysis offers many advantages for the elderly; for example, there is a shorter treatment time than with peritoneal dialysis and there is an opportunity to socialize with the staff and other patients. In addition, the patient receives continuous follow-up from the staff.

With peritoneal dialysis, which can be performed in the home or nursing home, fluid is placed directly into the abdominal cavity to wash out the toxins with special dialyzing solutions, and then it is drained out. This procedure can be done either continuously or overnight. It must be performed every day.

The dialysis process (whether performed through hemodialysis or peritoneal dialysis) can cause individuals to become weak, confused, fatigued, and lethargic. Alternatively, once patients become accustomed to the dialysis process, they may have few or no ill effects.

According to authors Pendse, Singh, and Zawada Jr., patients older than age 80 represent the fastest growing group of dialysis patients in the United States. Say these authors,

> Time constraints are not a problem, and these individuals often arrive eager for their treatments. Transportation is often available from assisted-living providers, retirement community staff, or

municipal programs. A high rate of compliance with all aspects of treatment often offsets a higher prevalence of comorbid (coexisting) (cardiac, vascular, malignancies) conditions in achieving a good outcome. As a result, many elderly patients placed on dialysis continue to enjoy a good quality-of-life and benefit from documented improvement in a variety of health outcome measures.

Risks and Complications

Older individuals receiving dialysis face increased risks compared to their younger counterparts, according to authors Dimkovic and Oreopoulos. For example, elderly individuals have an increased risk of infection from the dialysis due to their aging immune system, and infection is a major cause of death among elderly dialysis patients. Older individuals also have an increased risk for gastrointestinal bleeding, especially if they are taking any nonsteroidal anti-inflammatory medications (NSAIDs).

Dialysis patients have an increased risk for anemia. Malnutrition is another risk factor with hemodialysis, and as many as 20 percent of elderly patients may suffer from malnutrition and a decreased rate of survival. Hypotension (below-normal blood pressure) is another problem that occurs in at least 20–30 percent of patients receiving dialysis, according to Dimkovic and Oreopoulos.

There are also long-term risks to dialysis; for example CARDIOVASCULAR DISEASE may develop, as may blood loss leading to iron deficiency. Dialysis dementia may also occur, caused by aluminum poisoning, according to Nicholls, Benz, and Pressman in their chapter on the nervous system and dialysis in *Handbook of Dialysis.* Some early signs of dialysis dementia are stammering and stuttering. An electroencephalogram (EEG) of the brain can determine whether dialysis dementia is present. Dialysis patients with dementia who do not have aluminum poisoning may have other disorders that should be diagnosed and treated. Rarely, thiamine deficiency may cause dialysis dementia.

Emotional problems are also common among patients undergoing dialysis, particularly DEPRESSION. The procedure is long and very wearying to older patients, who also know that it will need to be repeated for the rest of their lives unless they have a kidney transplant.

Outlook and Lifestyle Modifications

Patients undergoing dialysis must make a plan to repeatedly visit the dialysis center or, in the case of peritoneal dialysis, have someone come to their home to perform the dialysis. Most people receiving dialysis have little energy and thus cannot perform numerous tasks that may have been easy for them to accomplish in the past, such as preparing meals, cleaning their home, and managing other ACTIVITIES OF DAILY LIVING.

Patients receiving dialysis should be careful to avoid wearing tight clothing over the access site for their dialysis, according to the National Institutes of Health. In addition, they should check the site after receiving dialysis and report on any bleeding, swelling, or infection. If access is on an arm, they should not allow anyone to take their blood pressure on that arm.

Number of Older People Receiving Dialysis

According to a 2007 article in the *Annals of Internal Medicine,* the number of octogenarians (people in their 80s) and nonagenarians (people in their 90s) receiving dialysis increased dramatically from 7,054 people in 1996 to 13,577 in 2003. Yet the overall survival did not change much, from less than half who survived over this seven-year period. The median survival was less than 16 months for patients ages 80 to 84 and less than 12 months for patients age 85 and older.

Looking at a younger population of elderly people, in a study reported in 2007 in the *Canadian Medical Association Journal,* the researchers analyzed data on 14,512 patients age 65 and older who had undergone dialysis between 1990 and 1999. The researchers found that the percentage of patients who were age 75 and older at the onset of their dialysis increased from 32.7 percent in the period 1990–1994 to 40.0 percent in the period 1995–1999. Clearly, treatment with dialysis has increased among older people.

According to the researchers, the survival rates for patients improved in the later time frame from the rate in the early 1990s, even though the older patients had more ailments. For example, the life expectancy of those aged 75 to 79 increased from an additional 2.73 years in the early 1990s to 3.19 years in the latter part of the 1990s. The survival rate for patients age 80 and older also increased.

See also HEALTH-CARE AGENT/PROXY; KIDNEY DISEASE.

Dimkovic, Nada, and Dimitrios G. Oreopoulos. "Substitutive Treatments of End-Stage Renal Diseases in the Elderly: Dialysis." In *The Aging Kidney in Health and Disease.* Macias Nunez, Juan F., J. Stewart Cameron, and Dimitrios G. Oreopoulos, eds. New York: Springer, 2008, pp. 443–463.

Jassal, Sarbjit Vanita, M.D., et al. "Changes in Survival among Elderly Patients Initiating Dialysis from 1990 to 1999." *Canadian Medical Association Journal* 177, no. 9 (October 23, 2007): 1033–1038.

Kurella, Manjula, et al. "Octogenarians and Nonagenarians Starting Dialysis in the United States." *Annals of Internal Medicine* 146 (2007): 177–183.

Nicholls, Anthony J., Robert L. Benz, and Mark R. Pressman. "Nervous System and Sleep Disorders." In *Handbook of Dialysis.* Fourth Ed. Daugirdas, John T., Peter G. Blake, and Todd S. Ing, eds. Philadelphia, Pa.: Wolters Kluwer, 2007, pp. 700–713.

Pendse, Shona, Ajay Singh, and Edward Zawada, Jr. "Initiation of Dialysis." In *Handbook of Dialysis.* Fourth Ed. Daugirdas, John T., Peter G. Blake, and Todd S. Ing, eds. Philadelphia, Pa.: Wolters Kluwer, 2007, pp. 14–21.

diapers, adult Disposable products that older adults may use when they have difficulty with or cannot reach the bathroom in time to use the toilet. URINARY INCONTINENCE refers to those who cannot hold their urine, and FECAL INCONTINENCE refers to those who cannot hold their stools at all or only minimally. Often bedridden patients may develop urinary or fecal incontinence, requiring the use of adult diapers.

Sometimes patients with advanced ALZHEIMER'S DISEASE or other forms of DEMENTIA will need adult diapers because they have forgotten the toilet training that they had learned long ago or are unaware of the need to use the toilet. In other cases, individuals could use the toilet but others decide for them that they should use adult diapers. This is an example of LEARNED HELPLESSNESS.

See also TOILETING.

disability Inability to perform tasks that many people can perform, such as ACTIVITIES OF DAILY

LIVING, that impedes normal life. According to the Administration on Aging, in a study in 2002, 52 percent of older individuals reported having some type of disability and 37 percent of the group said that they suffered from a severe disability. This study also revealed that the level of disability increased with age, and 57 percent of those who were older than 80 years old reported a severe disability. This makes sense, since older individuals are more likely to be burdened with debilitating diseases.

The Administration on Aging reported on another study on Medicare beneficiaries and their ability to perform specific activities of daily living. About 27 percent of elderly Medicare beneficiaries reported difficulty in performing one or more activities of daily living. In comparison, 91 percent of Medicare beneficiaries who resided in institutions (such as nursing homes) reported difficulty with one or more activities of daily living. The rate of limitations increase with age, and those who are age 85 and older are generally much more impaired than those who are ages 65 to 74.

It is interesting to note that some studies on aging BABY BOOMERS indicate that they may be less healthy than older individuals were at their age. This may be due to OBESITY and related factors.

See also ACCESSIBILITY TO FACILITIES; AMERICANS WITH DISABILITIES ACT; ASSISTIVE DEVICES/ASSISTED TECHNOLOGY; ELDERIZING A HOME; FAMILY AND MEDICAL LEAVE ACT; HEALTH-CARE AGENT/PROXY.

Administration on Aging. *A Profile of Older Americans: 2006.* Washington, D.C.: U.S. Department of Health and Human Services, 2006. Available online. URL: http://www.aoa.gov/PROF/Statistics/profile/2006/profiles2006.asp. Accessed September 11, 2007.

disaster, natural Disasters such as hurricanes, floods, and severe storms can cause severe CONFUSION and distress among elderly individuals, particularly among those with ALZHEIMER'S DISEASE or DEMENTIA, but also among older people with illnesses requiring supervision or medication, such as ARTHRITIS, DIABETES, HYPERTENSION, and so forth. They may be afraid that they will be unable to obtain their medications. They may also fear that the people who normally provide care will become unavailable to them. It is best for caregivers to attempt to maintain as calm an attitude as possible when dealing with older individuals who are worried or confused about natural disasters.

Older individuals are at a high risk for harm during a natural disaster; for example, the majority of the victims of Hurricane Katrina were older than age 60, and more than 70 percent of those who died were age 60 and older. In addition, after Hurricane Katrina hit, an estimated 200,000 people (including older people) could not get their usual medications, and they had no access to health care.

According to the Centers for Disease Control and Prevention (CDC), older individuals should have a plan for a disaster, or one should be made for them. For example, in addition to a basic emergency supply kit, older adults need an emergency plan that lists exactly where they should go in the event of an emergency, as well as what they need to bring with them (such as eyeglasses, medications, hearing aids, oxygen, medical records, and so forth). They also need a plan for how they will get there and who they should call for help. A list of medications, doctors, and pharmacies should be kept in a waterproof bag.

In developing an emergency plan the Administration on Aging suggests the following for the elderly and their families:

- Develop a family communication plan so that the whereabouts and well-being of every family member is reported to a key person during a disaster.

- Exchange cell phone numbers and contact information among family members and update it when necessary.

- Plan how to keep informed of developments in the disaster by telephone, cell phone, computer, radio, television, or newspaper.

- Determine a meeting place away from home that is reasonably familiar and convenient for all family members.

- Maintain an adequate supply of personal, health, and home supplies, including a two-week supply of prescription medications and enough ready-to-eat food and water to last three days.

- Prepare a "to-go kit" that is ready and accessible in case of a need for a quick departure and that includes a flashlight, extra batteries, a battery-operated radio, a first-aid kit, contact lenses or eyeglasses, medications, copies of prescriptions, photo identification, copies of essential documents (birth certificate, marriage certificate, Social Security card, and Medicare, Medicaid, and other insurance cards), and a small amount of cash (a maximum of $50).

In Florida, because of the high risk for hurricanes, the Department of Health has recommended that older adults pack a 30-day supply of medication and also a two-week supply of special food or supplements whenever a hurricane is expected. If a hurricane is approaching, the state of Florida waives state restrictions on obtaining more than a month's worth of medicine at one time.

If families have relatives living in a nursing home, assisted-living facility, or retirement community, they should ask about disaster planning, including

- How does the facility define an emergency?
- What emergency plans are in place?
- Are sufficient supplies and generators available?
- When will an evacuation occur, and how will it be carried out?
- Who will notify families that a resident has been evacuated?

See also ANXIETY AND ANXIETY DISORDERS.

doctors, changing to another one Older individuals may be distressed when they must change physicians, but this is a common problem that many face. Their doctors may retire, die, or relocate, and thus it becomes imperative to choose a new physician.

When others provide the older person with assistance in identifying a new doctor, it is best for family members or other caregivers to locate a doctor who is sympathetic to the needs of elderly people. Some doctors prefer to treat younger people, and they may become impatient in the face of slowed talk or any confusion evinced by the older

person (See AGEISM.) It may be helpful for family members to go with the elderly person to the appointment to meet the new physician to see if he or she appears to be a right fit for the older person and his or her health needs.

Some considerations in choosing a new doctor are the following:

- Is the doctor board-certified? Specialists should be board-certified in their field, such as neurology, rheumatology, psychiatry, and so forth.
- Does the doctor listen carefully? A visit to the doctor is necessary to make this determination.
- Does the doctor accept MEDICARE? Most physicians do accept Medicare, but some do not.
- Is the doctor's office relatively easy to get to?
- Does the doctor's office offer a laboratory to obtain tests or will the older person have to travel elsewhere to obtain blood tests?
- Who sees the doctor's patients if he or she is not available?
- Does the doctor see many older patients or is his or her practice primarily oriented to younger patients?
- Does the doctor treat older patients with the same health problems as the individual seeking a doctor? (Such as DIABETES, HYPERTENSION, etc.)
- Will the doctor refer patients with special problems to other physicians who are specialists?
- Does the doctor see patients with multiple health problems? (Many older people have multiple health issues.)

During the first visit with a doctor the older person is considering, he or she should ask the following questions:

- Are you willing to give me written instructions about my care?
- May I bring a family member, such as my spouse, son, or daughter to my office visits?
- Are you willing to discuss my condition with my family members, with my written permission?
- Will you maintain my privacy if I do *not* wish you to discuss my condition with others? Under what

conditions, if any, would you need to breach confidentiality?

See also ADULT CHILDREN/CHILDREN OF AGING PARENTS; FAMILY CAREGIVERS; MEDICAL RECORDS.

National Institute on Aging. "Choosing a Doctor." Washington, D.C.: U.S. Department of Health and Human Services, May 2006. Available online. URL: http://www.niapublications.org/agepages/choose.asp. Accessed August 25, 2007.

driving Operating a motor vehicle, usually a private car. About 75 percent of Americans age 65 and older have driver's licenses, and by the year 2025, it is anticipated that the number of older drivers will increase by 2.5 times over the number of elderly drivers in 1995. This increase will be largely driven by the aging of BABY BOOMERS.

However, some older drivers should not be driving at all because they have ALZHEIMER'S DISEASE, DEMENTIA, or other disorders that severely impede their reflexes and judgment. Yet it can be very difficult or even seemingly impossible for many adult children to tell their elderly parents that they should no longer drive because it is unsafe for themselves and for others on the road.

In her book *The Eldercare Handbook: Difficult Choices, Compassionate Solutions,* author Stella Mora Henry offered some suggestions on how to help an adult child decide if a parent should stop driving. For example, Mora Henry said that if a parent drives either too fast or too slow, this is one clear indicator of a problem. Another indicator is if an adult child feels compelled to call a parent to make sure that he or she arrived home safely. She also advises adult children to ask themselves if they would ride with their parent or if they would let their children ride with the parent. If the answers to these questions are "No," it is likely that the parent should stop driving.

Deaths from Car Crashes

According to the Centers for Disease Control and Prevention (CDC), 3,355 people age 65 and older died in motor vehicle crashes in 2004 in the United States. In addition, 177,000 older adults suffered nonfatal injuries in 2004.

In the 21st century, older drivers are much more likely to drive than in past years, possibly because of the decrease in mass transportation. However, crash rates are especially high among drivers age 80 and older, who also have the highest rate of fatalities of any age group. This high death rate is a result in part from the number of car crashes that individuals in this group experience, as well as from the physical frailty of seniors.

According to the CDC, most of the traffic deaths of older drivers occurred in the daytime (79 percent) or on weekdays (73 percent). Most of the car crashes (73 percent) that older drivers experienced involved another vehicle. Older men are more likely to die from a car crash than older women.

Delayed Responses and Declining Vision

As most individuals age, both their vision and response times decline. They may also suffer from cataracts or glaucoma, further impairing their vision. Visual acuity and depth perception diminish as well, and night vision may become much worse. Some older people suffer from a movement disorder, such as PARKINSON'S DISEASE, that may affect their response and reaction time. Others may suffer from arthritic joints and have difficulty with the mechanics of driving.

As a consequence of their diminished visual acuity and slower physical responses, many older people willingly limit their driving to daytime hours and non-rush-hour traffic. Yet they may still cause accidents and if they are in a car crash, they are more likely to be seriously injured than younger people.

Indications that Alzheimer's Disease Is Affecting Driving

Although some individuals with early Alzheimer's disease can continue driving, the National Highway Traffic Safety Administration (NHTSA) says there are some indications that the person with Alzheimer's should stop driving.

The following are some early warning signs that the person should stop driving:

- The individual needs more help than required in the past with understanding directions or with learning a new route.

- The individual has difficulty remembering where he or she is going or where the car was parked or left behind.
- The individual keeps getting lost on routes that were familiar in the past.
- The individual has trouble making turns, especially left turns.
- The individual feels confused when exiting the highway or with some traffic signs, such as a four-way stop.
- The individual receives traffic tickets for moving violations.
- The individual finds that other drivers are frequently honking at the individual for some reason.
- The individual stops at a green light or brakes inappropriately, thus confusing and frustrating other drivers.
- The individual drifts into other traffic lanes.
- The individual finds unexplained dents and scrapes on the car and cannot recall any minor accidents.
- The individual has trouble controlling emotions that affect and impair driving, such as anger or sadness.

Interventions to Stop Driving

Some family members intercede to try to stop the older driver from driving altogether, particularly if he or she has Alzheimer's or another form of dementia or is too physically frail to drive safely anymore. This action is often greatly resented by the older person, who may be angry at the potential loss of independence and may also feel very insulted that others feel that he or she is no longer competent to drive. Burkhardt and his colleagues in their article on mobility and independence say,

> When persons with diminished capabilities continue to drive, an increased safety risk is created for all members of society. But the older driver facing the prospect of reducing or terminating his or her driving (because of declining skills or for other reasons) often expects substantially reduced mobility. Such expectation leads in turn to reluctance among these older drivers, family members, and government agencies to terminate an older per-

son's driving privileges. Thus, the point at which older persons voluntarily give up or are forced to relinquish their driving privileges is often seen by elders and those around them as a watershed event with large implications regarding independence, self-sufficiency, and social responsibilities.

If the elderly person should stop driving, solutions should be presented to him or her; for example, if the individual will still live at home, a plan should be made for how he or she will get to doctor's appointments or to the supermarket and other places where the elderly person needs to go.

Burkhardt, Jon E. et al. "Mobility and Independence: Changes and Challenges for Older Drivers: Executive Summary." Administration on Aging (July 1998).
Mora Henry, Stella, R.N., with Ann Convery. *The Eldercare Handbook: Difficult Choices, Compassionate Solutions.* New York: Collins, 2006.

drug abuse Excessive use or misuse of medications, particularly such drugs as NARCOTICS. Often older people may not purposely misuse drugs, but instead they may misuse or abuse them because of CONFUSION. For example, if someone cannot remember whether he or she has already taken the drug, they may decide to take another dose and run the risk of overdosing.

Another common problem is that many older individuals share prescription drugs with others, usually thinking that they are being helpful and saving others money. This is both dangerous and illegal and can cause harm to others. It is unknown how common this form of drug abuse is, but some experts believe that it is prevalent. (See PRESCRIPTION DRUG ABUSE/MISUSE.) It is also possible to use over-the-counter drugs to excess; for example, chronic high doses of acetaminophen can be harmful to the liver.

Older Americans occasionally use illegal drugs such as marijuana, heroin, and so forth, but they abuse these drugs at a significantly lower rate than individuals of all other age groups. According to the Substance Abuse and Mental Health Services Administration in their annual report, only 1.1 percent of individuals age 65 and older abused illicit drugs in the past year and less than 1 percent abused illegal drugs in the past month.

See also ADVERSE DRUG EVENT; ALCOHOLISM; BINGE DRINKING; DIABETES; IRRITABILITY; MEMORY IMPAIRMENT; SUBSTANCE ABUSE AND DEPENDENCE.

Gwinnell, Esther, M.D., and Christine Adamec. *The Encyclopedia of Drug Abuse.* New York: Facts On File, 2007.
Substance Abuse and Mental Health Services Administration. *Results from the 2006 National Survey on Drug Use and Health: National Findings.* Rockville, Md.: Office of Applied Studies, 2007.

durable power of attorney (DPA)   A legal document that an adult creates in advance, usually with the assistance of an ATTORNEY, which transfers certain rights and responsibilities to another person. These rights and responsibilities are still effective in the event of the older individual's physical incapacity or mental incompetence. In contrast, a "regular" power of attorney presupposes the continued mental capacity of the individual, who is assumed to be capable of overseeing or providing input to the person who is acting on his or her behalf.

The key advantage of the DPA is that it empowers a trusted individual to act for another. The key disadvantage is that sometimes this trust is misplaced and the power is abused.

There are two types of durable powers of attorney. One is for health care, in which the older person names another person who can make medical decisions if he or she is unable to make them. The other allows the individual to name a person to act on their behalf for any legal purpose.

According to *The American Bar Association Legal Guide for Americans over 50,* the durable power of attorney can be terminated in one of four ways.

First, the durable power of attorney can be revoked at any time and for any reason, although it should be revoked only in writing and the person holding the DPA should be notified. Second, death terminates the DPA. Third, the durable power of attorney can include a specific termination date or event, such as September 30, 2011, or when a house or property is sold. Finally, if the agent representing the individual and to whom the durable power of attorney was given becomes incapacitated or dies, and no one else is appointed to fill this void, then the DPA is void.

All states in the United States and in the District of Columbia have statutes regarding the durable power of attorney. Each state has its own laws regarding how durable powers of attorney may be set up and the restrictions applied to them. Some states allow different types of durable powers of attorney, such as one for financial affairs only or one for health-care decisions only. Individuals should contact an attorney in their state to learn about the applicable laws.

Some states have a "springing power of attorney." This is a power of attorney that is planned for ahead of time and that can only be used at a specific future time or when a specific event occurs, such as if the individual becomes mentally incompetent or physically incapacitated.

See also END-OF-LIFE ISSUES; HEALTH-CARE AGENT/ PROXY; LEGAL GUARDIANSHIP; LIVING TRUST; LIVING WILL; WILLS.

American Bar Association. *The American Bar Association Legal Guide for Americans over 50.* New York: Random House Reference, 2006.

elder care The provision of assistance to individuals age 65 years and older in the United States, including assistance with such issues as health and medical care, health insurance, medication, HOME CARE, TRANSPORTATION, NUTRITION, a safe place to live, and the resolution of a variety of legal and family issues.

It is important for an older person's needs to be taken seriously, yet some individuals, including some doctors, have an attitude tainted by AGEISM toward older people, assuming that of course they are sick, since they are old. In fact, the risk for illness does increase with age, yet many diseases, disorders, and chronic ailments can be treated, enabling the elderly person to feel significantly better. It may become necessary for the elderly person to change doctors if he or she is not receiving good medical care. Of course, many physicians are compassionate and caring individuals, but the doctor may relocate to another area, choose to retire, or may die, necessitating a search for a new physician. (See DOCTORS, CHANGING TO ANOTHER ONE.)

Medical Issues

In the arena of medical issues, many family members and others who assist older people are concerned about such major health issues as HEART DISEASE and CANCER, which are the number one and two killers of older people in the United States. However, there are also many other areas of concern with regard to the health of the elderly, such as serious eye diseases (EYE DISEASES, SERIOUS) as well as BLINDNESS, CHRONIC OBSTRUCTIVE PULMONARY DISEASE, EMPHYSEMA, HEART ATTACK, KIDNEY DISEASE, KIDNEY FAILURE, OSTEOPOROSIS, PARKINSON'S DISEASE, PROSTATE DISEASES, SARCOPENIA, and SHINGLES. Some older people suffer from VITAMIN AND MINERAL DEFICIENCIES, which are important to identify

for many reasons; for example, a deficiency of vitamin B_{12} may be misdiagnosed as dementia. HEARING DISORDERS, many of which are treatable, are also common among older people.

Many older individuals require short- or long-term HOSPITALIZATION for their illnesses, sometimes needing care in the INTENSIVE-CARE UNIT (ICU). Older people are also at an increased risk for a variety of ACCIDENTAL INJURIES. Older people face an increased risk for FALLS, which can cause FRACTURES and lead to a temporary or long-term stay in a NURSING HOME. About 5 percent of the elderly population resides in nursing homes, but this percentage increases dramatically to 18.2 percent for those age 85 and older.

A significant percentage of older people suffer from ALZHEIMER'S DISEASE, and this disease, as well as other illnesses that cause DEMENTIA, are of concern to anyone who loves and/or cares for an older person. Alzheimer's disease and other forms of dementia may be associated with AGGRESSION, CONFUSION, DELUSIONS, HALLUCINATIONS, PSYCHOTIC BEHAVIOR, RAGE, and SUNDOWNING (day/night reversal).

It is important for older people who need medication to take their medicine, but many older people have a problem with MEDICATION COMPLIANCE, either because they forget to take their medicine or they simply refuse to take it. Sometimes they think they are "cured" because they feel better after taking one or two pills and do not realize that they must continue to take the medicine according to their doctor's orders. Medication compliance is crucial to older people and may mean the difference between life and death. Sometimes even an over-the-counter medication can help to sustain life, as with ASPIRIN THERAPY among those who have had or are at risk for having a STROKE.

Their doctors are also important to older people. In addition to their primary care physician who maintains the patient's MEDICAL RECORDS (and may be a GERIATRICIAN), many older people also see physicians who specialize in treating specific areas of the body and specific disorders and diseases.

It is also true that increasingly many segments of the population are turning to COMPLEMENTARY/ALTERNATIVE MEDICINE to treat their medical problems, and older people are no exception, often using herbs and vitamins and minerals to treat their ailments. It is important to notify the physician about every medication, including over-the-counter (OTC) drugs, and herbs and minerals that the older person takes, because sometimes these remedies lead to serious MEDICATION INTERACTIONS with his or her prescribed medications and/or medical conditions or even to an ADVERSE DRUG EVENT. It is also important that the patient has an effective MEDICATION MANAGEMENT plan in place.

Another matter of concern with regard to medications is INAPPROPRIATE PRESCRIPTIONS FOR THE ELDERLY, because some drugs are dangerous or risky for many older people. In addition, older people sometimes become involved with PRESCRIPTION DRUG ABUSE/MISUSE, often by accident or as a result of confusion.

Some older people have problems with issues of SUBSTANCE ABUSE AND DEPENDENCE, particularly with regard to ALCOHOLISM and sometimes with BINGE DRINKING. Although the substance abuse may be a problem of long standing, in some cases, particularly among older females, they may turn to substances in their elderly years because of DEPRESSION, loneliness, and pain from medical problems. In addition, HOLIDAYS can be depressing for elderly individuals whose spouse may have died and whose adult children may live faraway.

The older person suffering from severe pain may need to take NARCOTICS, and he or she as well as other family members should be aware of the risks and benefits associated with these drugs.

Although older people often look askance at seeking the help of mental health professionals, the reality is that problems such as depression are common among the elderly. Older people have a greater risk than younger people for facing MULTIPLE LOSSES in their lives, which can lead to depression. If the depression is severe, the older person may be at risk for SUICIDE. Rarely, elderly males even resort to suicide-homicide, especially when faced with a terminal diagnosis of a spouse. ANTIDEPRESSANTS may greatly improve the elderly person's outlook. Some older people are at risk for developing anxiety (see ANXIETY AND ANXIETY DISORDERS), which can make them very unhappy and distraught; however, treatment with therapy and with BENZODIAZEPINES can alleviate most or even all of this concern.

Coverage for medical care is an important issue, and most older people receive MEDICARE; however, Medicare generally covers only 80 percent of the health-care costs and the older person is responsible for paying the 20 percent balance. For this reason, many older people purchase MEDIGAP INSURANCE policies, while impoverished elderly individuals rely upon MEDICAID coverage. MEDICARE PRESCRIPTION DRUG COVERAGE is a boon to many older people, who previously could not afford the drugs they needed. MEDICARE PREVENTIVE SERVICES covers services for eligible recipients to detect current medical problems as well as predict potential future problems and includes tests such as screening for CHOLESTEROL, PROSTATE CANCER, a screening COLONOSCOPY, and immunizations against HEPATITIS B.

Many older people suffer from diseases common to a large portion of the elderly population, such as ARTHRITIS, BACK PAIN, DIABETES, HEADACHES, GOUT, HYPERTENSION, KIDNEY DISEASE, or other illnesses causing CHRONIC PAIN.

SLEEP DISORDERS are common among many older people, as are problems with TOILETING, such as FECAL INCONTINENCE or URINARY INCONTINENCE.

As much as possible, it is important for older people to EXERCISE (after consulting with their physicians) and to avoid the many medical risks surrounding OBESITY. It is also crucial for older people who still smoke to give up SMOKING, because smoking increases the risk for CARDIOVASCULAR DISEASE and many other ailments. It is also a good idea to maintain good health by obtaining annual FLU immunizations as well as an immunization for PNEUMONIA, as recommended by the physician.

Living Issues

Many older people choose INDEPENDENT LIVING and wish to remain at home. They prefer AGING

IN PLACE as long as possible but may find that ACTIVITIES OF DAILY LIVING, including BATHING AND CLEANLINESS and BILL PAYING, prove challenging. They need some assistance, but at the same time they may fear their LOSS OF INDEPENDENCE. If they choose to remain living independently, wearable IDENTIFICATION or a PERSONAL EMERGENCY DEVICE may provide some level of comfort and assurance of safety. Sometimes these individuals choose to have COMPANIONS live with them.

Elderly people living alone face FIRE RISKS and dangers from natural disasters and ENVIRONMENTAL HAZARDS. In very warm climates, it is important to frequently check on elderly individuals who could be at risk for HEAT STROKE/HEAT EXHAUSTION.

Sometimes older people relocate to live with a relative; however, MOVING IN WITH FAMILY MEMBERS involves advance planning to ease possible areas of disagreement or tension. For example, it is important to consider ELDERIZING A HOME and making necessary HOME MODIFICATIONS to alleviate problem areas that could be dangerous or unsafe for the older person.

Another alternative is moving to an ASSISTED-LIVING FACILITY where meals are provided, a nurse may be on staff, and transportation is provided to doctor's appointments, the supermarket, and other locations.

Many older people benefit from using ASSISTIVE DEVICES, ranging from canes and HEARING AIDS to computerized technology.

Sometimes older people are relatively healthy but they need extra care because they undergo a serious medical procedure, such as a JOINT REPLACEMENT or other form of surgery. As a result, they may be able to live with a family member temporarily, subsequently relocating to their own home or to assisted living. Often REHABILITATION in a nursing home is an interim step between the hospital and going home.

Elderly individuals sometimes have difficulty with ACCESSIBILITY TO FACILITIES despite the provisions outlined under the AMERICANS WITH DISABILITIES ACT, which requires that both public and private establishments provide reasonably accessible accommodations to disabled individuals.

If the older person is still DRIVING, health issues may increase his or her risk for accidental injuries incurred while operating it. (See ACCIDENTAL INJURIES.)

Legal Issues

There are a variety of legal issues involved with assisting older individuals, such as the POWER OF ATTORNEY, the HEALTH-CARE AGENT/PROXY, LEGAL GUARDIANSHIP, the LIVING TRUST, WILLS, and other issues associated with ESTATE PLANNING and the distribution of ASSETS. There is also a variety of family legal issues involved, such as who will care for the older person if care is needed and who will make medical and legal decisions should the older person become unable to make such decisions. If the older person becomes mentally incompetent, this must be adjudicated by a court. (See MENTAL COMPETENCY.)

Older individuals are sometimes the victims of CRIMES AGAINST THE ELDERLY, including violent crimes such as ASSAULT and ABUSE as well as nonviolent crimes such as fraud and identity theft. (See Appendix XIII for a list of state consumer protection offices.) In addition, some older people are victims of NEGLECT.

End-of-Life Issues

Few people wish to face it, but elderly people are at risk of DEATH from many illnesses. For this reason, it is best for an older person to make a plan for the medical care they wish to receive if they become at risk for death. The LIVING WILL provides guidance to relatives as to which life-sustaining measures, if any, that the older person wishes will occur if they become terminally ill. Decisions about PALLIATIVE CARE for individuals with terminal illnesses should be made ahead of time whenever possible; for example, the older person may need to move to a HOSPICE to receive appropriate care. Some older people set aside money in advance to pay for their FUNERAL arrangements and choose the CEMETERY in which they wish to be buried in order to ease the pain of others in making difficult decisions when suffering from BEREAVEMENT.

The older person may also decide that CREMATION is the best choice for him or her, and some older people make arrangements ahead of time for their own cremation upon their death.

Family Issues

Many families must help the elderly person make difficult decisions as the older person ages. The elderly person may wish to remain at home but be unable to provide himself or herself basic care, and thus home care may be the right solution. Sometimes the family member needs to work but may wish for the older person to live with him or her. In that case, considering ADULT DAY CENTERS may be the answer if the older person is still mobile yet requires care during the day. The FAMILY AND MEDICAL LEAVE ACT also allows for most adult children to take time off from work when an elderly parent is sick and needs them.

Often the ADULT CHILDREN of aging parents, many of whom are BABY BOOMERS, may feel overwhelmed about the many decisions they must help their elderly parents make about their care, and they may suffer from COMPASSION FATIGUE or CAREGIVER STRESS. It is important for every caregiver to realize that good care cannot be provided if the caregiver becomes too sick or exhausted. In these cases, the caregiver should consider taking advantage of local RESPITE SERVICES. Other relatives may live faraway, and they are unable to provide direct care; instead, they may provide LONG-DISTANCE CARE by hiring professionals or communicating with family members who live with or nearby the older person.

When there are two or more adult siblings, there is a considerable potential for SIBLING RIVALRY AND CONFLICT about many different issues involving the older person, and it is best for such issues to be resolved ahead of time whenever possible. The adult child may also have conflicts with the older person himself or herself about many issues. (See CONFLICTS, WITH ADULT CHILDREN/PHYSICIANS/OTHERS; TALKING TO ELDERLY PARENTS ABOUT DIFFICULT ISSUES.) Often the older person may be confused or forgetful and sometimes may have difficulty with DECISION MAKING.

Issues of Race, Ethnicity, and Gender

Older individuals differ in terms of their RACE AND ETHNICITY as well as their gender. For example, elderly AFRICAN AMERICANS and NATIVE AMERICANS are more likely to have diabetes than whites, while CAUCASIANS are more likely to be diagnosed with osteoporosis. African Americans are also more likely to be diagnosed with hypertension while whites are more likely to have Alzheimer's disease.

When comparing older men and women and their GENDER DIFFERENCES, women have a greater LIFE EXPECTANCY than males. Remarriage is significantly less likely among older women than older men, largely because older women generally outnumber and live longer than older men. There are also health differences; for example, older women are more likely to have RHEUMATOID ARTHRITIS and sleep disorders, and men are more likely to have hearing disorders.

Military Veterans

Most elderly military veterans are males who served in World War II, the Korean War, or the Vietnam War, although increasing numbers of baby boomer females are aging veterans. Some elderly veterans receive VETERAN BENEFITS, such as monthly payments, hospital and clinic services, and other options. Special services are provided for veterans who are blind or severely disabled, and the Veterans Administration also pays for nursing home services for some veterans. When the elderly veteran dies, the families of deceased military veterans may choose to bury the deceased veteran in a military cemetery.

elderizing a home   Making safety changes or modifications to a home or apartment so that it will be safer for an older person. Home modification and repair funds may be available through Title III of the OLDER AMERICANS ACT and distributed through the local area agency on aging. To identify the nearest agency, contact the Eldercare Locator at (800) 677-1116 or visit the Web site at http://www.eldercare.gov. In some cases, MEDICARE may pay for home modifications. (For more information, call Medicare at [800] 633-4227.)

Examples of elderizing a home are removing area rugs that can be slippery, installing nightlights so that the older person can easily find the bathroom at night, using nonskid bath mats in the bathroom, and installing grab bars and stools in shower stalls and bathtubs so that the older person will find it easier to stand and avoid slipping. It may be necessary to install higher toilets that are easier for the elderly person to sit on and stand up from, in contrast to the traditionally low toilet.

HOME MODIFICATIONS TO CONSIDER WHEN ELDERIZING A HOME

Kitchen

☐ Are all appliances and utensils conveniently and safely located?

☐ Are stove controls easy to use and clearly marked?

☐ Can the oven and refrigerator be opened easily?

☐ Are the cabinet doorknobs easy to use?

☐ Can you sit down while working?

☐ Is the kitchen counter height and depth comfortable for you?

☐ Would you benefit from having some convenience items, such as a handheld spray, a garbage disposal, or a trash compactor?

Bathroom

☐ Are there grab bars where needed?

☐ Can you get into and out of the bathtub or shower easily?

☐ Is the water temperature properly regulated in order to prevent scalding or burning?

☐ Would you benefit from having a handheld showerhead?

Closets, Storage Spaces

☐ Do you have enough storage space?

☐ Have you gotten the maximum use out of the storage space you have, including saving space with special closet shelf systems and other products?

☐ Are your closets and storage areas conveniently located?

☐ Can you reach items in the closet easily? Are your closet shelves too high?

Doors, Windows

☐ Are your doors and windows easy to open and close?

☐ Are your door locks sturdy and easy to operate?

☐ Are your doors wide enough to accommodate a walker or wheelchair?

☐ Do your doors have peepholes or viewing panels? If so, are they set at the correct height for you to use?

☐ Is there a step up or down at the entrance to your home? If so, is the door threshold too high or low for you to get in or out of easily?

☐ Is there enough space for you to move around while you are opening or closing your doors?

Driveway, Garage

☐ Does your garage door open automatically?

☐ Is your parking space walkway available?

☐ Is your parking space close to the entrance of your home?

☐ Is the lighting to your garage and outside area sufficient?

Electrical Outlets, Switches, Safety Devices

☐ Are light or power switches easy to turn on and off?

☐ Are electrical outlets easy to reach?

☐ Are the electrical outlets properly grounded to prevent shocks?

☐ Are your extension cords in good condition?

☐ Can you hear the doorbell in every part of the house?

☐ Do you have smoke detectors throughout the home?

☐ Do you have an alarm system? Do you understand how to operate it?

☐ Is the telephone readily available for emergencies? Do you have a cordless telephone that you keep nearby?

☐ Would you benefit from having an assistive device to make it easier to hear and talk on the telephone?

Floors

☐ Are all of the floors in your home on the same level?

☐ Are steps up and down marked in some way?

☐ Are all floor surfaces safe and covered with nonslip or nonskid materials?

☐ Do you have scatter rugs or doormats that could be hazardous?

Hallways, Steps, Stairways

☐ Are hallways and stairs in good condition?

☐ Do all of your hallways and stairs have smooth, safe surfaces?

☐ Do your stairs have steps that are big enough for your whole foot?

☐ Do you have handrails on both sides of the stairway?

☐ Are the handrails on your stairs wide enough for you to grasp them securely?

☐ Is the lighting sufficient on the steps and in hallways?

☐ Would you benefit from building a ramp to replace the stairs or steps inside or outside your home?

Lighting, Ventilation

☐ Do you have night-lights where they are needed?

☐ Is the lighting in each room sufficient for the use of the room?

☐ Is the lighting bright enough to ensure safety?

☐ Is each room well ventilated with good air circulation?

Source: Material adapted from Administration on Aging. "Housing: Home Remodeling." Available online. URL: http://www.aoa.gov/eldfam/housing/home_remodeling/home_remodeling.asp. Accessed February 13, 2008.

Installing lever handles at faucets in the kitchen and bathroom so that they can be gripped and manipulated easily by arthritic hands is another way to make a home safer. This will also help reduce the risk of scalding. It is also important to have a fully charged smoke detector in the kitchen, as well as a portable fire extinguisher that is readily available. Replace a teakettle with one that has an automatic shutoff device for individuals who may forget to turn off the stove.

Tack down or secure electrical cords so that the individual will not trip over them, since FALLS are a major problem for older people. Check the light-ing to ensure that it is bright enough for the individual to see. Also check the furniture to ensure that it is not too low and/or too awkward for elderly people to rise from. The furniture should not have sharp edges, nor should it obstruct easily moving about.

Closets are another major problem area for the older person. Items kept in closets should be well within reach, so that he or she does not have to strain to reach them or stand on a chair to access them and risk falling. Assistive devices such as tools that enable the older person to reach items can also be helpful; however, the overall clutter should be minimized so that the older person does not topple any items down upon himself or herself.

All stairs should have handrails. The stairs should also be free of clutter so that the elderly person will not trip. Mark the edges of steps with brightly colored electrical tape to prevent falls for older individuals with failing eyesight or who may not have their glasses on at night.

If there are any sliding glass doors in the home, affix brightly colored decals to them so that the older person does not walk into the door.

Many elderly people are at risk directly outside their homes, where there may be no handrails or there may be existing handrails that are precariously mounted. Any problematic handrails should be replaced. The outside lighting should also be checked to make sure it is adequate at night.

The Administration on Aging checklist of possible home modifications is a helpful resource when considering each area of the home from the older person's perspective (See pp. 102–03).

According to the Administration on Aging, more than 60 percent of older people live in homes that are more than 20 years old, and these homes often need repairs and modifications. Such changes could significantly increase the older person's comfort; for example, if the person has trouble getting in and out of the shower, grab bars and transfer benches could be installed.

If it is hard for the older person to turn the faucet handles or doorknobs, in the bathroom, they can be replaced with lever handles. If heating or ventilation is inadequate, insulation can be added, as well as new storm windows and air conditioning.

See also ACCESSIBILITY TO FACILITIES; ACCIDENTAL INJURIES; ALZHEIMER'S DISEASE; AMERICANS WITH DISABILITIES ACT; ASSISTIVE DEVICES/ASSISTED TECHNOLOGY; DEMENTIA; FAMILY AND MEDICAL LEAVE ACT; HOME CARE; HOUSING/LIVING ARRANGEMENTS; PERSONAL EMERGENCY DEVICE.

Adamec, Chris. *The Unofficial Guide to Eldercare.* New York: Macmillan, 1999.

Administration on Aging. "Housing: Home Remodeling." Available online. URL: http://www.aoa.gov/eldfam/housing/home_remodeling/home_remodeling.asp. Accessed February 13, 2008.

emergency department care   Many elderly people require emergency care in a hospital emergency department (also commonly known as "the emergency room") because they are more likely than younger individuals to experience HEART ATTACKS, STROKES, FRACTURES, and other life-threatening conditions requiring immediate treatment. They are also more likely to need attention from emergency medical technicians (EMTs) who provide the ambulance services. In some cases, they may need to be transferred to an intensive care unit because of the severity of their injury or disease.

Of older people who require emergency care, those who are age 85 and older are the most likely to need emergency assistance. As seen in Table 1, nearly a third of those age 85 and older, or 31.8 percent, went to the emergency room in the past 12 months over the period 2000–2003.

TABLE 1. PERCENTAGE OF ADULTS AGE 65 AND OLDER WHO USED EMERGENCY ROOM CARE, 2000–2003

Selected Characteristic	Number in Thousands	Percentage
Age 65 and older	**33,219**	**23.2**
Ages 65–74	17,876	20.6
Ages 75–84	12,075	24.9
Age 85 and older	3,268	31.8
Age 65 and older		
Men	14,147	22.6
Women	19,072	23.6
Race and Hispanic origin		
White, not Hispanic	27,529	22.7
Black, not Hispanic	2,685	27.5
Asian, not Hispanic	649	20.6
Hispanic	2,015	25.0
Poverty status, age 65 and older		
Poor	2,479	29.0
Near poor	6,083	26.8
Not poor	12,791	22.1

Source: Material adapted from Schoenborn, Charlotte A., Jackline L. Vickerie, and Eva Powell-Griner. "Health Characteristics of Adults 55 Years of Age and Over: United States, 2000–2003." *Advance Data from Vital and Health Statistics,* No. 370. Hyattsville, Md.: National Center for Health Statistics, 2006, pp. 22–23.

Older women and men need emergency room assistance at about the same rate. However, of all races, African Americans age 65 and older are the most likely to need emergency care. Among older blacks, in the period 2000–2003, 27.5 percent needed to go an emergency room, compared to the next highest group, Hispanics (25 percent). Poor people are more likely to seek emergency room care than are those who are near poor or not poor.

See also ACCESSIBILITY TO FACILITIES; ACCIDENTAL INJURIES; ADVERSE DRUG EVENT; AMERICANS WITH DISABILITIES ACT; DISASTER, NATURAL; FALLS; FAMILY AND MEDICAL LEAVE ACT; HEALTH-CARE AGENT/PROXY; HEART FAILURE; HOSPITALIZATION; PERSONAL EMERGENCY DEVICE.

emphysema A serious illness that damages the air sacs of the lungs and is caused by years of cigarette SMOKING. People with a deficiency of alpha-1 antitrypsin, a natural substance that occurs in the lungs, also have an increased risk for emphysema. Emphysema is not curable although it is treatable. The air sacs cannot deflate completely and thus they are also unable to fill with fresh air and provide a sufficient supply of oxygen.

Symptoms and Diagnostic Path

The most common symptoms of emphysema include

- chronic cough with or without sputum
- shortness of breath
- wheezing
- decreased ability to exercise

In addition, some individuals with emphysema experience an unintentional weight loss; swelling in the feet, ankles, and legs; and anxiety and fatigue.

Emphysema is diagnosed with a physical examination, which may show an exhaling (breathing out) that takes twice as long as inhaling. The individual with emphysema may have a barrel-shaped chest. There may also be indicators of insufficient blood levels of oxygen.

When emphysema is suspected, the physician may order a chest X-ray, pulmonary function tests,

and tests for arterial blood levels that show the levels of oxygen and carbon dioxide in the blood. Other tests may include a computerized tomography (CT) scan on the chest and a pulmonary ventilation/perfusion scan.

Treatment Options and Outlook

The most important action that anyone with emphysema can take is to stop smoking immediately in order to halt the further progression of the disease. Medications can also help individuals with emphysema, such as the use of nebulizers or hand-held inhalers, as well as the use of corticosteroid medications. If respiratory infections occur, antibiotics will be needed. Individuals with emphysema are also strongly encouraged to receive their INFLUENZA and PNEUMONIA vaccines each year, because they could become extremely ill if they received the full brunt of the flu and/or pneumonia.

Some patients with emphysema may undergo lung reduction surgery to remove the damaged portions of the lung and consequently enable the normal parts to work more efficiently.

The patient's prognosis depends on how severe the damage is to the air sacs. Physicians also consider the patient's level of shortness of breath as well as the results of their lung function tests.

Risk Factors and Preventive Measures

Individuals who smoke for years have a high risk of developing emphysema. Older men have a greater risk for emphysema than older women. According to the National Center for Health Statistics, an estimated 7 percent of older men had emphysema in 2004 compared with 4 percent of older women.

The best way to avoid emphysema altogether is to never smoke or to stop smoking immediately, well before the disease develops.

See also GENDER DIFFERENCES; HEALTH-CARE AGENT/PROXY; LUNG CANCER.

endocrinologist See CANCER; DIABETES; OSTEOPOROSIS; THYROID CANCER.

end-of-life issues Difficult issues that need to be decided when individuals are very old or may be near death (yet which are often ignored by older people and their family members), such as whether they wish heroic measures to be taken if they become severely ill or unconscious. An example of such a measure is the insertion of a feeding tube or a ventilator (breathing tube). Such decisions may be included in advance by the older person in a LIVING WILL.

If these decisions are *not* made in advance and an older person becomes severely ill and unable to communicate his or her wishes about health care, then others (such as the spouse or other family members) must make medical choices for him or her. Some older individuals may choose to have only PALLIATIVE CARE rather than heroic measures, which means that they may wish to have pain control but not extreme and possibly very painful efforts to save their lives. Others may wish every effort possible be made to sustain their lives.

Other end-of-life issues include the decision for how the individual's remains will be managed, whether through CREMATION or a traditional FUNERAL. Some individuals purchase contracts with crematoriums or funeral homes in advance of their deaths, so that their loved ones will not have to make such difficult decisions in a state of BEREAVE-MENT. Some individuals even plan their own funerals ahead of time, choosing the casket, who should speak, the site of the burial, and so forth.

Many individuals have stated that they would prefer to die at home and in their own beds rather than in a hospital and hooked up to many tubes and lines. Such a choice should be respected if it is possible.

It is very difficult for most family members to talk to older individuals about end-of-life issues, and they may try to stop older people from discussing what they want in the event of severe health problems or death. Most experts recommend that when older people wish to discuss such matters, their family members should respect their wishes and listen, instead of making irrational statements such as "You're going to be around forever," "You'll never die," and so on.

See also ADVANCE DIRECTIVE; BEREAVEMENT; CAR-DIOPULMONARY RESUSCITATION; DEATH; DEATH, FEAR OF; ESTATE PLANNING; HEALTH-CARE AGENT/PROXY; HOSPICE; TALKING TO ELDERLY PARENTS ABOUT DIF-FICULT ISSUES.

environmental hazards Some items and conditions in the environment can be harmful to older people with heart disease or DIABETES, such as secondhand smoke, carbon monoxide, some household products that are used improperly, and even drinking water, which may contain lead and other pollutants. (See WATER.)

Indoor Pollution

Older adults may spend up to 90 percent of their time indoors, but even in the home there are many potential environmental hazards according to the Environmental Protection Agency (EPA). For example, indoor air may contain fumes from household products, secondhand smoke, and even carbon dioxide. All of these contaminants can become dangerously toxic, especially to individuals at risk for heart disease or STROKE.

Secondhand Smoke

Secondhand smoke from tobacco smoke is one of the worst indoor pollutants according to the EPA. In addition, smoke from wood burning stoves and fireplaces can be dangerous, because they may generate smoke with fine carbon monoxide particles that can trigger palpitations and chest pain, shortness of breath and fatigue, particularly in older adults who have heart disease.

Household Products

If used improperly, some household products are extremely dangerous for those with heart problems; for example, fumes from paint solvents can stress the lungs and the heart. In addition, although lead-based paints are banned in the United States, many homes that were built before 1978 still have lead-containing paints. If renovations need to be done to the home, individuals should take care to minimize paint chips or dust generated from the renovation to avoid hazards to individuals with HYPERTENSION.

Carbon Monoxide

An odorless and invisible gas, carbon monoxide is very dangerous for those with heart disease or congestive heart failure because it decreases the ability to carry oxygen. Even low levels of carbon monoxide may cause a person with heart disease to have chest pain. Some sources of carbon monoxide are fumes from gas water heaters, ranges, dryers, furnaces, space heaters, fireplaces, and stoves. Cars should never be left idling in the garage—even if the garage is open—because they generate carbon monoxide.

Gas appliances should be adjusted as needed, and exhaust fans should be installed and used. Trained professionals should inspect and clean furnaces, flues, and chimneys every autumn. Carbon monoxide detectors should be installed throughout the home.

Outdoor Air Pollution

Individuals who have heart disease or who have had a stroke or are at risk for stroke should avoid contact with air that has particulates and exhaust from vehicles. Particle pollution refers to small soot products found in the outside air, originated from vehicles, power plants, fires, and industrial smokestacks. Particle pollution is especially dangerous for those with heart disease, CHRONIC OBSTRUCTIVE PULMONARY DISEASE, and asthma.

Pollutant Gases Ozone, sulfur dioxide, and nitrogen dioxide are gases in the air and can be dangerous. Ozone can cause chest pain that may be mistaken for a heart attack. Anyone who thinks he or she may be having a heart attack should call 911 and not worry about whether ozone could be causing the problem.

The air quality is important to people with diabetes. Some studies have found that when air pollution is high, there are also higher rates of hospitalization for people with diabetes.

Drinking Water Contaminated drinking water can contribute to heart disease. Lead exposure in drinking water can increase hypertension. Exposure to arsenic from a private well or small water system can be harmful to the heart.

Excessive Heat Heat stroke, characterized by hot, dry, and red skin, and a lack of perspiration, can be very dangerous for older people. Some warning signs of heat stroke are hallucinations and confusion. Heat stroke is a medical emergency. If untreated, it can cause permanent severe damage to organs, as well as disability. It can also be fatal.

People with heart disease and stroke are more vulnerable to excessive heat than others. In addition, some medications cause some older people to be more susceptible to very high air temperatures. People with diabetes are also sensitive to high temperatures, and excessive heat can make it harder for the body to regulate its temperature.

Air conditioning is the best defense against heat stress. Individuals may also take cool showers and wear light-colored and loose-fitting clothing. They should also ask their physicians if their medications could increase their vulnerability to heat-related illnesses.

In addition, when air temperatures are high, individuals should drink plenty of fluids but avoid beverages with caffeine or alcohol or those that have large amounts of sugar. These types of drinks can cause dehydration.

See also CARDIOVASCULAR DISEASE; DIABETES; ELDERIZING A HOME; HEAT STROKE/HEAT EXHAUSTION.

Environmental Protection Agency. *Fact Sheet: Diabetes and Environmental Hazards: Information for Older Adults and Their Caregivers.* Washington, D.C.: August 2007.
———. *Fact Sheet: Environmental Hazards Weigh Heavy on the Heart: Information for Older Americans and Their Caregivers.* Washington, D.C.: September 2005.
———. *Fact Sheet: "It's Too Darn Hot"—Planning for Excessive Heat Events: Information for Older Adults and Family Caregivers.* Washington, D.C.: October 2007.

estate planning A plan made by individuals, often elderly persons, to maximize the transfer of their assets to loved ones upon their death. For example, a LIVING TRUST is one legal means to transfer ownership of assets while the older person still lives, and this type of legal action also enables the elderly person to manage his or her own money and property unless or until he or she should become incapacitated.

Each state has its own laws that govern living trusts and other legal documents, and an attorney in the state where the older person resides should be consulted about such matters.

See ASSETS; ATTORNEYS; DURABLE POWER OF ATTORNEY; END-OF-LIFE ISSUES; HEALTH-CARE AGENT/PROXY; POWER OF ATTORNEY; WILLS.

exercise Active or moderate movement, whether through participating in sports, swimming, doing calisthenics, walking, or other actions or a combination of actions. Most older Americans should be able to perform at least some form of exercise; however, many people older than age 65 are very physically inactive.

According to the National Institute on Aging, more than two-thirds of older adults fail to exercise on a regular basis. Yet regular exercise can significantly improve their flexibility and also often decreases problems with ANXIETY AND ANXIETY DISORDERS or DEPRESSION, as well as improving chronic illnesses such as HYPERTENSION and DIABETES. Strength/resistance exercises can also improve problems with SARCOPENIA, or reduced skeletal muscle mass, a common problem among older individuals.

Exercise can also help resolve problems with being overweight and OBESITY, which are common among many older people. Even when the legs hurt due to peripheral ARTERIOSCLEROSIS (hardening of the arteries in the legs), physicians generally recommend exercise as a therapy.

Check with the Doctor First

Everyone should check with his or her doctor before beginning an exercise program. This is particularly important for older individuals with the following conditions:

- severe shortness of breath
- chest pain
- irregular or fluttery heartbeat
- infections with fever
- blood clot
- a hernia that is causing problems
- sores in the feet or ankles that do not heal
- some eye conditions such as bleeding in the retina or a detached retina

Categories of Exercise

According to the National Institute on Aging, there are several primary types of exercise that many older people can participate in. First are endurance exercises, which increase the heart rate and breathing and help improve the health of the circulatory system, lungs, and heart. Endurance exercises are also believed to either delay or prevent diabetes, heart disease, colon cancer, and stroke. Examples of endurance exercises are swimming, walking, raking, mopping the floor, and jogging. Sports that build up endurance are golf (without using a cart), tennis doubles, rowing, and volleyball. Vigorous activities that build up endurance are climbing stairs, bicycling uphill, downhill skiing, and jogging.

There are also strength exercises, such as the arm raise, the chair stand, the biceps curl, and others. Strength exercises help to build up muscles, and they can also increase the body's metabolism. Strength exercises may prevent OSTEOPOROSIS.

Individuals should check with their doctors before beginning any exercise program. The National Institute on Aging (NIA) booklet "Exercise: A Guide from The National Institute on Aging" includes a series of recommended strength and balance exercises for older individuals. Written descriptions and draw-

TABLE 1. EXERCISE TO THESE LIMITS EACH WEEK						
Sunday	**Monday**	**Tuesday**	**Wednesday**	**Thursday**	**Friday**	**Saturday**
Endurance	Endurance	Endurance	Endurance	Endurance	Endurance	Endurance
	Strength/balance, upper body	Strength/balance, lower body	Strength/balance, upper body	Strength/balance, lower body	Strength/balance, upper body	Strength/balance, lower body
Stretching	Stretching	Stretching	Stretching	Stretching	Stretching	Stretching
Anytime/anywhere balance	Anytime/anywhere balance	Anytime/anywhere balance	Anytime/anywhere balance	Anytime/anywhere balance	Anytime/anywhere balance	Anytime/anywhere balance

Source: National Institute on Aging. *Exercise: A Guide from the National Institute on Aging.* Washington, D.C.: U.S. Department of Health and Human Services, September 2006, p. 71.

TABLE 2. A SAMPLE WALKING PROGRAM

	Warm-up	Exercising	Cool Down	Total Time
Week 1				
Session A	Walk 5 min	Then walk briskly 5 min	Then walk more slowly 5 min	15 min
Session B	Repeat above pattern			
	Repeat above pattern			
Continue with at least three exercise sessions during each week of the program				
Week 2	Walk 5 min	Walk briskly 7 min	Walk 5 min	17 min
Week 3	Walk 5 min	Walk briskly 9 min	Walk 5 min	19 min
Week 4	Walk 5 min	Walk briskly 11 min	Walk 5 min	21 min
Week 5	Walk 5 min	Walk briskly 13 min	Walk 5 min	23 min
Week 6	Walk 5 min	Walk briskly 15 min	Walk 5 min	25 min
Week 7	Walk 5 min	Walk briskly 18 min	Walk 5 min	28 min
Week 8	Walk 5 min	Walk briskly 20 min	Walk 5 min	30 min
Week 9	Walk 5 min	Walk briskly 23 min	Walk 5 min	33 min
Week 10	Walk 5 min	Walk briskly 26 min	Walk 5 min	36 min
Week 11	Walk 5 min	Walk briskly 28 min	Walk 5 min	38 min
Week 12	Walk 5 min	Walk briskly 30 min	Walk 5 min	40 min
Week 13 on	Gradually increase your brisk walking time to 30–60 minutes, three or four times a week. Remember that your goal is to get the benefits you are seeking and enjoy your activity.			

Source: National Heart, Lung, and Blood Institute. *Aim for a Healthy Weight.* Washington, D.C.: National Institutes of Health, 2005, p. 28.

ings of these exercises are available on the NIA Web site at http://www.nia.nih.gov/HealthInformation/Publications/ExerciseGuide/chapter04b.htm.

Older individuals who do not already exercise regularly should start slowly with endurance exercises, performing them for about five minutes and building up stamina slowly. The goal of endurance exercises is to build up to 30 minutes per day.

Resistance exercises are good to prevent falls, a common problem among many older adults. Flexibility exercises keep the muscles limber, and stretching exercises may help patients recover more quickly from injuries and may prevent some injuries from occurring. Stretching exercises can improve flexibility, such as hamstrings stretches, alternative hamstrings stretches, and other exercises. Written descriptions and drawings of these stretching exercises are available on the NIA Web site at http://www.nia.nih.gov/HealthInformation/Publications/ExerciseGuide/chapter04a.htm

Individuals should build up exercising gradually. A good way to start is by doing simple chair exercise aerobics. Once the person feels like she or he is in better shape (and the physician agrees), then the NIA says many people can exercise up to the limits described in Table 1.

Walking is an excellent exercise for many people, and the National Heart, Lung, and Blood Institute provides a graduated walking program that many people can use. (See Table 2.)

Keep in mind the following tips when walking:

• Hold your head up and keep your back straight.

• Bend your elbows as you swing your arms.

• Take long, easy strides.

See also FRAILTY; NUTRITION; OBESITY.

Moran, S. A., C. J. Caspersen, G. D. Thomas, D. R. Brown, and The Diabetes and Aging Work Group (DAWG). *Reference Guide of Physical Activity Programs for Older Adults: A Resource for Planning Interventions.* Atlanta, Ga.: National Center for Chronic Disease Prevention and Health Promotion, Centers for Disease Control and Prevention, 2007.

National Heart, Lung, and Blood Institute. *Aim for a Healthy Weight.* Washington, D.C.: National Institutes of Health, 2005.

National Institute on Aging. *Exercise: A Guide from the National Institute on Aging.* Washington, D.C.: U.S. Department of Health and Human Services, September 2006.

extremely severe headaches The most dangerous headache is one that comes on suddenly, is the worst headache the person has ever experienced, and that is unlike any headache that he or she has ever had in the past. Such a headache could mean that the individual is undergoing a STROKE, which is a life-threatening event. According to Doctors Walker and Wadman in their article on headache and the elderly for *Clinics in Geriatric Medicine,* headache in an elderly person could be an indicator of a life-threatening disorder, and physicians should not exclude such conditions as subarachnoid hemorrhage, subdural hematoma, giant cell arteritis, or GLAUCOMA, as well as serious infections such as meningitis and encephalitis.

In the case of the unusually extreme headache, someone should call emergency services ("911"). The person should not try to drive himself or herself to the hospital because of the risk of unconsciousness and a serious car crash, not only risking the individual's life but also the lives of others on the road.

See also HEADACHE.

eye diseases, serious Disorders of the eye that may lead to difficulty with vision or even BLINDNESS. Most serious eye diseases and causes of blindness are age related. The most common eye diseases among older individuals are CATARACTS, GLAUCOMA, and AGE-RELATED MACULAR DEGENERATION (AMD). Annual eye examinations may enable the early discovery of eye disease and treatment that prevents or delays further deterioration. Some diseases such as DIABETES and HYPERTENSION increase the risk for serious eye diseases. As a result, individuals with diabetes and/or high blood pressure should be sure to have annual eye examinations.

There are an estimated 5.5 million elderly people in the United States who are either blind or visually impaired by a serious eye disease, such as blindness, LOW VISION, glaucoma, cataracts, or AMD. As seen in Table 2, the risk for blindness in 2004 was highest among those ages 80 and older, or 7 percent, compared to a risk of less than 1 percent for those ages 70 to 79. In addition, the risk for low vision was also the highest among those age 80 and older, or 16.7 percent, compared to only 3 percent for those ages 70 to 79.

In the most extreme cases, ASSISTIVE DEVICES are helpful to blind individuals; for example, according to the American Foundation for the Blind, about 107,000 people in the United States use long, white canes to help them move around. In addition, an estimated 7,000 blind Americans use dog guides, although this requires training of the blind person. Some elderly blind people learn to use braille, a method of writing in which letters and symbols are written using raised dots.

Low vision is a problem among older people who have trouble performing basic important daily tasks because their vision is so poor, even with the use of glasses or contact lenses; for example, they may have trouble reading, cooking, sewing, and selecting clothes that match. In addition, they have trouble recognizing their friends and family members. They also have an increased risk for FALLS.

Most people with low vision have a problem with age-related macular degeneration, cataracts, glaucoma, and/or diabetes. African Americans and Hispanics ages 65 years and older have a particularly high risk for low vision compared to individuals of other races and ethnicities.

People with low vision can benefit from using telephones and clocks with large numbers, large-print publications, magnifying glasses, and computer systems that talk, among some of the more common assistive devices.

According to the National Eye Institute, some questions that people with low vision should ask their eye care professionals are

• What changes can I expect in my vision?

• Will my vision get worse? How much of my vision will I lose?

- Will regular eyeglasses improve my vision?
- What medical/surgical treatments are available for my condition?
- What can I do to protect or prolong my vision?
- Will diet, exercise, or other lifestyle changes help me?
- If my vision cannot be corrected, can you refer me to a low vision specialist?
- Where can I get a low vision examination and evaluation? Where can I get vision rehabilitation?

Another serious eye disease is glaucoma. Glaucoma is an imbalance in eye fluid production, which often causes excessive eye fluid pressure; however, some people with glaucoma have normal eye pressure. As a result, the dilated eye examination is the best way to determine the presence of glaucoma. If glaucoma is untreated, it eventually leads to blindness in most cases. African Americans are more likely to develop glaucoma than whites, and they are also more likely to go blind from glaucoma than are whites. The risk for glaucoma increases with age, and those who are ages 80 and older have the highest risk, or 7.7 percent, compared to a risk of 3.9 percent for those ages 70 to 79 years. (See Table 1.)

Glaucoma is treated with eye drops that lower the pressure in the eye. If the eye drops fail to work, surgery may be needed in which a laser beam creates openings to help fluid drain out.

With age-related macular degeneration (AMD), the macula, the central part of the retina, breaks and prevents clear and sharp vision. Most people (about 90 percent) with this disease have the "dry" type of AMD, which is a less severe form than wet AMD. With dry AMD, the cells deteriorate but there is no bleeding; with the wet form of AMD, new blood vessels grow and leak both fluid and blood under the macula. AMD is the main cause of blindness among people ages 65 and older in the United States.

AMD is a painless eye disease, and its common symptoms are distorted vision, blurriness, and viewing straight lines as wavy ones. Nutritional supplements (vitamin E, vitamin C, beta-carotene, and zinc) may help some individuals with advanced AMD; however, smokers should avoid beta-carotene because it may increase their risk of lung cancer.

There are no treatments for dry AMD other than keeping aware of the problem. With wet AMD, laser surgery may improve vision and stop bleeding. The risk for AMD increases with age, and those with the greatest risk for both intermediate and advanced AMD are age 80 years and older. (See Table 1.)

Cataracts are another common problem that cloud the vision and can lead to blindness in older people if untreated. People with diabetes are at high risk for developing cataracts, as are smokers. Cataract surgery, in which the patient's clouded lens is replaced with an artificial one, is highly successful

TABLE 1. SUMMARY OF EYE DISEASE PREVALENCE DATA, 2004 PREVALENCE OF CATARACT, AGE-RELATED MACULAR DEGENERATION, AND OPEN-ANGLE GLAUCOMA AMONG ADULTS 40 YEARS AND OLDER IN THE UNITED STATES

Age	Cataract		Advanced AMD		Intermediate AMD		Glaucoma	
Years	Persons	%	Persons	%	Persons	%	Persons	%
40–49	1,046,000	2.5	20,000	0.1	851,000	2.0	290,000	0.7
50–59	2,123,000	6.8	113,000	0.4	1,053,000	3.4	318,000	1.0
60–69	4,061,000	20.0	147,000	0.7	1,294,000	6.4	369,000	1.8
70–79	6,973,000	42.8	377,000	2.4	1,949,000	12.0	530,000	3.9
80 and older	6,272,000	68.3	1,081,000	11.8	2,164,000	23.6	711,000	7.7
Total	**20,475,000**	**17.2**	**1,749,000**	**1.5**	**7,311,000**	**6.1**	**2,218,000**	**1.9**

Source: Adapted from National Eye Institute. "Statistics and Data: Summary of Eye Disease Prevalence Data: Prevalence of Cataract, Age-Related Macular Degeneration, and Open-Angle Glaucoma among Adults 40 Years and Older in the United States. Available online. URL: http://www.nei.nih.gov/eyedata/pbd_tables.asp. Accessed April 10, 2008.

TABLE 2. PREVALENCE OF BLINDNESS AND LOW VISION AMONG ADULTS AGE 40 AND OLDER IN THE UNITED STATES

Age	Blindness		Low Vision	
Years	Persons	%	Persons	%
40–49	51,000	0.1	80,000	0.2
50–59	45,000	0.1	102,000	0.3
60–69	59,000	0.3	176,000	0.9
70–79	134,000	0.8	471,000	3.0

Source: Adapted from National Eye Institute. "Prevalence of Blindness and Low Vision Among Adults 40 Years and Older in the United States." Available online. URL: http://www.nei.nih.gov/eyedata/pbd_tables.asp. Accessed April 10, 2008.

for most people. The surgery is performed on an outpatient basis. The risk for cataracts increases with age; for example, the risk is 2.5 percent for those ages 40 to 49 but increases to 42.8 percent for those ages 70 to 79 and increases further to 68.3 percent for those age 80 and older. (See Table 1.)

Diabetic retinopathy is another severe eye disease, and it primarily occurs among older people who have had diabetes for 30 years or more. Diabetic retinopathy leads to blindness if untreated. In the early stage of the disease, known as *non-proliferative diabetic retinopathy,* the blood vessels start to leak fluid into the retina, causing a clouding of vision. As the disease advances, the symptoms worsen. Symptoms of the early stage of diabetic retinopathy include poor night vision and "floaters" or tiny fragments that move across the eye in the line of vision.

In the late stage of diabetic retinopathy, or *proliferative diabetic retinopathy,* blood vessels grow into the eye and cause much worse vision and even blindness, if untreated. Laser surgery is used to treat diabetic retinopathy. In addition, good control of blood sugar and hypertension will improve the outcome of the disease.

See also BLINDNESS/SEVERE VISION IMPAIRMENT; GENDER DIFFERENCES.

National Eye Institute. *What You Should Know about Low Vision.* 2007. Available online: http://www.nei.nih. gov. Accessed February 13, 2008.

Prevent Blindness America and the National Eye Institute. *Vision Problems in the U.S.: Prevalence of Adult Vision Impairment and Age-Related Eye Disease in America.* 2002. Available online. URL: http://www.nei.nih.gov/eyedata. Accessed February 13, 2008.

fainting Losing consciousness for a few seconds or longer. Fainting may be caused by HYPOTENSION (low blood pressure), a severe INFECTION, malnutrition, extremely low blood sugar (hypoglycemia), or many other causes. Some medications or combination of medications may also induce fainting. The cause of the fainting should always be investigated to rule out the presence of any serious diseases so that the physician can treat any medical problems that may be present.

See also FALLS; INAPPROPRIATE PRESCRIPTIONS FOR THE ELDERLY; MEDICATION INTERACTIONS.

falls Accidental injuries caused by tripping or slipping, often because of a medical condition. In addition, falls may be caused by unsafe conditions in the home or at other sites. They may also be caused by medications that make the individual sedated or unsteady. Sometimes serious eye diseases impair the person's vision and may cause or contribute to falls. Falls are common among older individuals, particularly among older women. They are also very dangerous, and many older people who fall down risk painful bone fractures, and some even die as a result of a fall. Death may not be instant but may occur later as a result of injuries from the fall.

According to a 2006 article in *Morbidity and Mortality Weekly Report* on injuries and fatalities among older adults in the United States, about 30 percent of adults age 65 and older will ultimately experience unintentional falls that cause injuries or deaths.

Injuries and chronic disabilities often result from falls among older people. In 2003, 1.8 million older people were treated in emergency rooms for nonfatal injuries caused by falls. In addition, most hip fractures among older Americans are caused by falls, and in many cases, individuals require NURSING HOME care for a year or longer after their falls.

TABLE 1. AGE-ADJUSTED RATE OF NONFATAL FALLS AMONG PERSONS AGED 65 AND OLDER, BY SEX AND RACE— UNITED STATES, 2001–2005, RATE PER 100,000 POPULATION

Characteristic	Year				
	2001	2002	2003	2004	2005
Both sexes	**4,617.0**	**4,539.2**	**4,967.6**	**4,972.6**	**4,746.8**
Sex/Race					
Men overall	**3,590.0**	**3,490.6**	**3,859.4**	**3,847.6**	**3,674.0**
White	3.090.3	2,920.5	3,278.6	3,133.8	2,823.6
Black	2,813.8	3,270.4	3,114.4	3,521.6	3,033.6
Women overall	**5,283.0**	**5,238.0**	**5,697.8**	**5,712.2**	**5,466.7**
White	4,478.2	4,348.3	4,760.4	4,611.3	4,223.2
Black	4,914.3	4,828.8	4,752.5	4,220.3	4,595.7

Source: Centers for Disease Control and Prevention. "Fatalities and Injuries from Falls among Older Adults—United States, 1993–2003 and 2001–2005." *Morbidity and Mortality Weekly Report* 55, no. 45 (November 17, 2006): p. 1,223.

TABLE 2. STATE-BY-STATE VIEW OF UNINTENTIONAL FALL DEATHS AMONG ADULTS AGE 65 OR OLDER, 2004

State	Number of Deaths
Alabama	117
Alaska	7
Arizona	463
Arkansas	124
California	1,228
Colorado	265
Connecticut	185
Delaware	42
District of Columbia	36
Florida	1,236
Georgia	420
Hawaii	56
Idaho	94
Illinois	420
Indiana	216
Iowa	271
Kansas	178
Kentucky	125
Louisiana	111
Maine	42
Maryland	240
Massachusetts	204
Michigan	509
Minnesota	479
Mississippi	143
Missouri	468
Montana	82
Nebraska	141
Nevada	72
New Hampshire	74
New Jersey	263
New Mexico	203
New York	794
North Carolina	480
North Dakota	68
Ohio	568
Oklahoma	157
Oregon	303
Pennsylvania	803
Rhode Island	105
South Carolina	144
South Dakota	90
Tennessee	299
Texas	803
Utah	80
Vermont	85
Virginia	294
Washington	459
West Virginia	131
Wisconsin	697
Wyoming	25
Total	**14,899**

Source: Centers for Disease Control and Prevention. *The State of Aging and Health in America 2007.* Bethesda, Md.: National Institutes of Health, 2007, p. 28.

The rate of nonfatal falls is higher among women overall; for example, the nonfatal fall rate for all women over the period 2001–2005 was 5,466.7 per 100,000 compared to a rate of 3,674.0 for all men. However, the rate of nonfatal falls was higher among black men and black women when compared to their own gender. For example, the rate of nonfatal falls was 4,595.7 per 100,000 for black women compared to a rate of 4,223.2 for white women. Among black men, the rate was 3,033.6 per 100,000 compared to a rate of 2,823.6 for white men. (See Table 1.)

Deaths from Falls

Although women fall more often, men have a higher rate of death from falls than women. In 2003, the rate of death from falls for men was 46.2 per 100,000 compared to 31.1 per 100,000 for women. Among blacks, whites, and Pacific Islanders, both white women and white men had the greatest risks for experiencing fatal falls.

According to the Centers for Disease Control and Prevention (CDC), in looking at unintentional fall deaths among adults ages 65 and older in 2004, there were 14,899 deaths, with the greatest number of deaths occurring in Florida (1,236) and California (1,228), which are also states with large numbers of older individuals. (See Table 2.)

Hip Fractures Resulting from Falls

Many older people suffer from hip fractures caused by falls, and the rate of fatal falls or hospitalizations for hip fractures among older Americans

TABLE 3. RATES OF HOSPITALIZATIONS FOR HIP FRACTURES PER 100,000 POPULATION AMONG MEN AND WOMEN AGE 65 AND OLDER—UNITED STATES, 1993–2003

Hip fractures	Year										
	1993	**1994**	**1995**	**1996**	**1997**	**1998**	**1999**	**2000**	**2001**	**2002**	**2003**
Both sexes	917.6	900.3	875.6	990.5	929.1	930.8	919.3	877.3	866.3	804.8	775.7
Men	552.3	578.0	579.6	567.1	635.7	678.9	597.3	570.6	556.3	525.1	583.6
Women	1,118.9	1,078.4	1,033.1	1,239.2	1,096.4	1,071.0	1,098.4	1,042.2	1,038.6	971.4	886.2

Source: Centers for Disease Control and Prevention. "Fatalities and Injuries from Falls among Older Adults—United States, 1993–2003 and 2001–2005." *Morbidity and Mortality Weekly Report* 55, no. 45 (November 17, 2006): p. 1,223.

per 100,000 population was at its highest level in 2003, or 36.8, up from 23.7 in 1993. (See Table 3.) According to the CDC, this increase in the rate in falls may be due at least in part to an increased life expectancy among older Americans. Women had a markedly higher rate of suffering hip fractures than men: 886.2 per 100,000 for women compared to 583.6 for men.

Note that the rate of hip fractures has steadily fallen since 1993, when the rate was 917.6 per 100,000 population, to the rate of 775.7 in 2003 (nearly a 16 percent decrease). Better identification of and medical treatment for OSTEOPOROSIS (the cause for many fractures) is likely the reason for this improvement.

Risk Factors for Falls

Some factors increase the likelihood that an older person will fall. For example, the older the individual, the greater the risk for a fall, and thus an 85-year-old person has a greater risk of falling than a 75-year-old person. Individuals with chronic illness or disabilities, such as those who have had a STROKE or who have PARKINSON'S DISEASE or heart disease, have a greater risk of experiencing a fall. Individuals who are cognitively impaired are more likely to fall, such as those with ALZHEIMER'S DISEASE or another form of DEMENTIA.

A lack of exercise increases the risk for an older person falling, and those who have had previous falls have an increased risk of falling again. Individuals who abuse alcohol have a higher rate of falls than others. Some medications, particularly ANTIDEPRESSANTS and sedatives, as well as antianxiety drugs, such as BENZODIAZEPINES, also increase the risk of falls among elderly individuals. Older people who are malnourished or dehydrated have a higher risk of falling than others.

In Canada, falls are also a major problem for older individuals, and an estimated 62 percent of all injury-related hospitalizations of older individuals result from falls, and the injury rate from falls among senior citizens is nine times that of individuals younger than age 65. (See CANADA.)

See also ACCESSIBILITY TO FACILITIES; ACCIDENTAL INJURIES; ADVERSE DRUG EVENT; ALCOHOLISM; AMERICANS WITH DISABILITIES ACT; ASSISTIVE DEVICES/ASSISTED TECHNOLOGY; ELDERIZING A HOME; FAMILY AND MEDICAL LEAVE ACT; FRAILTY; GAIT DISORDERS; GENDER DIFFERENCES; HEALTH-CARE AGENT/PROXY; INAPPROPRIATE PRESCRIPTIONS FOR THE ELDERLY; OSTEOPOROSIS.

Centers for Disease Control and Prevention. "Fatalities and Injuries from Falls among Older Adults—United States, 1993–2003 and 2001–2005." *Morbidity and Mortality Weekly Report* 55, no. 45 (November 17, 2006): 1,221–1,224.
———. *The State of Aging and Health in America 2007.* Bethesda, Md.: National Institutes of Health, 2007.
Division of Aging and Seniors, Public Health Agency of Canada. *Report on Seniors' Falls in Canada.* Ottawa, Ontario: Minister of Public Works and Government Services, Canada, 2005.

Family and Medical Leave Act (FMLA) A federal law in the United States that provides for the circumstances under which employees at most companies must be allowed to take unpaid time off from work, either because of their own illness or the sickness of a child, spouse, or parent.

Some ADULT CHILDREN/CHILDREN OF AGING PARENTS use the provisions of the FMLA to take time off to care for their aging parents when they are ill or when their parents need to be accompanied to their doctor's appointments or medical treatments. In most cases (74.5 percent), other workers are temporarily assigned to cover the employee's job while he or she is away, and in an estimated 18 percent of cases, the company hires temporary outside replacement workers to do the work. In the balance of cases, the work is either put on hold or the employer uses some other method to cover the work of the absent employee.

Enacted by the U.S. Congress in 1993 and signed into law by President Clinton, the FMLA went into effect on August 5, 1993, and the initial regulations took effect on April 6, 1995. The law requires most employers in the United States (those with 50 or more workers) to allow employees who have worked for them for at least a year (and who have met other provisions of the law, such as having worked for at least 1,250 hours in the past year) to take up to 12 weeks of unpaid leave per year for their own medical problems or the problems of a spouse, child, or parent. The employee may also choose to combine their paid regular or sick leave from work with their FMLA leave.

According to the *Federal Register* in 2007, an estimated 76.1 million workers were covered by FMLA regulations in 2005. It was also estimated that between 6.1 to 13.0 million workers took FMLA leave in 2005. Leave may be taken for 12 consecutive weeks, or it may be split up into smaller increments, referred to as *intermittent leave,* according to the U.S. Department of Labor. It is the Department of Labor that enforces any violations of the FMLA. At least 25 percent of the workers who used FMLA in 2005 leave took at least part of it as intermittent leave.

A serious health condition in oneself or a family member is defined by the FMLA as "an illness, injury, impairment, or physical or medical treatment by a health-care provider." As a result, if a person is hospitalized and then needs to recuperate at home for some period, the FMLA would generally apply. However, hospitalization of oneself or a relative is not a prerequisite for using the provisions of the FMLA; many serious illnesses fulfill the conditions of the FMLA. For example, the FMLA specifically lists DIABETES under the law in 29 D.F.R.

§ 825.114(a)(1), (2), where it is one of five situations covered under "continuing treatment by a health-care provider."

That situation is defined as follows: "Any period of incapacity or treatment due to a chronic serious health condition requiring periodic visits for treatment, including episodic conditions such as asthma, diabetes, and epilepsy." Thus, if a person becomes ill or a child, spouse, or parent member becomes seriously ill, then the provisions to a spouse or a parent with a serious health condition would apply.

Many people do not use the entire 12 weeks, because unless the state law or company policy stipulates otherwise the leave is *unpaid,* and most people can afford to take only a few unpaid weeks off at most.

The employee has certain responsibilities under the law. For example, the employer must be notified of what the serious health condition is, although this can be reported confidentially. When the leave ends, the employer must allow the worker to come back to the same job or to a comparable job.

According to the *Federal Register* in June 2007, a family medical leave administrator reported:

> What I am seeing with increasing regularity are FMLA requests for employees to care for an elderly parent who is ill and not able to afford a caregiver to attend to his/her needs. These are usually for intermittent leaves that will allow the employee to chauffeur their parent to the doctor [or] attend to their parent post surgery.

To learn more about the FMLA, employees should contact their human resources departments.

See also AMERICANS WITH DISABILITIES ACT; DISABILTY; EMERGENCY DEPARTMENT CARE; FAMILY CAREGIVERS.

Lipnic, Victoria A., and Paul Decamp. "Family and Medical Leave Act Regulations: A Report on the Department of Labor's Request for Information." 2007 Update. June 2007. Available online. URL: http://www.dol.gov/esa/whd/fmla2007Report.htm. Downloaded February 14, 2008.

family caregivers Individuals, some of whom are retired themselves, who provide care and assistance to elderly people, usually a parent, grandparent, or other relative. The majority who provide caregiving (about 60 percent) are still working and must divide their time between the needs of their jobs, their immediate family, and their elderly relatives. Most family caregivers are female, but an increasing number are male relatives.

Family caregivers who provide care for a relative with DEMENTIA often suffer from considerable stress themselves. It is not only difficult to help a person with dementia, it is also emotionally painful because the family caregiver often remembers how vital and independent the person was before the dementia developed. Often they find themselves missing their mother, father, or other relative, because the person they are caring for now is very different and may not even recognize them.

In a study published in 2006 in the *Annals of Internal Medicine*, the researchers studied 642 in-home family caregivers of patients with dementia. The caregivers were Hispanic or Latino, white or black, and their relatives had ALZHEIMER'S DISEASE or a related disorder. The caregivers were divided into an intervention group or a control group.

The intervention group addressed such issues as caregiver depression, social support, self-care, and problem behaviors in the individual with dementia, while the control group did not receive this assistance. The caregivers in the control group received two brief phone calls during the six-month study period. The researchers also noted high levels of depressive symptoms among both groups of family caregivers when the study began.

The researchers found white or Hispanic/Latino family caregivers who were in the intervention group had a significantly improved quality of life compared to those in the control group, but the black caregivers in the intervention group did not have a significantly improved quality of life. Interestingly, the researchers found statistically significant quality-of-life improvements among blacks who provided caregiving to their spouse. The researchers also found that the prevalence of clinical depression was lower in the caregivers of all races/ethnicities in the intervention group when compared to the rate of depression in those in the control group.

See also ADULT CHILDREN/CHILDREN OF AGING PARENTS; BABY BOOMERS; COMPASSION FATIGUE; FAM-ILY AND MEDICAL LEAVE ACT; HEALTH-CARE AGENT/PROXY; LONG-DISTANCE CARE; SIBLING RIVALRY AND CONFLICT; TALKING TO ELDERLY PARENTS ABOUT DIFFICULT ISSUES.

Belle, Steven H., et al. "Enhancing the Quality of Life of Dementia Caregivers from Different Ethnic or Racial Groups: A Randomized Controlled Trial." *Annals of Internal Medicine* 145 (2006): 727–738.

fecal incontinence Difficulty or impossibility in managing daily bowel movements. This problem may be caused by a lactose intolerance. It may also be a side effect of some medications, or may be caused by a MEDICATION INTERACTION, or by many other medical problems. The individual with fecal incontinence should consult with a physician because in many cases, the cause of the problem can be identified and resolved. However, in some cases, the fecal incontinence cannot be controlled, and the older person will need to rely upon adult diapers.

See also DIAPERS, ADULT; URINARY INCONTINENCE.

fire risks and the elderly Fires are extremely dangerous and distressing for elderly individuals, especially when they have one or more disabilities and may find it difficult or impossible to leave a building rapidly. In addition, people who may have only recently lost their sight have not yet developed an increased reliance on their hearing and may revert to touching items in order to move about, a dangerous situation when a fire is present. Continuous high-decibel smoke alarms may also impede the hearing of many elderly individuals.

As is seen in Table 1, individuals ages 65 and older have a higher death rate than the risk for the entire population in the United States. For example, the death rate per million among all males in the United States in 2001 was 17.5, but the death rate for all older adults was 35.4 per million. The relative risk of dying in a fire was computed for all categories, and the rate for older African-American males was the highest or 9.7 times the risk compared to the relative risk for the overall population of 1.0 (See Table 1). It may be that African Americans are

TABLE 1. FIRE FATALITIES AND RELATIVE RISK FOR OLDER ADULTS, 2001

Gender/Race	2001 Fire Deaths	Death Rate per Million	Relative Risk
Total	4,007	14.0	1.0
Male	2,455	17.5	1.2
Female	1,552	10.7	0.8
White	2,908	12.6	0.9
African American	1,006	27.7	2.0
American Indian	49	18.1	1.3
Asian/Pacific	44	3.8	0.3
White male	1,777	15.6	1.1
African-American male	616	35.7	2.5
American Indian male	33	24.3	1.7
Asian/Pacific male	29	5.2	0.4
White female	1,131	9.7	0.7
African-American female	390	20.5	1.5
American Indian female	16	11.8	0.8
Asian/Pacific female	15	2.5	0.2
All older adults (Age 65+)			
Total	1,250	35.4	2.5
Male	638	43.6	3.1
Female	612	29.5	2.1
White	942	30.2	2.2
African American	283	97.1	6.9
American Indian	8	51.7	3.7
Asian/Pacific	17	18.8	1.3
White male	473	36.5	2.6
African American male	151	135.7	9.7
American Indian male	5	74.9	5.3
Asian/Pacific male	9	23.4	1.7
White female	469	25.8	1.8
African-American female	132	73.2	5.2
American Indian female	3	34.0	2.4
Asian/Pacific female	8	15.4	1.1

Source: Adapted from United States Fire Administration/National Fire Data Center. *Fire and the Older Adult.* Department of Homeland Security, January 2006, page 35. Available online. URL: http://www.usfa.dhs.gov/statistics/reports/older.shtm. Accessed February 20, 2008.

in poorer health and/or they are more likely to live in POVERTY, but further investigation is needed to determine the causes.

The risk for death from a fire increases with age. According to the U.S. Fire Administration report, individuals ages 65 to 74 years old were 1.8 times more likely than the general population to die in a fire in 2001. That risk increased to 2.8 times for those ages 75 to 84 years and further increased to 4.6 times more likely to die for adults age 85 years and older.

Elderly Individuals Have an Increased Risk for Injuries and Deaths

According to the United States Fire Administration report *Fire and the Older Adult*, about 1,000 Americans age 65 years and older die in a home fire every year and more than 2,000 elderly people are injured each year in fires. Older adults are 2.5 times more likely to die in a fire than are younger individuals. In addition, older men are more likely to die from a fire than older women. African Americans and American Indians have a higher risk of death from a fire than whites (see Table 1).

Sensory and cognitive impairments among older adults increase their risk for injury or death. For example, often people rely on their sense of smell to detect fire; however, this sense diminishes with age. In addition, older people may have an impaired sense of smell due to sinus disease or neurodegenerative diseases such as PARKINSON'S DISEASE or ALZHEIMER'S DISEASE. The sense of touch may be impaired among older people, who may also experience thinning of the skin. Some of the reasons for these skin changes include the following:

- more fragile blood vessels than in the past
- cumulative effects of sun exposure
- side effects of medications
- dehydration
- natural thinning of the skin's outer layer with aging
- changes in connective tissue that reduce the strength and elasticity of the skin

Impairments in sight and sound also contribute to the inadequate response to fires that the elderly may experience. For example, research by the Consumer Product Safety Commission in 2003 revealed that older adults had difficulty hearing or responding to the sound of smoke detectors.

EYE DISEASES, SERIOUS, contribute to difficulty in responding to fires, and many older people experience such eye problems as GLAUCOMA, CATARACTS, and macular degeneration.

Memory impairments and dementia contribute to a failure to respond to a fire emergency. According to the authors of *Fire and the Older Adult*, "Accidents, falls, and contact with dangerous substances are more prevalent among dementia patients, and for such patients, living quarters should be modified to remove anything within reach that could pose a potential fire risk."

DEPRESSION is another contributor to the failure to respond to a fire emergency. Older individuals who are depressed may be confused or fatigued. They may also be suicidal and see the fire as a sign that they should die. Untreated depression is very dangerous for older individuals.

Older individuals may also be impaired by ALCOHOLISM or SUBSTANCE ABUSE, including PRESCRIPTION DRUG ABUSE, and thus may fail to respond adequately or at all to a serious fire emergency.

Education and Preparation Are Key

Adult children and others can reduce the risk of harm to their elderly relatives by helping them obtain good medical care and ensuring their eyesight is as good as possible. In addition, they should practice escape routes in a fire drill manner with the older adult to ensure that the older person knows the quickest route to leave the area. It should be stressed that belongings are not as important as the individual's life, and personal possessions should be left behind.

See also EMERGENCY DEPARTMENT CARE; SUICIDE.

United States Fire Administration/National Fire Data Center. *Fire and the Older Adult.* Department of Homeland Security, January 2006. Available online. URL: http://www.usfa.dhs.gov/statistics/reports/older.shtm. Accessed February 20, 2008.

flu/influenza A highly contagious viral infection that occurs annually and has been a known problem since the 16th century. The virus was isolated for the first time in 1933. Transmission of the flu virus occurs through direct or indirect contact, such as by an individual touching a contaminated surface and then touching the mouth, nose, or eyes and transmitting the disease to himself, herself, and/or others.

Most elderly individuals are advised to be immunized against influenza each year because new versions of the flu develop annually, and also because older people have a greater risk than most other groups of suffering severe consequences up to and including death if they contract the flu. In fact, most of the people (90 percent) who die from the flu are age 65 and older. Older people also have the highest rates of hospitalizations and complications from the flu.

TABLE 1. PERCENTAGE OF ADULTS AGE 65 AND OLDER WHO REPORTED RECEIVING INFLUENZA VACCINE DURING THE PRECEDING 12 MONTHS, 2004–2005

State/Area	2004	2005
Alabama	66.2	60.8
Alaska	64.1	61.1
Arizona	66.2	62.5
Arkansas	68.7	65.2
California	70.9	65.9
Colorado	78.8	74.2
Connecticut	73.1	71.1
Delaware	69.3	65.8
District of Columbia	54.9	54.7
Florida	65.1	55.6
Georgia	64.4	60.8
Hawaii	unknown	72.1
Idaho	66.2	63.9
Illinois	65.4	55.9
Indiana	64.3	64.0
Iowa	74.1	71.7
Kansas	68.1	66.0
Kentucky	64.3	62.4
Louisiana	68.6	62.4
Maine	72.2	67.8
Maryland	64.6	59.3
Massachusetts	70.6	69.8
Michigan	66.9	67.1
Minnesota	78.3	78.2
Mississippi	66.9	61.5
Missouri	69.1	61.7
Montana	72.2	69.5
Nebraska	75.8	72.6
Nevada	59.0	53.0
New Hampshire	70.7	70.2
New Jersey	67.6	63.4
New Mexico	72.4	68.0
New York	65.9	61.8
North Carolina	67.0	65.5
North Dakota	74.3	70.1
Ohio	67.6	64.7
Oklahoma	75.0	73.2
Oregon	71.1	68.9
Pennsylvania	63.8	59.3
Rhode Island	73.0	67.2
South Carolina	66.0	60.9
South Dakota	76.9	76.3
Tennessee	66.4	61.6
Texas	67.1	61.6
Utah	75.5	69.6
Vermont	66.6	66.3
Virginia	68.6	66.8
Washington	67.9	67.8
West Virginia	67.9	63.6
Wisconsin	74.3	71.8
Wyoming	73.8	72.9
Puerto Rico	35.3	32.0
U.S. Virgin Islands	39.4	37.5
Median	**67.9**	**65.5**

Source: Adapted from Centers for Disease Control and Prevention, "Percentage of Adults Aged 65 Years and Older Who Reported Receiving Influenza Vaccine During the Preceding 12 Months and Percentage of Adults Aged 65 Year and Older Who Reported Ever Receiving Pneumococcal Vaccine, by State/Area, United States, Behavioral Risk Factor Surveillance System, 2004–2005." *Morbidity and Mortality Weekly Report* 55, no. 9 (October 6, 2006), Atlanta, Ga.: Centers for Disease Control and Prevention, p. 1,066.

Yet many older individuals still fail to receive the flu vaccine. According to the National Center for Health Statistics, older whites are much more likely to receive a flu shot than blacks or Hispanics/Latinos. For example, in 2004, 67.3 percent of whites age 65 and older received a flu shot compared to 54.6 percent of Hispanics/Latinos and less than half (45.7 percent) of blacks.

According to the Centers for Disease Control and Prevention (CDC), in 2005, a median of 65.6 percent of individuals age 65 and older received a flu shot, down from 67.9 percent in 2004. (A median is a statistic that means half the people were below this percentage and half were above. It is a middle point and a better measure than an average.)

The percentages of older individuals receiving flu shots in the states and U.S. territories ranged greatly in 2005, from a low of 32 percent in Puerto Rico to a high of 78.2 percent in Minnesota. (See Table 1.) The reason for this decease may have been a shortage of flu vaccine in 2005 because of a shortage of manufacturers, a problem that has since been corrected. According to the CDC, in most years, a great deal of unused flu vaccine is left over, indicating that many more people could have

TABLE 2. PERCENTAGE OF PEOPLE AGE 65 AND OLDER WHO REPORTED HAVING BEEN VACCINATED AGAINST INFLUENZA AND PNEUMOCOCCAL DISEASE, BY RACE AND HISPANIC ORIGIN, 2003–2004

Year	White	Black	Hispanic or Latino
Influenza			
2003	68.6	47.8	45.4
2004	67.3	45.7	54.6
Pneumococcal disease			
2003	59.6	37.0	31.0
2004	60.9	38.6	33.7

Source: Federal Interagency Forum on Aging Related Statistics. "Older Americans Update 2006: Key Indicators of Well-Being." Hyattsville, Md.: National Center for Health Statistics, 32, 2006.

been immunized against this potentially dangerous disease.

In considering the race of those who received a flu or pneumonia shot in 2004–2005, whites were the most likely to receive injections and blacks were the least likely. (See Table 2.)

Symptoms and Diagnostic Path

The flu is transmitted through the respiratory system, and it may cause an abrupt fever (of about 101°–102°F), chills, runny nose, lack of appetite, and severe fatigue. The affected individual may also have a cough, headache, and aches throughout the body, but especially in the back. Some people also have eye pain and become sensitive to light until they recover. The flu generally lasts two to three days.

Influenza is diagnosed by its symptoms in the individual. It is also diagnosed in part by the prevalence of influenza in the general area. The flu virus can be cultured from swabs of the throat or nose, but this procedure is rarely done because the culture takes 48 hours to grow and it takes another two days to determine the type of virus. As a result, it is not practical to take a culture, since most people will have recovered from their illness by the time the culture results become available.

Treatment Options and Outlook

Once the flu has been contracted, measures should be taken to keep down the fever and manage other symptoms. Acetaminophen or ibuprofen may be taken to reduce the fever and decrease pain from muscle aches. The patient may also be given a sponge bath to lower the fever. If the symptoms become severe, such as a very high fever or copious vomiting, the patient may need to be hospitalized.

Risk Factors and Preventive Measures

One common complication of the flu is infection with bacterial pneumonia, such as *Streptococcus pneumoniae* or *Staphylococcus aureus*. In addition, patients may have a worsening of chronic bronchitis or even experience inflammation of the heart (myocarditis).

As mentioned, immunization is recommended for individuals age 65 and older. The vaccine does not prevent all older people from catching the flu, according to the CDC. However, it does demonstrably reduce the risk for complications and death among those who contract the flu despite having been immunized. For example, the vaccine is 50 to 60 percent effective at preventing hospitalization and 80 percent effective at preventing death. In one flu outbreak in Michigan in 1982–83, the NURSING HOME residents who were not immunized for influenza were four times more likely to die than were the immunized residents.

It is also important for individuals to regularly wash their hands, particularly after using the bathroom, and whenever possible, avoiding others who are coughing and clearly seriously ill.

See also INFECTIONS; PNEUMONIA.

Centers for Disease Control and Prevention. *Epidemiology and Prevention of Vaccine Preventable Diseases*. 10th Edition. Washington, D.C.: National Institutes of Health, 2007, pp. 235–256.

———. "Percentage of Adults Aged 65 and Older Who Reported Receiving Influenza Vaccine During the Preceding 12 Months and Percentage of Adults Aged 65 Years and Older Who Reported Ever Receiving Pneumococcal Vaccine, by State/Area, United States, Behavioral Risk Factor Surveillance System, 2004–2005." *Morbidity and Mortality Weekly Report* 55, no. 9 (October 6, 2006), Atlanta, Ga.: Centers for Disease Control and Prevention.

fractures Breaks of a bone. Fractures can be very dangerous and debilitating for those age 65 and older. According to the Centers for Disease Control and Prevention (CDC), between 360,000 and 480,000 older adults experience fractures related to accidental FALLS in the home or elsewhere each year.

Fractures are more commonly found among individuals with OSTEOPOROSIS, and fractures that occur in the wrist, hip, forearm, or the back are the most common among individuals with osteoporosis. Fractures of the hip often lead to HOSPITALIZATION, and many who have broken a hip do not recover their former level of independence and may have to be relocated to a NURSING HOME. DEPRESSION is common among those who suffer a major fracture.

Fractures may also be caused by physical ABUSE, and sometimes physicians mistakenly attribute fractures to osteoporosis or to simple accidents when, in fact, the older individual has been abused by others. Doctors sometimes may even refuse to believe the older person who says that he or she was abused, assuming that such an accusation must be a sign of DEMENTIA. (See AGEISM.)

Genetics and Fractures

Some studies indicate there may be a genetic risk for fractures in the elderly, although no specific gene has been identified to date. In a study of thousands of Swedish twins born between 1896 and 1944 and published in the *Archives of Internal Medicine* in 2005, the researchers found the heritability of first hip fractures was the greatest among individuals before age 69, followed by the age range of 69 to 79 years.

The researchers found that one in five twins, or more than 6,000 individuals with fractures, had suffered a fracture after age 50, with a greater risk for fractures among females. More than half the fractures were associated with osteoporosis, and osteoporotic hip fracture was found in more than 1,000 of the twins. According to the researchers,

> The results of our study demonstrated that heritability for fracture is dependent on site and age. These findings are important for efforts to target effective interventions against osteoporotic fractures. Our results indicate that hip fracture preventure [sic] strategies should be focused on lifestyle intervention in the oldest elderly. On the

other hand, especially hip but even other types of osteoporotic fractures at younger ages seem to be strongly genetically influenced.

Fractures, Falls, and Limitations of Activity

It is estimated that 95 percent of all hip fractures experienced by elderly individuals are caused by falls, and at least three-fourths of all hip fractures are incurred by older females. Survivors of hip fractures often experience significant DISABILITY. In addition, the risk for death from hip fractures is high, and up to an estimated 20 percent of individuals with hip fractures die within a year.

As might be expected, fractures significantly limit the activities of those who experience them, and this limitation is the greatest among those aged 75 years and older. For example, 25.4 of 1,000 people ages 65 to 74 years experience limited activity because of fractures or joint injuries they have suffered. This rate increases to 48.6 per 1,000 for those age 75 years and older.

See also ABUSE; ACCIDENTAL INJURIES; AMERICANS WITH DISABILITIES ACT; ASSISTIVE DEVICES/ASSISTED TECHNOLOGY; FAMILY AND MEDICAL LEAVE ACT; FRAILTY; INAPPROPRIATE PRESCRIPTIONS FOR THE ELDERLY.

He, Wan, Manisha Sengupta, Victoria A. Velkoff, and Kimberly A. DeBarros. *65+ in the United States: 2005.* Washington, D.C.: U.S. Census Bureau, December 2005.

Michaelsson, Karl, et al. "Genetic Liability to Fractures in the Elderly." *Archives of Internal Medicine* 165 (September 12, 2005): 1,825–1,830.

frailty Chronic weakness. According to Doctors Boockvar and Meier, frailty in older adults has the following primary signs:

- slowed performance
- weight loss
- low activity levels
- poor endurance or fatigue
- loss of strength

When three or more of these features are present, the older person is at risk for FALLS, HOSPITALIZATION, and even DEATH. Frailty is linked with long-term disease, and if the frailty becomes severe, the individual may need PALLIATIVE CARE to provide pain relief for chronic health problems.

Some experts distinguish primary frailty from secondary frailty. Primary frailty refers to frailty when there is no apparent disease present. Secondary frailty refers to frailty when there are one or more known advanced and serious diseases. Those with secondary frailty are believed to have a worse prognosis.

Frail adults may have decreased endocrine function, such as low thyroid levels, and they may have an accelerated loss of muscle mass and strength, particularly after age 75. They may also have decreased levels of testosterone, estrogen, and growth hormone. According to Boockvar and Meier, frailty can be categorized into three stages: an early stage when the frailty is first recognized; a middle stage when the decline in function begins; and a late stage when the patient is suffering from life-threatening illnesses and death will occur soon.

Physical frailty may be seen as simply a sign of old age by doctors and family members, but it should be addressed so that the patient can be treated for underlying medical problems such as CANCER, chronic INFECTIONS, MEDICATION INTERACTIONS, or other causes that are readily treatable.

Specific signs, such as weakness, can be improved with exercise, while weight loss can be halted through the use of high-calorie nutritional supplements and frequent small meals. Care should be taken to ensure that the patient can eat and does not have problems with dentures. Often frail older adults are depressed, and ANTIDEPRESSANTS can improve these conditions. (Antidepressants are also associated with a risk for falls, however, so precautions should be taken.)

The physicians and families of patients who are frail should also talk to them about advance directives such as a LIVING WILL, so that the doctor and the relatives know what the patient wants should he or she become extremely ill and require tube feeding, CARDIOPULMONARY RESUSCITATION, or other heroic measures to stay alive.

See also ACCIDENTAL INJURIES; ACTIVITIES OF DAILY LIVING; AMERICANS WITH DISABILITIES ACT; ASSISTIVE DEVICES/ASSISTED TECHNOLOGY; END-OF-LIFE ISSUES; EXERCISE; FAMILY AND MEDICAL LEAVE ACT; FRACTURES; GERIATRICIAN; HEALTH-CARE AGENT/PROXY; HOME CARE; HOSPICE; MEDICATION MANAGEMENT; NURSING HOMES; NUTRITION; SARCOPENIA; TALKING TO ELDERLY PARENTS ABOUT DIFFICULT ISSUES.

Boockvar, Kenneth S., M.D., and Diane E. Meier, M.D. "Palliative Care for Frail Older Adults: 'There Are Things I Can't Do Anymore That I Wish I Could . . .'" *Journal of the American Medical Association* 296, no. 18 (November 8, 2006): 2,245–2,253.

fraud   See CRIMES AGAINST THE ELDERLY; MEDICARE.

frequent nightmares   See NIGHTMARES, FREQUENT.

funerals   Ceremonies and rituals that are meant to honor a deceased person as well as to provide comfort to bereaved surviving family members, friends, coworkers, and others. Funerals may be very elaborate and complex functions with hundreds or even thousands of attendees, or they may be very private and small family affairs, depending on the needs and wishes of the family. The funeral gives those who loved the deceased person an opportunity to express their feelings publicly and to share their sadness with others.

Related to the funeral are the many different ways that grieving family members decide to commemorate the death of their loved ones. For example, some individuals choose to plant a tree or a flowering bush in remembrance of the deceased. Others choose to give the funeral director specific meaningful items to include in the casket. In his 2004 article in *Generations* on remembrances of loved ones author Reiko Schwab says,

> In a loving farewell, we may place in the casket some of the items that the deceased kept close to the heart. Some of us may also wish to give something we value as a parting gift to the deceased—for example, an Eagle Scout badge from a son to his father, with whom the son enjoyed so many camping trips.

Schwab says that others try to improve the situation of whatever caused the death of their loved ones, such as with programs to prevent drunken driving if the deceased was killed by a drunk driver, or helping cancer patients if the deceased died of cancer. Others donate money and/or time for research on the cause of their loved one's death.

Funerals can be extremely difficult to plan for the grieving widows, widowers, and other family members, and they may need assistance from others in the family to make decisions about caskets, the funeral ceremony itself, and other choices. Sometimes individuals try to prevent their older family members or disabled family members from attending the funerals of their friends and family members in a misguided attempt to protect them from emotional pain. Experts say that it is usually better to allow elderly individuals and others to attend funerals and grieve their losses.

See also BEREAVEMENT; CEMETERY, CHOICE OF; CREMATION; DEATH; DEATH, FEAR OF; END-OF-LIFE ISSUES.

Cassell, Dana K., Robert C. Salinas, M.D., and Peter A. S. Winn, M.D. *The Encyclopedia of Death and Dying.* New York: Facts On File, 2005.

Schwab, Reiko. "Acts of Remembrance, Cherished Possessions, and Living Memorials." *Generations* 27, no. 11 (Summer 2004): 26–30.

gait disorders Difficulty or awkwardness in walking and movement, which may be caused by a variety of medical problems or other causes, including sedating medications, PARKINSON'S DISEASE, and other illnesses. Some individuals with ALZHEIMER'S DISEASE and other forms of DEMENTIA may exhibit gait disorders. Gait disorders significantly increase the risk of FALLS, which may in turn lead to serious injuries and FRACTURES. Gait disorders are important to diagnose and treat because victims are at considerable risk of further deterioration without treatment.

Many gait disorders are not detected, often because the physician does not observe the patient walking, and also because the patients themselves do not realize that they are walking abnormally. The patient also may mistakenly think that his or her abnormal gait is a normal part of aging.

Symptoms and Diagnostic Path

Gait disorders are manifested in difficulty with walking and pacing and in unusually slow walking. Often there will be a stooped posture. Some types of gait disorders are associated with difficulty with starting or stopping walking. Balance may also be impaired in a person with a gait disorder. Physicians observe the patient walking and they also have a variety of tests to check the patient's gait. For example, the doctor may have the person sit on a chair and then observe the patient standing and walking away from the chair. Neurological tests may be performed, such as having the patient walk (or try to walk) on the toes or heels or with a narrow or tandem stance or even stand with both feet close together with their eyes closed.

Treatment Options and Outlook

If a gait disorder is diagnosed, physical therapy can often improve the condition. Exercises have also been shown to reduce the risk of falls in those with gait disorders. Walking can improve mobility as well. One of the best exercises is walking in a pool, as often seniors with a gait disturbance will also develop a fear of falling, and being in the water eliminates that fear. Balance training is another excellent measure to correct impaired walking.

Risk Factors and Preventive Measures

Patients with PARKINSON'S DISEASE or degenerative joint disease are at risk for developing gait disorders. In addition, patients who have had a STROKE or who have peripheral neuropathy or a Vitamin B_{12} deficiency are also at risk for developing gait disorders. The use of alcohol and some medications, such as diuretics, antiarrhythmics, antihypertensive drugs, or sedating medications, can further amplify the risk.

See also ADVERSE DRUG EVENT; HEALTH-CARE AGENT/PROXY; VITAMIN AND MINERAL DEFICIENCIES/EXCESSES.

gambling Although many older Americans enjoy playing occasional games of bingo, cards, and other games of chance, as well as purchasing tickets from state lotteries, most of them do not have a serious problem with gambling. However, some elderly individuals do have such a problem, and they also have a higher rate of substance abuse and psychiatric disorders as well as health problems.

In a study published in the *American Journal of Geriatric Psychiatry* in 2006, the researchers discussed factors present in older adults who were non-gamblers, lifetime recreational gamblers, and disordered gamblers: Recreational gamblers enjoyed gambling but it was not harmful to their lives; disordered gamblers included problem gamblers, who met some, but not all, of the full diagnostic criteria for pathological gambling; and pathological gamblers, whose constant betting had impeded their family, social, and career pursuits. The researchers analyzed data from over 10,000 adults age 60 and older and found that less than 29 percent of the subjects were recreational gamblers and less than 1 percent were disordered gamblers.

The researchers compared older adult non-gamblers to both the recreational gamblers and the disordered gamblers. They found that recreational gamblers had higher rates of alcohol use disorders and nicotine use than the non-gamblers, and they also had higher rates of mood and anxiety disorders. Among the pathological gamblers, the situation was significantly worse, with much higher rates of alcohol use disorders and use of nicotine and higher percentages of psychiatric disorders than found in the two other categories. (See Table 1.)

As can be seen in Table 1, drug use disorders were not common among the elderly population studied in any of the categories that were considered. However, disordered gamblers had more than five times the risk for a drug use disorder (4.59 percent) than did non-gamblers (0.75 percent).

Many health problems were also more common among the disordered gamblers in this study. (See Table 2.) For example, the researchers found that pathological gamblers were significantly more likely to have a past-year diagnosis of angina and ARTHRITIS. For example, 44.3 percent of the non-regular gamblers had arthritis compared to 60.2 percent of the pathological gamblers. In addition, 8.8 percent of the non-regular gamblers had experienced angina compared to 22.7 percent of the pathological gamblers.

As can be seen in Table 2, in some cases the recreational gamblers had a slightly better health outlook than the non-gamblers; for example, about 5 percent of the recreational gamblers had ARTERIOSCLEROSIS compared to about 6 percent of the non-gamblers. In addition, about 8 percent of the recreational gamblers had angina (a heart condition) compared to about 9 percent of the non-gamblers.

However, the disordered gamblers fared significantly worse than the other two groups in every health category and had a much higher rate of health problems. According to the researchers,

> Previous studies have similarly noted increased cardiovascular and musculoskeletal symptoms among adult disordered gamblers. . . . Disordered gamblers may experience more stress, be more sedentary, and participate in fewer health-related activities than their nongambling or nondisordered gambling counterparts, which may increase the likelihood of their developing medical conditions such as angina and arthritis. Alternatively, individuals with physical limitations may be drawn to gambling insofar as it does not require much physical activity and provides entertainment.

The researchers concluded, "Because older adults rarely seek mental health services and treatment-seeking for gambling is particularly uncommon, screenings for lifetime gambling participation and problems in primary care settings may be warranted for some older adults."

See also ALCOHOLISM; ANXIETY AND ANXIETY DISORDERS; DEPRESSION; DRUG ABUSE; SUBSTANCE ABUSE AND DEPENDENCE.

TABLE 1. PERCENTAGES OF PSYCHIATRIC AND MEDICAL DISORDERS AMONG OLDER ADULTS WHO DO NOT GAMBLE, GAMBLE RECREATIONALLY, OR WHO ARE PATHOLOGICAL GAMBLERS

Category of Gambler	Any Alcohol Use Disorder	Any Drug Use Disorder	Use of Nicotine	Mood Disorders	Anxiety Disorders
Non-gamblers	12.8	0.75	8.0	11.0	11.6
Recreational Gamblers	30.1	1.18	16.9	12.6	15.0
"Disordered" Gamblers (Problem gamblers and pathological gamblers)	53.2	4.59	43.2	39.5	34.5

Source: Adapted from Pietrzak, Robert H., et al. "Gambling Level and Psychiatric and Medical Disorders in Older Adults: Results from the National Epidemiologic Survey on Alcohol and Related Conditions." *American Journal of Geriatric Psychiatry* 14, no. 1 (2006): 301–313.

TABLE 2. PREVALENCE OF HEALTH PROBLEMS AMONG OLDER NON-GAMBLERS, RECREATIONAL GAMBLERS, AND DISORDERED GAMBLERS, BY PERCENTAGE OF EACH POPULATION

Category of Gambler	Hypertension	Tachycardia	Arteriosclerosis	Angina	Myocardial Infarction	Arthritis
Non-gamblers	44	8	6	9	3	44
Recreational Gamblers	46	9	5	8	2	40
"Disordered" Gamblers (Problem gamblers and pathological gamblers)	51	17	8	23	5	60

Source: Adapted from Pietrzak, Robert H., et al. "Gambling Level and Psychiatric and Medical Disorders in Older Adults: Results from the National Epidemiologic Survey on Alcohol and Related Conditions." *American Journal of Geriatric Psychiatry* 14, no. 1 (2006): 301–313.

Pietrzak, Robert H., et al. "Gambling Level and Psychiatric and Medical Disorders in Older Adults: Results from the National Epidemiologic Survey on Alcohol and Related Conditions." *American Journal of Geriatric Psychiatry* 14, no. 1 (2006): 301–313.

gastroenterologist See CANCER; COLORECTAL CANCER; COLONOSCOPY; PANCREATIC CANCER; STOMACH CANCER.

gender differences Aging can affect men and women differently in many ways; for example, according to the National Center for Health Statistics, most women live longer than most men. However, in one unique study of older men who survived to at least age 90, reported in a 2008 issue of the *Archives of Internal Medicine*, the researchers studied 970 men who lived to age 90 or beyond to seek modifiable risk behaviors in these long-lived men. Concluded the researchers, "Modifiable healthy behaviors during early elderly years, including smoking abstinence, weight management, blood pressure control, and regular exercise, are associated not only with enhanced life span in men but also with good health and function during older age."

Some diseases are more common in women or in men. Women age 65 and older are more likely to suffer from and be limited in their activities by ARTHRITIS, according to the Centers for Disease Control and Prevention (CDC) in an analysis published in the *Journal of Women's Health* in 2007. In contrast, men are more likely to suffer from any form of cancer, according to the National Cancer Institute. The CDC reports that men are also more likely to suffer from heart disease than women. Yet women are more likely to develop rheumatoid arthritis, according to the National Institute of Arthritis and Musculoskeletal and Skin Diseases.

According to the National Center for Health Statistics, older men have a greater risk for heart disease than older women, and 37 percent of men ages 65 and older had heart disease in 2004 compared to 28 percent of older women.

Of course, some diseases and disorders are inherently gender based; for example, most people who get breast cancer are female, according to the National Cancer Institute, and all people who get prostate cancer or other prostatic diseases are male.

Women, especially those who are petite and/or Asian, are more likely than men to suffer from OSTEOPOROSIS, according to the National Institutes of Health, and women are also more likely to be diagnosed with PARKINSON'S DISEASE. Older women are also more likely to suffer from joint pain than older men, according to the CDC.

The National Eye Institute reports that women are more likely than men to suffer from age-related macular degeneration, a serious eye disease that can lead to blindness. Older women are also more likely than men to suffer from glaucoma, which may cause severe headaches.

In considering common headaches, according to Doctors Kandel and Sudderth in their book *The Headache Cure*, women are more likely to suffer from tension headaches and migraines, while men are more likely to suffer from cluster headaches.

(See EYE DISEASES, SERIOUS; HEADACHES.) Men have a greater risk for HEARING DISORDERS than women, according to the CDC. In considering all older men and women, the National Center for Health Statistics reports that 55 percent of women ages 65 and older had hypertension in 2004 compared to 48 percent of older men. (See HYPERTENSION.)

In considering accidental injuries, women are more likely to be injured from FALLS than men are; however, men are more likely to die from falls than women, according to the CDC. Women are also more likely to use HOME CARE than men, according to the National Center for Health Statistics, which also reports that women are more likely to have knee and hip replacements than men are. (See JOINT REPLACEMENT.) Men are more likely to develop ALCOHOLISM than women are, but women are more likely to become alcoholics at a later age than men. Older men are also more likely than older women to be admitted to treatment centers for substance abuse. (See SUBSTANCE ABUSE AND DEPENDENCE.)

Older women are more likely than older men to need assistance with daily activities, according to the CDC; for example, 53.4 percent of men and 60.7 percent of women in the age group of 75 to 79 years need assistance. Of those who are ages 80 and older, 68.2 percent of men and 76.7 percent of women need help with their daily activities. (See ACTIVITIES OF DAILY LIVING.)

In considering psychiatric illnesses, older women are more likely to suffer from DEPRESSION than men, according to the National Institute of Mental Health (NIMH). However, NIMH reports that older men are more likely to die from SUICIDE than are older women. Older men are more likely to be diagnosed with DIABETES than older women.

Older men also have a greater risk for EMPHYSEMA than older women, probably because more older men were smokers in their adult years than older women. Older men are more likely to die from a car crash than older women, according to the CDC. (See DRIVING.)

Older men are more likely to remarry than are older women, according to the National Center for Health Statistics (See MARRIAGE/REMARRIAGE.) In addition, older women are more likely to live alone than men, according to the Census Bureau. (See

HOUSING/LIVING ARRANGEMENTS.) According to the Census Bureau, older women are also more likely to live in NURSING HOMES than older men, in large part because most women live to an older age than most men.

According to the Department of Health and Human Services, older women were more likely to be impoverished (12.3 percent) than were older men (7.3 percent) in 2005. (See POVERTY.)

In considering aging military veterans, most are male because most people who served in World War II or the Korean War were male; however, increasing numbers of aging female veterans will be an issue since many female baby boomers served in the Vietnam War and thereafter. Individuals who are injured or became ill while on active duty may be eligible for long-term benefits through the Department of Veterans Affairs. (See VETERAN BENEFITS.)

See also RACIAL AND ETHNIC DIFFERENCES; SUBSTANCE ABUSE AND DEPENDENCE.

Kandel, Joseph, M.D., and David Sudderth, M.D. *The Headache Cure.* New York: McGraw-Hill, 2005.
Theis, Kristina A., Charles G. Helmick, M.D., and Jennifer M. Hootman. "Arthritis Burden and Impact Are Greater Among U.S. Women than Men: Intervention Opportunities." *Journal of Women's Health* 16, no. 4 (2007): 441–453.
Yates, Laurel B., M.D., et al. "Exceptional Longevity in Men: Modifiable Factors Associated with Survival and Function to Age 90 Years." *Archives of Internal Medicine* 168, no. 3 (February 11, 2008): 284–290.

geriatrician A physician who has obtained one or two years additional training in the medical and social needs of older people and who specializes in treating individuals age 65 and older. Many doctors who treat the elderly are not geriatricians, but instead they are general internists or specialists in the chronic medical problems of the particular patient, whether it is the neurologist for chronic HEADACHES or BACK PAIN, the rheumatologist for ARTHRITIS, the oncologist for CANCER, and so on. Some doctors prefer to treat younger patients, while other doctors like to treat people of all ages. The geriatrician treats only older people.

See also END-OF-LIFE ISSUES; PALLIATIVE CARE.

glaucoma   A disease that damages the optic nerve of the eye. Open-angled glaucoma is the most common form of this disease, and it is caused by a buildup of fluid in the eye, which causes the eye pressure to increase. According to the National Institutes of Health (NIH), glaucoma is the leading cause of BLINDNESS in the United States. About 3 million people in the United States have glaucoma.

Note that Medicare will pay for an annual dilated eye examination for these categories of individuals

- African Americans age 50 years and older
- individuals with a family history of glaucoma
- individuals with diabetes

Symptoms and Diagnostic Path

There are usually no symptoms in the early stages of glaucoma. As a result, annual eye checkups performed by an optometrist or ophthalmologist are recommended because these exams can detect the early stages of glaucoma before serious damage has occurred.

If untreated, as glaucoma progresses, the individual may experience fading side vision and, if the disease remains untreated, eventually the person will lose all peripheral vision. Ultimately blindness will occur.

The "air puff" test, in which a burst of air is applied to the eye, and other tests may be used to measure eye pressure during an eye examination; however, glaucoma is more frequently detected during an eye examination when the pupils have been dilated (enlarged) by chemical eye drops that the optometrist or ophthalmologist has inserted.

Treatment Options and Outlook

Prescription eye drops are frequently used to treat glaucoma. According to the National Eye Institute, eye drops or oral medications are the first line of treatment against glaucoma, and they may help to lower the eye pressure or cause the eye to make less fluid. If eye drops do not sufficiently lower eye pressure, then surgery may be indicated. For example, laser trabeculoplasty burns tiny holes in the eye and allows for fluid drainage. One eye is treated at a time, and treatments are performed four to six weeks apart.

Before this outpatient procedure, the doctor numbs the eye and then aims a laser at the eye to burn tiny holes in the eye and enable fluid drainage. The patient may see flashes of red or green light during this procedure. If the patient has glaucoma in both eyes, one eye is treated at a time, and treatments are scheduled at least four to six weeks apart.

Some eye professionals may use conventional surgery that is performed in an eye clinic or hospital. The doctor provides medication to help the patient relax and then makes tiny numbing injections around the eye. A small amount of tissue is removed to create a new passage for the fluid to drain. The patient is then given special eye drops to prevent inflammation and infection. However, conventional surgery may cause poorer vision than with laser surgery, and it may also cause side effects such as inflammation, infection, corneal problems, and CATARACTS.

Risk Factors and Preventive Measures

African Americans over age 40 have the greatest risk among all races in the United States for developing glaucoma; for example, glaucoma is five times more likely to occur in African Americans than in Caucasians and is four times more likely to cause blindness in African Americans than Caucasians. All individuals over age 60 are at risk, especially African Americans, Mexican Americans, and those of any race with a family history of glaucoma. Annual eye examinations can help with prevention by detecting the early signs of glaucoma.

See also BLINDNESS/SEVERE VISION IMPAIRMENT; EYE DISEASES, SERIOUS.

Prevent Blindness America and the National Eye Institute. *Vision Problems in the U.S.: Prevalence of Adult Vision Impairment and Age-Related Eye Disease in America,* 2002. Available online. URL: http://www.nei.nih.gov/eyedata. Accessed February 13, 2008.

gout   A form of ARTHRITIS that is acutely painful and is caused by excessive levels of uric acid. It is caused by a buildup of needle-shaped crystalline deposits of uric acid in the joints. Gout represents about 5 percent of all types of arthritis, according to the National Institute of Arthritis and Musculo-skeletal and Skin Diseases (NIAMS).

Most people with gout are male; however, among patients older than age 60 with newly diagnosed gout, about half are women, according to Doctors Rott and Agudelo in their article on gout for the *Journal of the American Medical Association*. In addition, in the case of women who are older than age 80, the dominance of the disease shifts, and more women than men have gout. Gout must be differentiated from pseudogout, which is the deposit of excessive crystals of calcium.

Uric acid is derived from substances that are called purines, which are naturally found in the body tissues. Purines are also found at high levels in particular foods, such as anchovies, dried beans, liver, and peas. Individuals with chronic gout should avoid foods that are high in purines.

Symptoms and Diagnostic Path

Gout is diagnosed by the individual's symptoms, family history, and personal medical history, as well as laboratory tests that reveal high levels of uric acid in the blood (hyperuricemia). Sometimes physicians withdraw fluid from the inflamed joint to check for the presence of gouty crystals.

Diagnosing gout may be difficult in older patients since it is sometimes misdiagnosed as rheumatoid arthritis because gouty tophi (hard buildups of gout in the joint) may resemble a similar condition seen with chronic rheumatoid arthritis. It is also possible for older individuals to have *both* gout and rheumatoid arthritis.

In addition, gout sometimes may present in an atypical fashion in elderly patients compared with younger patients, according to Rott and Agudelo. They report that "Gout in elderly patients may have an insidious onset and an unimpressive presentation, lacking the acute pain, swelling, and inflammation of classic gout." In addition, say the authors, "Multiple small joints of the hands may be involved, in contrast with the monoarthritis [one site] of classic gout." Of course, gout may also present in the typically classic manner of affecting only one joint severely.

Gout can be triggered by stress, alcohol, drugs, or other illnesses. Often attacks subside within three to 10 days, even if the individual is not treated. Other attacks may occur within months but may not recur for years.

The following are the four stages of gout:

1. Asymptomatic hyperuricemia—In this stage, there is no pain, but the blood shows elevated levels of uric acid. The patient in this stage usually does not require any treatment.
2. Gouty arthritis—In this stage, deposits of uric acid crystals collect in the joint spaces, and they cause severe pain and swelling. An attack of gout in this stage can be triggered by drugs, alcohol, stress, or another illness. Attacks last from three to 10 days, with or without treatment. As the disease progresses, attacks can occur more frequently and last for longer periods of time.
3. Interval gout—This is the stage between attacks, when there are no symptoms and no pain.
4. Chronic tophaceous gout—With this form of gout, the disease may have caused permanent damage to affected joints and may also have damaged the kidneys as well. Most people with gout who are treated do not experience this stage.

Often the first sign of gout is a reddish and painful swelling in the big toe, although other joints may be involved instead (or as well), such as the joints in the ankle, knee, fingers, wrists, elbows, ankles, and heels. The pain is extreme and can also cause swelling, heat, redness, and joint stiffness.

Physicians who have diagnosed gout in the past can often diagnose the disease on sight; however, laboratory tests such as the erythrocyte sedimentation rate (ESR) blood test will help to confirm their diagnosis. Tests for uric acid in the blood can be misleading because hyperuricemia (high levels of uric acid in the blood) may be found in some patients who do not have gout, while normal or even low levels of uric acid may occur in patients who actually do have gout.

Treatment Options and Outlook

Individuals with gout are often treated with nonsteroidal anti-inflammatory drugs (NSAIDs), such as indomethacin (Indocin) and naproxen (Anaprox, Naprosyn). However, indomethacin can be problematic for many elderly patients and cause gastric distress.

Patients with gout may also be treated with an oral or injected corticosteroid drug such as prednisone. In addition, they may also be treated with one of a variety of prescribed nonsteroidal anti-inflammatory drugs (NSAIDs) such as celecoxib (Celebrex). Allopurinol (Zyloprim) may also be given to prevent future attacks of gout by treating the hyperuricemia. Patients should be warned of the possible side effect of a rash or fever with allopurinol. If these side effects occur, allopurinol should be discontinued.

Dietary changes can also be very helpful for the person with gout. Patients with chronic gout are advised to avoid foods that are high in purines, such as anchovies, asparagus, dried beans and peas, herring, liver, mackerel, mushrooms, sardines, and scallops. They should also drink plenty of water.

Risk Factors and Preventive Measures

Men are more likely to develop gout than women, but some women also suffer from gout. Other risk factors are

- a genetic history—an estimated 20 percent of people with gout have a family history of this disease

- a high consumption of purine-rich foods
- overweight and obese
- an enzyme defect that causes difficulty with breaking down purines
- alcohol consumption
- exposure to lead in the environment
- other health problems, such as problems with the kidneys, heart disease, HYPERTENSION, Type 2 DIABETES, and hypothyroidism
- some medications or minerals, such as diuretics, aspirin-containing drugs, niacin, cyclosporine (an immune suppressant), and levodopa, a drug used to treat PARKINSON'S DISEASE
- a past history of organ transplant

See also OSTEOARTHRITIS; RHEUMATOID ARTHRITIS.

Rott, Keith T., M.D., and Carlos A. Agudelo, M.D. "Gout." *Journal of the American Medical Association* 289, no. 21 (June 4, 2003): 2,857–2,860.

guardianship See LEGAL GUARDIANSHIP.

gynecologist See BREAST CANCER; CANCER.

hallucinations Sensory experiences in which a person believes that he or she sees, hears, or feels experiences that are not actually occurring. An example of a hallucination is a person seeing bugs or monsters on the ceiling when there is nothing there.

Hallucinations may occur because of severe psychiatric disorders such as schizophrenia. They may also occur as a side effect of an individual receiving very high doses of NARCOTIC pain medications such as morphine, which may be given to patients with CANCER or other illnesses that cause severe pain. In addition, individuals with various forms of DEMENTIA such as ALZHEIMER'S DISEASE may experience hallucinations. Patients with PARKINSON'S DISEASE on a moderate to high dose of medication may experience visual hallucinations.

See also ADVERSE DRUG EVENT; AGGRESSION, PHYSICAL; COGNITIVE IMPAIRMENT; CONFUSION; DELUSIONS; IRRITABILITY; MEMORY IMPAIRMENT; RAGES.

headache Pain perceived to stem from some part of the head, although the cause may actually emanate from another part of the body, such as the cervical spine/neck (as with the CERVICOGENIC HEADACHE). Common types of headaches experienced by older patients include tension-type headaches, migraines, cluster headaches, sinus headaches, and cervicogenic headaches. Health issues such as high blood pressure, diabetes, or infection in the body can also be common causes of headache pain. In general, common (primary) headaches decline with age, and the individual who is 80 years old is less likely to have a common headache type than the person who is age 65.

According to authors Silberstein, Lipton, and Goadsby in their chapter on geriatric headaches in *Headache in Clinical Practice,* at age 70, 10 percent of women and 5 percent of men report suffering from headaches. In addition, the elderly have an increased likelihood compared to younger individuals of experiencing headaches caused by such serious conditions as giant cell arteritis, cerebrovascular disease, or PARKINSON'S DISEASE. Thus, headaches in an older person, particularly those of a new type or onset, should not be summarily dismissed by patients or doctors as "just a headache." This is particularly true if the headache is very severe.

According to Randolph W. Evans in his article on geriatric headaches in *Annals of Long-Term Care* in 2002, the risk of new-onset headaches among the elderly is 10 times greater than the prevalence among younger individuals, and some causes of these headaches may include subdural hematoma, stroke, temporal arteritis, trigeminal neuralgia, severe anemia, glaucoma, and angina.

An EXTREMELY SEVERE HEADACHE unlike a headache that has ever been experienced before should never be ignored in an older person because it could be a precursor to a stroke or aneurysm in the brain. The older person with such a headache should call "911" for emergency medical treatment because it could be a symptom of a life-threatening condition. The individual should not attempt to drive to the physician's office or the hospital emergency room, because he or she could become very disoriented or even unconscious on the way. In addition, time is of the essence in the treatment of an extremely severe headache, and rapid diagnosis and treatment may mean the difference between disability and no disability or life and death.

Primary headaches are caused by tension-type headaches, migraines, and cluster headaches, while secondary headaches are caused by other disorders; for example, disorders of the teeth or eyes may lead to the secondary symptom of headache. Some headaches can be either primary or secondary headaches, depending on the circumstances. For example, a headache caused by simple sinusitis is a primary headache; however, if there is bone inflammation of the sinuses or fluid pressure on pain-sensitive structures, then it is a secondary headache.

Headache is also a common symptom of fever and of many different illnesses, such as FLU/INFLUENZA. Some individuals develop headaches when they stop consuming caffeinated products, especially when they are heavy coffee, tea, or cola drinkers habituated to caffeine. Individuals who consume a great deal of alcohol may develop "hangover" headaches the day after excessive drinking.

Medications such as antihypertensives may also lead to chronic headaches, as may nitroglycerin (a medication used to treat the heart), calcium channel blockers, corticosteroids, estrogens, and other categories of commonly used medications.

In a study of elderly people with headaches reported by Lisotto et al. in 2004 in the *Journal of Headache Pain,* the researchers found that about 82 percent of the 282 patients over age 65 had primary headaches, and 15 percent had secondary headaches. (The other headaches could not be classified.) Of the secondary headaches, the most common causes were trigeminal neuralgia (pain emanating from the trigeminal nerve in the cheekbone), which represented about 26 percent of all the secondary headaches.

Symptoms and Diagnostic Path

The headache may be experienced on any part of the head, depending on the type of headache. The sinus headache may cause pain between the eyes (where the maxillary sinuses are located), while the migraine may be experienced at the area of the temples. Migraines may be preceded by an aura of the individual seeing flashing lights, although many elderly patients have no aura. (In addition, some elderly patients have migraine auras without headaches, a condition more common in older people than younger individuals.) Migraines may also be accompanied by nausea and vomiting. Migraines may cause a tearing up of the eyes, although sinus headaches may also cause this symptom. The person with a migraine is often photosensitive as well as sensitive to sound. There may be associated weakness or numbness on one side of the body, which may make the migraine appear to be a stroke. Fortunately, this is quite rare.

Cluster headaches are one-sided, very painful headaches that last from 15 to 90 minutes. The individual may wake up suddenly with a cluster headache. Patients with cluster headaches may also be sensitive to light, and for this reason, sometimes this headache is misdiagnosed as a migraine.

Giant cell arteritis, which is a headache type that is seen almost exclusively in the elderly, presents with headache, fatigue, and vision loss. Up to 90 percent of older patients with giant cell arteritis have headaches. They may also have scalp tenderness, such that it is painful for them to wear a hat or place their head on a pillow. Other symptoms of giant cell arteritis are night sweats, fever, and weight loss.

It is important for the doctor to be informed of the location of the headache and its severity. If the patient has experienced similar headaches in the past, this information should be provided as well.

The physician may order a computed tomography (CT) scan or a magnetic resonance imaging (MRI) scan of the brain to determine if there are any detectable serious problems that require immediate and urgent treatment.

The physician should ask the patient if the headache was preceded by a fall, since many older individuals have problems with falls, and a subdural hematoma may result from a fall, causing a headache.

Headaches may accompany strokes, and such headaches are usually extremely severe. If the patient says the headache is the worst of his or her life, it may be a subarachnoid hemorrhage (leaking blood from the blood vessels in the brain) causing the head pain. Patients with subarachnoid hemorrhage may also have nausea and vomiting, neck stiffness, and visual disturbances. A lumbar puncture is necessary to rule out subarachnoid hemorrhage. Often, an emergency angiogram of the blood vessels is necessary.

Treatment Options and Outlook

The treatment of headache depends on the diagnosis. If the headache does not appear to require emergency treatment and may be a tension-type headache or other common headache, often medication is given, such as acetaminophen. If the headache is a secondary headache, then the primary disorder should be identified and treated; for example, if the headache stems from a metabolic disorder, that disorder is treated, and often the headaches will resolve.

If the headache appears to stem from the use of a medication, the drug is either discontinued or the dosage is decreased, whenever possible.

Cluster headaches may be treated with the administration of oxygen, as long as the patient does not also have chronic obstructive pulmonary disease (which is often caused by years of smoking and is related to emphysema). Some patients improve with melatonin, although no supplements should be taken without consulting with the physician.

As mentioned earlier, extremely severe headaches require urgent treatment because if the headache is related to a stroke or brain aneurysm, the individual could suffer brain damage or even death if treatment is not administered rapidly.

Once the diagnosis is made, medication must be chosen with care because some drugs are less safe in geriatric patients than in younger patients; for example, "triptan" drugs that are prescribed for migraines are generally not recommended for older patients, particularly if elderly patients have uncontrolled hypertension, diabetes, coronary artery disease, or even if they are at risk for these diseases. If the headache is a tension-type headache, medications should be started at a lower dosage than among younger patients.

Cervicogenic headaches may be treated with injections of corticosteroids. A Lidoderm skin patch (a prescribed medication) may also reduce the pain of a cervicogenic headache.

In addition to medications, there are many other treatments for headaches. Sinus headaches may be treated with antibiotics and decongestants. Chronic tension-type headaches may be treated with massage therapy or acupuncture. Physical therapy as well as chiropractic treatments may also be quite beneficial in alleviating these types of headaches.

Some headaches may respond to progressive relaxation therapy, in which the patient learns to tighten and then relax specific muscles. Yoga and tai chi may be beneficial to some patients with chronic headaches. Electrical stimulation therapy that is provided by the physician's office improves the headaches of some patients. Neurofeedback is a procedure that allows patients to view their own brain waves on an electroencephalograph and to learn to change their brain waves through relaxation, thus also decreasing headache pain. This procedure may improve chronic headaches for some patients.

If patients can identify their own headache triggers, they may also be able to decrease the frequency and severity of their headaches. Stress is a very common headache trigger, but there are many other triggers, such as some foods, bright lights, and noise. Some patients are very sensitive to weather changes, and a rainy or snowy day may trigger a headache. A lack of sufficient sleep is a very common headache trigger, and the one best solution is to obtain sufficient hours of sleep (usually at least seven hours per night for most people).

Driving a car may trigger a cluster headache in some individuals, and driving may worsen an already existing migraine or cluster headache.

Some patients with chronic headaches obtain significant pain relief through Botox therapy. This is the same drug, Botulinum toxin Type A, that is given to some individuals to minimize their facial wrinkles, but it can also be effective in reducing headache pain. Botox must be administered by a physician or his or her assistant and should never be received from a nonmedical person.

Risk Factors and Preventive Measures

Older women have a greater risk for most types of headaches than men, while both older women and older men have about equal risk for cluster headaches. To prevent future headaches, individuals should not ignore their own pain and should report it to the physician for further evaluation. Underlying medical conditions that cause chronic headaches should be identified and treated.

Whenever possible, individuals should seek to identify their headache triggers, whether they are foods, the weather, medications, and other possible headache triggers.

Evans, Randolph W., M.D. "Geriatric Headache." *Annals of Long-Term Care* 10, no. 5 (May 2002). Available online. URL: http://www.annalsoflongtermcare.com/article/738. Downloaded June 30, 2008.

Kandel, Joseph, M.D., and David Sudderth, M.D. *The Headache Cure.* New York: McGraw-Hill, 2005.

Lisotto, C., et al. "Headache in the Elderly: A Clinical Study." *Journal of Headache Pain* 5 (2004): 36–41.

Silberstein, Stephen D., Richard B. Lipton, and Peter J. Goadsby. "Geriatric Headache." In *Headache in Clinical Practice.* 2nd ed. London: Martin Dunitz, 2002, pp. 269–281.

health-care agent/proxy (also known in some states as a health-care proxy) An individual who has been specifically designated in advance to make health-care decisions for another person if that person cannot make such decisions himself or herself. This person should be someone who the older person trusts with his or her life because broad authority is usually given to the person. The health-care agent should be an adult at least 18 years old and should not be the older person's doctor or an employee of the doctor, unless that person is a spouse or a close relative.

See also ADVANCE DIRECTIVE; LEGAL GUARDIANSHIP; POWER OF ATTORNEY; LIVING TRUST; LIVING WILL; WILLS.

Commission on Law and Aging. *Consumer's Tool Kit for Health Care Advance Planning.* Second Ed. Washington, D.C.: American Bar Association, 2005.

Health Maintenance Organization (HMO) See MEDICARE.

hearing aid Device that enables a person with a hearing impairment to hear better. See ASSISTIVE DEVICES/ASSISTED TECHNOLOGY; HEARING DISORDERS; HEARING LOSS.

hearing disorders Difficulty with hearing, ranging from a mild HEARING LOSS to relatively moderate problems with hearing and up to and including total DEAFNESS. An estimated one-third of individuals between ages 65 and 74 in the United States have some level of hearing impairment, and nearly half of those older than age 75 have some level of hearing loss to total deafness.

The risk for the development of hearing disorders increases with age, although not all older people lose their hearing. As a result, it should not be assumed that all elderly individuals are deaf, and older people should not be spoken to in overly loud tones unless and until it has been established that they actually do have a hearing impairment. (Many older people complain that others often shout at them, assuming that they are deaf when they are not.)

Older men and women represent about 13 percent of the population in the United States, but account for more than a third (37 percent) of all hearing-impaired individuals, according to the Centers for Disease Control and Prevention (CDC).

In general, older men are more likely than older women to have hearing disorders. According to the CDC, 47.5 percent of older men age 65 and older had some form of hearing impairment in 2003 compared to 31.9 percent of all older women of the same age. In addition, older white men and women are more likely than older black, Hispanic, or Asian men and women to have hearing disorders. For example, 41 percent of whites age 65 and older had hearing impairments compared to 34 percent of Asians, 24.5 percent of Hispanics, and 24.4 percent of blacks of the same age.

There is a link between age and hearing loss. According to the National Institute on Hearing Loss and Other Communication Disorders, 18 percent of Americans ages 45 to 64 have a hearing loss. The percentage of those with hearing loss increases to 30 percent of adults ages 65 to 74 and further to 47 percent of adults ages 75 and older.

Yet many times hearing disorders remain undiagnosed. Older men and women are significantly less likely to receive an evaluation for a hearing disorder than they are to be evaluated for a vision disorder. This may be caused in part to a reluctance and reticence to obtain a HEARING AID, which increases the denial that an individual may have about having a hearing impairment. According to the National Institute on Deafness and Other Communication Disorders, only one of every five people who would benefit from wearing a hearing aid will wear one. There is an element of vanity in the individual's refusal to consider that he or she may have a hearing impairment, which seems to imply that the person is "old." Yet many hearing aids are barely noticeable.

SMOKING increases the risk for the development of hearing disorders, as does continued exposure to very loud noises.

According to the National Institute on Deafness and Other Communication Disorders, individuals who answer "Yes" to three or more of the questions below may have a hearing disorder and should have their hearing checked by a doctor.

- Do I have a problem hearing on the telephone?
- Do I have trouble hearing when there is noise in the background?
- Is it hard for me to follow a conversation when two or more people talk at once?
- Do I have to strain to understand a conversation?
- Do I misunderstand when spoken to by women or children (who generally have higher voices)?
- Do many people I talk to seem to mumble (or not speak clearly)?
- Do I misunderstand what others are saying and respond inappropriately?
- Do I often ask people to repeat themselves?
- Do people complain that I turn the TV volume up too high?
- Do I often hear a ringing, roaring, or hissing sound?
- Do some sounds seem too loud?

Sometimes a hearing disorder can be diagnosed by the GERIATRICIAN or general practitioner, or the physician may refer the individual to an otolaryngologist, a physician who specializes in treatment of the nose, ear, and throat, or an audiologist, a health professional who is trained to assess hearing. An audiologist performs a series of painless tests to see if the individual is able to hear sounds of different pitch and loudness. He or she can also help the individual select the appropriate hearing aid device if necessary.

Other people can help the person who has trouble with hearing by doing the following:

- Avoid speaking while chewing gum or eating.
- Avoid covering your mouth with your hands while you are speaking.
- Face the person when speaking to him or her.
- Use gestures and facial expressions to provide clues as to what is being said.
- Be patient.
- Repeat what was said, if necessary, summarizing in different words.
- Be sure that lighting is in front of you when you speak. This allows a person with a hearing impairment to observe body language that provides communication clues.
- Turn off the radio or television during conversations.
- Speak slightly louder than normal, but do not shout. Shouting may distort your speech.
- Speak at your normal rate and do not exaggerate sounds.
- Rephrase statements into short, simple sentences if it appears you are not being understood.
- In restaurants and social gatherings, choose seats or conversation areas away from crowded or noisy areas.

Causes of Hearing Loss and Disorders

There are many possible causes of hearing loss and disorders, including aging itself, some medications, a STROKE, an inherited risk for hearing disorders, an ear infection, the exposure to very loud noise in the past, or a head injury.

In addition to hearing loss, there are also other hearing disorders that can be aggravating, such as TINNITUS and MÉNIÈRE'S DISEASE. Tinnitus is a problem with hearing a constant ringing in the ears, and at least 12 million Americans have tinnitus. It may have been caused by medications, ear damage, or extreme noise.

Ménière's disease is an inner ear problem that can cause dizziness, vertigo, and a feeling of disorientation. About 615,000 people have been diagnosed with Ménière's disease in the United States.

Presbycusis is another hearing disorder that causes sounds to seem less clear to the individual and also lower in volume. The individual also perceives the speech of others as slurred and distorted because of this hearing disorder. Presbycusis is a common hearing disorder among older individuals. It is caused by disorders of the inner ear and may also be caused by heart disease, HYPERTENSION, DIABETES, or circulatory problems.

See also HYPERACUSIS.

hearing loss A limited ability or an inability to hear or understand speech. Hearing loss is the most common impairment in the United States, affecting millions, including many older people. According to the National Institute on Deafness and other Communication Disorders (NIDCD), one in three people older than 60 and half of those older than 85 have hearing loss. Hearing loss may be temporary or permanent, partial or complete, and it may involve one or both ears.

Adaptive Aids for Hearing Impairments

The most commonly known adaptive device for those with hearing loss problems is the hearing aid, a tiny device worn on or inside the ear. Hearing devices are carefully fitted to the individual by an audiologist. Special masking devices that make a hissing or other noise are sometimes used to "drown out" the inner sound of tinnitus.

Other adaptive devices include a telephone amplifying device that makes sound louder. There are also alerts for doorbells, smoke detectors, and even alarm clocks that provide a visual signal or a vibration in addition to the sound; for example, if the doorbell is ringing, a flashing light may appear.

The NIDCD says that individuals should ask themselves the following questions if they want to know if they have a hearing problem. If the answer is "Yes" to three or more questions, the individual may have a hearing disorder and should consult with his or her physician.

- Do I have a problem hearing on the telephone?
- Do I have trouble hearing when there is noise in the background?
- Is it hard for me to follow a conversation when two or more people talk at once?
- Do I have to strain to understand a conversation?
- Do many people I talk to seem to mumble or not speak clearly?
- Do I misunderstand what others are saying and respond inappropriately?
- Do I often ask people to repeat themselves?
- Do I have trouble understanding the speech of women and children?
- Do people complain that I turn the TV volume up too high?
- Do I frequently hear a ringing, roaring, or hissing sound?
- Do some sounds seem too loud?

Symptoms and Diagnostic Path

Although hearing loss usually develops gradually and painlessly, some warning signs may include

- a ringing or buzzing in the ears (tinnitus) after an exposure to a loud noise
- experiencing a muffling of sounds after hearing an explosion
- difficulty understanding conversation after being in a noisy environment
- an inability to understand conversation except when reading lips in a quiet environment
- difficulty identifying the source of a sound

After determining that ear wax, infection, or illness are not responsible for the hearing loss, the doctor may evaluate the patient's ability to hear the ticking of a watch or to repeat or respond to something said in a whisper. If hearing problems are apparent or likely, the doctor may then refer the patient to an audiologist trained in measuring hearing loss. The doctor may also send the patient to an otolaryngologist, a physician who treats disease and conditions of the ear, nose, and throat.

Treatment Options and Outlook

Depending on the nature of the hearing loss, using warm water to remove ear wax, or medication to cure illness, or surgery to correct abnormalities can all significantly improve hearing in many cases. When hearing cannot be restored, adaptive devices can help amplify sounds and reduce background noises. The cochlear implant is another option. This is a device worn behind the ear, and it conveys sound to a speech processor that is kept in a pocket or worn on a belt. A small round receiver that is surgically implanted behind the ear sends sound signals to the brain.

Risk Factors and Preventive Measures

The primary environmental cause of hearing loss is exposure to noise loud enough to make the ears ring and to make it necessary to shout in order to be heard. More than 30 million Americans are regularly exposed to dangerously high noise levels, and about one-third of all hearing loss is at least partially caused by such exposure. Even a single brief exposure to loud noise can be hazardous.

People older than age 50 years may lose some hearing each year and may find it becomes increasingly difficult to follow a normal conversation. It is considered normal by many people for someone who is age 65 or older to need a hearing aid. Hearing loss affects one in three adults older than age 60 and half of those older than 85 years. Hearing loss is generally more severe in women than in men.

Some types of hearing loss run in families. Other causes of hearing loss include

- a head injury or other trauma
- heart disease
- stroke
- some chemotherapy drugs or other medications

- otosclerosis, a condition preventing sound from reaching the middle ear and the most common cause of hearing loss in older adults
- a cyst or flap of skin growing into the middle ear

See also ASSISTIVE DEVICES/ASSISTED TECHNOLOGY; HEARING DISORDERS.

heart attack (also known as myocardial infarction) A dangerous and potentially fatal spasm of the heart muscles that occurs when oxygen flow to the heart is blocked, often because a clot in the coronary artery blocks blood and oxygen to the heart. A heart attack is a major medical emergency.

According to the American Heart Association, sometimes the term *acute coronary syndrome* is used to describe individuals who have either an acute myocardial infarction or unstable angina, another form of heart disease. Sometimes heart attack is preceded by unstable angina, which refers to chest pain that feels like pressure or squeezing in the chest, and it does not follow any particular pattern, such as occurring after vigorous exercise. This pain does not go away with medication or rest. Anyone with any chest pain should consult their physician immediately. If the individual is experiencing heart attack symptoms, they or another person should call 911 and the person should travel to the hospital by ambulance, so that immediate treatment is given.

About a million people have a heart attack in the United States each year, and half die, according to the National Institutes of Health. About a third of individuals with a heart attack have had a heart attack before, according to the National Heart, Lung, and Blood Institute. The average age of a person having a first heart attack is 64.5 for men and 70.4 for women. Heart attack can lead to HEART FAILURE and immediate or eventual death.

The best way to avoid a heart attack is to act very quickly because artery-opening treatments and clot-busting drugs can often stop a heart attack if they are administered immediately by emergency personnel. The best chances of survival occur if these drugs are given within an hour of the start of the symptoms of a heart attack.

Symptoms and Diagnostic Path

Some symptoms may indicate a heart attack and "911" emergency medical personnel should be called immediately. In addition, the patient should travel to the hospital in an ambulance because oxygen and other lifesaving measures can be administered on the way to the hospital by trained people. According to the National Heart, Lung, and Blood Institute, about half the people who die from a heart attack die within one hour from having their first symptoms and before they reach the hospital. Any of the following symptoms may indicate the person is having a heart attack:

- pressure, squeezing, fullness, or pain discomfort in the chest. Sometimes chest pain is intense (crushing) and sometimes it is subtle. Sometimes it may resemble the pain of heartburn. (In fact, it may be heartburn; however, the risk is too high to wait and see.) Generally, pain occurs in the center of the chest and lasts for more than a few minutes.
- pain or discomfort in one or both arms, as well as the back, jaw, neck, or stomach
- shortness of breath
- discomfort/pain in the arms, shoulder, neck, or back
- nausea, vomiting, dizziness, or sweating
- lightheadedness

The physician may use an electrocardiogram (ECG) to detect whether the electrical activity of the patient's heart has a normal rhythm. Electrical leads are placed on the chest, and these leads transmit cardiac data to the machine. The test causes no pain, and it can detect heart attack as well as an irregular heartbeat or insufficient heart pumping.

Laboratory tests can determine if a heart attack has occurred, because in the course of a heart attack, high levels of some proteins are released by the body into the bloodstream. Tests for troponin and serum myoglobin are often used and may be repeated later to see if there are improvements with treatment.

A nuclear scan of the heart may be performed to detect areas of the heart where blood is not flowing correctly (or at all!) or areas that are damaged. It can also show problems with pumping of the heart. Radioactive material is injected into the vein, usually in the arm. A scanning camera detects whether the material is taken up by the heart (indicating health) or not (indicating damage to the heart).

A coronary angiography may be performed, which is an X-ray of the heart and blood vessels. A catheter is passed through an artery in the groin or arm and to the heart. Then a dye is injected so that the doctor can study the blood flow of the heart.

Treatment Options and Outlook

Drugs are used to treat a heart attack. Aspirin is administered to thin out the blood and also to decrease the size of a blood clot during a heart attack. Oxygen is administered to make breathing easier. Nitrates such as nitroglycerin are given to relax the blood vessels and stop the pain. Beta-blocker medications are given to reduce the nerve impulses to the blood vessels and the heart. This causes the heart to beat more slowly and less forcefully. Angiotensin-converting enzyme (ACE) inhibitors may be given to lower blood pressure and reduce heart strain. Anticoagulants other than aspirin may be given to thin the blood, such as heparin and warfarin (Coumadin). Other medications are given as needed by the patient, such as anti-anxiety medications or pain medicine.

Other procedures or surgery may be needed if medications do not stop the heart attack. Medical procedures may include the angioplasty or a coronary artery bypass graft. With an angioplasty, a catheter connected to a balloon is threaded through the blood vessel and into the blocked coronary artery. The balloon is then inflated to push out the plaque that is occluding the artery and to widen the blood flow. In addition, a small mesh tube known as a *stent* may be inserted within the artery to make it stay open.

With a coronary artery bypass graft, a surgical procedure, the surgeon removes arteries or veins from other parts of the patient's body and then sews them within the heart to bypass the blocked coronary arteries, making a new route for the blood to flow to the heart.

Risk Factors and Preventive Measures

Individuals with previous heart disease have an increased risk for suffering a heart attack, particularly those who have been diagnosed with HEART DISEASE. Men have an increased risk for heart attack after age 45, and women have an increased risk after age 55. A family history of heart disease, such as a father or brother who was diagnosed with heart disease before age 55 or a mother or sister who was diagnosed before age 65, increases the risk for a heart attack.

Other risk factors for a heart attack are

- SMOKING
- emotional stress or pain
- exposure to extreme cold
- high blood cholesterol
- high blood pressure (HYPERTENSION)
- physical inactivity
- thyroid disease
- DIABETES

Another risk factor for heart attack is the presence of *metabolic syndrome*. This is a clustering of symptoms that are associated with the presence of both cardiovascular disease and Type 2 diabetes. According to the American Heart Association, metabolic syndrome is diagnosed when three or more of the following risk factors are present in an individual:

- high-density lipoprotein (HDL) cholesterol (the "good" cholesterol) below 40 mg/dL in men or 50 mg/dL in women
- triglyceride blood levels of 150 mg/dL or greater
- a fasting plasma glucose level of 100 mg/dL or more
- a waist circumference of 40 inches (102 cm) or greater in men or 34.6 inches (88 cm) or more in women
- a systolic blood pressure of 130 mm Hg or higher or a diastolic blood pressure of 85 mm Hg or greater, or receiving drug treatment for hypertension

After a person recovers from a heart attack, the doctor may order cardiac rehabilitation, which includes assistance with exercise, as well as education and counseling. The cardiac rehabilitation team may include doctors, nurses, physical therapists, dieticians, and psychologists, as well as other specialists deemed necessary.

To lower the risk for another attack, ASPIRIN THERAPY in the form of a baby aspirin every day is often given to those who have survived a heart attack. (There are some risks with aspirin therapy, and patients should discuss these with their doctors before beginning an aspirin regimen.) Other actions that can lower the risk of a heart attack are to stop smoking, lower the blood pressure (if the individual has hypertension), reduce high blood CHOLESTEROL, manage DIABETES if it is present, lose weight if the individual is obese, and maintain a daily physically active lifestyle.

See also CARDIOVASCULAR DISEASE; HEART DISEASE; EMERGENCY DEPARTMENT CARE; FRAILTY; HEALTH-CARE AGENT/PROXY; HEART FAILURE; LIVING WILL; OBESITY.

American Heart Association. *Heart Disease and Stroke Statistics—2008 Update.* Dallas, Tex.: American Heart Association, 2008. Available online. URL: http://www.americanheart.org/presenter.jhtml?identifier=3037327. Accessed February 19, 2008.

heart disease   Refers to disease of the heart, particularly HEART ATTACK (myocardial infarction) and chest pains from heart disease (angina pectoris) due to blockages in the coronary arteries of the heart. Heart disease is the number-one killer of older people in the United States (CANCER is the number-two killer) according to the American Heart Association.

According to the Centers for Disease Control and Prevention (CDC), heart disease represents 33 percent of all the deaths of individuals age 65 and older in the United States. Most people who die from coronary heart disease (82 percent) are ages 65 years and older. Heart disease is also a common cause of disability and death among adults age 65 and older in the United States. It is also very expensive; according to the CDC, heart disease was projected to cost $151.6 billion in direct and indirect costs in 2007.

Symptoms and Diagnostic Path

An individual with heart disease may have no symptoms or they may have angina, which is pain in the chest that eventually subsides. However, there may be no symptoms until the onset of the symptoms of a heart attack occur. Individuals should be evaluated for possible heart disease if they have risk factors such as DIABETES, HYPERTENSION, and high cholesterol levels. Some studies have indicated that elderly depressed patients have an increased likelihood of heart disease.

The warning signs of a heart attack are

- pain and discomfort in the chest that lasts for more than a few minutes—it may be severe or mild and may come and go.

- discomfort in other parts of the upper body, such as one or both arms, the back, neck, jaw, or stomach

- shortness of breath, with or without chest pain

- nausea, lightheadedness, or a cold sweat

Heart disease is diagnosed with an electrocardiogram (EKG), which measures the heart's electrical activity and detects patterns of abnormality in the heartbeat, heart muscles, and blood flow of the arteries. A nuclear scan of the heart shows the muscles of the heart as they work. Radioactive material is injected into a vein (usually the arm), and a camera shows how much of that material is taken up by the heart.

Echocardiograms use ultrasound to show the size, shape, and movement of the heart and can detect abnormalities. A coronary angiography images the heart and shows any problems with blood flow or blockages.

An exercise stress test may be given to measure how well the heart pumps when needing more oxygen.

Treatment Options and Outlook

Depending on the cause of the heart disease, it is treated with medications and recommendations for lifestyle changes, such as weight loss, smoking cessation, and increased exercise. Medications may be given to treat hypertension, high blood cholesterol, and heart disease. If the individual has diabetes, then blood sugar levels should be kept under very tight control. Aspirin therapy may be recommended to reduce the risk of a heart attack.

Sometimes medication treatment and lifestyle changes are insufficient to reduce the risks of heart attack or heart failure, and the patient will require surgery. There are many different types of cardiac surgeries, including surgery to repair or replace the heart valves, surgery to implant pacemakers in order to regulate the heart rhythms, and surgery to bypass or widen the blocked or narrowed heart arteries. (There are other surgeries as well.) The most extreme heart surgery is a heart transplant, using an implanted heart from a deceased person whose heart was donated for that purpose.

Risk Factors and Preventive Measures

According to the National Center for Health Statistics, older men have a greater risk for heart disease than older women, and 37 percent of men age 65 and older had heart disease in 2004 compared to 28 percent of older women.

In considering age as a primary factor in angina/coronary heart disease, myocardial infarction (heart attack), or myocardial infarction and coronary heart disease, in each case, individuals ages 65 years and older had the highest risks of all ages, according to the CDC. For example, the risk for myocardial infarction among those ages 19 to 44 was less than 1 percent. This risk increased to 4.8 percent among those ages 45 to 64. It then escalated by almost three times to 12.9 percent among individuals ages 65 years and older. (See Table 1.)

It is also important to note that individuals with the following risk factors are at an increased risk for heart disease:

- angina, a recurring pain or discomfort in the chest when the heart temporarily does not receive enough blood (and usually relieved by taking prescribed medication for angina)

- hypertension

- race: whites and blacks have the highest risk for heart disease (Asians and Hispanics have a lower risk for heart disease). However, note that blacks (both males and females) have the highest rates

TABLE 1. PERCENTAGE OF RESPONDENTS AGES 18 YEARS AND OLDER WHO REPORTED A HISTORY OF MYOCARDIAL INFARCTION OR ANGINA/CORONARY HEART DISEASE, BY AGE, UNITED STATES, 2005

Age	Number of Respondents	MI (%)	Angina/CHD (%)	MI or Angina/CHD (%)
19–44	128,328	0.8	1.1	1.6
45–64	137,738	4.8	5.4	7.7
65 and older	87,351	12.9	13.1	19.6

Source: Centers for Disease Control and Prevention. "Prevalence of Heart Disease—United States, 2005." *Morbidity & Mortality Weekly Report* 56, no. 6 (February 16, 2007): 113–118. Available online. URL: http://www.cdc.gov/mmwr/preview/mmwrhtml/mm5606a2.htm. Accessed February 19, 2008.

of death from heart disease compared with other races.

- SMOKING
- OBESITY
- men (although women with coronary heart disease have a greater risk of fatalities than men)
- individuals with high levels of low-density lipoproteins (also known as bad CHOLESTEROL)

In an analysis of more than 122,000 patients in 14 international clinical trials on heart disease, reported in 2003 in the *Journal of the American Medical Association*, the researchers found that 80 to 90 percent of patients with heart disease had a prior exposure to at least one of the following four risk factors:

- high total blood cholesterol levels
- current smoking
- diabetes
- hypertension

In this study, when considering age and gender only, the presence of hypertension was the most important factor for those age 65 years and older, followed by hyperlipidemia (high cholesterol levels).

Individuals with heart disease should consult with their physicians on individualized preventive measures to reduce their risk for a heart attack. ASPIRIN THERAPY is one preventive measure used successfully by many people. It is also important for people with hypertension to get their blood pressure under control the best they can to reduce their risk for heart disease. Obese individuals should lose weight to reduce their risk of a heart attack. Smokers should stop smoking immediately to decrease their risk of heart attack or heart failure.

See also ARTERIOSCLEROSIS; CARDIOVASCULAR DISEASE; CHOLESTEROL; FAMILY AND MEDICAL LEAVE ACT; GENDER DIFFERENCES; HEALTH-CARE AGENT/PROXY; HEART ATTACK; HEART FAILURE; HYPERTENSION; LIVING WILL; STROKE.

American Heart Association. *Heart Disease and Stroke Statistics—2008 Update.* Dallas, Tex.: American Heart Association, 2008. Available online. URL: http://www.americanheart.org/presenter.jhtml?identifier=3037327. Accessed February 19, 2008.

Centers for Disease Control and Prevention. "Prevalence of Heart Disease—United States, 2005." *Morbidity & Mortality Weekly Report* 56, no. 6 (February 16, 2007): 113–118.

Khot, Umesh N., M.D., et al. "Prevalence of Conventional Risk Factors in Patients with Coronary Heart Disease." *Journal of the American Medical Association* 290, no. 7 (August 20, 2003): 898–904.

heart failure A condition of the heart being unable to pump enough blood and oxygen to meet the needs of the body, especially under stress. Heart failure is also known as congestive heart failure. The heart does not usually actually stop, nor does the person die immediately, although death is a risk. (A better name for this condition might be "failing heart.") Instead, the condition is usually a chronic one. Heart failure is a chronic and extremely serious condition because heart failure eventually can lead to death. More than 287,000 people in the United States die each year from heart failure, according to the Centers for Disease Control and Prevention (CDC).

The CDC reports that about 5 million Americans have heart failure, and most (about 75 percent) are age 65 or older, while at least half are age 75 years and older. According to the CDC, about 550,000 new cases of heart failure are diagnosed per year.

Heart failure is also a leading cause of HOSPITALIZATION, and there were more than a million hospitalizations for heart failure in 2004. Heart failure is also the most costly illness that is paid for by MEDICARE as well as the most common cause for hospitalization among Medicare patients. More blacks on Medicare are hospitalized for heart failure than whites, according to the CDC.

The most common causes of heart failure are coronary artery disease, HYPERTENSION, and DIABETES, and according to the CDC, about seven of 10 people with heart failure had hypertension before they were diagnosed with heart failure. Nearly half (46 percent) of women who have had a heart attack will develop heart failure within six years compared to 22 percent of men.

According to Thomas and Rich in their article in *Generations* in 2006 on heart failure in older people, heart failure usually results from injury to the heart muscle caused by heart attack (myocardial infarction), or by viruses, chemotherapy, excessive consumption of ALCOHOL, OBESITY, or abnormality of the heart valves. Older individuals are more likely to suffer from heart failure because the heart becomes stiffer and less efficient with age. In addition, many older people have hypertension, increasing the risk for heart failure.

Many people with heart failure develop DEPRESSION, especially female patients.

Symptoms and Diagnostic Path

Many people with heart failure have no symptoms. When symptoms occur, they may include

- shortness of breath (dyspnea)
- extreme fatigue
- difficulty breathing when lying down
- pronounced neck veins
- decreased urine production and a need to urinate at night
- decreased alertness or concentration

- weight gain with swelling in the legs, ankles, or lower back
- chronic coughing
- irregular or rapid heartbeat
- edema (swelling) of the legs, feet, or ankles (more common in women than men)
- loss of appetite
- mental confusion or irritability
- abdominal swelling

According to the National Institutes of Health, some patients have no symptoms of heart failure unless they have one or more of the following conditions:

- anemia
- infections accompanied by high fever
- abnormal heart rhythms (arrhythmias)
- hyperthyroidism
- kidney disease

Pain may or may not be present, although there may be abdominal or chest pain if the heart failure is extensive and severe. The liver may be enlarged. A chest X-ray may reveal an enlarged heart and fluid around the lungs. An echocardiogram is used to determine the level of heart function. Other tests that are used to diagnose heart failure include a heart catheterization (a procedure in which a catheter is threaded to the heart), a chest X-ray, a cardiac magnetic resonance imaging (MRI) scan, nuclear heart scans, and an electrocardiogram (ECG).

Treatment Options and Outlook

The prognosis is poor if heart failure is advanced. Patients are treated with medications, such as diuretics (water pills), angiotensin-converting enzyme (ACE) inhibitors, beta-blockers, angiotensin receptor blockers (ARBs), nitrates, and digoxin. Patients may also be treated with a combination of hydralazine and nitrates. Blood thinners and calcium channel blockers may also be prescribed.

Diuretics rid the body of excess fluid and salt. ACE inhibitors decrease blood pressure and improve symptoms. ARBs act similarly to ACE inhibitors. Beta-blockers decrease blood pressure and heart rate and improve heart arrhythmias. Digoxin increases the force of the heart's pumping. If the patient is near death, pain may be treated with NARCOTICS or sedatives.

Patients with heart failure may need heart surgery. They may also need implanted devices, such as pacemakers (to speed up the heart) or implantable defibrillators that slow down an overly rapid heartbeat.

Patients with heart failure may be advised to prepare a living will and assign a durable power of attorney to a trusted person.

According to Thomas and Rich,

> The primary objectives of heart failure therapy are to improve survival, enhance quality of life, preserve independence, and reduce hospitalizations. Optimal treatment involves an individualized program comprising lifestyle and behavioral modifications, tailored drug therapy, and, in some cases, consideration of surgery and implanted devices.

Lifestyle recommendations are usually given, such as quitting smoking, staying active, and losing weight if the patient is obese. Limiting the intake of salt and sodium is also important. Patients may also need hospitalization and the intravenous administration of drugs to improve the ability of the heart to pump blood, such as dobutamine and milrinone.

If the individual with heart failure is extremely ill, they may need to have the excess fluid removed through kidney DIALYSIS. Some patients are treated with pacemakers or intra-aortic balloon pumps. At some point, a heart transplant may become the only way to sustain life.

Risk Factors and Preventive Measures

Common risk factors for heart failure are a prior heart attack, hypertension, and diabetes. Obese patients may need to reduce their weight substantially through exercise and decreased calories.

See also APPETITE, CHRONIC LACK OF; CARDIOVASCULAR DISEASE; HEART DISEASE; DEATH; DEATH, FEAR OF; EMERGENCY DEPARTMENT CARE; HEALTH-CARE AGENT/PROXY; HEART ATTACK; HEART DISEASE; LIVING WILL; STROKE; TALKING TO ELDERLY PARENTS ABOUT DIFFICULT ISSUES.

Thomas, Sabu, and Michael W. Rich. "Heart Failure in Older People." *Generations* 30, no. 4 (Fall 2006): 25–32.

heat stroke/heat exhaustion   Conditions that are caused by severe heat. According to the Centers for Disease Control and Prevention (CDC), heat stroke is a very serious condition that causes the body to be unable to perspire and also unable to cool itself down. Elderly people are at risk for heat stroke and heat exhaustion in very hot weather because they are more likely to take prescription medications that may impede sweating, and they are also more likely to suffer from chronic health conditions that interfere with the body's response to high temperatures. In addition, older people's bodies do not respond as rapidly to extremes of temperature as younger people's bodies.

The Environmental Protection Agency reports that more people die from excessive heat events than from lightning, hurricanes, tornadoes, floods, and earthquakes combined. The effect is disproportionately greater in cities where roads and buildings absorb and retain the sun's energy and create "heat islands." In contrast, the houses of people who live in rural areas cool off at night.

With heat stroke, the body temperature can rise to 106°F. or more within just 10 to 15 minutes. Without emergency treatment, heat stroke causes death or permanent disability. Some older individuals have died in their cars without air conditioning when they have ALZHEIMER'S DISEASE or another form of DEMENTIA.

The signs and symptoms of heat stroke are

- dizziness
- nausea
- a very high body temperature (greater than 103°F)
- hot, red, and dry skin without sweating
- HALLUCINATIONS, CONFUSION
- aggressive behavior

Heat exhaustion is a milder form of heat illness that can be caused by several days of exposure to high temperatures and an insufficient intake of fluids. Some signs and symptoms of heat exhaustion include

- fast and shallow breathing
- nausea or vomiting
- muscle cramps
- headache
- heavy sweating
- dizziness
- fast and weak pulse rate

The following steps can help protect against heat stroke or heat exhaustion:

- taking a cool shower or bath
- wearing lightweight clothing
- avoiding strenuous activity
- drinking noncaffeinated and nonalcoholic beverages
- remaining indoors in the heat of the day
- visiting older relatives at risk twice a day or more for signs of heat stroke or heat exhaustion
- taking older individuals to air-conditioned locations if they cannot transport themselves

If there are any indications of heat stroke or heat exhaustion, the following actions should be taken:

- Cool the person down in a cool shower.
- Move the person to a cool and shady area.
- Locate medical assistance as soon as possible.
- If emergency help is delayed, call the hospital emergency room for instructions.

See also EMERGENCY DEPARTMENT CARE; ENVIRON-MENTAL HAZARDS.

Environmental Protection Agency. *Fact Sheet: "It's Too Darn Hot"—Planning for Excessive Heat Events: Information for Older Adults and Family Caregivers.* Washington, D.C.: October 2007.

hepatitis B (HBV), chronic   A serious INFECTION that targets the liver and increases the risk for cirrhosis and liver cancer. An estimated 5,000 people die each year of liver cancer or cirrhosis caused by HBV. People who are at risk for infection with hep-

atitis B are also at risk for infection with hepatitis C, an even more serious form of hepatitis.

About 1.25 million people of all ages in the United States are infected with hepatitis B virus (HBV). The number of new infections has declined from about 260,000 per year in the 1980s to approximately 60,000 per year in 2004. The decline has primarily been due to the vaccination of children and adolescents.

Medicare provides payments for immunizations against hepatitis to older individuals who have not previously been vaccinated.

Hepatitis B can be transmitted through sex as well as through contact with infected blood. The individual with HBV should not share toothbrushes or razors or anything that may have blood on it. The individual also should not donate blood to blood banks, nor should he or she donate any tissues or body organs or even sperm.

HBV is not contracted by kissing or hugging, sharing eating utensils or drinking glasses, or by casual contact.

Symptoms and Diagnostic Path

Many people with HBV (about 30 percent) have no symptoms and do not know that they are ill. When symptoms do occur they may include

- jaundice
- fatigue
- abdominal pain
- loss of appetite
- nausea and vomiting
- joint pain

Patients with HBV should avoid alcohol (which can harm the liver further) and should see their physician on a regular basis. People with liver damage caused by HBV should be tested for hepatitis C and should also be vaccinated against hepatitis A.

Treatment Options and Outlook

Hepatitis is primarily treated with medications, and the individual is monitored by his or her primary care physician. A variety of drugs approved by the U.S. Food and Drug Administration (FDA) are used to treat HBV. For example, interferon-alfa (Intron

A) is an injected drug. Pegylated interferon (PEgasys) is also an injected medication. However, there are potentially serious risks with this medication, and patients should be thoroughly briefed before they start taking it. Lamivudine (Epivir-HBV) is an oral medication. Other oral medications include adefovir dipivoxil (Hepsera), entecavir (Baraclude), and telbivudine (Tyzeka and Sebivo).

Risk Factors and Preventive Measures

People who have or have had multiple sex partners or have been diagnosed with a sexually transmitted disease have an increased risk for contracting HBV. Illegal injection drug users are at risk for transmission, because they often use shared needles. Men who have sex with other men have an increased risk for contracting HBV.

The Centers for Disease Control and Prevention (CDC) recommend the following preventive steps:

- Vaccination against HBV is the best protection.
- Those who currently have or have ever had hepatitis B should not donate blood, organs, or any body tissue.
- Health care and public safety workers should be vaccinated against HBV.
- Individuals should not share with others personal items that could have blood on them, such as razors or toothbrushes.
- Condoms should be used when having sex. With older people, condoms are not used for contraception but rather to avoid sexually transmitted disease.
- Never share needles or syringes with others.
- If infected with HBV, avoid alcohol because it can worsen liver disease.

See also APPETITE, CHRONIC LACK OF; MEDICARE PREVENTIVE SERVICES.

HIPAA (Privacy Rule of the Health Insurance Portability and Accountability Act of 1966) See MEDICAL RECORDS.

hip replacement See JOINT REPLACEMENT.

Hispanics Individuals of Latin American or Spanish descent, including individuals whose families originated in Spain, South America, Mexico, Cuba, or other countries. According to the Administration on Aging, in 2005 people of Hispanic origin represented 6.2 percent of the older population in the United States. In 2006, there were 2.4 million Hispanics age 65 and older living in the United States, and the Hispanic population comprised 6.4 percent of the older population. By 2028, Hispanics age 65 and older will be the largest racial/ethnic minority in this age group.

Most older Hispanics lived in four states in 2006: California, Texas, Florida, and New York. An estimated 69 percent of older Hispanic men lived with their spouses in 2006, and 12 percent lived with nonrelatives. Seventeen percent of older Hispanic men lived alone. Among older Hispanic women, 40 percent lived with spouses, 34 percent lived with nonrelatives, and 25 percent lived alone. Older Hispanics are about twice as likely to live with other relatives than are individuals in the total older population.

The poverty rate for older Hispanics was 19.4 percent in 2006, which was more than twice the rate for non-Hispanic whites (7 percent). In general, older Hispanics have an increased risk for some diseases, such as CANCER, PNEUMONIA, and DIABETES. They also have an increased risk of losing all of their natural teeth. After blacks, Hispanics have the next highest rate of needing EMERGENCY DEPARTMENT CARE (19.5 percent).

In 2006, only about a third of older Hispanics received a pneumonia vaccination compared with 62 percent of non-Hispanic whites and 36 percent of non-Hispanic blacks.

About 11 percent of older Hispanics needed help from others for personal care in 2006, the same percentage for non-Hispanic blacks. The rate was 5.3 percent for non-Hispanic whites in 2006.

See also AFRICAN AMERICANS; ASIAN AMERICANS; CAUCASIANS; NATIVE AMERICANS.

Administration on Aging. *Snapshot: A Statistical Profile of Hispanic Older Americans Aged 65+.* U.S. Department of Health and Human Services. September 10, 2007.

holidays, effect on elders The impact of major national holiday celebrations on individuals who are age 65 and older. Holidays such as Thanksgiving, Christmas, Hanukkah, Easter, or New Year's Day can be very difficult for older people whose spouses, partners, or adult children have died and who may have also lost many other (or even all) their family members and friends. They may be reminded by the holidays of their past happy times with their loved ones, which sometimes can accentuate their BEREAVEMENT and cause them to feel even more lonely.

Older people may be living alone or residing in a NURSING HOME environment rather than living with their families as in the past during the holiday season. Being separated from family and loved ones during the holidays can be hard on anyone. However, it can be an especially difficult time for senior adults who may not have adequate support systems to cope with their feelings.

Their adult children may live too far away to visit easily, and they may feel sad or depressed that they cannot be with them or with their grandchildren. The heavy media emphasis on happy families during holidays can be highly anxiety invoking.

In addition, personal holidays may be problematic; for example, their own birthdays may be sad times for some older people who live alone and have no one with whom they can celebrate—few people will buy a birthday cake for themselves to eat alone. They may become extremely lonely and may also suffer from DEPRESSION.

home health/home care Care that is provided to elderly individuals within their own homes. The care may be limited to providing meals and minor assistance or it may include providing virtually all the needs of a severely disabled patient, such as cleaning catheters, providing tube feedings, and checking the individual's pulse and blood pressure. Search for home health-care agencies in an individual's local area on the Web site www.medicare.gov and follow the "Home Health Compare" link.

Some individuals pay for the cost of home care themselves; however, many individuals age 65 and older in the United States who are homebound and under a physician's care may receive coverage from MEDICARE or MEDICAID, depending on their situations. If the individual is at least 50 percent disabled and is a military veteran, he or she may receive home health-care coverage through the Veterans Administration.

Some individuals who receive home care, particularly those with a terminal illness such as CANCER, also receive HOSPICE services.

According to the National Center for Health Statistics, home health-care expenditures have grown from less than 1 percent of all health expenditures in 1960 (0.2 percent) to 2.3 percent in 2004. There are an estimated 7,500 home health-care agencies in the United States who provide home health care.

Who Needs Home Care?

According to the National Center for Health Statistics, over 2000–2003 individuals age 85 years and older (there were 3,268,000 people in this group) were the most likely of older individuals to need home health care, and 17 percent of this group needed care, compared to 7.9 percent of those who were ages 75 to 84 and to 3.9 percent of those who were ages 65 to 74 years old. (See Table 1.)

Older women used home care more than older men (7.6 percent of older women compared to 5.4 percent of older men). Among races and ethnicities, blacks were more likely to need home care (9 percent) compared to 6.5 percent each for whites and Hispanics. Asians were the least likely to need home care (5.0 percent).

Poor individuals were more likely to need home care than the near-poor or those who were not poor. Married people were least likely to need home care, among married, formerly married, or never married.

Quality of Home Care

Family caregivers and others who wish to check on the quality of a home health-care agency should ask the following questions:

- How long has this agency been serving the local community?

- Does the agency provide any brochures that describe its services and fees?

TABLE 1. NUMBER AND PERCENTAGE OF ADULTS AGE 65 AND OLDER WHO USED HOME CARE IN THE UNITED STATES, 2000–2003

Selected Characteristic	Population in Thousands	Percentage
Age 65 and older	**33,219**	**6.7**
65–74 years	17,876	3.9
75–84 years	12,075	7.9
85 years and older	3,268	17.0
Age 65 and older		
Sex		
Men	14,147	5.4
Women	19,072	7.6
Race and Hispanic origin		
White, not Hispanic	27,529	6.5
Black, not Hispanic	2,685	9.0
Asian, not Hispanic	649	5.0
Hispanic	2,015	6.5
Poverty status		
Poor	2,479	10.8
Near poor	6,083	7.6
Not poor	12,791	5.6
Marital status		
Currently married	18,456	4.8
Formerly married	13,160	9.2
Never married	1,177	8.4

Source: Adapted from Schoenborn, Charlotte A., Jackline L. Vickerie, and Eva Powell-Griner. "Health Characteristics of Adults 55 Years of Age and Over: United States, 2000–2003." *Advance Data from Vital and Health Statistics,* No. 370. Hyattsville, Md.: National Center for Health Statistics, 2006, pp. 22–23.

- Is the agency an approved Medicare provider?
- Is the care certified by a national accrediting agency such as the Joint Commission for the Accreditation of Healthcare Organizations?
- If required in your state, does the home health-care agency have a state license? Family members and/or caregivers should ask to see a copy of this document.
- Does the agency offer a "Patients' Bill of Rights" to seniors that describes both the rights and responsibilities of the agency and the senior?
- Does the agency prepare a written plan of care for the patient, which takes input from the doctor, the family, and the patient? If so, does the agency update the plan on an as-needed basis?
- How closely do supervisors oversee the patient's care to ensure high quality?
- Are agency staff members available on a 24-hour/7-day-a-week basis?
- How are agency caregivers hired and trained? How are potential employees screened?
- What is the procedure to handle any complaints or problems?
- How is billing handled?
- Will the agency provide a list of references for its caregivers?
- If the home health-care worker is unavailable, who does the agency call to fill in?

Note that if the responses to the questions are vague or inadequate, this is a red flag to a possible problem and that home-care service should not be used until the issue is cleared up. It may be that the person who is responding to the questions is new to the job. It may also be true that the home-care agency is inadequate or incompetent.

Individuals using home health care (or their relatives) should be sure to give the provider the following types of written and verbal information to maximize the experience for the older person:

- illnesses or signs of an emergency medical situation
- likes and dislikes
- medications and how and when they should be taken
- the need for canes, walkers, dentures, or other adaptive devices
- possible behavioral problems that may occur and the best way to handle them
- any problems in getting about (such as getting in and out of a wheelchair)
- special diets
- therapeutic exercises
- special clothing that the older person may need
- who to contact in the case of an emergency, and how to contact them

Medicare does not cover payment for some services that may be given to individuals in their

HOME HEALTH-CARE CHECKLIST

When I get my home health care	Yes	No	Comments
1. The staff is polite and treats me and my family members with respect.			
2. The staff explains my plan of care to me and my family, lets us participate in creating the plan of care, and lets us know ahead of time of any changes.			
3. The staff is properly trained and licensed to perform the type of health care that I need.			
4. The agency explains what to do if I have a problem with the staff or the care I am getting.			
5. The agency responds quickly to my requests.			
6. The staff checks my physical and emotional status at each visit.			
7. The staff responds quickly to changes in my health or behavior.			
8. My home is checked and suggestions are made to meet my special needs and to ensure my safety.			
9. The staff has told me what to do if I have an emergency.			
10. My privacy is protected.			

Source: Centers for Medicare and Medicaid Services. *Medicare and Home Health Care.* Washington, D.C.: Department of Health and Human Services, 2004, p. 21.

homes. Some examples of services that Medicare does not pay for include

- 24-hour-a-day care
- meals delivered to the home
- homemaker services such as shopping, cleaning, and laundry
- personal care given by home health aides such as bathing, dressing, and using the bathroom if this is the only care needed

To monitor existing home health care, the individual and family members should use the above checklist that was created by the Center for Medicare and Medicaid Services (CMS).

See also ASSISTED LIVING; ASSISTIVE DEVICES/ASSISTED TECHNOLOGY; GENDER DIFFERENCES; INDEPENDENT LIVING; NURSING HOMES; OMBUDSMAN.

homelessness   Lack of a formal home to live in, whether this lack is due to an individual's indi-gence, mental illness, SUBSTANCE ABUSE AND DEPENDENCE, or another cause. Some of the homeless live in emergency shelters, while others wander through the streets and parks. Some have ALZHEIMER'S DISEASE or another form of DEMENTIA. They may have no family members to care for them or they may refuse assistance from family members.

According to the *Annual Homeless Assessment Report to Congress* in 2007 (reported by the Department of Housing and Urban Development), based on a single day in 2005, less than 2 percent of the homeless population of people was age 62 or older compared with 15 percent of the total population who are homeless and 62 or older. Elderly people represented about 7 percent of population who were poverty-stricken in 2005.

See also HOUSING/LIVING ARRANGEMENTS.

Office of Community Planning and Development. *The Annual Homeless Assessment Report to Congress.* Washington, D.C.: U.S. Department of Housing and Urban Development. February 2007.

home modifications   See ELDERIZING A HOME.

hormone replacement therapy (HRT)   The use of medications with hormones, particularly medications such as estrogen or progesterone among women. (Some hormonal replacements combine hormones.) The drug may be given to improve the woman's vaginal dryness as well as problems with the urethra, which may begin to close, requiring dilatation by a urologist to resolve. Some women have been taken hormone replacement therapy for many years without a reevaluation of the need for this therapy.

Research on HRT is constantly evolving and changing, and every woman should discuss this issue with her doctor, including women who have been on HRT for years with no apparent problems. Some research, such as the Women's Health Initiative (WHI) study, has indicated that taking estrogen with or without progesterone is associated with a small but increased risk for heart disease, stroke, breast cancer, and the development of blood clots. The risk for blood clots is higher among women who also smoke. There is also an increased risk for developing gallstones.

On the other hand, HRT often provides relief from hot flashes, sleep problems, and vaginal dryness. It also decreases the risk for fractures; for example, the WHI study results showed that the women on HRT had 34 percent fewer hip fractures and 24 percent fewer total fractures than those not on hormones. However, this positive effect goes away after age 75.

Older men may also use hormone replacement therapy such as testosterone if they are low in this hormone, but they are much less likely to do so than are postmenopausal women to take female hormones.

Some research has indicated that the use of hormone replacement therapy, particularly the use of estrogen alone, may increase the risk for the development of breast CANCER. The decision for or against hormone replacement therapy should be made only after a careful consultation with the primary care physician in consultation with the individual's gynecologist and taking into account the woman's health history.

hospice   Hospice or hospice care is a concept of care that seeks to provide for the physical and emotional needs of terminally ill individuals, although it is sometimes also used for severely ill individuals who are not terminally ill. Hospice has been used for many years in Europe. The Connecticut Hospice, the first hospice in the United States, opened in 1974 and was funded by the National Cancer Institute for the first three years of its operation. MEDICARE began covering hospice payments in the United States in 1983, and MEDICAID started paying for hospices in some states in 1986. (The majority of states offer Medicaid hospice coverage.) Many private health insurance companies also cover hospice care.

Much of hospice care is provided to patients in their own homes by workers who travel to the home, although some hospice care is provided at inpatient facilities. Today the hospice provides no lifesaving measures to its patients; instead, hospice care encompasses an array of other services, such as providing pain medication and other treatments for pain management, counseling, spiritual guidance, and so forth.

Hospice patients may use services that are provided by physicians, nurses, home health aides, social workers, physical therapists, and others. However, the largest percentage of providers are nurses, followed by social workers/mental health specialists and then home health-care aides. (See Table 1.)

Characteristics of Hospice Care

According to *The Encyclopedia of Death and Dying,* hospice care is primarily characterized by these features:

(1) the patient's disease is terminal (approximately six months or less until death) and no aggressive efforts to prolong life are used; (2) the patient and family are treated as an integrated unit; (3) services are provided by an interdisciplinary team with in-patient and home care components coordinated; (4) hospice care services are available 24 hours per day, seven days per week; and (5) pain control and psychological well-being are prominent goals.

In a study to determine the self-identified needs of elderly patients who were receiving end-of-life

TABLE 1. NUMBER OF HOSPICE DISCHARGES AND PERCENT OF DAYS IN HOSPICE ACCORDING TO PROVIDERS, UNITED STATES, 2000

| | | | Length of Service in Days | | | |
| | | | Percentage Distribution | | | |
Discharges	Number	Percentage	Total	Less than 30 days	30 days or more	Average length of service
All discharges	621,000		100.0	62.8	37.2	46.9
Type of provider						
Nurses	598,700	96.4	100.0	63.5	36.5	45.8
Social workers/mental health specialists	470,000	75.8	100.0	61.0	39.0	45.6
Home health aides/nursing aides/attendants	427,500	68.8	100.0	58.5	41.5	49.7
Chaplains	328,400	52.9	100.0	64.5	35.5	43.2
Volunteers	102,900	31.1	100.0	50.4	49.6	64.2
Physicians	153,000	24.6	100.0	69.0	31.0	37.3
Homemakers/personal caretakers	40,900	6.6	100.0	58.3	41.7	77.4
Other[1]	116,700	18.8	100.0	60.7	39.3	40.8
Number of providers seen						
0–1[2]	65,500	10.6	100.0	76.0	24.0	47.4
2	91,900	14.8	100.0	67.5	32.5	33.1
3	120,300	19.4	100.0	60.3	39.7	50.5
4	118,600	19.1	100.0	54.7	45.3	55.9
5 or more	224,800	36.2	100.0	62.6	37.4	45.7

[1] A discharge is counted only once even though the patient may have seen more than one type of provider in this category, which includes dietitians or nutritionists, occupational therapists, physical therapists, respiratory therapists, speech pathologists or audiologists, and other providers.
[2] Includes a small number of discharges for whom no providers were reported.

Source: Adapted from National Center for Health Statistics. "Hospice Discharges and Their Length of Service." *Vital and Health Statistics Series* 13, no. 154 (August 2003), p. 13.

care in a Swedish palliative hospital ward, the researchers studied 15 men and 15 women with an average age of 79. The patients had a primary diagnosis of cancer. Although this study was performed in Sweden, these findings are also relevant to a North American audience.

The researchers found that the elimination of their physical pain was the primary need or goal in half the patients. In fact, some patients expressed a strong fear of pain. According to the researchers,

> To have the opportunity to speak about one's fear of being in pain and to have it confirmed that pain relief could be guaranteed seemed to dominate the physical picture of need and was just as prominent as the need for pain relief itself. These findings may suggest that adequate pain relief was accomplished but that the memory of the pain itself was very dominating and strong.

Perhaps it points to a need for assurance of relief of recurrent pain.

When the pain was alleviated, other needs presented, such as psychological, social, and spiritual needs.

The researchers found that most patients (61 percent) said that they wanted to spend their final days at home, while the rest preferred to stay in the hospital. Before their admission to the hospital palliative care ward, the most common symptoms of these patients were pain, appetite loss, anxiety, sleep difficulties, fatigue, shortness of breath, and vomiting.

Some patients reported that they were unhappy with their inability to take care of their physical or dental hygiene, which made some of them reportedly feel like they were in a condition of "physical decay." Others were cold. Psychologically, the patients were anxious, uncertain, and insecure. Some wanted seclusion. According to the researchers,

There was a need for seclusion to get some peace and quiet, maybe to have the opportunity to see relatives, and to be freer to express emotions and reactions to the situation. A common wish was to think back on their lives, maybe to recapitulate. Some of the patients pointed to psychosocial needs,

for example, to restore broken relationships and becoming [sic] reconciled before it was too late.

Among the primary social needs was the desire to visit with family and friends.

Hospice Care Users

More than 621,000 people used hospice services in 2000, and according to the National Center for

TABLE 2. NUMBER AND PERCENT DISTRIBUTION OF HOSPICE CARE DISCHARGE BY LENGTH OF SERVICES, ACCORDING TO SELECTED PATIENT CHARACTERISTICS: UNITED STATES, 2000

| | Discharges | | Length of Service in Days | | | |
| | | | Percentage Distribution | | | |
Discharge characteristic	Number	Percentage distribution	Total	Less than 30 days	30 days or more	Average length of service
Total	621,100	100.0	100.0	62.8	37.2	46.9
Sex						
Male	309,300	49.8	100.0	66.7	33.4	42.8
Female	311,800	50.2	100.0	58.9	41.1	50.9
Age at discharge						
Under 65	126,900	20.4	100.0	64.1	35.9	43.9
65 and older	494,300	79.6	100.0	62.4	37.6	47.7
65–74 years	153,100	24.7	100.0	65.0	35.0	41.2
75–84 years	176,400	28.4	100.0	62.3	37.7	50.6
85 years and older	164,800	26.5	100.0	60.2	39.8	50.5
Race						
White	522,500	84.1	100.0	62.6	37.4	46.7
Black or African American and other races	64,300	10.3	100.0	68.5	31.5	53.6
Black or African American	50,100	8.1	100.0	66.8	33.2	61.1
Unknown	34,400	5.5	100.0	55.5	44.5	36.7
Primary source of payment						
Medicare	488,000	78.6	100.0	61.5	38.5	48.1
All other sources	133,200	21.4	100.0	67.6	32.4	42.4
Medicaid	31,400	5.1	100.0	73.7	26.3	24.3
Private	80,600	13.0	100.0	64.4	35.6	49.4
Other	21,100	3.4	100.0	70.9	29.1	42.5
Reason for discharge						
Died	531,000	85.5	100.0	66.7	33.3	42.4
Did not die	90,200	14.5	100.0	39.5	60.5	73.1
Services no longer needed from agency	49,000	7.9	100.0	29.2	70.8	86.2
Transferred to inpatient care	14,500	2.3	100.0	Not enough data	63.9	81.7
Other and unknown	26,700	4.3	100.0	60.2	39.8	44.5

Source: National Center for Health Statistics. "Hospice Discharges and their Length of Service." *Vital and Health Statistics Series* 13, no. 154 (August 2003), p. 10.

Health Statistics, most individuals who were receiving these services were white and elderly, and they lived in a private or semiprivate residence. Only about 20 percent of the hospice care users were younger than age 65.

Hospice care was about evenly used by both men and women. Hospice services were not used by patients for long periods, and about two-thirds of hospice patients used their hospice services for less than 30 days (62.8 percent). In most cases (85.5 percent), the reason for the discharge from hospice services was death. (See Table 2.) The most common reason for admission to a hospice was cancer (58 percent), followed by heart disease, dementia, and other conditions.

Most people (71 percent) received help with at least one activity of daily living; for example, 71 percent were incontinent, 82 percent had a mobility limitation, 70 percent used a hospital bed, and 51 percent relied upon oxygen use.

The majority of patients (58 percent) using hospice services in 2000 had CANCER. Other primary diagnoses of hospice patients were HEART DISEASE, DEMENTIA, cerebrovascular disease, and CHRONIC OBSTRUCTIVE PULMONARY DISEASE. Most patients received three or more services from three or more providers, such as skilled nursing services, social services, personal care services, or spiritual care.

Medicare, Medicaid, or private health insurance covered most of the costs that were associated with hospice care, with Medicare providing the greatest percentage of hospice coverage.

According to the Administration on Aging, family caregivers should consider calling a hospice when

- They have questions about what to expect physically, emotionally, and spiritually as the person's end of life approaches.

- They need information about resources that can help them manage caregiver responsibilities.

- They have questions about how to have sensitive conversations about treatment choices, living arrangements, and personal care.

- They need help preventing and managing symptoms related to an illness or its treatment.

- They want guidance in finding the opportunities for hope, comfort, and meaning that are part of this time of life.

- They suffer feelings of loss, sadness, or grief, associated with the illness or death of a loved one.

See also ADVANCE DIRECTIVE; CREMATION; DEATH; DEATH, FEAR OF; END-OF-LIFE ISSUES; FRAILTY; FUNERALS; HEALTH-CARE AGENT/PROXY; HEART FAILURE; LIVING WILL; PALLIATIVE CARE; TALKING TO ELDERLY PARENTS ABOUT DIFFICULT ISSUES; TRANSPORTATION.

Administration on Aging. *Caring for Someone in the Last Years of Life.* U.S. Department of Heath and Human Services, November 1, 2004.

Cassell, Dana K., Robert C. Salinas, M.D., and Peter A. S. Winn, M.D. *The Encyclopedia of Death and Dying.* New York: Facts On File, 2005.

National Center for Health Statistics. "Hospice Discharges and Their Length of Service." *Vital and Health Statistics Series* 13, no. 154 (August 2003).

Wijk, Helle, and Agneta Grimby. "Needs of Elderly Patients in Palliative Care." *American Journal of Hospice & Palliative Medicine* 25, no. 2 (2008): 106–111.

hospitalization Admission to a hospital facility for the treatment of an illness, for surgery, or for a medical procedure. Hospitalizations may be planned, as with a scheduled surgical procedure, or they may result from emergencies, such as a STROKE or a HEART ATTACK or an accidental injury. Some groups of individuals are more likely to receive hospitalization than others; for example, individuals with ALZHEIMER'S DISEASE or other forms of DEMENTIA as well as those with DIABETES have a high rate of hospitalization.

Individuals with OSTEOPOROSIS may suffer from a FALL that leads to a FRACTURE and then to hospitalization. Some older people are hospitalized because they are very ill from INFLUENZA or PNEUMONIA (or both). For example, individuals age 65 and older represented 60 percent of all the hospitalizations for pneumonia in 2004.

According to the National Center for Health Statistics, the average hospital stay length for individuals age 65 and older was 5.6 days in 2004. Older people comprised 12 percent of the population of the United States in 2004, but they represented 38 percent of all hospital discharges and used 44 percent of total hospital days of care. About 12 million people age 65 and older were hospitalized for short stays in 2004 compared to 8 million people ages 45 to 64 in the same period.

In their book *The Encyclopedia of Death and Dying,* Cassell, Salinas, and Winn report that most terminally ill elderly people are cared for in hospitals, where there is a high risk of hospital-based INFECTIONS, BED SORES, and general disorientation of the patient. However, other sources report that increasing numbers of hospitals offer PALLIATIVE CARE, which concentrates on pain management rather than on continuing the patient's life. Many elderly patients have stated that they would prefer to die at home, an option that may be available through a HOSPICE program.

See also ACCIDENTAL INJURIES; ADVANCE DIRECTIVES; ADVERSE DRUG EVENT; EMERGENCY DEPARTMENT CARE; END-OF-LIFE ISSUES; FRAILTY; HEALTH-CARE AGENT/PROXY; HEART FAILURE; INAPPROPRIATE PRESCRIPTIONS FOR THE ELDERLY; LIVING WILL; LONG-TERM CARE; NURSING HOMES.

Cassell, Dana K., Robert C. Salinas, M.D., and Peter A. S. Winn, M.D. *The Encyclopedia of Death and Dying.* New York: Facts On File, 2005.
DeFrances, Carol J., and Michelle N. Podgornik. "2004 National Hospital Discharge Survey." *Advance Data from Vital and Health Statistics,* Centers for Disease Control and Prevention (CDC) no. 371 (May 4, 2006): 1–19.

housing/living arrangements   Elderly individuals may live in a variety of housing arrangements. Many continue to live in their own homes, with or without a spouse, and often despite steadily increasing problems with DISABILITY. Others move

TABLE 1. LIVING ARRANGEMENTS OF THE POPULATION AGE 65 AND OLDER: 2003 (NUMBER AND PERCENTAGE)

Age and Living Arrangement	Number			Percentage		
	Total	Men	Women	Total	Men	Women
65 and older	34,216	14,251	19,695	100.0	100.0	100.0
Alone	10,549	2,725	7,824	30.8	18.8	39.7
With spouse	18,427	10,341	8,086	53.9	71.2	41.1
With other relatives	4,462	1,026	3,436	13.0	7.1	17.4
With nonrelatives only	780	430	350	2.3	3.0	1.8
65 to 74	18,099	8,268	9,831	100.0	100.0	100.0
Alone	4,202	1,291	2,911	23.2	15.6	29.6
With spouse	11,398	6,141	5,257	63.0	74.3	53.5
With other relatives	1,965	523	1,442	10.9	6.3	14.7
With nonrelatives only	536	314	222	3.0	3.8	2.3
75 to 84	12,571	5,051	7,520	100.0	100.0	100.0
Alone	4,650	1,072	3,578	37.0	21.2	47.6
With spouse	6,060	3,525	2,535	48.2	69.8	33.7
With other relatives	1,682	357	1,325	13.4	7.1	17.6
With nonrelatives only	180	97	83	1.4	1.9	1.1
85 and Older	3,546	1,202	2,344	100.0	100.0	100.0
Alone	1,697	362	1,335	47.9	30.1	57.0
With spouse	969	675	284	27.3	56.2	12.5
With other relatives	815	146	669	23.0	12.1	28.5
With nonrelatives only	64	19	45	1.8	1.6	1.9

Source: He, Wan, Manisha Sengupta, Victoria A. Velkoff, and Kimberly A. DeBarros. *65+ in the United States: 2005.* Washington, D.C.: U.S. Census Bureau, December 2005, p. 152.

in with their family members, particularly an adult child. Many older individuals, especially older women who are widows, relocate from their homes to ASSISTED-LIVING FACILITIES. Contrary to popular opinion, most older people do not reside in NURSING HOMES.

According to the Census Bureau, in 2003, 10.5 million people age 65 and older in the United States lived alone, and of these, about 75 percent were women. Men age 65 and older are significantly more likely than older women to be living with a spouse. (See MARRIAGE/REMARRIAGE.)

Among older women, the most common arrangement was to live with a spouse (41.1 percent), followed by living alone (39.7 percent). Among older men, the most common arrangement was to live with a spouse (71.2 percent), followed by living alone (18.8 percent). The least most common arrangement for both men and women was to live with nonrelatives.

As men and women age, they are more likely to live alone, but the percentage of men who are living with a spouse is still far greater than the percentage of women living with a spouse. For example, among elderly people age 65 and older, 12.5 percent of women and 56.2 percent of men live with a spouse. The next most common arrangement for women is to live with other relatives (28.5 percent), while the next most common arrangement for older men is to live alone (30.1 percent). (See Table 1.)

See also AMERICANS WITH DISABILITIES ACT; CONGREGATE LIVING; CONTINUING CARE RETIREMENT CENTERS; FAMILY AND MEDICAL LEAVE ACT; GENDER DIFFERENCES; INDEPENDENT LIVING.

He, Wan, Manisha Sengupta, Victoria A. Velkoff, and Kimberly A. DeBarros. *65+ in the United States: 2005.* Washington, D.C.: U.S. Census Bureau, December 2005.

Huntington's disease   Huntington's disease is a hereditary disorder that causes the nerve cells in the brain to degenerate, leading to dementia. Huntington's disease is caused by a defect on chromosome four, and if one parent has had the disease, a child has a 50 percent risk of also developing the disease. George Huntington, an American physician, first described this disease in 1872. According to the National Institute of Neurological Disorders and Stroke, about 30,000 people in the United States have HD and about 150,000 have a 50 percent risk of developing HD.

There are two primary forms of Huntington's disease, including adult onset Huntington's, which usually develops when the person is in his or her 30s or 40s, and early onset Huntington's, which occurs in childhood or adolescence; however, some individuals do not develop HD until after age 55. According to the National Institute of Neurological Disorders and Stroke, this late-developing form of HD is particularly difficult to diagnose because the symptoms may be masked by other health problems, or the individual may show symptoms of DEPRESSION rather than the characteristic irritability and anger of the patient with HD.

The illness is not curable, and the individual may live from 10 to 30 years from its onset. Most patients with HD die from such infections as pneumonia or from injuries related to a fall.

Symptoms and Diagnostic Path

Huntington's disease is characterized by symptoms such as uncontrolled movements, an unsteady gait, and facial movements such as grimaces. The person may exhibit paranoia, antisocial behavior, and irritability. As the dementia worsens, there is memory loss as well as loss of judgment, personality changes, and disorientation.

Physical tests such as a magnetic resonance imaging (MRI) scan or a positronic emission tomography (PET) scan will show the loss of brain tissue that characterizes Huntington's disease.

Treatment Options and Outlook

There is no treatment for Huntington's disease, although medications are used to treat the symptoms; for example, dopamine blockers are given to reduce abnormal movements and behaviors. Most people with Huntington's disease die within about 20 years, and as a result, there are few elderly individuals with the disease.

Risk Factors and Preventive Measures

Individuals with at least one parent with the HD gene are at risk for developing HD. There are no preventive measures other than the decision to get tested ahead of time for the disease if one's parent has the genetic mutation. This is a difficult choice for most people, knowing that there is no cure for HD if the gene is found to be present.

See also DEMENTIA.

hyperacusis This disorder can transform sounds that do not annoy most people into sources of irritation or even pain. Some people with hyperacusis are unable to tolerate ordinary noises such as a drawer opening or water running. This extreme heightened sensitivity to sound, which rarely affects people who do not have TINNITUS, also affects 20 to 45 percent of those who do have tinnitus.

Symptoms and Diagnostic Path

Occurring in people with normal hearing as well as in those whose hearing is impaired, hyperacusis can become painful enough to restrict normal activities.

Hyperacusis usually results from one-time or the repeated exposure to excessive noise. Once the condition is present, silence aggravates hyperacusis. Hyperacusis may also stem from the following:

- an autoimmune disorder
- Lyme disease
- a head injury
- Bell's palsy
- chronic fatigue syndrome
- medication
- infection
- temporomandibular joint syndrome (TMJ)

Treatment Options and Outlook

Hyperacusis management involves providing earplugs, advising the patient to avoid loud noises, and recommending that the patient replace or disable their doorbells, telephone ringer, and other annoying noisemakers. A low frequency "pink noise" protocol may slowly improve noise tolerance by training patients to become accustomed to listening to sounds in a range slightly below their comfort level.

Risk Factors and Preventive Measures

Patients exposed to very loud noises are at risk for developing hyperacusis. Other conditions that are associated with hyperacusis include Lyme disease, post-traumatic stress disorder (PTSD), head injury, migraine and depression, according to David M. Baguley in his article for the *Journal of the Royal Society of America*. In addition, shingles, or the recurrence of chicken pox (herpes zoster), is another risk factor for hyperacusis.

Underlying factors for hyperacusis should be identified and treated and resolved whenever possible. In most cases, however, the hyperacusis cannot be cured and must be dealt with on a daily basis.

There are no known preventive measures for hyperacusis other than avoiding loud noises.

See also ADVERSE DRUG EVENT; AMERICANS WITH DISABILITIES ACT; ASSISTIVE DEVICES/ASSISTED TECHNOLOGY; DISABILITIES; FAMILY AND MEDICAL LEAVE ACT; GENDER DIFFERENCES; HEARING DISORDERS; HEARING LOSS.

Baguley, David M. "Hyperacusis." *Journal of the Royal Society of Medicine* 96 (December 2003): 582–585.

hypertension High blood pressure, which is defined as a systolic pressure (the first number or the numerator in a blood pressure reading) of greater than 140 and a diastolic pressure of greater than 90 (the second number, or denominator). Normal blood pressure is 120/80. Individuals whose systolic blood pressure is between 120 and 139 are said to have prehypertension. This is also true if the diastolic pressure is 80–89.

In general, the systolic pressure is a more important reading, particularly among older people. High blood pressure is a risk factor for the development of ALZHEIMER'S DISEASE and other forms of DEMENTIA. However, some studies have shown that antihypertensive therapy (such as medications) can reduce this particular risk.

Hypertension is a common problem among many older people, and according to the National Center for Health Statistics, about 30 percent of all nursing home residents have hypertension. It is extremely important that it be treated. Uncontrolled hypertension can lead to KIDNEY DISEASE and coronary HEART DISEASE as well as STROKE, HEART FAILURE, HEART ATTACK, BLINDNESS, and many other health problems such as DIABETES.

According to Mark A. Supiano, M.D., in his article on hypertension for *Generations,* more than 75 percent of women older than age 75 have hypertension. More dramatically, in one study, almost 90 percent of women who had normal blood pressure at age 65 developed hypertension by age 85.

Hypertension is a greater problem among older women than older men, and blacks are particularly affected by the problem of high blood pressure. In considering those age 65 and older, the prevalence of hypertension is the highest among women age 75 and older; about 85 percent of this group has hypertension compared with 71 percent of men in the same age group. In considering all older men and women, the National Center for Health Statistics reports that 55 percent of women age 65 and older had hypertension in 2004 compared with 48 percent of older men.

Symptoms and Diagnostic Path

Blood pressure is routinely measured by most physicians during an office visit. This is one way that hypertension is initially detected. The individual may experience a racing heart or mild headache or may have no symptoms at all, which is the reason why high blood pressure is often called "the silent killer." Individuals experiencing nausea and vomiting, perspiration, pale or red skin, visual changes, fatigue, crushing chest pain, or confusion should see a doctor right away, because the blood pressure may be dangerously high, possibly leading to a heart attack.

Treatment Options and Outlook

The goal for many people is to decrease the systolic pressure to less than 140 mm Hg. If patients with hypertension also have diabetes or kidney disease, a better goal would be 130. Weight loss can decrease hypertension in many cases. Increasing exercise can also help. Medications are often needed, and two or more drugs may be required before the blood pressure is within acceptable levels.

Drugs in the angiotensin-converting enzyme (ACE) inhibitor category are often used to treat high blood pressure. Some examples of such drugs are perindopril (Aceon), quinapril (Accupril), enalapril (Vasotec), and lisinopril (Zestril). ACE inhibitors can cause headache, fatigue, and insomnia, as well as a rapid heartbeat. Patients with chest pain, problems breathing or swallowing, and facial swelling should contact their doctor and emergency personnel for assistance immediately.

Diuretics (also often known as "water pills" because they increase the elimination of fluids and thus increase urination) are also used to treat hypertension, including such drugs as spironolactone (Aldactazide, Aldactone), furosemide (Lasix), and metolazone (Zaroxolyn). Diuretics may cause frequent urination, headache, upset stomach, and muscle cramps. Patients who take these drugs and develop a severe rash, GOUT, or problems with breathing or swallowing should contact emergency personnel and their doctors immediately.

Beta-blocker medications are often used to treat hypertension, including such drugs as propranolol (Inderal and Inderal LA), metoprolol (Lopressor), and labetalol (Trandate). Beta-blockers can cause numerous side effects, including fatigue, upset stomach, HEADACHE, dizziness, and lightheadedness. Individuals who take beta-blocker drugs and experience either chest pain or trouble breathing should notify emergency personnel and their physicians immediately so that they can be evaluated.

The calcium channel blocker is another type of drug that is used to treat hypertension, including such medications as diltiazem (Cardizem, Dilacor XR), verapamil (Calan, Coversa HS, Isoptin, and Verelan), and amlodipine (Norvasc). Calcium channel blockers should not be used by patients with heart problems or those taking nitrates. In addition, patients with kidney or liver problems should take care with these drugs.

The most common side effects of calcium channel blockers are drowsiness, headache, upset stomach, feeling flushed, and ankle swelling. Patients taking a calcium channel blocker who experience chest pain, severe rashes, fainting or irregular heartbeat should contact emergency personnel and their physicians immediately.

Angiotensin II antagonists are also medications that are used to control hypertension, including such drugs as losartan (Cozaar), candesartan (Altacand), and olmesartan (Benicar). Common side effects with angiotensin II antagonists are sinus problems, sore throat, heartburn, back pain, and diarrhea. Patients who take a drug in this category should notify their physicians if they have any problems with fainting, breathing, or facial swelling or swelling of other parts of the body.

In one unique study on the effect of foods containing cocoa in elderly men, researchers studied 470 men in the Zutphen Elderly Study in the Netherlands. The men were free of diseases at the onset of the study and were followed up five years later. The causes of their deaths were determined 15 years later.

The researchers found that consumption of food with cocoa was inversely associated with blood pressure and cardiovascular and all-cause mortality; that is, those who ate cocoa had lower risks for hypertension and death from cardiovascular or other diseases than non-cocoa eaters. Some of the cocoa-containing foods were chocolate bars, chocolate cookies, and chocolate candies. Two-thirds of the men consumed plain chocolate or chocolate bars. The researchers believed that a substance that is known as flavan-3-ols, which is in cocoa-containing foods, was probably responsible for the reduction in blood pressure. Cocoa is also a source of antioxidants. It was not necessary to consume a lot of chocolate to obtain the benefit. (It is also inadvisable for people to consume large quantities of chocolate because of the risk of obesity.)

According to the researchers,

The present study indicates that men with a usual daily cocoa intake of about 4.2 g, which is equal to 10 g of dark chocolate per day, had a lower systolic and diastolic blood pressure compared with men with a low cocoa intake. Although this amount is one tenth of the dose that is used in most intervention studies, it suggests that long-term daily intake of a small amount of cocoa may lower blood pressure.

The researchers added, "In conclusion, to our knowledge, this is the first observational study that found that habitual cocoa intake was inversely associated with blood pressure in cross-sectional analysis and with cardiovascular and all-cause mortality in prospective analysis."

Risk Factors and Preventive Measures

A family history of hypertension is predictive of high blood pressure in many people. OBESITY further increases the risk for hypertension, and thus weight loss often improves blood pressure considerably. Other risk factors are male gender, African-American race, and being age 65 and older.

People with high blood pressure should avoid smoking and drinking alcohol and should also avoid foods that are high in table salt. In addition, they should be sure to EXERCISE on a regular basis.

See also CARDIOVASCULAR DISEASE; DIABETES; GENDER DIFFERENCES.

Buijsse, Brian, Edith J. M. Feskens, Frans J. Kok, and Daan Kromhout. "Cocoa Intake, Blood Pressure, and Cardiovascular Mortality: The Zutphen Elderly Study." *Archives of Internal Medicine* 166 (February 27, 2006): 411–417.

He, Wan, Manisha Sengupta, Victoria A. Velkoff, and Kimberly A. DeBarros. *65+ in the United States: 2005.* Washington, D.C.: U.S. Census Bureau, December 2005.

Supiano, Mark A. "Hypertension in Later Life." *Generations* 30, no. 3 (Fall 2006): 11–16.

hypotension Unusually low blood pressure. Hypotension may be caused or worsened by illnesses or by some medications. The person may feel dizzy when suddenly moving from a lying-down to a sitting-up position or from a sitting to a standing position. Hypotension can lead to an increased risk for FALLS. Studies have shown that hypotension that occurs after eating a meal (postprandial hypotension) is a high-risk indicator for falls, particularly among people who have DIABETES or those who take three or more medications.

Orthostatic hypotension refers to a sudden drop in blood pressure (about 20 mm Hg in the systolic blood pressure) that occurs when a person changes from a lying-down to a sitting-up position or from a sitting-up to a standing position.

See also HYPERTENSION.

identification, wearable Necklaces, bracelets, watches, or other items that include personal identification that a person wears on some exposed part of the body. These forms of identification are very valuable for individuals with chronic severe diseases, such as DIABETES, HEART ATTACK, and STROKE, and who may be unable to provide vital information about themselves in case of an emergency. Some individuals wear devices that they can activate by pressing a button, and emergency services will be alerted. Individuals in ASSISTED-LIVING FACILITIES are the most likely to have such devices.

Wearable identification is also valuable for older people who are suffering from ALZHEIMER'S DISEASE or other forms of DEMENTIA, and who are prone to wandering off, and thus could become easily lost and confused. Wearable identification also provides important information regarding medication allergies (such as to penicillin) or medications that can have serious interactions with other drugs, such as warfarin (Coumadin), a blood thinner, and can prove lifesaving if the individual is unconscious or confused and cannot respond for himself or herself in an emergency.

Wearable identification is better for medical purposes than information that is kept in a purse or wallet, because individuals may become separated from their purses or wallets in the event of an emergency. Also it may take too long for others to search for and locate such identification in an emergency situation.

Wearable identification provides the person's medication and treatment needs, as well as his or her name and address, the name of the physician, and a name and phone number of the person to call if the older person needs assistance.

Some individuals may resist wearing medical ID bracelets or necklaces, but the lifesaving importance of such items cannot be overestimated.

See also ASSISTIVE DEVICES/ASSISTED TECHNOLOGY; EMERGENCY DEPARTMENT CARE; PERSONAL EMERGENCY DEVICE.

identity theft See CRIMES AGAINST THE ELDERLY.

inappropriate prescriptions for the elderly Because older people often metabolize drugs at a slower rate than middle-aged or younger people, and they often take multiple medications, they frequently need a lower dosage of some drugs or should avoid some drugs altogether. Physicians, however, sometimes fail to take into account the older person's age when prescribing a medication and they prescribe a potentially dangerous dosage and/or drug. As a result, older people as well as family members should ask the physician if he or she has taken into account the older person's age in determining both the drug and the dosage.

Drugs that are considered dangerous or inappropriate for older individuals living in nursing homes were originally identified by physician and researcher Mark Beers, et al., in 1991, and the list is periodically updated, most recently in 2003, and is now used by doctors to consider drugs to avoid as well as lower dosages of some drugs to prescribe for all people age 65 and older. Drugs that are considered inappropriate for the elderly according to the BEERS CRITERIA are not covered by the Medicare Part D prescription drug benefit.

According to a study reported in the *Archives of Internal Medicine* in 2004, a retrospective study was done of more than 765,000 subjects age 65 and older and who were prescribed one or more prescription drugs in 1999. The authors found that 21 percent of the subjects were given prescriptions for one or more drugs of concern. The most commonly prescribed drug types were psychiatric drugs (alone accounting for 45 percent of the drugs on the Beer list) and neuromuscular medications. Residents in the south of the United States were the most likely to be prescribed an inappropriate drug.

The doctors who prescribe these drugs to the elderly are not necessarily acting out of ignorance. According to the researchers in the *Archives of Internal Medicine* study, older patients may be on complicated drug regimens because of multiple chronic illnesses, and the doctor may be reluctant to take them off drugs that seem to help them. Also, the doctor may have determined that a specific drug, even if deemed inappropriate for the elderly by the Beers criteria, is best for the patient and the benefits outweigh the risks.

As mentioned, in 2003, the drugs listed on the Beers criteria were revised. Some drugs given a rating of a high risk for severity included most muscle relaxants, such as methocarbamol (Robaxin), carisoprodol (Soma), chlorzoxazone (Parflex), metaxalone (Skelaxin), and cyclobenzaprine (Flexeril). Many benzodiazepines (antianxiety drugs) were listed as having a high severity, particularly chlordiazepoxide (Librium), chlordiazepoxide-amitriptyline (Limbitrol), clidinium-chlordiazepoxide (Librax), diazepam (Valium), quazepam (Doral), halazepam (Paxipam), and clorazepate (Tranxene). The antidepressant fluoxetine (Prozac) is also on the list as a high-severity drug. For more information, individuals should contact their physicians.

See also HOSPITALIZATION; MEDICARE; MEDICATION COMPLIANCE; MEDICATION MANAGEMENT; NURSING HOMES.

Curtis, Lesley H., et al. "Inappropriate Prescribing for Elderly Americans in a Large Outpatient Population." *Archives of Internal Medicine* 164, no. 23 (August 9, 2004): 1,621–1,625.

Fick, Donna M., et al. "Updating the Beers Criteria for Potentially Inappropriate Medication Use in Older Adults: Results of a U.S. Consensus Panel of Experts." *Archives of Internal Medicine* 163, no. 22 (December 8, 2003): 2,716–2,724.

Jano, Elda, and Rajender R. Aparasu. "Healthcare Outcomes Associated with Beers Criteria: A Systematic Review." *The Annals of Pharmacotherapy* 41 (March 2007): 438–448.

independent living The situation of the older person who lives in a home, apartment, mobile home, or other facility where assistance is not provided on a regular basis. The individual may use some services, such as HOME HEALTH/HOME CARE or delivered meals, but he or she does not receive the higher level of assistance that is provided in an ASSISTED-LIVING FACILITY, CONTINUING CARE RETIREMENT CENTER, or a NURSING HOME.

Some assisted-living facilities are divided into particular areas for independent living and other areas for those individuals requiring additional care, such as assisted living or both assisted living and nursing home care. Individuals who live in an independent living complex may choose to participate in a variety of planned social activities, and they are often provided meals, but they do not require the higher level of care that is provided in the other sections of the facility.

See also CONGREGATE LIVING.

infections Bacterial or viral invasions of the body that cause minor to major illnesses. Some people are more susceptible to developing infections than others, such as individuals who have DIABETES, CANCER patients receiving immunosuppressant drugs, or those whose immune systems are weakened for any reason.

Preventable Infections

PNEUMONIA and FLU/INFLUENZA are still dangerous infections in the United States and Canada, and they may become extremely serious for older people, even leading to death. Yet these infections are largely preventable with immunizations. For this reason, doctors recommend that most people older than age 50 receive annual immunizations for flu and a one-time immunization for pneumonia. However, many older people fail to receive these immunizations, despite the fact that MEDICARE provides payment coverage for them both. Even if an immunized person contracts flu or pneumonia, their symptoms are less severe than if they had not received the vaccine.

In general, infections may cause back pain and other aches and pain throughout the body. They can weaken individuals and make them more likely to develop serious subsequent infections, further weakening the person. Infections are also often accompanied by fever higher than 99°F.

Sometimes, infections can be difficult to detect in older people, according to Dr. Mouton and his colleagues in their 2001 article for *American Family Physician.* Physicians and caregivers must look for subtle indicators. For example, a change in the individual's mental status sometimes may be the only sign of an infection, yet this indicator is often ignored. The authors state,

> Many signs and symptoms of infection that are common in younger adults, particularly fever and leukocytosis [high white-blood-cell count] present less frequently or not at all in older adults. While 60 percent of older adults with serious infections develop leukocytosis, its absence does not rule out an infectious process. Because frail older adults tend to have poorer body temperature response, elevations in body temperate of 1.1° (2°F.) from their normal baseline temperature should be considered a febrile [feverish] response. Fevers higher than 38.3° (101°F.) often indicate severe, life-threatening infections in older adults, and hospitalization should be considered for these patients.

See also HEPATITIS B; HOSPITALIZATION; PNEUMONIA.

Mouton, Charles P., M.D., et al. "Common Infections in Older Adults." *American Family Physician* 63 (2001): 257–268.

insomnia Difficulty getting to sleep that may become a chronic problem and a SLEEP DISORDER. Insomnia is a common problem among adults age 65 and older. It may stem from the use of some medications or may be caused by DEPRESSION, anxiety disorders, or other physical or mental health problems. It may also be related to losses, such as the death of a beloved spouse or friend.

If the insomnia becomes a chronic problem, then the individual's physician should review the medications that the person takes to see if they could be causing or contributing to the sleep problem. The doctor should also review the current circumstances of the person's life to try to determine if there may be an underlying psychological problem causing the insomnia that can be treated.

Therapy may help with insomnia. There are also over-the-counter and prescription sleep medications that can improve insomnia. A complete regimen of appropriate sleep habits and hygiene may help remedy this problem.

See also ANXIETY AND ANXIETY DISORDERS; BEREAVEMENT.

intensive-care unit (ICU) Special section of the hospital that provides a higher level of care for seriously or critically ill individuals who need constant attention and observation, such as the victims of a serious car crash or those who have had a HEART ATTACK or STROKE and are at risk for their condition worsening or for dying. Special monitors regularly take the patient's temperature, pulse, and blood pressure, and alarms go off if these readings fall below or go above certain predetermined levels. If patients' conditions improve significantly, they are usually moved to another part of the hospital, where the care is not so intensive.

Visits to patients in the intensive-care unit are usually restricted to family members only, and visits must generally be brief unless the patient is dying.

The ratio of nurse to patient is very high in intensive-care units, and it often is one to one or one to two, with aides available as well. This guarantees the opportunity for constant supervision over the very ill patient.

See also HEALTH-CARE AGENT/PROXY; HOSPITALIZATION.

irritability Easily annoyed and aggravated. Older individuals who are suffering from disorders that cause CHRONIC PAIN may have a problem with irritability, including such disorders as ARTHRITIS, BACK PAIN, and so forth. Patients with various forms of DEMENTIA (including ALZHEIMER'S DISEASE, the most common form of dementia) may also be extremely irritable. Such behavior can become very difficult for caregivers to cope with.

Sometimes chronic irritability is a sign of a clinical DEPRESSION, and the physician should investigate this possibility.

See ADULT CHILDREN/CHILDREN OF AGING PARENTS; AGGRESSION, PHYSICAL; COGNITIVE IMPAIRMENT; COMPANIONS; CONFUSION; DELUSIONS; DEMENTIA; HALLUCINATIONS; MEMORY IMPAIRMENT; RAGE.

joint replacement   Total joint replacements of the knee, hip, or other joints. As can be seen from Tables 1 and 2, knee replacement is about twice as common a procedure as is hip joint replacement among older people. In addition, women are more likely than men to have knee and/or hip replacements.

About 97 percent of these procedures in older people are necessary because of years of damage caused by OSTEOARTHRITIS, although some patients suffer from rheumatoid arthritis or other problems. The key complaint of patients who have joint replacements is severe pain caused by the action of bone rubbing on bone, and the patient may also be disabled. In the case of knee replacements, studies have shown a positive relationship between surgeons and hospitals that performed a large number of these procedures and successful outcomes, and it is likely that the same is true in the case of hip replacements. In addition, patients who see a physical therapist *before* surgery to learn exercises often have a quicker recovery than those who do not see a physical therapist until after surgery has occurred.

According to the National Institute of Arthritis and Musculoskeletal and Skin Diseases (NIAMS), the new joint may be made of plastic, metal, or both and is called a *prosthesis*. Sometimes the prosthesis is cemented into place; other times it is not cemented so that the bone will grow into it. In general, the cemented joint is used more frequently for older people.

Procedure

Patients generally go home from the hospital three to five days following surgery for hip or knee joint replacement, while the time in the hospital for other joint replacements may vary. Elderly patients may be discharged to a rehabilitative facility to recover for several weeks before returning home, depending on their physicians' recommendations.

With knee replacement, also known as *knee arthroplasty,* the procedure is performed under general anesthesia, and the ends of the femur (thigh bone) and the tibia (shin bone), as well as the undersurface of the kneecap, are cut so that the prosthetic knee can be fitted into place.

With hip replacement, also known as *hip arthroplasty,* the surgery is performed under general anesthesia, and the surgeon removes damaged bone and cartilage from the hip joint and replaces them with artificial parts. As with knee replacement, the hip prosthesis may be cemented or uncemented, although cemented replacements are often used for elderly individuals.

Physical therapy begins soon after surgery, sometimes the next day. The physical therapist helps the patient perform range-of-motion exercises.

Risks and Complications

Joint surgery is successful in about 90 percent of the cases, and problems are usually treatable. In general, some problems that may occur with joint replacement surgery include

- infection to the wound or around the new joint—minor infections are treated with antibiotics but deeper infections may require a second surgery

- blood clots that cause swelling and pain in the legs after knee or hip surgery—the doctor may recommend blood thinners and/or special stockings or boots to increase blood flow

- loosening of the new joint, causing pain—if the loosening is severe, a second surgery may be needed

- dislocation of the ball of the prosthesis—this can usually be fixed without further surgery but the patient may need to wear a brace for a period of time

- wearing down of the replacement—excessive wearing can lead to loosening, and if the prosthesis comes loose more surgery may be needed; however, sometimes the physician can replace just the plastic part of the replacement rather than the whole joint

- nerve and blood vessel injury caused by damage during the surgery—this is rare

Problems that may occur with knee replacements include

- blood clots in the legs (deep vein thrombosis [DVT])
- PNEUMONIA
- an infection that necessitates the removal of the joint
- a loosening or displacement of the prosthesis

According to the National Institutes of Health, the most common problem that may occur with hip replacements is hip dislocation. Other problems include blood clots and infections.

Outlook and Lifestyle Modifications

On average, the new joint will last from 10 to 15 years; however, in some cases, an earlier joint replacement may be needed.

With knee replacement, contact sports should be avoided, but activities such as swimming and golf are encouraged after recovery.

After hip surgery, the National Institutes of Health recommends the following to avoid displacing the joint:

- Do not cross the feet or ankles at any time.
- Keep feet about six inches apart when sitting.
- Avoid low chairs.
- Avoid bending at the waist and consider a long-handled shoehorn to help put on shoes and socks and an extension "grabber" to pick up objects too low to reach.
- When in bed lying down, place a pillow between the legs to keep them properly aligned.
- Consider purchasing an elevated toilet seat to keep the knees lower than the hips when sitting on the toilet.

TABLE 1. HOSPITAL DISCHARGES FOR KNEE REPLACEMENT SURGERY AMONG ADULTS AGE 65 AND OLDER, BY SEX AND AGE, 1992–2004

	1992–1993	1992–1993	2003–2004	2003–2004
	Average number of hospital discharges with procedure performed in thousands	Hospital discharges with procedure performed per 10,000 population	Average annual number of hospital discharges with procedure performed in thousands	Hospital discharges with procedure performed per 10,000 population
Sex and age				
Both sexes	124	38.6	263	72.9
65 and older	74	40.4	145	78.7
75 and older	50	36.1	118	66.9
Men				
65–74	40	30.7	94	62.3
75 and older	15	30.8	42	63.7
Women				
65–74	84	43.9	169	80.5
75 and older	35	39.1	76	68.7

Source: Adapted from National Center for Health Statistics. *Health, United States, 2006, with Chartbook on Trends in the Health of Americans.* Hyattsville, Md.: National Institutes of Health, 2006, p. 121.

TABLE 2. HOSPITAL DISCHARGES FOR NONFRACTURE HIP REPLACEMENT SURGERY AMONG ADULTS 18 YEARS OF AGE AND OLDER, BY SEX AND AGE: UNITED STATES, 1992–1993 AND 2003–2004

	1992–1993	1992–1993	2003–2004	2003–2004
	Average number of hospital stays with procedure performed in thousands	Hospital stays with procedure performed per 10,000 population	Average annual number of hospital stays with procedure performed in thousands	Hospital stays with procedure performed per 10,000 population
Sex and age				
Both sexes				
65 and older	81	25.2	142	39.5
65–74	44	24.0	72	39.2
75 and older	37	26.7	70	39.7
Men				
65–74	16	20.3	28	33.8
75 and older	11	22.8	26	39.2
Women				
65–74	28	27.0	44	43.7
75 and older	26	28.9	44	40.0

Source: National Center for Health Statistics. *Health, United States, 2006, with Chartbook on Trends in the Health of Americans.* Hyattsville, Md.: National Institutes of Health, 2006, p. 122.

Statistics on Joint Replacements

According to the National Center for Health Statistics, in 2003–2004, there were 263,000 knee replacements for individuals age 65 and older. Women had more knee replacements than men. (See Table 1.) The numbers of knee replacements increased dramatically since 1993, more than doubling from 74,000 for men and women ages 65 to 74 to 145,000 for this same age group by 2003. In addition, the numbers of knee replacements among individuals age 75 and older also more than doubled, increasing from 50,000 procedures in 1993 to 118,000 in 2003.

Non-fracture hip replacements in individuals with arthritis are also much more common than in the past. For example, in 1992–1993, there were 25.2 procedures for every 10,000 people age 65 and older. By the 2003–2004 period, this rate had significantly increased to 39.5 per 10,000 people. (See Table 2.) As can be seen from the table, older women had more hip replacements than older men, or a rate of 36.2 per 10,000 men and 41.8 per 10,000 women.

See also AMERICANS WITH DISABILITIES ACT; ARTHRITIS; ASSISTIVE DEVICES/ASSISTED TECHNOLOGY; DISABILITY; END-OF-LIFE ISSUES; FAMILY AND MEDICAL LEAVE ACT; FRACTURES; FRAILTY; GENDER DIFFERENCES; HOSPITALIZATION; NURSING HOMES.

Defrances, C. J., M. J. Hall, and M. N. Podgornik. "2003 National Hospital Discharge Survey." *Advanced Data from Vital and Health Statistics* 359. Hyattsville, Md.: National Center for Health Statistics.

National Center for Health Statistics. *Health, United States, 2006, with Chartbook on Trends in the Health of Americans.* Hyattsville, Md.: National Institutes of Health, 2006.

National Institute of Arthritis and Musculoskeletal and Skin Diseases. *Joint Replacement Surgery and You: Information for Multicultural Communities.* Washington, D.C.: National Institutes of Health, 2005.

kidney cancer According to the American Cancer Society, there were an estimated 51,190 new cases of cancer in the kidney and renal pelvis in 2007, and 12,890 people died of kidney cancer in 2007. Of the new kidney cancer cases in 2007, 31,590 were men and 19,600 were women. Of the deaths from kidney cancer in 2007, 8,080 were men and 4,810 were women.

Symptoms and Diagnostic Path

Some symptoms that commonly appear with kidney cancer are

- blood in the urine (hematuria that causes the urine to be rusty-looking or red)
- continuous pain in the side
- a mass or lump in the side or the abdomen
- weight loss
- fever
- extreme fatigue

Note that the above symptoms may occur in individuals who do not have kidney cancer; however, anyone with any of these symptoms should see a physician.

The doctor will check for general health signs and for the presence of high blood pressure. She or he will also feel the patient's abdomen and side for any sign of tumors. Urine tests will check for blood and other indicators of disease.

The doctor may order an intravenous pyleogram (IVP), which is a test in which dye is injected into the arm. The dye goes throughout the body, and it is excreted through the kidneys, making the kidneys show up clearly on X-rays. If there is a kidney tumor or other kidney diseases, the IVP will often reveal this information.

The doctor may also order a computerized tomography (CT) scan or an ultrasound test. A biopsy of the kidney will be performed if cancer is suspected. The doctor inserts a thin needle through the skin and into the kidney to remove the tissue to be biopsied. The pathologist will check the tissue for cancer cells.

If kidney cancer is present, the doctor will use imaging tests such as an MRI or CT scan to stage the cancer. There are four stages: Stage I, II, III, and IV.

Treatment Options and Outlook

Treatment may include surgery, arterial embolization, radiation therapy, biological therapy, or chemotherapy. Some people will receive a combination of treatments. The most common form of treatment is surgery, including either a radical nephrectomy, in which the entire kidney is removed along with the adrenal gland and some tissue surrounding the kidney, or a simple nephrectomy, in which only the kidney is removed.

Another option is a partial nephrectomy, in which only the part of the kidney with the tumor is removed, as when the person has only one kidney or the cancer is affecting both kidneys. People with small kidney tumors may also have a partial nephrectomy.

People with kidney cancer should ask the following questions before surgery:

- What kind of operation do you recommend for me?
- Do I need any lymph nodes removed? Why?
- What are the risks of surgery? Will I have any long-term effects? Will I need DIALYSIS?
- Should I store some of my own blood in case I need a transfusion?

- How will I feel after the operation?
- How long will I need to stay in the hospital?
- When can I get back to my normal activities?
- How often will I need checkups?
- Would a clinical trial be appropriate for me?

An arterial embolization is a procedure that shrinks the tumor, and it may be done before the surgery occurs. The doctor inserts a catheter into a blood vessel in the leg and moves it up to the renal artery, the main blood vessel supplying blood to the kidney. The doctor then injects a substance to block the blood flow to the kidney to prevent the tumor from receiving oxygen to grow. Some patients have back pain, nausea, or vomiting after the arterial embolization procedure.

Radiation therapy may be used to treat kidney cancer, and sometimes it is used before surgery to help shrink the tumor. Radiation therapy can also be used to relieve cancer pain. However, radiation therapy for kidney cancer can cause nausea and vomiting, diarrhea, and urinary discomfort.

Biological therapy is another form of therapy for kidney cancer. If patients have cancer that has spread to other parts of the body, the doctor may suggest substances such as interferon alpha or interleukin-2 be taken. Biological therapy may induce flulike symptoms, such as fever, chills, and muscle aches. These side effects end when treatment ends.

Chemotherapy is another form of therapy to fight kidney cancer. These anticancer drugs may cause hair loss, poor appetite, nausea and vomiting, bruising or easy bleeding, and extreme fatigue. Many side effects can be controlled with other drugs.

Risk Factors and Preventive Measures

A key risk factor for kidney cancer is cigarette SMOKING, and smokers have twice the risk for developing kidney cancer as nonsmokers. People who are obese also have an increased risk for developing kidney cancer. Men are more likely to develop kidney cancer than women.

High blood pressure (HYPERTENSION) also increases the risk for kidney cancer. Individuals on long-term dialysis also have an increased risk for kidney cancer.

See also CANCER.

kidney disease Diseases and disorders of the kidney, ranging from kidney INFECTIONS to KIDNEY FAILURE. The kidneys are also affected by health problems that are very common among elderly individuals, such as HYPERTENSION, HYPOTENSION, and DIABETES. In addition, many years of ALCOHOLISM may lead to kidney disease. Kidney disease is also often associated with ANEMIA. In some cases, ASPIRIN THERAPY (used to prevent heart attack) may lead to kidney disease and thus should be monitored very carefully by physicians. Patients with kidney disease may be treated by a urologist, a specialist physician who treats diseases and disorders of the urinary tract and kidneys, as well as diseases of the male prostate gland, such as PROSTATE CANCER or other PROSTATE DISEASES. The urologist is also a surgeon.

The two kidneys filter the blood of impurities, and they are vitally important organs. It is possible to live without one kidney or even with one part of the kidney, but if kidney function is completely gone, then the individual needs either DIALYSIS or the transplantation of a kidney in order to stay alive. Older African Americans have a higher rate of kidney failure than individuals of other races and ethnicities.

Dialysis is an artificial procedure in which a machine removes the impurities from the blood (since the kidney is no longer able to do this), while kidney transplantation provides a healthy kidney that is implanted in the patient. The donated kidney may come from a recent cadaver (dead person) or from a healthy and living donor who is a match.

Symptoms and Diagnostic Path

Often individuals with kidney disease have no symptoms. However, they may have mild symptoms or even severe pain, particularly BACK PAIN. For example, kidney stones cause severe pain, causing most people to contact their physicians or head quickly to the nearest hospital for EMERGENCY DEPARTMENT CARE.

Kidney disease is diagnosed based on the patient's symptoms as well as on laboratory findings. A 24-hour urine collection test is usually ordered if the physician suspects kidney disease. A simple urinalysis can detect bacteria in the urine, and the urine can also be cultured to determine the presence of bacteria as well as the type of bacteria.

Doctors can also order a blood urea nitrogen (BUN) test. BUN is a waste product produced by the kidneys, and increased levels of BUN may be an early warning sign of kidney disease that should be followed up. It may also indicate dehydration.

Treatment Options and Outlook

The treatment of kidney disease depends entirely on the cause. If the illness is bacterial, then antibiotics will be administered. In other cases, medications can be given to treat chronic kidney disease. If the illness is very advanced and has led to kidney failure, the only therapy that will work is kidney dialysis and eventually a kidney transplant.

See also HOSPITALIZATION.

kidney failure　The most serious form of KIDNEY DISEASE. Kidney failure is also known as end stage renal disorder (ESRD). With kidney failure, the kidneys can no longer remove impurities from the blood, and this failure drastically increases the risk of INFECTIONS that could rapidly overwhelm the body and kill the person. Also, when the kidneys fail, the balance of electrolytes (such as potassium, sodium, and chloride) can become severely disturbed, leading to illness and death.

Kidney failure may occur after years of long-term kidney disease. It may also result from chronic severe infections, long-term ALCOHOLISM or SUBSTANCE ABUSE AND DEPENDENCE, or be caused by a variety of other medical problems. African Americans have a higher rate of kidney failure than individuals of other races and ethnicities.

Kidney failure leads to death unless the patient undergoes either DIALYSIS, an artificial means to remove impurities from the blood, or has a kidney transplant. Individuals with kidney disease are treated by nephrologists, physicians who are specialists in treating diseases of the kidney.

See also CANCER; HEALTH-CARE AGENT/PROXY; HYPERTENSION; LIVING WILL.

knee replacement　See JOINT REPLACEMENT.

laxatives Over-the-counter or prescribed medications for individuals with CONSTIPATION. Some people who have difficulty maintaining regular bowel movements (daily or every other day) may also have a problem with passing very hard stools, and they may use stool softeners to facilitate their bowel movements. Other individuals take laxatives that are combined with stool softeners. Some non-laxative prescribed medications may be helpful to the person with chronic constipation.

Some people seek alternative remedies such as herbs or supplements to resolve their constipation problem; however, they should consult their physicians before taking these medications to make sure they will not cause any harmful effects together with other medications the older person already takes.

It is possible to become physically dependent on laxatives; seniors should consult with their physicians if they feel that they must always take a laxative in order to have a bowel movement at all. People who have chronic problems with constipation should increase their fiber intake by eating more fruits and vegetables. Improving their daily exercise and activity regimen can be a great help. In addition, their doctors should also look at their medications to see if the dosages should be adjusted, in the event that the medications that were prescribed are constipating. (Some medications, such as NARCOTICS, are very constipating.)

Certain chronic medical conditions have a known effect on bowel function, such as DIABETES or PARKINSON'S DISEASE. Adjustments in their daily activity levels, their medications, dietary changes, and even the timing of taking the medication can make a big difference in bowel habits for some seniors.

See also FECAL INCONTINENCE.

learned helplessness An induced feeling of powerlessness that often leads to real powerlessness. The key premise of the idea behind learned helplessness is that when people are treated as if they are completely helpless (even though they are capable of performing at least some tasks), they often will eventually take on the attributes of helplessness and, as a result, they will become helpless.

For example, if individuals are constantly urged to rest, even though they are capable of at least some physical activity, then some people may adopt the idea that they are weak and need to rest constantly and give up on any exercise, eventually causing them to become weaker than they would otherwise be. If people are fed, even though they can feed themselves, they may give up on attempting to self-feed.

These various acts of a relinquishment of independence often lead to DEPRESSION and an overall deterioration of the individual's health. Note that learned helplessness is usually not caused by others who seek to be cruel to the older person, and even very well-meaning relatives and other caregivers may unknowingly induce learned helplessness in others.

When people in a NURSING HOME or other facility are capable of using the toilet if they receive some assistance in getting to the bathroom, but that assistance is never or rarely received, then the affected people will become incontinent.

It is also true that learned helplessness in one task may generalize to an overall helplessness at many tasks. This means that if people feel that they cannot feed themselves, for example, they may also feel that they cannot perform other activities, including those they actually can perform.

Sometimes well-meaning caregivers or attendants try to do many or most things for an older person, but study after study shows that the people who are the healthiest and the happiest are those who can perform at least some ACTIVITIES OF DAILY LIVING on their own.

As a result, whenever possible, older people should be encouraged to maintain some level of control over their daily lives, even though they may take a much longer time or it causes some inconvenience to a facility or a caregiver.

See also ADULT CHILDREN/CHILDREN OF AGING PARENTS; COMPASSION FATIGUE; FAMILY CAREGIVERS; TALKING TO ELDERLY PARENTS ABOUT DIFFICULT ISSUES; SIBLING RIVALRY; TOILETING.

legal guardianship Process whereby an individual, often a family member, is appointed by the court to represent the interests of another person. Sometimes legal guardianship is known as conservatorship.

In the case of older individuals, the legal guardian is usually one who acts for a person who has been determined by a court to be mentally incompetent and thus is incapable of managing his or her own life and making major decisions about medical treatment, financial affairs, or other issues. This is a different situation than when the DURABLE POWER OF ATTORNEY is used, in which a person makes advance arrangements for another person to manage his or her affairs if and when the individual should later become mentally incompetent or physically incapacitated.

According to Peter J. Straus and Nancy M. Lederman in their book, *The Complete Retirement Survival Guide*, the power and the responsibility of a guardian vary from state to state. These powers may include the rights to

- consent to medical treatment
- decide where to live
- make a nursing home placement
- ensure clothing, food, housing, medical care, and personal needs are met
- initiate divorce or separation proceedings when it is in the ward's best interests
- make contracts

- bring and defend lawsuits
- apply for government benefits

In addition, the authors state that the guardian may be given power over the individual's financial affairs, including the power to enter into agreements with others on the individual's behalf, as well as manage property, invest their assets, rent or sell their home, control their money, receive income, make gifts or dispose of property, and enter into lawsuits on the behalf of the individual.

According to *The American Bar Association Legal Guide for Americans over 50*, a person may need a guardian when

- he or she can no longer manage his or her affairs because of serious incapacity;
- no other voluntary arrangements for decision making and management (such as durable powers of attorney) have been set up ahead of time, or when such arrangements are not working well;
- serious harm will come to the individual if no legally authorized decision maker is appointed.

According the American Bar Association book, the steps for appointing a guardian are

- Guardianship is initiated through a formal petition to the court, with notice provided to all interested parties.
- The individual who is alleged to be incapacitated has the opportunity for a full hearing.
- The court may appoint a guardian *ad litem* to represent the best interests of the alleged incapacitated person during the proceeding. In some states the judge appoints a court visitor or a team of valuators to investigate and report back to the court. In some states, a court-appointed lawyer may represent the rights and wishes of the alleged incapacitated person.
- Generally, the alleged incapacitated person must submit to an examination by a physician, psychologist, or other clinician.
- The judge weighs the evidence and crafts an order appointing the guardian and outlining the scope of the guardian's powers.

See also ATTORNEYS; ASSETS; COGNITIVE IMPAIR-MENT; END-OF-LIFE ISSUES; HEALTH-CARE AGENT/ PROXY; LIVING TRUST; LIVING WILL.

American Bar Association. *The American Bar Association Legal Guide for Americans over 50.* New York: Random House Reference, 2006.

Straus, Peter J., and Nancy M. Lederman. *The Complete Retirement Survival Guide. Second Edition.* New York: Checkmark Books, 2003.

life expectancy The time frame that an average person can expect to live. Due to numerous medical and technological advances, life expectancies have dramatically increased from past years, and consequently, many individuals in the 21st century may live until their 70s, 80s, or older; for example, CENTENARIANS are individuals who have lived to age 100 or older. The life expectancy of individuals age 65 and older has increased dramatically since 1900, when the average 65-year-old male had an additional life expectancy of 11.5 more years (or to 76.5), and the average 65-year-old female had an average life expectancy of 12.2 more years (or age 77.2).

In 2003 (the latest figures available as of this writing), the average 65-year-old male could expect to live 16.8 more years (or until age 81.8), and the average 65-year-old female could expect to live 19.8 more years (or until age 85.8). (See Table 1.)

Death Rates Have Changed for Heart Disease and Cancers

One reason life expectancies have increased is that death rates have dropped for nearly all age groups and races with regard to diseases of the heart, although they have risen for malignant cancers. For example, according to the National Center for Health Statistics, in 1960, the death rate for diseases of the heart for black males ages 65 to 74 was 2,281.4 per 100,000 people. By 2000, that rate had dropped to 1,212.8, a major reduction of 46.8 percent. Death rates dropped even further for white males and females, but not as much for black females. (See Table 2.)

However, death rates from malignant cancers have increased with age; for example, in 1960, the

TABLE 1. ADDITIONAL YEARS LIFE EXPECTANCY AT AGE 65, BY SEX: UNITED STATES, 1900–2003

Year	Male	Female
1900–1902	11.5	12.2
1909–1911	11.2	12.0
1919–1921	12.2	12.7
1929–1931	11.7	12.8
1939–1941	12.1	13.6
1949–1951	12.7	15.0
1959–1961	13.0	15.8
1969–1971	13.0	16.8
1979–1981	14.2	18.4
1989–1991	15.1	19.0
1997	15.9	19.2
1998	16.0	19.2
1999	16.1	19.1
2000	16.2	19.3
2001	16.4	19.4
2002	16.6	19.5
2003	16.8	19.8

Source: Adapted from National Center for Health Statistics. *Health, United States, 2006, with Chartbook on Trends in the Health of Americans.* Hyattsville, Md.: National Institutes of Health, 2006, p. 113.

rate for black males ages 75 to 84 was 1,053.3 per 100,000. By 2000, that rate had increased to 2,283.6, a 116.8 percent rate increase. (See Table 2.)

Life Expectancy Lower in the United States than in Some Other Countries

In comparing the life expectancy in the United States with that of other countries, the United States is far from first; for example, according to the Census Bureau, elderly male individuals in the following countries all had an average greater life expectancy at age 65 than did older males in the United States in 2000: Sweden, Japan, Singapore, Australia, Hong Kong, Switzerland, Israel, Italy, Canada, Spain, France, and Taiwan. (See Appendix X.)

Among females age 65 and older, women in Puerto Rico and the following countries had a greater life expectancy than older women in the United States in 2000: Japan, Singapore, Canada, Australia, France, Switzerland, Spain, Hong Kong, Sweden, Italy, Norway, Austria, Finland, Germany,

TABLE 2. DEATH RATES OF DISEASES OF THE HEART AND CANCER BY AGE, RACE, AND SEX, 1960 AND 2000 (DEATHS PER 100,000 POPULATION)

Cause of death, age, race, and sex	Death Rates		Percentage Change
	1960	2000	1960 to 2000
Diseases of the heart			
Age			
65 to 74			
White male	2,297.9	891.2	-61.2
Black male	2,281.4	1,212.8	-46.8
White female	1,229.8	451.3	-63.3
Black female	1,680.5	805.9	-52.0
75 to 84			
White male	4,839.9	2,209.6	-54.3
Black male	3,533.6	2,522.4	-28.6
White female	3,629.7	1,475.2	-59.4
Black female	2,926.9	2,004.2	-31.5
85 and older			
White male	10,135.8	6,257.6	-38.3
Black male	6,037.9	5,198.6	-13.9
White female	9,280.8	5,824.0	-37.2
Black female	5,650.0	5,489.0	-2.8
Malignant cancers			
Age			
65 to 74			
White male	887.3	999.3	+12.6
Black male	938.5	1,303.5	+38.9
White female	562.1	674.7	+20.0
Black female	541.6	744.5	+37.5
75 to 84			
White male	1,413.7	1,797.1	+20.8
Black male	1,053.3	2,283.6	+116.8
White female	959.3	1,080.1	+15.0
Black female	696.3	1,177.6	+69.1
85 and older			
White male	1,791.4	2,569.2	+43.4
Black male	1,155.2	3,012.7	+160.8
White female	1,304.9	1,464.7	+12.2
Black female	728.9	1,582.6	+117.1

Source: Adapted from He, Wan, Manisha Sengupta, Victoria A. Velkoff, and Kimberly A. DeBarros. *65+ in the United States: 2005.* Washington, D.C.: U.S. Census Bureau, December 2005, p. 44.

Belgium, New Zealand, the Netherlands, and Israel. (See Appendix X for more detail.)

See also DEATH; DEATH, FEAR OF.

He, Wan, Manisha Sengupta, Victoria A. Velkoff, and Kimberly A. DeBarros. *65+ in the United States: 2005.* Washington, D.C.: U.S. Census Bureau, December 2005.

liver cancer   The liver is the largest organ in the human body and is located behind the ribs and on the right side of the abdomen. An estimated 19,160 people were newly diagnosed with cancer of the liver and intrahepatic bile duct in 2007, and there were an estimated 16,780 deaths. Of the new cases in 2007, 13,650 were men and 5,510 were women. Of the deaths from liver cancer in 2007, 11,280 were men and 5,500 were women.

The risk for liver cancer increases with age. Sometimes cancer spreads from other parts of the body to the liver, but in that case, liver cancer is a secondary cancer.

Symptoms and Diagnostic Path

Often there are no symptoms of liver cancer; however, as the cancer grows larger, symptoms appear. Some symptoms may include

- bloated abdomen
- pain in the upper abdomen on the right side
- weight loss
- loss of appetite and feelings of fullness
- weakness and fatigue
- nausea and vomiting
- jaundice: yellowed skin and eyes and dark urine
- fever

Patients with these symptoms may have another medical problem but should see the doctor for a checkup. A hepatologist is a physician specialist who treats liver diseases.

To diagnose the possible presence of liver cancer, the doctor feels the abdomen to check the liver, spleen, and surrounding organs. He or she also checks for any abnormal buildup of fluid in the abdomen. The skin and eyes are checked for jaundice.

Blood tests can be used to detect liver problems, such as the alpha-fetoprotein (AFP). High AFP levels may indicate the presence of liver cancer.

Imaging tests such as a CT scan and ultrasound may be used.

A biopsy is done using a fine-needle aspiration, sometimes using the CT or ultrasound to help the doctor guide the needle.

If liver cancer is present, the doctor needs the cancer staged to determine whether the tumor can be surgically removed.

Treatment Options and Outlook

If it is found in the early stages, liver cancer can be surgically treated if the patient is healthy enough. If the cancer has spread or the disease cannot be controlled, doctors usually recommend palliative therapy to control pain and other symptoms of the disease. Because liver cancer is so hard to control, doctors may recommend that patients enroll in a clinical trial, which is a study of patients with the same disease, testing new treatments.

If part of the liver is removed, this is called a partial hepatectomy. In some patients, liver transplantation is performed. Patients cannot live without a liver.

If the liver cancer is localized, it may be treated with radiofrequency ablation, using a special hot probe to kill cancer cells. Other treatments include:

- percutaneous ethanol injection—an injection of alcohol directly into the liver tumor to kill the cancer cells
- cryosurgery—a metal probe is used to freeze and destroy cancer cells
- hepatic arterial infusion—a catheter is inserted into the hepatic artery, the artery that supplies blood to the liver; anticancer drugs are injected into the catheter
- chemoembolization—a tiny catheter is inserted into the leg and anticancer drugs are injected

If the liver cancer is advanced, anticancer therapy will be given to slow the cancer's growth, although the patient cannot be cured. Chemotherapy may be given to kill the cancer cells, as may radiation therapy.

Risk Factors and Preventive Measures

Chronic HEPATITIS is a risk factor for liver cancer, including infection with hepatitis B or C. Cirrhosis of the liver is another risk factor. Cirrhosis means that the live cells are damaged and replaced with scar tissue. Alcoholism, some parasites, and some drugs cause cirrhosis, and an estimated 5 percent of people with cirrhosis will develop liver cancer.

Men are about twice as likely to develop liver cancer as women. People with a family history of liver cancer are more likely to develop the disease. Liver cancer occurs more commonly in people older than 60 years.

See also CANCER.

living trust   A concept that is based on state law as well as a document that is usually prepared by an attorney to protect the individual's ASSETS. Both the concept and the document are designed so that the individual's financial assets and personal property will be held jointly with one or more trustees who are selected during the older person's lifetime, and then these assets will be inherited by the survivors upon death. A living trust is very different from a LIVING WILL, which is a document that stipulates what (if any) heroic measures should be taken if an individual is near death.

The living trust is often created to avoid probate court after the death of the individual, because the probate court may take a percentage of the assets of a deceased person and may also freeze these assets for a lengthy time (a year or longer) until the court adjudicates the disposition of the assets. The advantages and disadvantages of a living trust should be discussed with an experienced estate-planning attorney practicing in the state where the elderly person lives.

See also DURABLE POWER OF ATTORNEY; END-OF-LIFE ISSUES; HEALTH-CARE AGENT/PROXY; LEGAL GUARDIANSHIP; WILLS.

living will   A legal document, governed by state law, in which individuals declare whether and under what conditions they wish to have their life extended should they become critically ill and in danger of death. For example, some individuals may choose to avoid a respirator (breathing machine) if physicians believe that the patient cannot recover, or they may wish to avoid a feeding tube if they cannot be fed normally or intravenously.

State laws on living wills vary considerably. A living will is very different from a LIVING TRUST, which is a legal document that enables individuals to shelter their financial assets while alive. Many individuals state that they support the concept of a living will, but large numbers never follow through and actually create one.

In one study on advance care planning published in 1998 in the *Archives of Internal Medicine,* the researchers studied 48 individuals and their attitudes toward living wills. These individuals had an average age of 48 years, but the study findings were revealing and illustrative of likely views of individuals in other age groups.

The researchers found that the participants considered advance care planning as a means to prepare for their incapacity as well as for their death. In addition, they stated that their main goals were to maintain control and to relieve the emotional burden on their loved ones about making difficult medical treatment decisions if they were no longer able to make these decisions themselves.

The majority of the participants (69 percent) involved their loved ones in the advanced planning process. Of those who did not involve their loved ones, they cited the following reasons:

- The older person would become too upset or refuse to discuss the subject.
- The older person had never gotten around to it or it was a low priority.
- The older person was too uncomfortable with the subject to talk about it with loved ones.

Many of the study subjects failed to talk to their doctors about the issues, either because they thought the subject was too personal or because they felt that the physicians were too busy. This finding was problematic in that it is the physician who needs to know what actions, if any, the patient wants taken in the event of their incapacity and a medical emergency.

See also ATTORNEYS; CARDIOPULMONARY RESUSCITATION; DEATH, FEAR OF; END-OF-LIFE ISSUES; HEALTH-CARE AGENT/PROXY; PALLIATIVE CARE; TALKING TO ELDERLY PARENTS ABOUT DIFFICULT ISSUES.

Singer, Peter A., M.D., et al. "Reconceptualizing Advance Care Planning from the Patient's Perspective." *Archives of Internal Medicine* 158 (April 27, 1998): 879–884.

long-distance care   Assistance and advice, usually provided by a relative who does not live locally. Long-distance caregivers can arrange for professional caregivers, hire home health or nursing aids, and locate an ASSISTED-LIVING FACILITY or a NURSING HOME for the older person.

The situation is a frustrating one, and often the relative must rely on others, related or hired, to provide major caregiving. It is estimated that more than 7 million adults in the United States provide long-distance care for their aging relatives, primarily their elderly parents who live at least an hour away. Many long-distance caregivers are female, although it is estimated that up to 40 percent are male.

The long-distance caregiver may first notice the need for care during a visit to a relative. According to the National Institute on Aging, caregivers should ask themselves the following questions during the visit:

- Are the stairs manageable or does the older person need a ramp?
- Are there any tripping hazards at exterior entrances or inside the house (such as throw rugs)?
- Can the house be modified if the older person needs a walker or wheelchair?
- Is there enough food in the refrigerator? Are there basic staple foods in the kitchen cabinets?
- Does it appear that bills are being paid or is mail piling up unattended?
- Does the house appear to be sufficiently clean?
- Does the older person appear depressed or anxious?
- Is the older person taking medications? Does he or she appear able to manage these medications?
- If the older person is still driving, how would you assess the individual's driving skills?

Other suggestions for the long-distance care-giver include the following:

- Help your relative stay in contact with you. One option is to purchase a cell phone and teach the individual how to use it.
- Learn as much as you can about your relative's condition and medical problems, so you can talk to physicians and others with some basic knowledge.
- Plan visits ahead of time with goals that you hope to achieve and prioritize them.
- Obtain a phone book for your relative's local area so that you can find resources in the neighbor-hood. The reference department at the local public library often has city phone books for major cities around the country.

Some long-distance caregivers hire a geriatric care manager to assess their relative's needs and coordinate local care. The National Association of Professional Geriatric Care Managers can provide a referral or individuals may contact the Elder Care Locator. Sometimes local chapters of the Alzheimer's Association can recommend geriatric care managers.

Some questions to ask a geriatric care manager before hiring him or her are

- Are you a member of the National Association of Professional Geriatric Care Managers?
- How long have you been providing care-man-agement services?
- Are you available in the event of an emergency?
- Does your company also provide home-care services?
- How will you communicate with me?
- What are your fees? Can you provide this infor-mation in writing before services start?

If the long-distance caregiver goes with the older person to a doctor's visit, the following tips may help, according to the National Institute on Aging:

- Before the appointment, ask your parent, sib-lings, and the primary caregiver what questions or concerns they would like you to bring up. (If they initially say "nothing," wait a few minutes, because many times after a brief period people do think of something they would like to know.)
- Take a prioritized list of questions to the office visit and take notes on what the doctor recommends.
- Take a list of all medications that the parent is taking (or better yet, bring all of the containers to the doctor visit), including prescribed drugs, over-the-counter medications, and any "natural" remedies, such as supplements, vitamins, herbs, or homeopathic remedies.
- Do not answer for your parent when the doctor asks a question unless you have been asked to do so.
- Respect your parent's privacy and leave the room when necessary, such as when a physical examination will be done.
- Ask the physician to recommend any community resources that might be helpful to your parent.
- If the medical practice has a social worker on staff, ask to speak with her or him. The social worker may have valuable information that could be both helpful and time-saving.

Signs of Self-Neglect

When they visit, long-distance caregivers should consider signs that the older person is neglecting him or herself. Some signs that further action is needed are

- The older person is wearing unsuitable clothes for weather conditions, such as wearing summer clothes in freezing weather.
- The individual is hoarding items.
- The person cannot attend to basic housekeeping and a once clean home is extremely dirty and messy.
- The individual frequently leaves a hot stove unattended.
- The individual seems dehydrated.
- The individual seems very confused.

See also ACTIVITIES OF DAILY LIVING; ADULT CHIL-DREN/CHILDREN OF AGING PARENTS; AMERICANS WITH

DISABILITIES ACT; FAMILY AND MEDICAL LEAVE ACT; HEALTH-CARE AGENT/PROXY; LEGAL GUARDIANSHIP; LIVING WILL; NEGLECT; PALLIATIVE CARE; TALKING TO ELDERLY PARENTS ABOUT DIFFICULT ISSUES.

National Institute on Aging. *So Far Away: Twenty Questions for Long-Distance Caregivers.* National Institutes of Health. Available online. URL: http://www.nia.nih.gov/HealthInformation/Publications/LongDistance Caregiving. Accessed October 14, 2007.

long-term care Generally refers to the skilled care that is provided in a NURSING HOME setting. This term may, however, also refer to the requirement of a senior adult to receive help from an ongoing aide or to obtain assistance in his or her home or another location.

In some cases, long-term care may refer to rehabilitative care in a nursing home facility; for example, if the older person has an injury that requires less care than needed in a hospital but the individual needs more care than could be provided at a home, such as daily medical care, frequent physical therapy, and other services. Such an injury may have been caused by a fall. However, rehabilitative care is not considered permanent, while skilled nursing home care is considered to be the place where the individual is likely to live for the remainder of his or her life.

See also HOSPITALIZATION; LONG-TERM CARE INSURANCE.

long-term care insurance Refers to insurance that is purchased ahead of time, usually to pay for NURSING HOME care in the future should it be needed. There are many different companies that sell this form of insurance. It has many different pros and cons to take into consideration.

For example, on the plus side, if the long-term care insurance policy was created by a legitimate and trustworthy organization, it may provide needed benefits in the future so that a person can move to a nursing home without needing to liquidate most of his or her financial assets.

On the negative side, most older Americans ultimately do not need to live in nursing homes, and

thus, the payments for long-term care insurance may be made with no eventual gain. The individual might have been better advised to invest his or her money in other ventures. There are also some companies that have behaved in a disreputable manner and have bilked seniors of their life savings.

See also LONG-TERM CARE.

loss of independence, fear of One concern among many older people, particularly those who are diagnosed with serious illnesses, is that they will lose their ability to manage their own lives. For example, a physical injury may prevent them from DRIVING, and they will need to depend on others for TRANSPORTATION for some period of time. They may not wish to seek help from others, including their own adult children or other relatives, because they fear they will be perceived as helpless or needful and thus a burden to others.

Some older people are so fearful of losing their independence that they will conceal their very serious medical problems from their relatives who they believe (often rightfully so) might curtail their activities if they knew about these problems.

A primary fear of many older people is that they will become so incapacitated that they may have to be placed in a nursing home. They may elicit promises from others that they will never put them in a nursing home, yet the individual may become so chronically ill and frail that there is no alternative except a nursing home. Then the relative feels guilt about the placement, and if the older person is cognitively aware, he or she may be angry with the person who made the now-broken promise.

See also AGEISM; EXERCISE; LEARNED HELPLESSNESS; TALKING TO ELDERLY PARENTS ABOUT DIFFICULT ISSUES.

Lou Gehrig's disease See AMYOTROPHIC LATERAL SCLEROSIS (ALS); DEMENTIA.

low vision The National Eye Institute (NEI) recognizes another eye problem of the elderly called low vision. According to the NEI, low vision is a problem among people who have trouble performing everyday tasks, even with glasses, contact lenses, medications, or surgery. Just reading the mail can become a challenge for these individuals.

Symptoms and Diagnostic Path

According to the NEI, some signs of low vision are

- difficulty recognizing the faces of friends and relatives
- difficulty doing things that require seeing up close, such as sewing, reading, cooking, or making repairs around the house
- trouble picking out and matching the colors of clothing items
- trouble with performing activities at home because lights seem much dimmer than they used to be
- difficulty with reading street and bus signs or the names of stores

Treatment Options and Outlook

Individuals with any of these listed problems should see an eye care professional for a complete eye examination, such as an optometrist or an ophthalmologist. The eye specialist will be able to offer the best solution to low vision problems.

Risk Factors and Preventive Measures

Many older people are at risk for low vision, and this is why it is best for all older people to obtain an annual eye examination, as a preventive measure to act before their vision worsens.

See also EYE DISEASES, SERIOUS.

National Eye Institute. *What You Should Know about Low Vision.* Available online. URL: http: www.nei.nih.gov. Accessed February 13, 2008.

Prevent Blindness America and the National Eye Institute. *Vision Problems in the U.S.: Prevalence of Adult Vision Impairment and Age-Related Eye Disease in America.* 2002. Available online. URL: http://www.nei.nih.gov/eyedata. Accessed February 13, 2008.

lung cancer   Smoking cigarettes is responsible for the majority (an estimated 87 percent) of all deaths from lung cancer. Most people with lung cancer have smoked cigarettes for many years; however, some individuals who do not smoke have been exposed to passive smoking (also known as secondhand smoke) by being in the presence of others who smoke. As a result of this exposure to secondhand smoke, they may also suffer from negative health effects. In addition, exposure to radon gas may damage the lungs and cause lung cancer, such as from working in mines. An exposure to asbestos, such as from years of exposure in some jobs in construction and chemical industries, can also lead to the development of lung cancer.

According to the National Cancer Institute, there were an estimated 213,380 new cases of lung cancer in the United States in 2007. Of the new cases of lung cancer in 2007, 114,760 were men and 98,620 were women. It was anticipated that there would be 160,390 deaths from lung cancer in 2007, including the deaths of 89,510 men and 79,880 women. Most cases of lung cancer occur among people age 65 and older.

There are two primary types of lung cancer, including non–small cell lung cancer and small cell lung cancer. The majority (about 87 percent) of all cases of lung cancer are the non–small cell lung cancers. This type of lung cancer spreads more slowly than does small cell lung cancer.

Symptoms and Diagnostic Path

According to the National Institutes of Health, the most common symptoms of lung cancer include the following:

- a cough that does not go away and that worsens over time
- constant chest pain
- coughing up blood
- shortness of breath or hoarseness
- repeated bouts of pneumonia or bronchitis
- facial or neck swelling
- loss of appetite and weight loss
- fatigue
- night sweats

During the physical examination, the doctor listens to the patient's breathing and checks for the presence of any fluid in the lungs. A pulmonologist is a physican who specializes in treating diseases of the lungs. The physician may also check for the presence of swollen lymph nodes. If the doctor suspects lung cancer, he or she may order a chest X-ray as well as a computerized tomography (CT) scan of the chest to check for a tumor or abnormal fluid.

There are a variety of tests to confirm that lung cancer is present. For example, a sputum sample may be taken to check for cancer cells. In addition, fluid may be removed from the chest and checked for cancer cells. This procedure is known as thoracentesis. The doctor may also perform a bronchoscopy, which is a procedure in which an inserted tube passes through the lungs and enables the physician to remove samples of cells. A fine-needle aspiration is another test using a very thin needle to remove tissue from the lung or lymph node.

The National Cancer Institute recommends that patients who have lung cancer ask their doctors the following questions before a biopsy tissue sample is taken:

- Which procedure do you recommend? How will the tissue be removed?
- Will I have to stay in the hospital for this procedure? If so, for how long?
- Will I have to do anything to prepare for the procedure? If so, what?
- How long will the procedure take? Will I be awake? Will it hurt?
- Are there any risks? What are the chances of infection or bleeding after the procedure?
- How long will it take me to recover?
- How soon will I know the results? Who will explain them to me?
- If I do have cancer, who will talk to me about the next steps? When?

Treatment Options and Outlook

As with other forms of cancer, the treatment for lung cancer depends on how advanced and invasive the cancer is. The cancer must also be staged, which is an attempt to find out whether the cancer has spread to other parts of the body, and if it has, where it has moved to. When lung cancer spreads to other parts of the body, it is still called lung cancer, even if it has spread to the liver or other organs.

A bone scan may be performed to determine if the cancer has spread to the bones. The doctor may also order a magnetic resonance imaging (MRI) scan of the brain and other tissues to detect any spread (as different cancers have a tendency to spread to different organs).

Surgery may be indicated, as may radiation treatment. Other possible treatments may include radiation therapy, chemotherapy, or a combination of treatments. Targeted therapy is another option, in which medication is given either intravenously or by mouth. Targeted therapy is not the same as chemotherapy because it uses drugs to block the growth and spread of cancer cells.

According to the National Cancer Institute, patients with lung cancer should ask their doctors the following questions before any treatment starts:

- What is the stage of my disease? Has the cancer spread from my lung? If so, to where?
- What are my treatment choices? Which treatment do you recommend for me and why?
- Will I have more than one type of treatment?
- What are the expected benefits of each kind of treatment?
- What are the risks and possible side effects of each treatment? What can we do to control the side effects?
- What can I do to prepare for treatment?
- Will I need to stay in the hospital? If so, for how long?
- How will treatment affect my normal activities?
- How often should I have checkups after treatment?

Risk Factors and Preventive Measures

Age is a risk factor for lung cancer; most people with lung cancer are older than age 65. A family history of lung cancer is another risk factor. The most dominant risk factor for lung cancer, however, is smoking cigarettes for many years.

The most effective preventive measure against lung cancer is to never smoke or, if the person already smokes, to stop immediately.

See also CANCER.

macular degeneration   See AGE-RELATED MACULAR DEGENERATION; EYE DISEASES, SERIOUS.

magnetic resonance imaging (MRI)   A diagnostic tool that is considered by many health-care professionals to be the single greatest advance in diagnostic medicine in the last century. This unique tool is a noninvasive way to image healthy and damaged tissue without incurring the risk of radiation. A magnetic field is set up and special magnetic pictures are created. These images enable a physician to better diagnose and treat the patient.

Originally brought to the United States in 1985, MRI technology has been used extensively to diagnose all sorts of disease processes, including brain tumors, joint or tissue damage (in the knees, shoulders, hips, and wrists), and jaw joint derangement, as well as neck and back disc herniations. New protocols are advancing this technology all the time, to the point that dementias and recurrent tumors can be identified.

Initially, the magnet strength of the MRI equipment was significantly weaker than today, and the computer technology was not as elaborate or sophisticated. In addition, most MRIs were closed devices, such that the body part to be studied needed to be inserted into the scanner. Individuals who were claustrophobic and whose head, neck, or shoulders required imagery had considerable difficulty tolerating the scanner without taking anxiety medications ahead of time.

With recent breakthroughs, magnetic scanners are now much more open and "patient friendly," and the scanning times have also been drastically reduced. As a result, most patients find the MRI to be only a brief and minor inconvenience, if they even mind the procedure at all.

mania   Hyperexcited state of agitation. Some forms of the DEMENTIA that are associated with ALZHEIMER'S DISEASE may cause an individual to behave in a hyperactive and out-of-control manner. This behavior is very disruptive and difficult to handle for most people, including many experienced mental health professionals. This is also a key reason why it is very difficult for family members to provide care in their homes or by themselves for elderly relatives suffering from Alzheimer's disease or another form of dementia. Often with such diseases, there can be dramatic and rapid mood swings, making even the most mild patients quite challenging at times and sometimes even dangerous to deal with.

The individual may be delusional or paranoid, mistakenly thinking that he or she is being threatened or that someone is trying to take away something that is theirs. In general, delusional people cannot be talked out of their delusion, and at best, they can be distracted from their delusions by something else. Talking to the manic person in a calm and steady voice often can be helpful.

Some individuals will require sedating medication to control their mania, although whether and how much to drug older people is a controversial issue. This also leads to the issue of chemical restraints, or medications that are used for sedation. These types of drugs, as with physical restraints, are meant to safeguard patients and prevent them from hurting themselves or others. However, caution should be taken to avoid the abuse of either chemical or physical restraints.

See also AGGRESSION, PHYSICAL; COGNITIVE IMPAIRMENT; CONFUSION; DELUSIONS; HALLUCINATIONS; INAPPROPRIATE PRESCRIPTIONS FOR THE ELDERLY; IRRITABILITY; MEMORY IMPAIRMENT; RAGE.

marriage/remarriage In considering all older people age 65 and older, more than half (56 percent) were married in 2000, according to the U.S. Census Bureau. Most had been married at some point in time; 32 percent were widowed and 7 percent were divorced. Less than 5 percent of the elderly population had never been married. Note that many older people in the 21st century choose to live together rather than to remarry to avoid possible inheritance issues among their children and also to avoid losing the retirement income they receive from the Social Security Administration. (This action may also scandalize their adult children, who may assume that older people never engage in sexual activities, although this is an incorrect assumption.)

In 2005, about 11 percent of older people were divorced or separated, up from about 5 percent in 1980. In general, currently married people are in better health than other groups. (See EMERGENCY DEPARTMENT CARE and HOME HEALTH CARE.)

Older men are more likely to be married than older women, and they are also more likely to remarry, largely because there are so many more older women available to marry than older men. (In general, women live significantly longer than men. See LIFE EXPECTANCY.) According to the U.S. Census Bureau, about 31 percent of women age 65 and older were married in 2005 compared to 71 percent of older men in the same age group. In addition, men age 75 and older are more than twice as likely to be married than are older women (67.2 percent for men compared to 28.7 percent for women).

Women are also much more likely to be widowed than men; for example, among individuals age 65 and older, only 14.3 percent of men are widowed, while that percentage was more than three times greater (44.3 percent) for women. Black men and women are less likely to be married and more likely to be widowed than white men and women. (See Table 1.)

The likelihood of being married decreases with age for both men and women; for example, for those individuals ages 75 to 84, 69.8 percent of men and 33.7 percent of women were married. However, among those age 85 and older, only 56.1 percent of men and 12.5 percent of women were married.

TABLE 1. POPULATION AGE 65 AND OLDER BY MARITAL STATUS, AGE, SEX, RACE, AND HISPANIC ORIGIN, 2003 (IN PERCENTAGE)

Age, race, and Hispanic origin	Married Spouse, Present		Widowed	
	Men	Women	Men	Women
65 and Older	71.2	41.1	14.3	44.3
Non-Hispanic white alone	72.9	42.9	14.0	44.0
Black alone	56.6	25.4	19.3	50.8
Asian alone	68.6	42.7	13.6	39.7
Hispanic (any race)	68.8	39.9	12.3	39.5
65 to 74	74.3	53.5	8.8	29.4
Non-Hispanic white alone	76.4	56.5	8.3	28.8
Black alone	59.2	33.4	14.3	36.2
Asian alone	70.2	51.8	9.6	27.1
Hispanic (any race)	72.5	48.4	7.6	25.9
75 to 84	69.8	33.7	18.4	53.3
Non-Hispanic white alone	71.3	35.3	18.1	52.3
Black alone	54.9	19.3	23.2	62.7
Asian alone	69.7	35.1	16.6	53.7
Hispanic (any race)	65.7	31.4	17.1	53.5
85 and Older	56.1	12.5	34.6	78.3
Non-Hispanic white alone	57.8	13.1	33.6	77.8
Black alone	39.7	4.2	47.7	87.2
Asian alone	39.2	10.7	48.8	75.5
Hispanic (any race)	49.8	17.4	33.2	74.2

Source: He, Wan, Manisha Sengupta, Victoria A. Velkoff, and Kimberly A. DeBarros. *65+ in the United States: 2005.* Washington, D.C.: U.S. Census Bureau, December 2005, p. 147.

Remarriage of Elderly Parents

The remarriage of a parent sometimes can create considerable family friction. Sometimes adult children are jealous or resentful of the new spouse when a parent remarries. They may worry that they will lose their inheritance should their parent die before the new spouse dies and believe that the new spouse could then inherit everything.

This is especially worrisome to adult children if the new spouse also has adult children who may then inherit the entire estate. They may believe that their father or mother spent many years building up the inheritance.

They may also be jealous of the new spouse for the attention that he or she receives compared to the greater attention the adult children received before the remarriage. In addition, they may feel that the parent's remarriage is a rejection of their other parent, even when the other parent has been deceased for many years and was clearly a cherished person.

In one case, the bereaved adult children appeared at a garage sale at their stepparent's house, trying to buy a memento from their parent's belongings that were for sale. This case clearly illustrates that it is best for adult children and their parents to discuss such issues as the disposition of personal items in advance of the death of their parent, with both their parents and their stepparents. When possible, treasured items and their disposition should be listed in the older person's will.

Some issues that adult children might wish to consider that are in favor of a parent's remarriage are that the parent's health may improve and that the parent's dependency on the adult child, which may have been burdensome, is likely to decrease. In addition, most studies show that older married people are healthier and live longer than non-married or never-married individuals.

See also ADULT CHILDREN/CHILDREN OF AGING PARENTS; GENDER DIFFERENCES.

Adamec, Christine. "When Parents of Parents Remarry." *Single Parent* 27, no. 9 (October 1984): 20–21.

Gist, Yvonne J., and Lisa I. Hertzel. *We the People: Aging in the United States.* Washington, D.C.: U.S. Census Bureau, December 2004.

He, Wan, Manisha Sengupta, Victoria A. Velkoff, and Kimberly A. DeBarros. *65+ in the United States: 2005.* Washington, D.C.: U.S. Census Bureau, December 2005.

Medicaid The federal medical insurance program in the United States that was first enacted in 1965. This program is both federally and state funded in its mission to provide medical benefits to poor individuals who are disabled and elderly (as well as some other groups, such as dependent children and younger people who are disabled and poor). Medicaid pays for most medications for individuals who are eligible for this service.

At the federal level Medicaid is overseen by the Centers for Medicare and Medicaid Services (CMS). To qualify for Medicaid, individuals must be "categorically eligible," which means that low income in itself is not sufficient to guarantee eligibility. Instead, the person must qualify in some other way, such as by being older, disabled, and poor. Individuals receiving Supplemental Security Insurance (SSI) payments from the Social Security Administration are automatically eligible for Medicaid. It also pays for NURSING HOME care in many cases when the individual's private funds have been depleted.

Medicaid provides coverage for the following types of medical services:

- inpatient hospital care
- outpatient hospital care
- doctor visits
- medications
- laboratory and X-ray services
- skilled nursing facility services

Some states also include dental and optometric care in their Medicaid plans, as well as other services. Another option chosen by many states is a form of managed care or health maintenance organization (HMO) coverage for Medicaid enrollees, in which a particular physician or group provides most of the care. This service has proven cost-effective for both states and the federal government, because it diverts individuals on Medicaid from seeking their routine care at hospital emergency rooms.

See also ASSETS; DISABILITY; MEDICARE.

medical records Documents that are maintained by physicians that record key health information on their patients. Medical records not only aid doctors in reviewing their own patients' past history and treatments but these records may also serve to provide information to any other doctors or to new physicians whom the patient sees.

Most medical records are held in paper form, but increasing numbers of records are now computerized, particularly in larger clinics or hospitals.

Medical records in the United States are now protected by the Privacy Rule of the Health Insurance Portability and Accountability Act of 1996

(HIPAA), which created national standards for patient privacy. As a result, if an adult child or another person wishes to obtain medical information about an elderly person, they need a release signed by that person granting access unless they have been appointed a guardian or the older person has been found mentally incompetent, as a result of some form of DEMENTIA. (Physicians and medical staffs are very familiar with the provisions of this act and can provide further information.)

According to the U.S. Department of Health and Human Services (HHS), the HIPAA Privacy Rule accomplishes the following:

- provides patients more control over their health information
- sets boundaries on the use and release of health records
- establishes appropriate safeguards that health-care providers (such as doctors, nurses, and others) must achieve to protect the privacy of health information
- holds violators accountable, with civil and criminal penalties that can be applied if they violate the patient's privacy
- strikes a balance when public responsibility supports the disclosure of some forms of medical data, such as when it is needed to protect public health

 Patients can make more informed choices with access to this information, and according to HHS, the HIPAA rule

- enables patients to discover how their medical information may be used and certain disclosures of their information that have been made
- generally limits the release of information to the minimum that is reasonably needed for the purpose of disclosure
- generally gives patients the right to examine and obtain a copy of their health records and request corrections (note that some doctors will charge a fee for photocopies of medical records)
- empowers individuals to correct certain uses and disclosures of their health information

When senior adults travel, they should ask their doctor for a condensed copy of their medical records to carry with them. Taking the time to write down their chronological history of major health events also may be quite helpful, particularly if multiple physicians are involved in a patient's care. At a minimum, patients should have the names, addresses, phone, and fax numbers of their physicians with them at all times. In addition, any medications that older individuals take on a regular basis, including the name of the medication, dosage, and frequency, should be included.

See also MEDICATION COMPLIANCE.

U.S. Department of Health and Human Services. "What Does the HIPAA Privacy Rule Do?" Available online. URL: http://www.hhs.gov/hipaafaq/about/187.html. Accessed February 24, 2008.

Medicare A comprehensive federal health insurance program that is offered to elderly recipients of Social Security payments who are age 65 and older as well as to some disabled individuals who are eligible for the program; for example, individuals of any age with end-stage renal disease (KIDNEY FAILURE) are automatically eligible for Medicare coverage. The Medicare program is run by the Centers for Medicare and Medicaid Services (CMS), formerly known as the Health Care Financing Administration. It also administers the End-Stage Renal Disease Program that pays for DIALYSIS and kidney transplants for Medicare patients whose kidneys fail them.

Medicare provides medical coverage for an estimated 95 percent of the elderly in the United States, and it also provides medical coverage for many disabled adults.

Individuals can initially sign up for the Medicare seven-month period that begins three months before they turn 65 and ends three months after their 65th birthday. Individuals who are not yet age 65 can apply for Medicare up to three months before they turn 65. For further information, go to http://www.medicare.gov/Basics/Socialsecurity.asp.

Most doctors accept Medicare, but there are a few who do not. If the doctor accepts Medicare, he or she must accept the rate that Medicare sets for services and cannot charge more than that rate.

Medicare Parts A, B, C, and D

There are different parts to Medicare, including Parts A, B, C, and D. Part A covers mostly inpatient hospital services, although it also covers skilled nursing facilities (not long-term care), hospice care services, and home health care under certain conditions. It also covers some HOME HEALTH/HOME CARE and HOSPICE care, such as hospice care for people with a terminal illness who are not expected to live more than six months.

Part B provides medically necessary services, such as doctor visits, outpatient care, and some preventive services. In most cases, Medicare pays for 80 percent of the rate it deems reasonable for doctor visits, and the individual must pay the balance unless he or she has MEDIGAP insurance that pays for all or most of the remaining 20 percent. Most people pay a monthly premium for Medicare. In 2007 the monthly premium was $93.59.

Some individuals have TRICARE/TRICARE for Life coverage, which is the coverage that is provided to an active duty military member and his or her dependents, or to retired military members and their dependents.

Medicare Part B also partially covers items that are considered medically necessary by Medicare or that are regarded as preventive services, such as laboratory tests or examinations to diagnose, prevent, or manage a medical problem.

Some items that are covered in part under Part B are

- ambulance services to a hospital
- ambulatory surgery center fees
- blood received as an outpatient
- bone mass measurement
- colorectal cancer screenings
- diabetes screenings
- flu shots
- GLAUCOMA tests
- hearing and balance examinations
- HEPATITIS B immunizations
- kidney DIALYSIS services and supplies
- mammogram screenings
- pap tests and pelvic examinations for women

- physical therapy
- some injectable cancer drugs or immunosuppressive drugs
- smoking cessation counseling
- PROSTATE CANCER screenings
- cardiovascular screenings
- limited chiropractor services

In addition, part B covers part of the cost for foot examinations and treatments in those with diabetes-related nerve damage. Part B also covers all or some costs of durable medical equipment, such as oxygen, walkers, wheelchairs, and hospital beds needed at home. Part B also covers emergency room (also known as the emergency department) services.

Some items and services that are *not* covered by either Part A or Part B Medicare are

- acupuncture
- cosmetic surgery
- dental care
- routine eye care
- routine foot care
- hearing aids
- orthopedic shoes
- hearing tests not ordered by the doctor

Medicare Advantage Plans

Part C combines Part A and Part B and is provided through Medicare Advantage plans, such as health maintenance organizations (HMOs) or preferred provider organizations (PPOs). Individuals choose either the "original" Medicare or they choose a Medicare Advantage plan. There is also a special needs plan (SNP) for individuals who fit certain criteria, such as living in a nursing home or needing nursing care at home, being eligible for both Medicare and Medicaid, and having a chronic disabling condition, such as diabetes, congestive heart failure, mental illness, human immunodeficiency virus (HIV), or acquired immune deficiency syndrome (AIDS).

Prescription Medications

Part D covers part of the cost of prescription medications. Coverage is available through private companies that work with Medicare. Each Medicare drug plan has a list of covered drugs in their formulary, or the medications for which they provide coverage. (See MEDICARE PRESCRIPTION DRUG COVERAGE.)

Individuals who join a Medicare Advantage Plan usually get prescription drug coverage through the plan; however, some Advantage Plans do not include prescription drug coverage, so this aspect of coverage should be verified. It is also important to note that some prescription drug plans cover only certain medications, and patients need to be aware of this before choosing a particular plan.

Programs of All-Inclusive Care for the Elderly (PACE)

Another Medicare program is Programs of All-Inclusive Care for the Elderly (PACE), which combines medical, social, and long-term care services for elderly people who are frail and receive health care in the community. PACE is a joint Medicare and Medicaid program available in states that have chosen it as an optional benefit.

To qualify for PACE, individuals must

- be at least 55 years old
- live in a PACE service area
- be certified by the state as eligible for nursing home care

Medicare Rights

People receiving Medicare, no matter what type, have the right

- to obtain a decision about their health-care payment or services
- to appeal certain decisions about their health-care payment or services or prescription drug coverage
- to receive information on covered services and costs
- to receive emergency room or urgently needed care services
- to see doctors and specialists (including women's health specialists) and to go to Medicare-certified hospitals
- to participate in treatment decisions

- to know the available treatment choices
- to file complaints, including complaints about the quality of care
- to not be discriminated against
- to have personal and health information kept private

Decisions That Can Be Appealed

If the person on Medicare does not agree with a decision, in most cases it can be appealed. Examples of appeals include the following situations:

- a service, item, or prescription drug that the individual needs is not covered but the individual thinks it should be paid for by Medicare
- a service, item, or prescription drug that the individual wants is denied and he or she thinks it should be provided
- a service the individual receives is ending too soon
- the individual questions the amount that Medicare paid for a service or item received

Fighting Fraud May Pay Off

In some circumstances, if an individual on Medicare reports fraud, he or she may receive a reward of up to $1,000. Medicare fraud can be reported by phone at (800) 447-8477, e-mail at HHSTips@oig.hhs.gov, or by mail: Office of the Inspector General, HHS Tips Hotline, P.O. Box 23489, Washington, D.C. 20026. All of the following conditions must be met:

- The individual has reported suspected Medicare fraud.
- The Inspector General's Office has reviewed this suspicion.
- The suspected fraud is not already under investigation.
- The report made by the individual leads to the recovery of at least $100 of Medicare money.

See also INAPPROPRIATE PRESCRIPTIONS FOR THE ELDERLY; MEDICAID; MEDICAL RECORDS; MEDICARE PRESCRIPTION DRUG COVERAGE; MEDICARE PREVENTIVE SERVICES.

Centers for Medicare and Medicaid Services. *Medicare and You: 2008.* Washington, D.C.: Department of Health and Human Services, 2007.

Medicare Advantage Plans   See MEDICARE.

Medicare prescription drug coverage   Provision for at least a partial payment on prescribed drugs for those individuals who receive MEDICARE coverage. The benefit is provided to individuals through local pharmacies that Medicare has preselected and that participate in the prescription drug program. There is no income or asset requirement test, and everyone who receives Medicare is automatically eligible to receive prescription drug coverage. (For further information on the Medicare prescription drug program, contact Medicare officials at [800] 633-4227 or online at http://www.medicare.gov/pdphome.asp.)

Individuals sign up for the Medicare prescription drug coverage when they become eligible for Medicare. If individuals fail to sign up when they are first eligible, a penalty may be imposed. The signup may occur three months before the person turns age 65 to three months after the 65th birthday. If the individual is eligible for Medicare due to a disability, the individual may sign up for the program from three months before to three months after receiving cash disability payments for 25 months.

Individuals may join a Medicare prescription drug plan, or they may opt to join another Medicare health plan that also offers drug coverage. In most cases, individuals pay a monthly premium and must meet an annual deductible. As of 2007, the annual deductible ranged from zero to $265, depending on the particular circumstances of the individual.

Older individuals who have a very low income can apply to receive nearly all of their prescription medications at a greatly reduced cost. For further information, contact the Social Security Administration at (800) 772-1213, or go to the Social Security Web site at http://www.socialsecurity.gov.

See also INAPPROPRIATE PRESCRIPTIONS FOR THE ELDERLY; MEDICARE PREVENTIVE SERVICES.

Medicare preventive services   The services that Medicare covers for eligible recipients in order to detect current medical problems or potential future medical problems. For example, a one-time preventive physical examination is covered within the first six months that an individual receives Part B of Medicare. (Part B covers physician visits.) At this visit, the doctor will take the patient's medical history and also check the individual's height, weight, and blood pressure. A simple eye test is given or ordered as well as an electrocardiogram (EKG). The doctor will also determine if the patient needs any immunizations. Laboratory tests will be ordered as needed.

In addition, as of 2007, individuals at risk for abdominal aortic aneurysms may have a one-time ultrasound screening. Those who are at risk are individuals with a family history of abdominal aortic aneurysms, those who have smoked at least 100 cigarettes, and men ages 65 to 75.

Other Preventive Services

Medicare covers general screening tests for CHOLESTEROL, lipid, and triglyceride levels once every five years. For women only, Medicare covers annual mammograms to screen for BREAST CANCER and also covers a Pap test and pelvic examination every 24 months. (For women who are at risk for cervical or vaginal cancer, more frequent screenings are covered by Medicare.)

To test for COLORECTAL CANCER, Medicare provides coverage for the fecal occult blood test once every 12 months.

A flexible sigmoidoscopy, a test that examines a major part of the colon, is covered once every 48 months or every 120 months when it is used instead of a colonoscopy for those not at high risk for colorectal cancer. A screening COLONOSCOPY, which studies the entire colon, is covered by Medicare once every 120 months, but it is covered every 24 months if the patient is at high risk for colorectal cancer. A barium enema is covered once every 48 months or every 24 months if the patient is at high risk and the test is used instead of a sigmoidoscopy or a colonoscopy. Medicare pays the full cost for the fecal occult blood test and 80 percent of the Medicare-approved amount for the other tests if they are done in a hospital. If the tests are done in a hospital outpatient department or ambulatory surgical center, Medicare pays 75 percent of the Medicare-approved amount.

Medicare pays for the cost of a digital rectal examination to screen for PROSTATE CANCER once every 12 months and covers a Prostate Specific Antigen (PSA) test once very 12 months.

Medicare also pays the full cost for a FLU/INFLU-ENZA shot once a season, in fall or winter, as long as the doctor or health-care provider accepts assignment of benefits. The pneumococcal shot (for PNEUMONIA) is given once in a lifetime, and it is payable by Medicare.

As of this writing, Medicare also pays the cost of immunizations against HEPATITIS B for those individuals whose doctors say they are at medium to high risk for contracting hepatitis B, such as those with end-stage renal disease (KIDNEY FAILURE), hemophilia, or another condition that lowers the person's resistance to infection. Three shots are needed to immunize a person against hepatitis B. Medicare pays 80 percent of these costs.

Medicare also pays for bone mass measurements to screen for the presence of OSTEOPOROSIS for those at risk, covered once every 24 months and more frequently if medically necessary. Some groups of individuals who are considered at high risk for osteoporosis include

- those who are age 50 or older
- women
- those with a family history or personal history of broken bones
- white or Asian
- small-boned individuals
- individuals of low body weight (less than 127 pounds)
- individuals who smoke or drink to excess
- those with a low calcium diet

DIABETES screening with the fasting blood glu-cose test is covered by Medicare (up to two tests per year) for those individuals considered at risk for diabetes, such as those with HYPERTENSION (high blood pressure), who are obese, and/or those with a history of high blood sugar. In addition, Medicare

covers the test if individuals answer "Yes" to two or more of the following questions:

- Are you age 65 or older?
- Are you overweight?
- Do you have a family history of diabetes (such as parents, brothers, sisters)?
- Do you have a history of gestational diabetes (diabetes during pregnancy) or delivered a baby weighing more than nine pounds.

For those who have been diagnosed with dia-betes, Medicare covers 20 percent of the Medi-care-approved amount after the annual Part B deductible for such items as glucose monitors, test strips, and lancets.

See also MEDICARE; MEDICARE PRESCRIPTION DRUG COVERAGE; MEDIGAP INSURANCE.

Medicare supplemental insurance See MEDIGAP INSURANCE.

medication compliance Refers to following the specific directions of the physician and the pharma-cist with regard to the dosage, frequency, and timing of taking a prescribed medication. Unfortunately, medication compliance is a huge problem for many older people, because many older individuals take three or more different medications per day, and often they may become confused about whether they have taken a medication or not. If one or more new medications are added to their existing medica-tions, the CONFUSION may increase even further.

Sometimes older people do not take their medi-cation because they simply choose not to take it, which is yet another form of noncompliance with their medication regimen. They may think about the reasons why they are not taking the drug, or they may decide that they do simply not feel like taking it. This noncompliance can be very danger-ous for many older people with chronic diseases such as DIABETES or HYPERTENSION, which require medication to keep the disease under control.

In one study of cost-related medication non-adherence, or medications not filled because of their cost (prior to the implementation of Medicare Part D), reported in 2006 in the *Archives of Internal Medicine,* the researchers found that individuals who were in fair to poor health and with multiple illnesses and no prescription benefit coverage were at the greatest risk for not complying with the medications that their physician ordered. Some individuals took a smaller dose of their medication or they skipped a dose to make it last longer. It will be interesting to see research subsequent to the passage of Medicare Part D to see if medication adherence improves.

Common Errors with Medications

There are several common medication errors that many older people make that can have serious consequences. One is failing to work with their doctors to develop a plan to take their medication, such as linking taking the medication to mealtimes or before bed, upon arising, or linked to some other event that the person can remember. Without such a plan, it is likely a dosage could be missed.

Another common error is using several different pharmacies to obtain prescribed medications. Because many older people see more than one physician, they may inadvertently be prescribed some medications that could negatively interact with each other. If only one pharmacy is used, the pharmacist can usually detect any possible medication interactions and notify the physician and/or the patient ahead of time before any problems occur.

A third common error is for patients to assume that they no longer need the medication once they feel better. Feeling better may indicate that the medication is working and should be continued. In the case of an infection, the bacteria are often still present even when the patient starts feeling better, and if the medication is suddenly stopped, the infection may spiral out of control and the patient could become even sicker than he or she was in the first place.

Some medications may cause major or minor side effects and patients may stop taking them. However, in many cases, side effects abate within a day or two. A common error associated with side effects is to fail to advise the physician that the patient does not wish to take the medication any more. If the doctor knows that the patient is expe-

riencing a side effect, the physician can take several courses of action, such as lowering the dose, advising the patient to take the medication with meals (or without food), or even change the time of day that the medication is to be taken.

The doctor may also tell the patient to continue taking the drug because the side effects are mild and will go away or because the drug is necessary and the side effects must be tolerated. Of course, the doctor may also decide to end the medication altogether, but it is important to consult with the physician in the first place.

Another error is to take vitamins, minerals, or other supplements without telling the doctor. Often medications can have negative interactions with supplements. For example, patients taking warfarin (Coumadin), a blood thinner, should avoid supplements such as St. John's Wort or Vitamin E, which can also thin the blood. Some patients experience severe bleeding problems because they take these or other supplements without first alerting their doctors. Often they reason that supplements are safe because they are not prescribed drugs and are considered "natural." However, nearly any substance can cause harm under certain circumstances.

See also INAPPROPRIATE PRESCRIPTIONS FOR THE ELDERLY; MEDICATION MANAGEMENT; PAINKILLING MEDICATIONS; PRESCRIPTION DRUG ABUSE/MISUSE.

Soumerai, Stephen B., et al. "Cost-related Medication Nonadherence among Elderly and Disabled Beneficiaries: A National Survey 1 Year Before the Medicare Drug Benefit." *Archives of Internal Medicine* 166 (September 25, 2006): 1,829–1,835.

medication interactions The effect that medications may have on each other when they are taken by a person at about the same time. Some medications may potentiate (boost) the impact of other drugs, while others may weaken the effects of other drugs. Some medications, when taken together, can result in medical problems with serious or even fatal outcomes.

Medication interactions are a potential problem for any person who takes medicines, including over-the-counter drugs. Even alternative remedies can cause a problem. For example, ginkgo biloba and vitamin E can cause serious blood thinning, and they can also boost the impact of prescribed blood thinners such as warfarin (Coumadin). Even some seemingly benign over-the-counter medications, such as aspirin or acetaminophen (Tylenol), can cause a medication interaction.

If a physician does not know that the patient is taking an herbal remedy, the doctor cannot alert the patient to the risk of a medication interaction. This is a problem particularly with older patients, because some studies indicate that they often fail to tell their physicians about the supplements or vitamins they are taking. Many people mistakenly assume that since supplements are "natural," then they must be safe. This is a dangerous assumption to make.

Many older people are likely to be taking more than two or three medications for chronic conditions, such as high blood pressure and cardiac problems. It is a good idea for patients to use just one pharmacy so that the pharmacist can help them avoid possible drug interactions by keeping track of his or her various medications. It is also a good idea for patients to keep a complete list of all their medications and supplements so that this information can be provided to new physicians or pharmacists.

See also ADVERSE DRUG EVENT; INAPPROPRIATE PRESCRIPTIONS FOR THE ELDERLY; MEDICATION COMPLIANCE; MEDICATION MANAGEMENT; PRESCRIPTION DRUG ABUSE/MISUSE; VITAMIN AND MINERAL DEFICIENCIES/EXCESSES.

medication management A plan to ensure that medications are taken by a patient on a regular basis, in the right dosage, and at the right time. The patient may make the medication management plan or someone else, such as a relative or a nurse, may make the plan for the person. (Such as when the older person is in an early stage of DEMENTIA, for example.)

Many older people take three or more medications per day, and they may find it difficult to remember whether they took their morning or evening dose or even took the medication at all that day. Weekly pill containers and other devices can make medication management much simpler

for the older person. However, when the individual has ALZHEIMER'S DISEASE or another form of dementia, at some point in time it will become impossible for him or her to manage the medications, and others will need to take over.

See also INAPPROPRIATE PRESCRIPTIONS FOR THE ELDERLY; MEDICATION COMPLIANCE, MEDICATION INTERACTIONS.

Medigap insurance Supplemental insurance that pays for that part of the cost of a medical service or physician that is not covered by MEDICARE. The individual must either purchase Medigap insurance to cover additional costs or must pay the fees for the 20 percent balance himself or herself. For example, Medicare usually pays for 80 percent of outpatient physician visits, which means that the patient must either pay the remaining 20 percent or use Medigap insurance to cover the balance. In many states, individuals may choose from up to 12 different policies. Each Medigap plan must follow both state and federal laws.

memory impairment Difficulty with the recall of recent events or events long past, or with both types of events. Memory impairment is a common problem for those who have DEMENTIA or ALZHEIMER'S DISEASE. However, some memory lapses are common for all people of all ages, such as forgetting where one has left the car keys or forgetting to send a card on someone's birthday. In contrast, the person with severe memory impairment may forget how to get home from a familiar place or he or she may even forget the purpose of the watch on his or her wrist.

People suffering from DEPRESSION or anxiety disorders are more likely to have memory problems than those who are not depressed or anxious. In such cases, individuals are distracted or overwhelmed by their emotional problems. Pseudodementia is the term used to describe parents who have a memory dysfunction due to severe depression. When the depression or anxiety is removed or at least improved, in most cases, the person's memory will return to normal.

Many adult children of parents with Alzheimer's disease or other forms of dementia worry that they may too develop these diseases and may see every minor memory lapse as a sign that they have Alzheimer's.

See ADULT CHILDREN/CHILDREN OF AGING PARENTS; AGGRESSION, PHYSICAL; ANXIETY AND ANXIETY DISORDERS; COGNITIVE IMPAIRMENT; CONFUSION; DELUSIONS; HALLUCINATIONS; IRRITABILITY; MANIA; RAGE.

Ménière's disease Ménière's disease is a disorder of the inner ear. It is a distressing disorder because it affects the individual's balance. It is usually characterized by a sensation of spinning (vertigo) and may be accompanied by nausea and vomiting. In about one patient in five, Ménière's disease involves both ears. Often the second ear becomes affected two or three years after symptoms first appear.

In later stages of the disease, violent attacks of vertigo occur less often and then stop altogether. Sporadic bouts of tinnitus may become permanent. Doctors call these changes "Ménière's burnout." The patient may also feel pressure inside one or both ears and experience fluctuating hearing loss.

Many experts believe that Ménière's disease is caused by a tear in the membranous labyrinth, the site that regulates hearing and balance. Other suspected risk factors are

- stress
- excessive salt consumption
- endocrine or thyroid problems
- an abnormal sugar metabolism
- high CHOLESTEROL and/or triglyceride levels
- excessive levels of alcohol, caffeine, and nicotine

Symptoms and Diagnostic Path

The early stages of Ménière's disease may last more than a year. During that time, symptoms may appear and subside unpredictably, with months or more between attacks. Symptoms of dizziness, nausea, or tinnitus that affect one ear may abate within 10 minutes, or the symptoms may last all day. In general, an overall unsteadiness is a more persistent problem than other symptoms, and it may last for days.

The diagnosis usually involves confirming the presence and cause of edema, measuring changes in

sound recognition after the patient drinks glycerine, and observing eye movements to evaluate balance (electronystagmography). Electronystagmography is also used to evaluate dizziness. Another diagnostic tool involves having the patient stand on a special platform and, as the platform moves, the patient's body sway is measured.

Treatment Options and Outlook

Although it cannot be cured, medical management can control or eliminate the vertigo symptoms in the majority of patients. Eliminating tobacco, alcohol, caffeine, and monosodium glutamate (MSG, a food additive) can also improve the symptoms. Other beneficial approaches include medication to reduce the retention of salt and water and control the symptoms of dizziness and nausea and vomiting.

If the symptoms remain uncontrolled after two months of medical treatment, surgery may be indicated.

See HEARING DISORDERS.

meningitis A viral or bacterial infection of the brain, often acquired by individuals in an immune-compromised or weakened condition. The most common form of meningitis is pneumococcal meningitis, caused by pneumococcus, or the pneumonia virus. According to the National Institute of Neurological Diseases and Stroke, about 6,000 cases of pneumococcal meningitis occur each year in the United States. Enteroviruses are another common cause of meningitis. Varicella zoster, the virus that causes chicken pox and that can reappear many years later as SHINGLES, is another cause of meningitis.

More than half of all meningitis acquired as an infection occurs in people age 50 and older. The death rates for older patients with meningitis are 50 to 70 percent, so it is very important to rapidly diagnose and treat this disease. According to the Centers for Disease Control and Prevention, enteroviruses are small viruses comprised of ribonucleic acid (RNA) and protein, and there are about 62 enteroviruses that make humans ill. They are also very common and can be spread through respiratory secretions (cough or nasal mucus) of an ill person as well as through the stool. An enterovirus can also be contracted through touching contaminated surfaces, such as a door handle, a remote control device, a telephone, or a water glass. Many people infected with enterovirus do not become ill, but those who are weakened are more likely to become sick.

Symptoms and Diagnostic Path

The common symptoms of meningitis are fever, a sudden and severe headache, nausea and vomiting, and a stiff neck. Sometimes a pink rash develops. The person may also have photophobia (aversion to light). In extreme cases, the patient may suffer stroke, seizures, brain damage, and death.

Note that elderly patients may not have the classic meningitis symptoms of severe headache and fever. Instead, they are more likely to complain of confusion and experience nausea and vomiting. They may also be drowsy. A lumbar puncture of spinal fluid can determine whether the patient has meningitis. A neurological examination will help the doctor assess nerve and motor function. Laboratory screening of the blood and urine can help detect an infection of the brain and/or the spinal cord.

Treatment Options and Outlook

If bacterial meningitis is present, patients are treated aggressively with the appropriate antibiotics. Sometimes oral antibiotics are followed by intravenous antibiotics. Corticosteroids may be used to relieve brain pressure and swelling. If the patient has viral meningitis, this is treated with bed rest, pain medicine, and encouragement of fluids. Anticonvulsants may be prescribed to prevent seizures.

The prognosis depends on how sick the individual is and how rapidly treatment is given. If the meningitis is mild, most people can make a full recovery within two to four weeks. Bacterial meningitis may cause complications, such as hearing loss, blindness, and permanent brain and nerve damage.

Risk Factors and Preventive Measures

Individuals who are in a weakened state because of having the human immunodeficiency virus (HIV) or who are taking immunosuppressant medications are more likely to develop severe infections such as meningitis than others. In addition, sometimes hospitalized patients have a greater risk for meningitis because of problems with sanitation.

To prevent contracting meningitis, good personal hygiene and frequent hand washing are recommended. Individuals should avoid sharing food with others. There are also some vaccines that can prevent pneumonia and pneumococcal meningitis.

mental competency   A legal term that refers to an individual's ability to make rational decisions on a daily basis about his or her life, such as where to live, what medical treatment to receive (or refuse to receive), and many other decisions. State courts apply state laws to determine the legal mental competency of individuals, and laws vary considerably from state to state. This determination is usually made based on medical information that is provided by one or more physicians (often a neurologist or a psychiatrist).

People with ALZHEIMER'S DISEASE, DEMENTIA, or other ailments that cause mental impairments may be regarded as mentally incompetent by their family or other individuals. Concerned individuals may obtain a court order stipulating the mental incompetence of the patient, based on the physicians' findings. The court may then appoint an individual to be the guardian of the mentally incompetent person. The guardian will make decisions on behalf of that person, such as financial and medical decisions.

In general, mentally incompetent people do not retain their civil rights to vote or to marry. They may not drive a car, and they may not have complete (or any) access to their funds. The guardian may also receive access to the individual's monthly pension funds or other assets. To protect the mentally incompetent person, most courts require periodic reports from the guardian, and some states divide the guardianship responsibilities among several different people. For example, one person may oversee the financial assets of the mentally incompetent person, while another person may make medical decisions or day-to-day choices for the individual.

A person can have mild dementia yet he or she may continue to be mentally competent. It is important to remember that being declared mentally incompetent is a legal decision, whereas a diagnosis of dementia is a medical decision. The legal decision that a person is no longer mentally competent affects an individual's income, as well as who controls his or her assets and so forth.

See also AGGRESSION, PHYSICAL; COGNITIVE IMPAIRMENT; CONFUSION; DURABLE POWER OF ATTORNEY; GUARDIANSHIP; HALLUCINATIONS; IRRITABILITY; MANIA; MEMORY IMPAIRMENT; RAGE.

migraine headaches Migraines are extremely severe headaches that may be preceded by warning symptoms in some people (also called the migraine aura), such as a suddenly runny nose or the patient seeing flashing lights. However, for many people, migraines appear suddenly and with no advance warning.

Symptoms and Diagnostic Path

The migraine causes extreme pain and often causes extreme sensitivity to both light and sound. Some people with migraines are also sensitive to odors. Many people with a migraine seek to isolate themselves until the pain has passed. The condition is diagnosed based on symptoms as well as ruling out other conditions through laboratory tests and magnetic resonance imaging (MRI) scans. Often there is a strong family or genetic history for this type of headache.

Treatment Options and Outlook

Migraines are usually treated with medications, such as drugs in the triptan class including sumatriptan (Imitrex), zolmitriptan (Zomig), rizatriptan (Maxalt), almotriptan (Axert), frovatriptan (Frova), and eletriptan (Relpax). In 2008, Treximet was approved by the U.S. Food and Drug Administration to treat migraines. Treximet includes sumatriptan and naproxensodium (Ibuprofen). In some cases, drugs such as Fiornal or Fiorcet are used to treat migraines. These drugs contain a combination of headache medicine with acetaminophen and caffeine. Sometimes ANTIDEPRESSANTS or antiseizure drugs are used to treat chronic migraines.

In addition, alternative remedies such as the herb feverfew and supplemental magnesium have brought relief to some people with chronic migraines.

Risk Factors and Preventive Measures

Migraine headaches are often an inherited problem. Women generally suffer from more migraines than men. Individuals should determine their particular triggers (weather, stress, certain foods, etc.) and avoid them as much as possible to limit the number of migraines.

See also EXTREMELY SEVERE HEADACHES; HEADACHE; TENSION HEADACHES.

motor vehicle accidents See ACCIDENTAL INJURIES; DRIVING.

moving in with family members In many cases, older family members who can no longer live independently yet do not need NURSING HOME care will move in with adult children, grandchildren, or other relatives. The family dynamics are markedly changed by this move because the older person is not the individual in charge of the home anymore, and the adult child or other person is now the person who must make the major decisions about the home. However, whenever possible, it is important to try and maintain as much independence as possible for the older person.

Having an older person move into the home will cause major changes, even when everyone gets along well. If there are still teenage or younger children in the home, they will be affected by having an older relative move in and may express some resentment, especially if they are told they must give up a room or share a room. They may also resent receiving less attention. Spouses, partners, roommates, and others will have similar reactions. There are many issues to consider before making the decision to have an older relative move in, and sometimes there is very little time to make the decision.

According to the National Family Caregiver Support Program of the Administration on Aging, the major advantages of having an older relative move in include the following:

- Nursing homes and other long-term facilities can be very expensive, and if the relative lives with a family member, considerable money can be saved. (Note, however, that the relative may be eligible for MEDICAID payment for nursing home care if she or he has no or few assets, in terms of money in the bank, stocks, bonds, and so forth.)

- If the relative lives with the family, they can oversee the care that is provided, such as home care.

- The relative of the older person can be involved with major decisions affecting the relative when the older person lives in the home.

- When the relative lives in the home, family members can spend more time with the older person.

- Children still living in the home will have an opportunity to know their grandparent or other older relative and learn both compassion and a sense of responsibility, as well as of family continuity.

- If the relative is reasonably healthy, he or she may be able to help with household tasks or with children living in the household.

According to the National Family Caregiver Support Program of the Administration on Aging, the major disadvantages of having an older relative move in include the following:

- Relative caregivers may have less time for themselves and for other family members and may also experience conflicts between what their job requires and the older person needs. (Although some workers resolve this issue by doing some or all of their work by telecommuting from home.)

- The relative and/or the older person may resent changes in the relationship that may take place as a result of the relative moving in with the family.

- The relative caregiver will lose at least some privacy.

- There may be less space for other family members when an older relative moves in.

- Caregiving for an older relative may prove to be physically and/or emotionally demanding.

The National Family Caregiver Support Program recommends that anyone considering intergenerational living ask themselves the following questions:

- Is the home large enough so that everyone can have privacy when they want it?

- Is there a separate bedroom and bath for the older family member, or can an accessory apartment be created?

- Are rooms available on the first floor for the older relative? If not, can the relative climb stairs safely?

- If not available, is it possible to add to or remodel a home to provide a bedroom and bath to the first floor?

- Are safety features needed, such as ramps and better lighting?

- Does the bathroom have a shower? If so, is it large enough to accommodate a wheelchair, if needed? Can safety features such as grab bars or seats be installed to prevent falls?

- Are door openings wide enough for a wheel chair?

See also ADULT CHILDREN/CHILDREN OF AGING PARENTS; ELDERIZING A HOME; FAMILY CAREGIVERS; HOUSING/LIVING ARRANGEMENTS; INDEPENDENT LIVING; LEARNED HELPLESSNESS.

National Family Caregiver Support Program. "Because We Care: When Your Care Receiver Lives with You." Administration on Aging, 2004. Available online. URL: http://www.aoa.gov/prof/aoaprog/caregiver/carefam/taking_care_of_others/wecare/lives-with-you.asp. Accessed February 24, 2008.

multi-infarct dementia (MID) Multi-infarct dementia (MID) is caused by multiple strokes that damage the brain tissue.

Symptoms and Diagnostic Path

Some strokes may occur without anyone—including the individual—noticing that anything is wrong. These silent strokes are particularly the types of strokes that cause MID. The main causes of strokes are untreated HYPERTENSION (high blood pressure), DIABETES, high CHOLESTEROL levels, and HEART DISEASE.

As more strokes occur and, consequently, even more areas of the brain become damaged, the symptoms of multi-infarct dementia become much more noticeable. These symptoms may include confusion, problems with short-term memory, difficulty following instructions, inappropriate laughing or crying, and frequently getting lost. In fact, these symptoms often may be difficult for physicians to differentiate from Alzheimer's disease.

Treatment Options and Outlook

Brain damage that was caused by a stroke cannot be reversed. The treatment concentrates on the prevention of any further strokes, as well as control of diseases that increase the risk for stroke.

The outlook for those with MID is poor, and death may be caused by a stroke, heart disease, or PNEUMONIA.

See also DEMENTIA.

multiple losses   Refers to the experience of suffering two or more serious personal or health losses within the same time frame. For example, an older individual might need to have surgery (such as a JOINT REPLACEMENT), which is a traumatic event for most people, and then a spouse may become ill or die, all within the same year or within an even shorter time frame. Medical crises are more likely to occur among older individuals, and multiple losses increase their risk of DEPRESSION as well as the risk for the development of various anxiety disorders, such as generalized anxiety disorder or post-traumatic stress disorder.

Multiple losses may also decrease the amount of sleep that the individual obtains, thus weakening the overall immune system and causing the person to be more prone to contracting illnesses and infections.

See also ANXIETY AND ANXIETY DISORDERS; BEREAVEMENT; SLEEP DISORDERS.

myocardial infarction   See HEART ATTACK.

narcotics Drugs that are scheduled (controlled) by the Drug Enforcement Administration (DEA) in the United States because of their risk for becoming habit-forming or addictive. Narcotics are highly effective painkillers, but they are also sometimes abused or misused by the general population, particularly among those seeking the euphoric "high" of a drug. Examples of some narcotics that are abused include morphine, oxycodone, OxyContin (a timed-release form of oxycodone), and hydrocodone.

Narcotics should only be used by the specific individuals for whom they are prescribed, and they should never be given to others. Many older individuals do not realize this and may swap drugs with each other to save money or to try to help a friend. Such an act would be illegal as well as extremely dangerous, since the reactions of others to narcotics may vary considerably depending on other medications that they take, their current medical condition, their age, and many other intervening factors.

Some individuals taking medications for severe pain have reactions to narcotics, ranging from CONSTIPATION to HALLUCINATIONS, anxiety, or DELUSIONS. Such a reaction may mean that a lower dosage of the drug should be used or that a different narcotic altogether should be employed.

According to the Centers for Disease Control and Prevention (CDC), the self-reported use of narcotics was greatest among older individuals during the period 1999–2002 (5.7 percent), and older women were more likely to use narcotics than older men or 6.8 percent of older women compared to 4.1 percent of older men. (See Table 1.)

See also ANXIETY AND ANXIETY DISORDERS; CHRONIC PAIN; DIABETES; DRUG ABUSE; GENDER DIFFERENCES; MEDICATION COMPLIANCE; PAINKILLING MEDICATIONS; PRESCRIPTION DRUG ABUSE/MISUSE; SUBSTANCE ABUSE AND DEPENDENCE.

Chartbook on Trends in the Health of Americans. Hyattsville, Md.: National Institutes of Health, 2006.

Gwinnell, Esther, M.D., and Christine Adamec. *The Encyclopedia of Drug Abuse.* New York: Facts On File, 2008.

Native Americans A racial and ethnic designation that indicates that the individual is a member of an Indian tribe in the United States. In 2005, less than one percent of individuals age 65 and older were American Indian or Native Alaskan.

Native Americans may or may not choose to live on a reservation. Native Americans have a greatly increased risk for some specific health problems, particularly DIABETES and HYPERTENSION. These problems are also often linked to high rates of OBESITY, which is a common problem among

TABLE 1. ADULTS 18 YEARS OF AGE AND OLDER AND PERCENTAGE OF REPORTED NARCOTIC USE IN THE MONTH PRIOR TO INTERVIEW, BY SEX AND AGE, 1999–2002

Both sexes	
18–44 years	3.6
45–64 years	4.6
65 and older	5.7
Men	
18–44 years	2.5
45–64 years	3.4
65 and older	4.1
Women	
18–44 years	4.6
45–64 years	5.7
65 and older	6.8

Source: Adapted from *Chartbook on Trends in the Health of Americans.* Hyattsville, Md.: National Institutes of Health, 2006, p. 120.

Native Americans of all ages, including the elderly. ALCOHOLISM is also a frequently occurring problem among large numbers of Native Americans of all ages.

See also AFRICAN AMERICANS; ASIAN AMERICANS, CAUCASIANS; HISPANICS.

neglect/self-neglect Another form of maltreatment, neglect is the omission or failure to provide necessary food, shelter, medical care, medications, or other necessities of life. Neglect differs from abuse, which is the commission of harmful acts up to and including homicide. Self-neglect is the failure of the older person himself or herself to obtain necessary items or medical care.

As with abuse, neglect can result in the death of the older person. Neglectful acts against seniors may be illegal according to particular state laws, and neglect can be reported to state authorities. Some older people are severely neglected by their families, who may undervalue them or even openly or secretly wish for them to die so that they may inherit their money or simply not be "burdened" with their care anymore. More often, family members turn a blind eye to the problem, not wishing to intercede.

Neglect may also occur inadvertently when family members who live in distant locations are entirely unaware of the deterioration in the condition of an elderly person. The elderly person may have actively sought to conceal his or her problems, so as not to worry the relative or because the older person clings to independence and fears that if medical problems are identified, he or she may be sent to live in a nursing home.

Sometimes family members themselves actively deny that there is anything wrong with a parent or relative, even in the face of obvious evidence that there is a problem, because they do not wish to acknowledge a problem or work on solutions. One family member may see that there is a problem, while others insist that everything is "just fine."

For example, a very disheveled parent or other relative who was formerly very neat and clean may be explained away as sick or tired. A person who is now extremely thin may be said to be on a "diet," when to most other people, it is obvious that the individual needs medical attention and an improved diet. Some family members are very adept at denying the obvious to avoid taking action, and this situation will continue unless someone else intercedes, such as a physician or another relative.

According to the National Center on Elder Abuse, some key signs of neglect in an elderly person include the following:

- dehydration, malnutrition, untreated bed sores, and poor personal hygiene
- unattended or untreated health problems
- hazardous or unsafe living condition/arrangements (such as improper wiring, no heat, or no running water)
- unsanitary and unclean living conditions (such as dirt, fleas, lice on person, soiled bedding, fecal/urine smell, inadequate clothing)
- an elder's report of being mistreated

Risk Factors for Maltreatment

According to Gorbien and Eisenstein in their 2005 article in *Clinics in Geriatric Medicine* on elder abuse and neglect, studies have shown that key risk factors for mistreatment (including abuse and neglect) include low income, social isolation, minority status, a lack of access to resources, a low level of education, substance abuse by the older person or the caregiver, a previous history of family violence, a history of psychological problems, caregiver stress, cognitive impairment, functional impairment, and older age. Most studies also show that women are more likely to be maltreated than men.

With regard to those who abuse and neglect, offenders often fall into one or more categories, according to Gorbien and Eisenstein. These include the overwhelmed, who are generally well intentioned. Another group is the impaired, who are also well intentioned but have problems that make it impossible for them to provide proper care. They are more often likely to neglect rather than to abuse their elders.

Gorbien and Eisenstein say, "These caregivers may suffer from mental or physical problems that serve as barriers to providing adequate care.

They may be unaware of the deficits in their care delivery."

Another group of caregivers are the narcissists, who are nonrelatives whose form of maltreatment is to neglect seniors or steal from them. Gorbien and Eisenstein say, "They see the relationship as a means to an end and may be attracted to nursing homes or centers where they can enter into relationships with vulnerable adults."

The bully is another form of caregiver who is neglectful and may also sexually abuse the older person. According to Gorbien and Eisenstein,

> This group may feel entitled to exert power and authority. They may have narcissistic tendencies and often feel that the victim deserved the maltreatment. This type of offender may honor limits in other settings and has insight into the nature of the maladaptive behavior.

The last type of perpetrator is the sadist, who is a sociopath and enjoys mistreating the older person, which makes him or her feel powerful and important.

Self-Neglect

Sometimes self-neglect is the primary problem, as older people fail to eat meals or go to their doctors' appointments. (Often untreated DEPRESSION may be the cause of this behavior; depression is highly treatable.) Gorbien and Eisenstein state that many of the same factors for abuse and neglect are also relevant in those who self-neglect, such as alcohol or drug abuse, older age, isolation, psychiatric illnesses, and functional dependence. Some studies have also shown that POVERTY, cognitive impairment, and being nonwhite are also risk factors for self-neglect.

According to a 2007 article on self-neglecting elders in the *Journal of the American Medical Association*, self-neglect is a risk factor for early death, and when it occurs it is often exhibited by older people living alone. According to the authors, "They [elders] display behaviors such as piling garbage inside the home, allowing food to spoil, failing to maintain utilities in the home, ignoring serious medical issues, and even lying in their own excrement." The authors say the behavior is on a continuum and some self-neglect is relatively mild,

such as failing to throw away old mail or keep the house normally clean. For others, however, they "live in abject squalor without electricity and other utilities."

According to an article in 2006 in the *Journal of Elder Abuse & Neglect*, vitamin D deficiency is common in the elderly, but it is particularly common among those who self-neglect. These older people have impaired physical performance and inadequate living skills, which could be improved by treating the vitamin D deficiency (as well as the self-neglectful behavior).

In another study of self-neglect, based on more than 500 patients studied by a geriatric medicine team (reported in 2007 in the *American Journal of Public Health*), the researchers analyzed patient charts of patients who had been referred to a protective services agency. In this study, 86 percent of the subjects were age 65 or older. Most (72 percent) were females. The most frequent type of diagnosis was cardiovascular disease with hypertension. Next most common (53 percent) were mental disorders, such as dementia (16 percent), depression (14 percent), and delirium (7.3 percent). Endocrine disorders were also frequently diagnosed, such as diabetes (25 percent). About half the patients were taking no medications. The researchers concluded:

> Self-neglect among the elderly results in a failure to perform activities of daily living, which is manifested by some combination of poor hygiene, squalor in and outside their dwellings, a lack of utilities, an excess numbers of pets, and inadequate food stores. We found that 77.6% of patients had impairment in some of the activities of daily living evidenced by abnormal physical performance scores. . . . We believe elders who self-neglect are those with impairment in activities of daily living, who lack the needed support services, and who fail to recognize the danger. These older persons lose the cognitive capacity for self-protection. Of course, there are social issues beyond access to support such as lack of family, lack of transportation, and insufficient funds that likely also impact self-neglect.

See also ABUSE; LONG-DISTANCE CARE.

Aung, Koko, et al. "Vitamin D Deficiency Associated with Self-Neglect in the Elderly." *Journal of Elder Abuse & Neglect* 18, no. 4 (2006): 63–78.

Bitondo Dyer, Carmel, et al. "Self-Neglect among the Elderly: A Model Based on More Than 500 Patients Seen by a Geriatric Medicine Team." *American Journal of Public Health* 97, no. 9 (September 2007): 1,671–1,676.

Bitondo Dyer, Carmel, M.D., Sabrina Pickens, and Jason Burnet. "Vulnerable Elders: When It Is No Longer Safe to Live Alone." *Journal of the American Medical Association* 298, no. 12 (September 26, 2007): 1,448–1,449.

Gorbien, Martin J., M.D., and Amy R. Eisenstein. "Elder Abuse and Neglect: An Overview." *Clinics in Geriatric Medicine* 21 (2005): 279–292.

National Center on Elder Abuse, Administration on Aging. "Major Types of Elder Abuse." Available online. URL: http://www.ncea.aoa.gov/ncearoot/Main_Site/FAQ/Basics/Types_Of_Abuse.aspx. Accessed March 26, 2008.

nephrologist   See CANCER; KIDNEY CANCER; KIDNEY DISEASE.

neurologist   See DEMENTIA; HEADACHE; BACK PAIN.

nightmares, frequent   Some elderly individuals are able to get to sleep but then they frequently suffer from terrifying nightmares. In one study published in the Netherlands of more than 6,000 subjects, some elderly men and women had "rather often" or very frequent nightmares, with women having a greater percentage of nightmares than men. Of the men, 6.9 percent had rather often nightmares and 2.1 percent had nightmares very often. Of the women, 9.6 percent had rather often nightmares and 2.3 percent had nightmares very often. The researcher found that cardiac symptoms, such as irregular heartbeats or spasmodic chest pain, were associated with nightmares that occurred very often.

Commenting on the findings, the researcher said, "The results of the present study show that very frequent nightmares are associated with an increase in irregular heart beats independent of the detrimental effect of poor sleep." He added:

> There are case reports on persons with no previously known heart disease in whom nightmares have occurred immediately before they have fallen ill with coronary artery dissection and other life-threatening cardiac events. It therefore seems reasonable to assume that nightmares precede rather than succeed cardiac symptoms in the majority of cardiac events. This may indicate that nightmares and also other sleep complaints in the elderly are important health problems and should receive more attention, and that sleep-improving therapeutic measures may be one way of protecting cardiac health in the elderly.

See also SLEEP DISORDERS.

Asplund, R. "Nightmares, Sleep and Cardiac Symptoms in the Elderly." *Netherlands, the Journal of Medicine* 61, no. 7 (July 2003): 257–261.

nursing homes   Facilities that provide rehabilitative and/or long-term care to individuals. There are about 1.5 million people residing in 16,100 nursing homes nationwide in the United States, based on statistics from 2004. This is a drop from 1999, when 1.6 million residents lived in 18,000 nursing homes. (See Table 1.) Although many people continue to believe that most of the elderly live in nursing homes, the reality is that the majority of older individuals live independently, with family members, or in an ASSISTED-LIVING FACILITY or some other type of housing arrangement.

Short-Term v. Long-Term Care

Rehabilitative nursing homes are facilities that provide temporary assistance to individuals who are injured or ill. For example, after recovering from a fall, the individual may be transferred from a hospital to a rehabilitative facility. These individuals ultimately return to their homes or other housing arrangements, while some are transferred to skilled nursing facilities, or long-term nursing home care.

Some nursing homes provide short-term rehabilitative assistance to individuals who are recovering from HEART ATTACKS, STROKES, or other medical problems that do not (or no longer) require hospital care, yet the individual still needs more care than can be provided at home.

Other nursing homes, often called skilled nursing facilities, provide long-term care to elderly individuals who can no longer function at home because of their physical and/or psychiatric problems, such as DEMENTIA or ALZHEIMER'S DISEASE.

TABLE 1. NUMBER OF NURSING HOMES, BEDS, CURRENT RESIDENTS, AND DISCHARGES, UNITED STATES, SELECTED YEARS 1973–2004

Type of estimate	1973–74	1977	1985	1995	1997	1999	2004
Homes	15,700	18,900	19,100	16,700	17,000	18,000	16,100
Beds	1,177,300	1,402,400	1,624,200	1,770,900	1,820,800	1,879,600	1,730,000
Current residents	1,075,800	1,303,100	1,491,400	1,548,600	1,608,700	1,628,300	1,492,200
Discharges	1,077,500	1,117,500	1,223,500	Not available	2,369,000	2,522,300	Not available

Source: Centers for Disease Control/National Nursing Home Survey, selected years.

Only about 5 percent of the entire elderly population reside in nursing homes, but this percentage increases dramatically to 18.2 percent for those age 85 years and older.

MEDICARE pays for rehabilitative nursing care for those who are eligible but does not pay for long-term care in a nursing home. However, MEDICAID does pay for long-term care for those who are financially eligible.

Some nursing homes are hospital-like, with nurses stationed on each floor and one or two people living in a room. The staff often provides physical therapy, occupational therapy, and speech therapy, as well as other forms of therapy as needed. Nursing homes often have trained social workers on their staff. These are individuals who work with senior citizens and their families to help resolve issues regarding relationships, housing, transportation, and long-term care as well as other issues. Some nursing homes offer a homelike environment, and the daily routine is less fixed and rigid than it is in a hospital-like facility. In such nursing homes, the kitchen is open to the residents, and the staff tries to create a homey atmosphere.

Residents of Nursing Homes

In considering all the residents of nursing homes in the United States, according to the Census Bureau, people age 85 years and older represent about 45 percent of all residents, while those ages 75 to 84 represent about 34 percent of all residents. Thus, together, they represent the majority, or 79 percent, of all nursing home residents. In considering race alone, blacks ages 65 to 84 are significantly more likely than whites to live in a nursing home. Most nursing home residents (75 percent) are female, according to the Centers for Disease Control and Prevention (CDC).

There are also regional differences. For example, 2.7 percent of elderly residents age 65 and older live in nursing homes in the West compared with a high of 5.5 percent who live in nursing homes in the Midwest. In considering individuals age 85 and older, the largest percentage of elderly people (22.7 percent) who lived in nursing homes resided in the Midwest, followed by 19.9 percent who lived in the Northeast.

In considering gender, older women are much more likely to live in nursing homes than older men; for example, according to the Census Bureau, in 1999, about 21 percent of white and black women age 85 and older lived in nursing homes compared with 7.5 percent of very elderly black men and 4.9 percent of very elderly white men.

Rights of Nursing Home Residents

According to the Long-Term Care Ombudsman Program, nursing home residents have the right to

- be treated with respect and dignity
- be free from chemical and physical restraints
- manage their own finances
- voice grievances without fear of retaliation
- associate and communicate privately with any person of their own choice
- send and receive personal mail
- have personal and medical records kept confidential
- apply for state and federal assistance without discrimination
- be fully informed prior to admission of their rights, services available, and all charges; and be given advance notice of transfer or discharge

NURSING HOME CHECKLIST

Name of Nursing Home _____

Date of Visit _____

	Yes	No	Comments
Basic Information			
The nursing home is Medicare-certified.			
The nursing home is Medicaid-certified.			
The nursing home has the level of care needed (such as skilled, custodial), and a bed is available.			
The nursing home has special services, if needed, in a separate unit (such as dementia, ventilator, or rehabilitation), and a bed is available.			
The nursing home is located close enough for family and friends to visit.			
Resident Appearance			
Residents are clean, appropriately dressed for the season or time of day, and well groomed.			
Nursing Home Living Spaces			
The nursing home is free from overwhelming unpleasant odors.			
The nursing home appears clean and well-kept.			
The temperature in the nursing home is comfortable for residents.			
The nursing home has good lighting.			
Noise levels in the dining room and other common areas are comfortable.			
Smoking is not allowed or may be restricted to certain areas of the nursing home.			
Furnishings are sturdy yet comfortable and attractive.			
Staff			
The relationship between the staff and the residents appears to be warm, polite, and respectful.			
All staff wear name tags.			
Staff knock on the door before entering a resident's room and refer to residents by name.			
The nursing home offers a training and continuing education program for all staff.			
The nursing home does background checks on all staff.			
The guide on your tour knows the residents by name and is recognized by them.			
There is a full-time registered nurse (RN) in the nursing home at all times, other than the administrator or director of nursing.			
The same team of nurses and certified nursing assistants (CNAs) work with the same resident four to five days per week.			
CNAs work with a reasonable number of residents.			
CNAs are involved in care-planning meetings.			

	Yes	No	Comments
There is a full-time social worker on staff.			
There is a licensed doctor on staff. Is he or she there daily? Can he or she be reached at all times?			
The nursing home's management team has worked together for at least a year.			
Residents' Rooms			
Residents may have personal belongings and/or furniture in their rooms.			
Each resident has storage space (closet and drawers) in his or her room.			
Each resident has a window in his or her bedroom.			
Residents have access to a personal telephone and television.			
Residents have a choice of roommates.			
Water pitchers can be reached by residents.			
There are policies and procedures to protect resident's possessions.			
Hallways, Stairs, Lounges, and Bathrooms			
Exits are clearly marked.			
There are quiet areas where residents can visit with friends and family.			
The nursing home has smoke detectors and sprinklers.			
All common areas, resident rooms, and doorways are designed for wheelchair use.			
There are handrails in the hallways and grab bars in the bathroom.			
Menus and Food			
Residents have a choice of food items at each meal. (Ask if your favorite foods are served.)			
Nutritious snacks are available upon request.			
Staff help residents eat and drink at mealtimes if help is needed.			
Activities			
Residents, including those who are unable to leave their rooms, may choose to take part in a variety of activities.			
The nursing home has outdoor areas for resident use, and staff help residents go outside.			
The nursing home has an active volunteer program.			
Safety and Care			
The nursing home has an emergency evacuation plan and holds regular fire drills.			
Residents get preventive care, like a yearly flu shot, to help keep them healthy.			
Residents may still see their personal doctors.			
The nursing home has an arrangement with a nearby hospital for emergencies.			

(Continues)

	Yes	No	Comments
Care-plan meetings are held at times that are convenient for residents and family members to attend whenever possible.			
The nursing home has corrected all deficiencies (failure to meet one or more federal or state requirements) on its last state inspection report.			

Source: Medicare, Nursing Home Checklist. Available online. URL: http://www.medicare/gov/nursing/overview.asp. Downloaded on August 1, 2007.

Antipsychotic Medications and Nursing Home Residents

Despite one of the rights listed by the Long-Term Care Ombudsman Program, some nursing homes continue to rely on administering antipsychotic medications to residents.

According to a 2007 study in the *Archives of Internal Medicine,* some nursing homes are three times more likely to prescribe antipsychotic medications to their residents without regard for their clinical needs. Antipsychotics are known to increase the risk for FALLS and hip FRACTURES. They are also associated with movement disorders. The researchers said that the current use of antipsychotics was greater than those that caused the development of past federal regulations to limit the use of antipsychotics.

In the 2007 study, 15,317 subjects, who were nursing home residents in Canada, were prescribed an antipsychotic medication. This was about a third of the residents. (It is likely this is a problem in the United States as well as in Canada.)

The researchers found that nursing homes ranged from prescribing antipsychotics to an average of about 21 percent of the residents to others prescribing these drugs to an average of 44 percent of the residents. Most of the residents had dementia or psychosis, although 17 percent had neither diagnosis. However, even for those residents with no diagnosis of psychosis or dementia, if they resided in a nursing home that relied heavily on antipsychotic drugs, they were at risk for being medicated with such a drug. According to the researchers:

> The marked variation in the rate of antipsychotic prescribing between the facilities with high and low antipsychotic prescribing rates remained strong even among the group of residents for who[m] we identified no clinical indication for the use of an antipsychotic therapy. Specifically, we found that residents residing in facilities with the highest antipsychotic prescribing rates were 3 times more likely to be dispensed an antipsychotic therapy even when there was no diagnosis of psychosis or dementia that might support the need for these agents. Prescribing an antipsychotic therapy to a resident with no clinical indication for the therapy has been identified by the Centers for Medicare and Medicaid Services as a measure of poor quality of care.

Emotional Distress and Moving to a Nursing Home

It should be noted that individuals who are compelled to move to a nursing home because of their failing health and who are aware of their situation (and do not have ALZHEIMER'S DISEASE or another form of DEMENTIA) can become depressed and distressed about the extreme loss of independence. It is important for family and friends to visit the individual as frequently as possible to maintain his or her link with the outside world and decrease the risk of the development of a clinical DEPRESSION.

Risks for Nursing Home Admission

In a study that looked at the risk factors for admission to nursing homes in middle-aged and elderly people, published in *Archives of Internal Medicine* in 2006, the researchers found that for those ages 45 to 64, DIABETES increased the odds of being moved to a nursing home by a factor of three. However, among older people ages 65 to 74, OBESITY was a risk factor to admission to a nursing home; it was not a risk factor for younger individuals.

Finding a Nursing Home

Individuals considering a nursing home for an elderly relative (or themselves) may wish to use the checklist (developed by the federal government) on pages 198–200 when visiting nursing homes.

See also ADVERSE DRUG EVENT; AGGRESSION, PHYSICAL; AMERICANS WITH DISABILITIES ACT; ASSISTED-LIVING FACILITIES; COGNITIVE IMPAIRMENT; CONFUSION; DELUSIONS; END-OF-LIFE ISSUES; GENDER DIFFERENCES; HALLUCINATIONS; HEALTH CARE AGENT/PROXY; HOME HEALTH CARE; INAPPROPRIATE PRESCRIPTIONS FOR THE ELDERLY; IRRITABILITY; MANIA; MEMORY IMPAIRMENT; OMBUDSMAN; RAGE; TALKING TO ELDERLY PARENTS ABOUT DIFFICULT ISSUES.

Administration on Aging. *Fact Sheet: The Long-Term Ombudsman Program.* Washington, D.C.: U.S. Department of Health and Human Services, 2006.

He, Wan, Manisha Sengupta, Victoria A. Velkoff, and Kimberly A. DeBarros. *65+ in the United States: 2005.* Washington, D.C.: U.S. Census Bureau, December 2005.

Lau, Denys T., et al. "Hospitalization and Death Associated with Potentially Inappropriate Prescriptions among Elderly Nursing Home Residents." *Archives of Internal Medicine* 165 (January 10, 2005): 68–74.

Rochon, Paula A., et al. "Variation in Nursing Home Antipsychotic Prescribing Rates." *Archives of Internal Medicine* 167 (April 9, 2007): 676–683.

Valiyava, Elmira, et al. "Lifestyle-Related Risk Factors and Risk of Future Nursing Home Admission." *Archives of Internal Medicine* 166 (May 8, 2006): 985–990.

nutrition   A balanced diet is very important for older people, yet many elderly individuals fail to eat well. As a result, older people may become malnourished and underweight, increasing their risk for developing INFECTIONS and diseases, such as ANEMIA. They may also become obese and increase their risk for DIABETES and some forms of CANCER.

Some diseases are directly affected by good or bad nutrition, most prominently diabetes. If the person with diabetes consumes excessive quantities of carbohydrates, he or she could suffer from severe hyperglycemia and even coma and death. Daily monitoring of the blood glucose is essential for all people with diabetes, but many may be unwilling or unable to perform this monitoring. In such a case, caregivers will need to take over this task.

According to the National Institute on Aging, the average woman age 50 and older needs to consume 1,600 calories if she has a low physical activity level. If her activity level is moderate, she needs 1,800 calories, and if she has an active lifestyle, she needs 2,000–2,200 calories per day. Men need more calories than women, and the average man older than age 50 needs 2,000 calories for a low physical activity, 2,200–2,400 calories for moderate levels of physical activity, and 2,400–2,800 calories if he has an active life.

Common Eating Problems and Solutions

In the article "Eating Well as We Age," researchers at the U.S. Food and Drug Administration (FDA) described common problems that many older people have with eating well and also discussed possible solutions. For example, one common problem is that older people have trouble chewing their food. This may cause considerable difficulty with eating meat, vegetables, and fruits, so the older person may simply stop eating these foods.

The FDA researchers recommended that instead of trying to eat fresh fruit that is difficult to chew, older individuals should instead try eating soft canned fruits such as applesauce or drink fruit juices. "Juicing" may be an alternative for some senior adults to get their required fruits, vegetables, and even proteins. Some people who have trouble with chewing may need to have their dentures adjusted or their teeth and gums checked by a dentist.

If older individuals have trouble eating raw vegetables, they can drink vegetable juices or eat creamed or mashed cooked vegetables. If meat is difficult to chew, older people can eat ground meat, as well as eggs, cheese, yogurt, milk, and foods with milk, such as creamed soup or pudding. If sliced bread is too hard to eat, older people can eat bread pudding, cooked cereal, or rice.

According to the FDA, another problem is that some older people fear that they will get a stomachache or gas from certain foods. There are solutions for this problem too. For example, if milk is a problem for the older person, then the individual may try related foods that may not bother them, such as yogurt or cheese. If vegetables such as cabbage or broccoli cause too much gas, older people can drink vegetable juices and eat vegetables such as carrots, green beans, and potatoes.

Some older individuals do not eat well because it may be too hard for them to cook or they may be unable to stand for a long time. One solution is to eat microwaveable foods and purchase ready-to-eat foods. Older people can also participate in senior citizen food programs.

Some organizations such as Meals on Wheels and related organizations provide assistance by delivering meals to the home. The National Elderly Nutrition program, which is funded by the Administration on Aging, provides meals to impoverished older persons and their spouses. Some individuals live in ASSISTED-LIVING FACILITIES where they can obtain all or most of their meals in a dining room.

Lack of appetite is another problem for many older people, sometimes because of the effects of medications they take or because they are sad or depressed because they must eat alone. A solution is to eat with friends and family or participate in group meal programs. Sometimes medications could be affecting appetite, and if so, check with the doctor to see if the medication or the dosage could be changed. Adding herbs and spices to foods could make them more appetizing.

Healthy Eating Tips

According to the Weight-control Information Network, the following are tips for older people who wish to eat in a healthy manner:

- Select high-fiber foods such as whole-grain breads and cereals, vegetables, beans, and fruit. These foods help avoid constipation and also reduce the risk for Type 2 diabetes and heart disease.

- Avoid skipping meals. This practice could slow down the metabolism and cause a person to eat more high-calorie and high-fat foods at their next meal.

- Eat three servings of vitamin D–fortified low-fat or fat-free milk, cheese, or yogurt every day. These products are high in vitamin D and calcium, and they help to keep the bones strong. If a person has trouble with milk products (as with lactose intolerance), he or she can try soy-based beverages or reduced-lactose milk products. The physician may recommend that the older person also take a calcium and vitamin D supplement.

- Select lean turkey breast, beef, fish, or chicken with the skin removed to reduce the amount of calories and fat in the diet.

- Drink plenty of water or fluids high in water. Often people feel less thirsty as they age, but they still need fluids to remain healthy. Fluids high in water are caffeine-free tea and coffee, as well as soup and low-fat or skim milk.

- Select foods that are fortified with vitamin B_{12}, such as breakfast cereals. Check with the physician to see if the older person should take a vitamin B_{12} supplement as well.

- Keep snacks such as low-fat cheese, low-sodium soup, and whole wheat crackers on hand. Limit the consumption of cake, potato chips, candy, and soda.

See also APPETITE, CHRONIC LACK OF; CONSTIPATION; EXERCISE; HYPERTENSION; VITAMIN AND MINERAL DEFICIENCIES/EXCESSES.

Food and Drug Administration. *Eating Well as We Age.* Rockville, Md.: Department of Health and Human Services. (Undated.) Available online. URL: http://www.fda.gov/opacom/lowlit/eatage.pdf. Accessed November 2, 2007.

Weight-control Information Network. *Healthy Eating & Physical Activity across Your Lifespan: Young at Heart.* Bethesda, Md.: National Institute of Diabetes and Digestive and Kidney Diseases, January 2007.

obesity Excessive weight, as defined in terms of one's height and weight and also by the body mass index (BMI), a measure that takes into account both height and weight. (See the body mass index tables in this entry.) Many older people are overweight or obese. This condition is dangerous, and obesity is a significant health risk factor for a large number of major and serious diseases, such as HEART DISEASE, DIABETES, OSTEOARTHRITIS, HYPERTENSION, gall bladder disease, and even some forms of CANCER, particularly breast cancer, colon cancer, and prostate cancer. In addition, some forms of SLEEP DISORDERS, such as SLEEP APNEA, are more prevalent among the obese.

Although many frail older individuals are slender or underweight, some obese elderly individuals are also frail. In a study of 27 frail obese older people reported in 2006 in the *Archives of Internal Medicine,* the researchers found that weight loss and exercise improved the frailty of the subjects. The study group, who received six months of weekly behavioral training and exercise training three times a week, lost as much as 8 percent of their body weight compared to no weight loss in the control group. The treated subjects experienced improved strength and walking speed and improved in other measures. According to the researchers:

> It has been suggested that successful weight loss is difficult to achieve in the older population because of ingrained, lifelong diet and activity habits, and attempts to change these habits will cause distress and anxiety. In contrast, we found that most of our subjects looked forward to the weekly group meetings and regular exercise sessions, and embraced lifestyle change. However, these results may not necessarily apply to the general obese older adults population because we selected subjects who volunteered for the study and were able to participate in a weight loss and exercise program. Neverthe-less, our results provide evidence that successful weight loss and adherence with exercise training are feasible in the obese older adults, and a group intervention program may provide important social interactions that enhance compliance.

Obesity Varies by Age among the Elderly

Obesity is a problem for some groups of older people more than other groups. For example, according to a 2005 research report by the Agency for Healthcare Research and Quality, in 2002 people age 75 and older were the least likely of all age groups to be obese (14.3 percent); however, among those ages 65 to 74, 25.6 percent were obese. The near elderly, ages 55 to 64, had the highest rate of obesity (27.5 percent) of those who were older than age 55. The reason for this finding is unknown, but it may be that unhealthy obese elderly people die before they reach the age of 75.

Body Mass Index and Obesity

As mentioned, obesity is measured in terms of the body mass index, which takes into account both the height and weight of the person in order to derive a BMI number. In general, those who have a BMI of less than 18.5 are considered underweight, while those with a BMI in the range of 18.5–24.9 are normal weight. Individuals who have a BMI above 25 and up to 29.9 are overweight, while those whose BMI is equal to or exceeds 30.0 are obese. If the BMI is equal to or greater than 40.0, the person is classified as extremely obese.

The BMI measure does not distinguish between males and females. Also, it should be noted that very muscular and athletic people may have a higher BMI than the average person, without necessarily being overweight. In addition, note that the BMI tables are used for adults of all ages.

TABLE 1. CLASSIFICATION OF OVERWEIGHT AND OBESITY BY BODY MASS INDEX (BMI), WAIST CIRCUMFERENCE, AND ASSOCIATED DISEASE RISK

	BMI	Obesity Class	Disease Risk (Relative to Normal Weight and Waist Circumference)	
Underweight	< 18.5		Men < or = to 40 in (102 cm)	> 40 in (102 cm)
			Women < or = to 35 in (88 cm)	> 35 in (88 cm)
Normal	18.5–24.9			
Overweight	25.0–20.9		Increased	High
Obesity	30.0–34.9	I	High	Very high
	35.0–39.9	II	Very high	Very high
Extreme Obesity	> or = to 40	III	Extremely high	Extremely high

Source: National Heart, Blood, and Lung Institute. *The Practical Guide: Identification, Evaluation, and Treatment of Overweight and Obesity in Adults.* Bethesda, Md.: National Institutes of Health, October 2000, p. 10.

As an example of how BMI is used, in a person who is 5'9", if he or she weighs 124 pounds or less, the BMI of the individual is below 18.5, and that person is considered underweight and should gain more weight to be healthy. According to the Centers for Disease Control and Prevention (CDC), a healthy weight for an adult of this height is a very broad range of between 125 to 168 pounds, or a BMI of 18.5 to 24.9. In contrast, for a person who is 5'9" and weighs from 169 to 202 pounds, he or she would be considered overweight; if the person weighed 203 pounds or more, obese.

Abdominal obesity is another issue, and if most of the individual's fat is located around the waist, this means the individual has a greater risk for heart disease or diabetes. The risk increases when the waist measurement is greater than 35 inches for women and 40 inches for men.

Overweight Women May Be Healthier Than Underweight or Obese Women

There are some studies indicating that overweight is not always a health problem among older people, although obesity continues to cause serious health risks. In an interesting study published in 2007 in the *American Journal of Public Health,* researchers found that older women with BMIs in the range of 25 to 29.9 had the lowest level of mortality, despite the label of "overweight" for this range using the BMI measure. This study of more than 8,000 women age 65 and older, drawn from the Study of Osteoporotic Fractures, looked at the deaths of the women over an eight-year period.

The researchers found that women at either extreme of BMIs, both high and low, whether underweight or obese, had a significantly greater death risk than women in the 25 to 29.8 BMI range, despite the label of "overweight." According to the researchers:

Perhaps a certain amount of adiposity [fat] confers a survival advantage in elderly women. Some studies have suggested that the association between body size and mortality in older women is explained either by preexisting poor health status or weight loss. We found that the U-shaped relation between body size and mortality remained when we adjusted for self-reported health status or excluded early deaths as well as when we excluded women who had lost more than 10% of their body weight since they were aged 50 years.

Further research is indicated to determine if the findings reported in this study are valid for other older women as well as for older men.

Groups with Obesity Problems

According to the National Center for Health Statistics, nearly a third (29.7 percent) of people age 65 and older in the United States were obese in 2004. Older women have a slightly higher rate of obesity (30.4 percent) than older men (28.9 percent). One of the reasons for obesity among the elderly is a sedentary lifestyle. Experts say that most of the elderly, including those who are disabled, can perform some level of physical activity that will help reduce their risk for obesity.

CALCULATED BODY MASS INDEX, 40.5"–60" AND 78 LBS.–94 LBS.

Weight

Height (Cm)	(In)	35.4	35.8	36.3	36.7	37.2	37.6	38.1	38.6	39.0	39.5	39.9	40.4	40.8	41.3	41.7	42.2	42.6
Kg →	Lb →	78	79	80	81	82	83	84	85	86	87	88	89	90	91	92	93	94
101.6	40	34.3	34.7															
102.9	40.5	33.4	33.9	34.3	34.7													
104.1	41	32.6	33.0	33.5	33.9	34.3	34.7											
105.4	41.5	31.8	32.2	32.7	33.1	33.5	33.9	34.3	34.7									
106.7	42	31.1	31.5	31.9	32.3	32.7	33.1	33.5	33.9	34.3	34.7							
108.0	42.5	30.4	30.8	31.1	31.5	31.9	32.3	32.7	33.1	33.5	33.9	34.2	34.6					
109.2	43	29.7	30.0	30.4	30.8	31.2	31.6	31.9	32.3	32.7	33.1	33.5	33.8	34.2	34.6	35.0		
110.5	43.5	29.0	29.4	29.7	30.1	30.5	30.8	31.2	31.6	32.0	32.3	32.7	33.1	33.4	33.8	34.2	34.6	34.9
111.8	44	28.3	28.7	29.1	29.4	29.8	30.1	30.5	30.9	31.2	31.6	32.0	32.3	32.7	33.0	33.4	33.8	34.1
113.0	44.5	27.7	28.0	28.4	28.8	29.1	29.5	29.8	30.2	30.5	30.9	31.2	31.6	32.0	32.3	32.7	33.0	33.4
114.3	45	27.1	27.4	27.8	28.1	28.5	28.8	29.2	29.5	29.9	30.2	30.6	30.9	31.2	31.6	31.9	32.3	32.6
115.6	45.5	26.5	26.8	27.2	27.5	27.8	28.2	28.5	28.9	29.2	29.5	29.9	30.2	30.6	30.9	31.2	31.6	31.9
116.8	46	25.9	26.2	26.6	26.9	27.2	27.6	27.9	28.2	28.6	28.9	29.2	29.6	29.9	30.2	30.6	30.9	31.2
118.1	46.5	25.4	25.7	26.0	26.3	26.7	27.0	27.3	27.6	28.0	28.3	28.6	28.9	29.3	29.6	29.9	30.2	30.6
119.4	47	24.8	25.1	25.5	25.8	26.1	26.4	26.7	27.1	27.4	27.7	28.0	28.3	28.6	29.0	29.3	29.6	29.9
120.7	47.5	24.3	24.6	24.9	25.2	25.6	25.9	26.2	26.5	26.8	27.1	27.4	27.7	28.0	28.4	28.7	29.0	29.3
121.9	48	23.8	24.1	24.4	24.7	25.0	25.3	25.6	25.9	26.2	26.5	26.9	27.2	27.5	27.8	28.1	28.4	28.7
124.5	49	22.8	23.1	23.4	23.7	24.0	24.3	24.6	24.9	25.2	25.5	25.8	26.1	26.4	26.6	26.9	27.2	27.5
127.0	50	21.9	22.2	22.5	22.8	23.1	23.3	23.6	23.9	24.2	24.5	24.7	25.0	25.3	25.6	25.9	26.2	26.4
129.5	51	21.1	21.4	21.6	21.9	22.2	22.4	22.7	23.0	23.2	23.5	23.8	24.1	24.3	24.6	24.9	25.1	25.4
132.1	52	20.3	20.5	20.8	21.1	21.3	21.6	21.8	22.1	22.4	22.6	22.9	23.1	23.4	23.7	23.9	24.2	24.4
134.6	53	19.5	19.8	20.0	20.3	20.5	20.8	21.0	21.3	21.5	21.8	22.0	22.3	22.5	22.8	23.0	23.3	23.5
137.2	54	18.8	19.0	19.3	19.5	19.8	20.0	20.3	20.5	20.7	21.0	21.2	21.5	21.7	21.9	22.2	22.4	22.7
139.7	55	18.1	18.4	18.6	18.8	19.1	19.3	19.5	19.8	20.0	20.2	20.5	20.7	20.9	21.2	21.4	21.6	21.8
142.2	56	17.5	17.7	17.9	18.2	18.4	18.6	18.8	19.1	19.3	19.5	19.7	20.0	20.2	20.4	20.6	20.8	21.1
144.8	57	16.9	17.1	17.3	17.5	17.7	18.0	18.2	18.4	18.6	18.8	19.0	19.3	19.5	19.7	19.9	20.1	20.3
147.3	58	16.3	16.5	16.7	16.9	17.1	17.3	17.6	17.8	18.0	18.2	18.4	18.6	18.8	19.0	19.2	19.4	19.6
149.9	59	15.8	16.0	16.2	16.4	16.6	16.8	17.0	17.2	17.4	17.6	17.8	18.0	18.2	18.4	18.6	18.8	19.0
152.4	60	15.2	15.4	15.6	15.8	16.0	16.2	16.4	16.6	16.8	17.0	17.2	17.4	17.6	17.8	18.0	18.2	18.4

CALCULATED BODY MASS INDEX, 61"–71" AND 78 LBS.–94 LBS.

Height Cm	In	Weight Kg 35.4 / Lb 78	35.8 / 79	36.3 / 80	36.7 / 81	37.2 / 82	37.6 / 83	38.1 / 84	38.6 / 85	39.0 / 86	39.5 / 87	39.9 / 88	40.4 / 89	40.8 / 90	41.3 / 91	41.7 / 92	42.2 / 93	42.6 / 94
154.9	61	14.7	14.9	15.1	15.3	15.5	15.7	15.9	16.1	16.2	16.4	16.6	16.8	17.0	17.2	17.4	17.6	17.8
157.5	62	14.3	14.4	14.6	14.8	15.0	15.2	15.4	15.5	15.7	15.9	16.1	16.3	16.5	16.6	16.8	17.0	17.2
160.0	63	13.8	14.0	14.2	14.3	14.5	14.7	14.9	15.1	15.2	15.4	15.6	15.8	15.9	16.1	16.3	16.5	16.7
162.6	64	13.4	13.6	13.7	13.9	14.1	14.2	14.4	14.6	14.8	14.9	15.1	15.3	15.4	15.6	15.8	16.0	16.1
165.1	65		13.1	13.3	13.5	13.6	13.8	14.0	14.1	14.3	14.5	14.6	14.8	15.0	15.1	15.3	15.5	15.6
167.6	66				13.1	13.2	13.4	13.6	13.7	13.9	14.0	14.2	14.4	14.5	14.7	14.8	15.0	15.2
170.2	67							13.2	13.3	13.5	13.6	13.8	13.9	14.1	14.3	14.4	14.6	14.7
172.7	68									13.1	13.2	13.4	13.5	13.7	13.8	14.0	14.1	14.3
175.3	69												13.1	13.3	13.4	13.6	13.7	13.9
177.8	70														13.1	13.2	13.3	13.5
180.3	71																	13.1

CALCULATED BODY MASS INDEX, 44"–68" AND 95 LBS.–112 LBS.

		Weight																
Kg		43.1	43.5	44.0	44.5	44.9	45.4	45.8	46.3	46.7	47.2	47.6	48.1	48.5	49.0	49.4	49.9	50.8
Lb		95	96	97	98	99	100	101	102	103	104	105	106	107	108	109	110	112
Height Cm	In																	
111.8	44	34.5	34.9															
113.0	44.5	33.7	34.1	34.4	34.8													
114.3	45	33.0	33.3	33.7	34.0	34.4	34.7											
115.6	45.5	32.3	32.6	32.9	33.3	33.6	34.0	34.3	34.6	35.0								
116.8	46	31.6	31.9	32.2	32.6	32.9	33.2	33.6	33.9	34.2	34.6							
118.1	46.5	30.9	31.2	31.5	31.9	32.2	32.5	32.8	33.2	33.5	33.8	34.1	34.5	34.8				
119.4	47	30.2	30.6	30.9	31.2	31.5	31.8	32.1	32.5	32.8	33.1	33.4	33.7	34.1	34.4	34.7		
120.7	47.5	29.6	29.9	30.2	30.5	30.8	31.2	31.5	31.8	32.1	32.4	32.7	33.0	33.3	33.7	34.0	34.3	34.9
121.9	48	29.0	29.3	29.6	29.9	30.2	30.5	30.8	31.1	31.4	31.7	32.0	32.3	32.7	33.0	33.3	33.6	34.2
124.5	49	27.8	28.1	28.4	28.7	29.0	29.3	29.6	29.9	30.2	30.5	30.7	31.0	31.3	31.6	31.9	32.2	32.8
127.0	50	26.7	27.0	27.3	27.6	27.8	28.1	28.4	28.7	29.0	29.2	29.5	29.8	30.1	30.4	30.7	30.9	31.5
129.5	51	25.7	25.9	26.2	26.5	26.8	27.0	27.3	27.6	27.8	28.1	28.4	28.7	28.9	29.2	29.5	29.7	30.3
132.1	52	24.7	25.0	25.2	25.5	25.7	26.0	26.3	26.5	26.8	27.0	27.3	27.6	27.8	28.1	28.3	28.6	29.1
134.6	53	23.8	24.0	24.3	24.5	24.8	25.0	25.3	25.5	25.8	26.0	26.3	26.5	26.8	27.0	27.3	27.5	28.0
137.2	54	22.9	23.1	23.4	23.6	23.9	24.1	24.4	24.6	24.8	25.1	25.3	25.6	25.8	26.0	26.3	26.5	27.0
139.7	55	22.1	22.3	22.5	22.8	23.0	23.2	23.5	23.7	23.9	24.2	24.4	24.6	24.9	25.1	25.3	25.6	26.0
142.2	56	21.3	21.5	21.7	22.0	22.2	22.4	22.6	22.9	23.1	23.3	23.5	23.8	24.0	24.2	24.4	24.7	25.1
144.8	57	20.6	20.8	21.0	21.2	21.4	21.6	21.9	22.1	22.3	22.5	22.7	22.9	23.2	23.4	23.6	23.8	24.2
147.3	58	19.9	20.1	20.3	20.5	20.7	20.9	21.1	21.3	21.5	21.7	21.9	22.2	22.4	22.6	22.8	23.0	23.4
149.9	59	19.2	19.4	19.6	19.8	20.0	20.2	20.4	20.6	20.8	21.0	21.2	21.4	21.6	21.8	22.0	22.2	22.6
152.4	60	18.6	18.7	18.9	19.1	19.3	19.5	19.7	19.9	20.1	20.3	20.5	20.7	20.9	21.1	21.3	21.5	21.9
154.9	61	17.9	18.1	18.3	18.5	18.7	18.9	19.1	19.3	19.5	19.7	19.8	20.0	20.2	20.4	20.6	20.8	21.2
157.5	62	17.4	17.6	17.7	17.9	18.1	18.3	18.5	18.7	18.8	19.0	19.2	19.4	19.6	19.8	19.9	20.1	20.5
160.0	63	16.8	17.0	17.2	17.4	17.5	17.7	17.9	18.1	18.2	18.4	18.6	18.8	19.0	19.1	19.3	19.5	19.8
162.6	64	16.3	16.5	16.6	16.8	17.0	17.2	17.3	17.5	17.7	17.9	18.0	18.2	18.4	18.5	18.7	18.9	19.2
165.1	65	15.8	16.0	16.1	16.3	16.5	16.6	16.8	17.0	17.1	17.3	17.5	17.6	17.8	18.0	18.1	18.3	18.6
167.6	66	15.3	15.5	15.7	15.8	16.0	16.1	16.3	16.5	16.6	16.8	16.9	17.1	17.3	17.4	17.6	17.8	18.1
170.2	67	14.9	15.0	15.2	15.3	15.5	15.7	15.8	16.0	16.1	16.3	16.4	16.6	16.8	16.9	17.1	17.2	17.5
172.7	68	14.4	14.6	14.7	14.9	15.1	15.2	15.4	15.5	15.7	15.8	16.0	16.1	16.3	16.4	16.6	16.7	17.0

CALCULATED BODY MASS INDEX, 69"–77" AND 95 LBS.–112 LBS.

Height Cm	In	Weight Kg 43.1	43.5	44.0	44.5	44.9	45.4	45.8	46.3	46.7	47.2	47.6	48.1	48.5	49.0	49.4	49.9	50.8
		Lb 95	96	97	98	99	100	101	102	103	104	105	106	107	108	109	110	112
175.3	69	14.0	14.2	14.3	14.5	14.6	14.8	14.9	15.1	15.2	15.4	15.5	15.7	15.8	15.9	16.1	16.2	16.5
177.8	70	13.6	13.8	13.9	14.1	14.2	14.3	14.5	14.6	14.8	14.9	15.1	15.2	15.4	15.5	15.6	15.8	16.1
180.3	71	13.2	13.4	13.5	13.7	13.8	13.9	14.1	14.2	14.4	14.5	14.6	14.8	14.9	15.1	15.2	15.3	15.6
182.9	72		13.0	13.2	13.3	13.4	13.6	13.7	13.8	14.0	14.1	14.2	14.4	14.5	14.6	14.8	14.9	15.2
185.4	73					13.1	13.2	13.3	13.5	13.6	13.7	13.9	14.0	14.1	14.2	14.4	14.5	14.8
188.0	74								13.1	13.2	13.4	13.5	13. 6	13.7	13.9	14.0	14.1	14.4
190.5	75											13.1	13.2	13.4	13.5	13.6	13.7	14.0
193.0	76													13.0	13.1	13.3	13.4	13.6
195.6	77																13.0	13.3

CALCULATED BODY MASS INDEX, 48"–76" AND 114 LBS.–146 LBS.

Weight

Height (Cm)	In	Kg: 51.7	52.6	53.5	54.4	55.3	56.2	57.2	58.1	59.0	59.9	60.8	61.7	62.6	63.5	64.4	65.3	66.2
Lb:		114	116	118	120	122	124	126	128	130	132	134	136	138	140	142	144	146
121.9	48	34.8																
124.5	49	33.4	34.0	34.6														
127.0	50	32.1	32.6	33.2	33.7	34.3	34.9											
129.5	51	30.8	31.4	31.9	32.4	33.0	33.5	34.1	34.6									
132.1	52	29.6	30.2	30.7	31.2	31.7	32.2	32.8	33.3	33.8	34.3	34.8						
134.6	53	28.5	29.0	29.5	30.0	30.5	31.0	31.5	32.0	32.5	33.0	33.5	34.0	34.5				
137.2	54	27.5	28.0	28.4	28.9	29.4	29.9	30.4	30.9	31.3	31.8	32.3	32.8	33.3	33.8	34.2	34.7	
139.7	55	26.5	27.0	27.4	27.9	28.4	28.8	29.3	29.7	30.2	30.7	31.1	31.6	32.1	32.5	33.0	33.5	33.9
142.2	56	25.6	26.0	26.5	26.9	27.3	27.8	28.2	28.7	29.1	29.6	30.0	30.5	30.9	31.4	31.8	32.3	32.7
144.8	57	24.7	25.1	25.5	26.0	26.4	26.8	27.3	27.7	28.1	28.6	29.0	29.4	29.9	30.3	30.7	31.2	31.6
147.3	58	23.8	24.2	24.7	25.1	25.5	25.9	26.3	26.8	27.2	27.6	28.0	28.4	28.8	29.3	29.7	30.1	30.5
149.9	59	23.0	23.4	23.8	24.2	24.6	25.0	25.4	25.9	26.3	26.7	27.1	27.5	27.9	28.3	28.7	29.1	29.5
152.4	60	22.3	22.7	23.0	23.4	23.8	24.2	24.6	25.0	25.4	25.8	26.2	26.6	26.9	27.3	27.7	28.1	28.5
154.9	61	21.5	21.9	22.3	22.7	23.0	23.4	23.8	24.2	24.6	24.9	25.3	25.7	26.1	26.4	26.8	27.2	27.6
157.5	62	20.9	21.2	21.6	21.9	22.3	22.7	23.0	23.4	23.8	24.1	24.5	24.9	25.2	25.6	26.0	26.3	26.7
160.0	63	20.2	20.5	20.9	21.3	21.6	22.0	22.3	22.7	23.0	23.4	23.7	24.1	24.4	24.8	25.2	25.5	25.9
162.6	64	19.6	19.9	20.3	20.6	20.9	21.3	21.6	22.0	22.3	22.7	23.0	23.3	23.7	24.0	24.4	24.7	25.1
165.1	65	19.0	19.3	19.6	20.0	20.3	20.6	21.0	21.3	21.6	22.0	22.3	22.6	23.0	23.3	23.6	24.0	24.3
167.6	66	18.4	18.7	19.0	19.4	19.7	20.0	20.3	20.7	21.0	21.3	21.6	22.0	22.3	22.6	22.9	23.2	23.6
170.2	67	17.9	18.2	18.5	18.8	19.1	19.4	19.7	20.0	20.4	20.7	21.0	21.3	21.6	21.9	22.2	22.6	22.9
172.7	68	17.3	17.6	17.9	18.2	18.5	18.9	19.2	19.5	19.8	20.1	20.4	20.7	21.0	21.3	21.6	21.9	22.2
175.3	69	16.8	17.1	17.4	17.7	18.0	18.3	18.6	18.9	19.2	19.5	19.8	20.1	20.4	20.7	21.0	21.3	21.6
177.8	70	16.4	16.6	16.9	17.2	17.5	17.8	18.1	18.4	18.7	18.9	19.2	19.5	19.8	20.1	20.4	20.7	20.9
180.3	71	15.9	16.2	16.5	16.7	17.0	17.3	17.6	17.9	18.1	18.4	18.7	19.0	19.2	19.5	19.8	20.1	20.4
182.9	72	15.5	15.7	16.0	16.3	16.5	16.8	17.1	17.4	17.6	17.9	18.2	18.4	18.7	19.0	19.3	19.5	19.8
185.4	73	15.0	15.3	15.6	15.8	16.1	16.4	16.6	16.9	17.2	17.4	17.7	17.9	18.2	18.5	18.7	19.0	19.3
188.0	74	14.6	14.9	15.1	15.4	15.7	15.9	16.2	16.4	16.7	16.9	17.2	17.5	17.7	18.0	18.2	18.5	18.7
190.5	75	14.2	14.5	14.7	15.0	15.2	15.5	15.7	16.0	16.2	16.5	16.7	17.0	17.2	17.5	17.7	18.0	18.2
193.0	76	13.9	14.1	14.4	14.6	14.8	15.1	15.3	15.6	15.8	16.1	16.3	16.6	16.8	17.0	17.3	17.5	17.8
195.6	77	13.5	13.8	14.0	14.2	14.5	14.7	14.9	15.2	15.4	15.7	15.9	16.1	16.4	16.6	16.8	17.1	17.3
198.1	78	13.2	13.4	13.6	13.9	14.1	14.3	14.6	14.8	15.0	15.3	15.5	15.7	15.9	16.2	16.4	16.6	16.9

CALCULATED BODY MASS INDEX, 55"–78" AND 148 LBS.–180 LBS.

Height Cm	In	Kg 67.1 / Lb 148	68.0 / 150	68.9 / 152	69.9 / 154	70.8 / 156	71.7 / 158	72.6 / 160	73.5 / 162	74.4 / 164	75.3 / 166	76.2 / 168	77.1 / 170	78.0 / 172	78.9 / 174	79.8 / 176	80.7 / 178	81.6 / 180
139.7	55	34.4	34.9															
142.2	56	33.2	33.6	34.1	34.5	35.0												
144.8	57	32.0	32.5	32.9	33.3	33.8	34.2	34.6										
147.3	58	30.9	31.3	31.8	32.2	32.6	33.0	33.4	33.9	34.3	34.7							
149.9	59	29.9	30.3	30.7	31.1	31.5	31.9	32.3	32.7	33.1	33.5	33.9	34.3	34.7				
152.4	60	28.9	29.3	29.7	30.1	30.5	30.9	31.2	31.6	32.0	32.4	32.8	33.2	33.6	34.0	34.4	34.8	
154.9	61	28.0	28.3	28.7	29.1	29.5	29.9	30.2	30.6	31.0	31.4	31.7	32.1	32.5	32.9	33.3	33.6	34.0
157.5	62	27.1	27.4	27.8	28.2	28.5	28.9	29.3	29.6	30.0	30.4	30.7	31.1	31.5	31.8	32.2	32.6	32.9
160.0	63	26.2	26.6	26.9	27.3	27.6	28.0	28.3	28.7	29.1	29.4	29.8	30.1	30.5	30.8	31.2	31.5	31.9
162.6	64	25.4	25.7	26.1	26.4	26.8	27.1	27.5	27.8	28.2	28.5	28.8	29.2	29.5	29.9	30.2	30.6	30.9
165.1	65	24.6	25.0	25.3	25.6	26.0	26.3	26.6	27.0	27.3	27.6	28.0	28.3	28.6	29.0	29.3	29.6	30.0
167.6	66	23.9	24.2	24.5	24.9	25.2	25.5	25.8	26.1	26.5	26.8	27.1	27.4	27.8	28.1	28.4	28.7	29.1
170.2	67	23.2	23.5	23.8	24.1	24.4	24.7	25.1	25.4	25.7	26.0	26.3	26.6	26.9	27.3	27.6	27.9	28.2
172.7	68	22.5	22.8	23.1	23.4	23.7	24.0	24.3	24.6	24.9	25.2	25.5	25.8	26.2	26.5	26.8	27.1	27.4
175.3	69	21.9	22.2	22.4	22.7	23.0	23.3	23.6	23.9	24.2	24.5	24.8	25.1	25.4	25.7	26.0	26.3	26.6
177.8	70	21.2	21.5	21.8	22.1	22.4	22.7	23.0	23.2	23.5	23.8	24.1	24.4	24.7	25.0	25.3	25.5	25.8
180.3	71	20.6	20.9	21.2	21.5	21.8	22.0	22.3	22.6	22.9	23.2	23.4	23.7	24.0	24.3	24.5	24.8	25.1
182.9	72	20.1	20.3	20.6	20.9	21.2	21.4	21.7	22.0	22.2	22.5	22.8	23.1	23.3	23.6	23.9	24.1	24.4
185.4	73	19.5	19.8	20.1	20.3	20.6	20.8	21.1	21.4	21.6	21.9	22.2	22.4	22.7	23.0	23.2	23.5	23.7
188.0	74	19.0	19.3	19.5	19.8	20.0	20.3	20.5	20.8	21.1	21.3	21.6	21.8	22.1	22.3	22.6	22.9	23.1
190.5	75	18.5	18.7	19.0	19.2	19.5	19.7	20.0	20.2	20.5	20.7	21.0	21.2	21.5	21.7	22.0	22.2	22.5
193.0	76	18.0	18.3	18.5	18.7	19.0	19.2	19.5	19.7	20.0	20.2	20.4	20.7	20.9	21.2	21.4	21.7	21.9
195.6	77	17.6	17.8	18.0	18.3	18.5	18.7	19.0	19.2	19.4	19.7	19.9	20.2	20.4	20.6	20.9	21.1	21.3
198.1	78	17.1	17.3	17.6	17.8	18.0	18.3	18.5	18.7	19.0	19.2	19.4	19.6	19.9	20.1	20.3	20.6	20.8

CALCULATED BODY MASS INDEX, 61"–78" AND 182 LBS.–214 LBS.

Height			Weight																	
		Kg	82.6	83.5	84.4	85.3	86.2	87.1	88.0	88.9	89.8	90.7	91.6	92.5	93.4	94.3	95.3	96.2	97.1
Cm	In	Lb	182	184	186	188	190	192	194	196	198	200	202	204	206	208	210	212	214
154.9	61		34.4	34.8															
157.5	62		33.3	33.7	34.0	34.4	34.8												
160.0	63		32.2	32.6	32.9	33.3	33.7	34.0	34.4	34.7									
162.6	64		31.2	31.6	31.9	32.3	32.6	33.0	33.3	33.6	34.0	34.3	34.7						
165.1	65		30.3	30.6	31.0	31.3	31.6	32.0	32.3	32.6	32.9	33.3	33.6	33.9	34.3	34.6	34.9		
167.6	66		29.4	29.7	30.0	30.3	30.7	31.0	31.3	31.6	32.0	32.3	32.6	32.9	33.2	33.6	33.9	34.2	34.5
170.2	67		28.5	28.8	29.1	29.4	29.8	30.1	30.4	30.7	31.0	31.3	31.6	32.0	32.3	32.6	32.9	33.2	33.5
172.7	68		27.7	28.0	28.3	28.6	28.9	29.2	29.5	29.8	30.1	30.4	30.7	31.0	31.3	31.6	31.9	32.2	32.5
175.3	69		26.9	27.2	27.5	27.8	28.1	28.4	28.6	28.9	29.2	29.5	29.8	30.1	30.4	30.7	31.0	31.3	31.6
177.8	70		26.1	26.4	26.7	27.0	27.3	27.5	27.8	28.1	28.4	28.7	29.0	29.3	29.6	29.8	30.1	30.4	30.7
180.3	71		25.4	25.7	25.9	26.2	26.5	26.8	27.1	27.3	27.6	27.9	28.2	28.5	28.7	29.0	29.3	29.6	29.8
182.9	72		24.7	25.0	25.2	25.5	25.8	26.0	26.3	26.6	26.9	27.1	27.4	27.7	27.9	28.2	28.5	28.8	29.0
185.4	73		24.0	24.3	24.5	24.8	25.1	25.3	25.6	25.9	26.1	26.4	26.7	26.9	27.2	27.4	27.7	28.0	28.2
188.0	74		23.4	23.6	23.9	24.1	24.4	24.7	24.9	25.2	25.4	25.7	25.9	26.2	26.4	26.7	27.0	27.2	27.5
190.5	75		22.7	23.0	23.2	23.5	23.7	24.0	24.2	24.5	24.7	25.0	25.2	25.5	25.7	26.0	26.2	26.5	26.7
193.0	76		22.2	22.4	22.6	22.9	23.1	23.4	23.6	23.9	24.1	24.3	24.6	24.8	25.1	25.3	25.6	25.8	26.0
195.6	77		21.6	21.8	22.1	22.3	22.5	22.8	23.0	23.2	23.5	23.7	24.0	24.2	24.4	24.7	24.9	25.1	25.4
198.1	78		21.0	21.3	21.5	21.7	22.0	22.2	22.4	22.6	22.9	23.1	23.3	23.6	23.8	24.0	24.3	24.5	24.7

CALCULATED BODY MASS INDEX, 66"–78" AND 216 LBS.–250 LBS.

Height			Weight																
Cm	In	Kg	98.0	98.9	99.8	100.7	101.6	102.5	103.4	104.3	105.2	106.1	107.0	108.0	108.9	109.8	110.7	111.6	112.5	113.4
		Lb	216	218	220	222	224	226	228	230	232	234	236	238	240	242	244	246	248	250
167.6	66		34.9																	
170.2	67		33.8	34.1	34.5	34.8														
172.7	68		32.8	33.1	33.5	33.8	34.1	34.4	34.7											
175.3	69		31.9	32.2	32.5	32.8	33.1	33.4	33.7	34.0	34.3	34.6	34.9							
177.8	70		31.0	31.3	31.6	31.9	32.1	32.4	32.7	33.0	33.3	33.6	33.9	34.1	34.4	34.7				
180.3	71		30.1	30.4	30.7	31.0	31.2	31.5	31.8	32.1	32.4	32.6	32.9	33.2	33.5	33.8	34.0	34.3	34.6	34.9
182.9	72		29.3	29.6	29.8	30.1	30.4	30.7	30.9	31.2	31.5	31.7	32.0	32.3	32.5	32.8	33.1	33.4	33.6	33.9
185.4	73		28.5	28.8	29.0	29.3	29.6	29.8	30.1	30.3	30.6	30.9	31.1	31.4	31.7	31.9	32.2	32.5	32.7	33.0
188.0	74		27.7	28.0	28.2	28.5	28.8	29.0	29.3	29.5	29.8	30.0	30.3	30.6	30.8	31.1	31.3	31.6	31.8	32.1
190.5	75		27.0	27.2	27.5	27.7	28.0	28.2	28.5	28.7	29.0	29.2	29.5	29.7	30.0	30.2	30.5	30.7	31.0	31.2
193.0	76		26.3	26.5	26.8	27.0	27.3	27.5	27.8	28.0	28.2	28.5	28.7	29.0	29.2	29.5	29.7	29.9	30.2	30.4
195.6	77		25.6	25.9	26.1	26.3	26.6	26.8	27.0	27.3	27.5	27.7	28.0	28.2	28.5	28.7	28.9	29.2	29.4	29.6
198.1	78		25.0	25.2	25.4	25.7	25.9	26.1	26.3	26.6	26.8	27.0	27.3	27.5	27.7	28.0	28.2	28.4	28.7	28.9

According to a research report by the Agency for Healthcare Research and Quality, blacks were the most likely of all races to be obese (33.9 percent). People of multiple races were the least likely to be obese (12.2 percent).

The risk for obesity varies drastically from state to state in the United States, according to the Centers for Disease Control and Prevention (CDC). For example, the CDC estimated that 25.6 percent of older adults in Louisiana were obese (the worst state in the country for obesity) compared with only 10.2 percent of the elderly in Hawaii (the best state) who were obese. The CDC goal is for only 15 percent of the elderly to be obese, but few states have met this target.

Dementia and Obesity

Some studies have found that obese elderly individuals have a greater risk of developing DEMENTIA. In a review of eight longitudinal studies on weight dementia, published in a 2007 issue of *Age and Ageing,* the researchers evaluated the findings. The studies covered 1,688 patients with dementia of more than 28,000 subjects. In four of these studies, the researchers found a significant risk of developing dementia that was associated with obesity as defined by BMI. According to the researchers, "There is a prevailing assumption that obesity is not a major risk factor for age-related cognitive decline. This review suggests that increased BMI is likely to be an independent risk factor for dementia." The researchers also found that smoking might be a risk factor for dementia, although smokers are generally thinner than nonsmokers.

Resolving Obesity

Obesity can be treated by increasing exercise and decreasing calorie intake, and many physicians can offer dietary suggestions or refer obese patients to nutritionists. It is also a good idea to check the patient for hypothyroidism, because many older people have low thyroid levels, and this condition may make weight loss difficult for them. Hypothyroidism is easily treatable with a thyroid pill.

There are prescribed and over-the-counter drugs for those who are obese. Alli, formerly called orlistat (Xenical), is a currently available over-the-counter weight reduction medication. Alli limits the absorption of fatty foods and can lead to FECAL INCONTINENCE in some people. Some individuals use sibutramine (Meridia), another medication to decrease appetite. Sibutramine increases the blood pressure and heart rate and is not recommended for people with hypertension or a history of stroke or heart arrhythmias. Most experts report, however, that there are currently no drugs that are effective for most people who are obese, although many such drugs are under development.

Some individuals resort to bariatric surgery, or having their stomach surgically made smaller; however, this surgery is not recommended for most elderly people because of its risks. According to Doctors Abell and Minocha in their 2006 article on gastrointestinal complications of bariatric surgery in the *American Journal of Medical Sciences,* the top five complications of such procedures include dumping, vitamin/mineral deficiencies, vomiting/nausea, staple line failure, and infection. "Dumping" refers to the very rapid emptying of the contents of the gut into the small intestines. This process can cause nausea, pain, and diarrhea, and treatment for dumping can be difficult. The most commonly reported vitamin and mineral deficiencies were of iron, vitamin B_{12}, vitamin D, and calcium. (Note that a deficiency of vitamin B_{12} can cause apparent symptoms of dementia.)

In addition, as many as 70 percent of patients who have bariatric surgery and who lose weight very rapidly (as is commonly expected) will develop gallstones. Other complications from the surgery may include ulceration, bleeding, injury to the spleen, and even death.

According to an article on the risks for death from bariatric surgery, published in the *Archives of Surgery* in 2007, 2.6 percent of more than 16,000 patients died after having bariatric surgery during the period 1995–2004. The risk for death increased significantly among those older than age 65, and the leading cause of death was coronary heart disease, which killed 19 percent of the patients. An earlier article published in the *Journal of the American Medical Association* in 2005 discussed the finding that among Medicare beneficiaries, the risk of death among those ages 65 and older was substantially higher than the risk among younger individuals. As a result of these serious surgical risks, few doctors will perform bariatric surgery on elderly patients.

In general, only individuals who are more than 100 pounds overweight are considered for bariatric surgery.

There are numerous diet plans and clubs to help people lose weight, but most are only temporarily effective, if they work at all. In addition, some forms of behavior therapy may help individuals lose weight. For example, stress management, social support, and cognitive restructuring are all forms of psychotherapy that have been demonstrated as effective at helping individuals lose weight. Occasionally, hypnotherapy may be effective as well.

Often a combination of therapies is effective, such as psychotherapy, medication, and exercise.

See also CANCER; CHOLESTEROL; EXERCISE; HEART FAILURE; HYPERTENSION; NUTRITION; VITAMIN AND MINERAL DEFICIENCIES/EXCESSES.

Abell, Thomas L., M.D., and Anil Minocha, M.D. "Gastrointestinal Complications of Bariatric Surgery: Diagnosis and Therapy." *American Journal of the Medical Sciences* 331, no. 4 (2006): 214–218.

Bohannon, Richard W., et al. "Adiposity of Elderly Women and Its Relationship with Self-reported and Observed Physical Performance." *Journal of Geriatric Physical Therapy* 28, no. 1 (2005): 10–13.

Centers for Disease Control and Prevention. *The State-by-State Report Card on Healthy Aging.* Available online. URL: http://www.cdc.gov/aging/pdf/saha_2007.pdf. Accessed April 7, 2008.

Flum, David R., M.D., et al. "Early Mortality among Medicare Beneficiaries Undergoing Bariatric Surgical Procedures." *Journal of the American Medical Association* 294, no. 15 (October 19, 2005): 1,903–1,908.

Gorospe, Emmanuel, and Jatin K. Dave. "The Risk of Dementia with Increased Body Mass Index." *Age and Ageing* 36 (2007): 23–29.

Matkin Dolan, Chantal, et al. "Associations Between Body Composition, Anthropometry, and Mortality in Women Aged 65 Years and Older." *American Journal of Public Health* 97, no. 5 (2007): 913–918.

National Heart, Lung, and Blood Institute. *Aim for a Healthy Weight.* Bethesda, Md.: National Institutes of Health, August 2005.

———. *Clinical Guidelines on the Identification, Evaluation, and Treatment of Overweight and Obesity in Adults: The Evidence Report.* Bethesda, Md.: National Institutes of Health, September 1998.

———. *The Practical Guide: Identification, Evaluation, and Treatment of Overweight and Obesity in Adults.* Bethesda, Md.: National Institutes of Health, October 2000.

Omalu, Bennett I., M.D., et al. "Obesity, Mortality, and Bariatric Surgery Death Rates." *Archives of Surgery* 142, no. 10 (2007): 923–928.

Rhoades, J. A. *Overweight and Obese Elderly and Near Elderly in the United States, 2002: Estimates for the Noninstitutionalized Population Age 55 and Older.* Rockville, Md.: Agency for Healthcare Research and Quality. Available online. URL: http://www.meps.ahrq.gov/papers/st68/stat68.pdf. Accessed October 25, 2007.

Villareal, Dennis T., M.D., et al. "Effect of Weight Loss and Exercise on Frailty in Obese Older Adults." *Archives of Internal Medicine* 166 (April 24, 2006): 860–866.

obsessive-compulsive disorder (OCD) See ANXIETY AND ANXIETY DISORDERS.

Old Age Survivors/Disability Insurance Program (OASDI) A money payment program administered by the Social Security Administration that provides benefits to many older individuals and disabled people of all ages who are eligible. About 96 out of 100 workers in paid employment or self-employment are covered or eligible for coverage. In addition, family members of the beneficiary, such as their spouses and minor children, may also be eligible to receive benefits.

The overwhelming majority of Americans age 65 and older are recipients of OASDI benefits. According to the Office of the Chief Actuary of the Social Security Administration, as of June 30, 2007, about 91 percent of the population age 65 and older were receiving benefits. As of that date, there were about 31 million retired people receiving retirement benefits from the Social Security Administration, and the average monthly amount was $1,050. There were also about 2.5 million spouses receiving benefits, and the average monthly amount was $519. In addition, 499 children received benefits based on the retired workers' eligibility, and the average monthly payment was $523.

One problem that government officials are beginning to worry about is that the oldest BABY BOOMERS (born 1946–1964) have become eligible for Social Security early retirement benefits, and it may be difficult to fund this expense out of payments deducted from current workers. The oldest baby boomers were age 62 in 2008 and will become eligible for full retirement benefits at age 66, which will occur in 2012. It is believed that many will choose to retire as soon as they can.

Office of the Chief Actuary, Social Security Administration. *Fact Sheet on the Old-Age, Survivors, and Disability Insurance Program.* Baltimore, Md.: Social Security Administration. Available online. URL: http://www.ssa.gov/OACT/FACTS. Accessed November 21, 2007.

Older Americans Act   An act that was originally passed in 1965 and which established the Administration on Aging. Later amendments provided for programs for Native-American elders, services for low-income minority elders, home-care services for very ill elders, and the establishment of the long-term care OMBUDSMAN program and other services.

The act was reauthorized and amended in 2000 and signed into law by President Bill Clinton in 2000. The reauthorized act included a new program, the National Family Caregiver Support Program, and as of 2007, the program is funded at $162 million and has served an estimated 750,000 caregivers nationwide. In addition, funding of $6.3 million was provided in fiscal year 2007 to support caregivers of Native Americans.

The National Family Caregiver Support Program called for all states to offer the following five basic services for family caregivers:

- information about available services
- assistance in gaining access to services
- organization of support groups, individual counseling, and caregiver training to help caregivers make decisions and solve problems related to their caregiving roles
- respite care so that caregivers could be temporarily relieved from caregiving responsibilities
- limited supplemental services to complement the care that is provided by caregivers

The National Family Caregiver Support Program also provided funding of grants to state agencies so that the states could provide information and assistance to family caregivers of older people. In addition, the reauthorized act included an acknowledgment of the needs of older people with development disabilities. In 2006, President George Bush signed the Older Americans Act of 2006, which was basically a reauthorization of the provisions of the 2000 law.

See also ADULT CHILDREN/CHILDREN OF AGING PARENTS.

oldest old   Refers to very old individuals, such as those older than age 85. Centenarians are individuals who have attained their one-hundredth birthday. The oldest old are more likely than younger individuals to have medical problems as well as mental health issues. They have a high risk of developing ALZHEIMER'S DISEASE, OSTEOARTHRITIS, and vision impairments or HEARING DISORDERS. They also have a higher risk of developing other forms of dementia, as well as heart disease and CANCER.

The numbers of the oldest old are growing rapidly in the United States and in the world. They will need help with TRANSPORTATION (although some are still DRIVING) and many other aspects of life. Most people age 85 and older cannot work and must rely on others for assistance. In some cases, the fixed income they receive from Social Security or private pensions barely meets their financial needs. As a result, some resort to GAMBLING or succumb to scams that can strip them of their life savings.

The challenge for countries around the world is to appreciate and enjoy the benefits and wisdom of its oldest citizens and at the same time provide the assistance and medical services they need as well as the emotional care that is often required.

See also CRIMES AGAINST THE ELDERLY; DEATH; DEATH, FEAR OF.

ombudsman   An individual at the state level who advocates primarily for elderly people residing in NURSING HOMES and sometimes for those living in ASSISTED-LIVING FACILITIES and other long-term care facilities. The Ombudsman Program was launched in 1972 as a demonstration project with the Public Health Service and was transferred to the Administration on Aging in 1974. All states have an ombudsman program under the federal OLDER AMERICANS ACT. (See Appendix III for a listing of state agencies managing the ombudsman program.)

Ombudsmen investigate specific complaints about nursing homes, and an estimated 1,000 paid ombudsmen and 14,000 volunteers investigate more than 260,000 complaints each year, according to the Administration on Aging. Ombudsmen also provide information and advice to an estimated 280,000 people per year on many topics, including how to locate a nursing home as well as help people determine how to pay their expenses for the facility. According to ombudsmen, the most frequent nursing home complaints are a lack of resident care due to inadequate staffing.

Ombudsman responsibilities include

- identifying, investigating, and resolving complaints made by or on behalf of residents
- providing information to residents about long-term care services
- representing the interests of residents before governmental agencies and seeking administrative, legal, and other remedies to protect residents
- analyzing, commenting on, and recommending changes in laws and regulations pertaining to the health, safety, welfare, and rights of residents
- educating and informing consumers and the general public regarding issues and concerns related to long-term care and facilitating public comment on laws, regulations, policies, and actions
- promoting the development of citizen organizations to participate in the program
- providing technical support for the development of resident and family councils to protect the well-being and rights of residents
- advocating for changes to improve residents' quality of life and care

See also ABUSE; INAPPROPRIATE PRESCRIPTIONS FOR THE ELDERLY; RESTRAINTS.

Administration on Aging. *Fact Sheet: The Long-Term Ombudsman Program.* Washington, D.C.: U.S. Department of Health and Human Services, 2006.

oncologist See CANCER.

ophthalmologist See BLINDNESS; CATARACTS; EYE DISEASES, SERIOUS.

oral cancer According to the American Cancer Society, there were 34,360 new cases of cancer in the oral cavity and pharynx (throat) in 2007, including 24,180 men and 10,180 women. An estimated 7,550 people died of oral cancer in 2007, including 5,180 men and 2,370 women. Most oral cancers start in the tongue or the floor of the mouth.

Symptoms and Diagnostic Path

Some symptoms of oral cancer include

- patches inside the mouth or on the lips that are white, a mixture of red and white, or red (white patches are the most common, but mixed red and white or red patches are more likely to become malignant)
- a sore on the lip or mouth that does not heal
- bleeding in the mouth
- loose teeth
- pain or difficulty with swallowing
- difficulty wearing dentures
- a lump in the neck
- an earache

Note that these symptoms can be found in people who do not have cancer, but individuals with these symptoms should see their physicians.

The dentist may be the first person to notice the symptoms of oral cancer, or the physician may notice them. The dentist or doctor will also move the tongue to check its sides and underneath the tongue. The floor of the mouth will also be checked. If an abnormality is found, a small tissue sample can be biopsied, often under local anesthesia.

Oral cancer will be staged to determine its extent. The doctor may use an endoscope to check the throat, windpipe, and lungs. This procedure is done under local anesthesia and sometimes under general anesthesia.

Dental X-rays of the entire mouth can show if the cancer has spread to the jaw. Chest X-rays can show whether the cancer has spread to the chest and lungs. Other tests such as CT scans or MRI scans will provide information about whether oral cancer has spread.

Treatment Options and Outlook

Treatment for oral cancer may include surgery and/or radiation therapy. Surgery is a common treatment for oral cancer. If surgery is considered, the patient should ask the surgeon the following questions:

- What kind of operation do you recommend for me?

- Do I need any lymph nodes removed? Why?

- How will I feel after the operation? How long will I be in the hospital?

- What are the risks of surgery?

- Will I have trouble speaking, swallowing, or eating?

- Where will the scars be? What will they look like?

- Will I have any long-term effects?

- Will I look different?

- Will I need reconstructive or plastic surgery? When can that be done?

- Will I lose my teeth? Can they be replaced? How soon?

- Will I need to see a specialist for help with my speech?

- When can I get back to my normal activities?

- How often will I need checkups?

- Would a clinical trial be appropriate for me?

Radiation therapy may be used for patients who cannot have surgery or to treat small tumors. It may also be used before surgery to shrink the tumor or after the surgery to kill any remain-ing cancer cells. For oral cancer, patients may be treated with external radiation from a machine or internal radiation from an implanted pellet. The internal radiation is performed in the hospital, and the pellets are removed before the patient goes home after a few days. Some patients have both types of radiation therapy.

Radiation therapy for oral cancer may cause serious tooth decay problems, and the dentist may suggest using a fluoride gel toothpaste. It may also cause sore or bleeding gums, so flossing should be done gently. Sometimes radiation therapy also causes infections due to dry mouth and damage caused to the lining of the mouth. Sores or other changes should be reported to the nurse or doctor.

Radiation therapy may also cause denture problems, jaw stiffness, changes in the voice, and changes in the sense of food and smell. It may also affect the thyroid gland.

Before receiving radiation therapy for oral cancer, patients should ask the doctor the following questions:

- Which type of radiation therapy do you recommend for me? Why do I need this treatment?

- When will the treatments begin? When will they end?

- Should I see my dentist before I start treatment? If I need dental treatment, how much time does my mouth need to heal before radiation therapy starts?

- What are the risk and side effects of this treatment? What can I do about them?

- How will I feel during therapy?

- What will my mouth and face look like afterward?

- Are there any long-term effects?

- Can I continue my normal activities?

- Will I need a special diet? For how long?

- How often will I need checkups?

- Would a clinical trial be appropriate for me?

Chemotherapy treatment by injection may also be given, usually at the doctor's office or in an outpatient area of the hospital. Chemotherapy may cause similar side effects to radiation therapy and may also cause pain that feels like a toothache. It may also cause hair loss, poor appetite, nausea and vomiting, mouth and lip sores, and diarrhea.

During treatment, sharp or crunchy foods like tortilla chips should be avoided, as well as foods high in citrus fruits or that are hot or spicy. Alcohol should also be avoided. Since the teeth are already at risk for cavities from treatment, sugary foods should be limited.

Risk Factors and Preventive Measures

Smoking is a risk factor for oral cancer. Alcohol is another risk factor, and people who smoke and drink have an elevated risk for developing this form of cancer. Excessive sun exposure can also lead to oral cancer.

Individuals who have had cancer in the head or neck are at risk for oral cancer, and smoking increases the risk.

See also CANCER.

osteoarthritis The most common form of ARTHRITIS. Osteoarthritis is a degenerative disease of the joints of the body that causes joint pain and reduces motion, and it is particularly common among older people, who are the most likely age group to suffer from this disease. It is also the most common cause of the eventual need for JOINT REPLACEMENTS. Osteoarthritis most frequently occurs in the spine, hands, knees, and hips, although any joint can be affected.

Osteoarthritis has various causes, although often the cause cannot be determined and the primary goal of the doctor is to treat the symptoms of the disease. Osteoarthritis cannot be cured, but its symptoms (particularly pain and stiffness) can be treated. Some causes of osteoarthritis are joint injuries, a genetic defect in the joint cartilage, obesity, joints that are improperly formed, stresses on the joints from sports and some occupations, and aging.

Symptoms and Diagnostic Path

In the initial stages of osteoarthritis, there may be no symptoms. Later, the individual may experience pain and swelling, and degenerative changes are noted in X-rays of the bones. After many years, physicians may visually note arthritic changes in the individual's fingers and toes without needing an X-ray.

Some warning signs of osteoarthritis are

- swelling or tenderness around one or more joints
- the sound of bone rubbing against bone or a crunching feeling as the person moves about
- the feeling of stiffness in a joint after sitting for a long time or when getting out of bed in the morning

Physicians diagnose osteoarthritis based on the patient's medical history and a physical examination as well as with tests (such as X-rays and laboratory tests) that rule out other arthritic diseases, such as RHEUMATOID ARTHRITIS and GOUT.

Treatment Options and Outlook

Medications and exercise are the mainstay treatments for osteoarthritis. Patients with osteoarthritis may be treated with over-the-counter or prescribed nonsteroidal anti-inflammatory drugs (NSAIDs). Unfortunately, these drugs can cause gastrointestinal upset in some patients and may also lead to gastric ULCERS in others. Some patients find temporary relief with prescribed transdermal patches of lidocaine (Lidoderm).

Doctors also strongly encourage overweight or obese patients with osteoarthritis to lose weight, which will, in turn, usually decrease the individual's pain from osteoarthritis because of decreased stress on the bones. Regular exercise may help loosen up the joints as well. Some patients will also improve with physical therapy.

The application of heating pads or ice may reduce the painful inflammation that may be present with osteoarthritis. Sometimes massage therapy will also help. Some patients report temporary relief with acupuncture. In some cases, patients will need surgery to treat their arthritis, as with joint replacements.

Risk Factors and Preventive Measures

Osteoarthritis commonly occurs among related family members. Although osteoarthritis cannot be prevented altogether, keeping one's weight at a normal level and exercising regularly can limit the damage that is caused by osteoarthritis. Individuals who smoke should stop smoking, because smoking worsens the pain and stiffness.

See also CHRONIC PAIN; GENDER DIFFERENCES; PAINKILLING MEDICATIONS; NARCOTICS.

osteoporosis The progressive loss of bone strength, which results in an increased risk of serious FRACTURES, even from relatively minor FALLS. Osteoporosis more commonly presents in the elderly rather than in younger people. An endocrinologist is often the physician that diagnoses and treats calcium disorders such as osteoporosis. An endocrinologist is a medical doctor who specializes in treating diseases and major medical problems involving the endocrine glands. When the osteoporosis affects the bones of the spinal column, neurologists or neorosurgeons may be the first ones to diagnose this condition.

According to the National Institute of Arthritis and Musculoskeletal and Skin Diseases (NIAMS), about 10 million people older than age 50 in the United States have osteoporosis. In addition, another 34 million people in the United States have a condition of below-normal bone mass that does not reach the diagnostic level of osteoporosis. This condition is called osteopenia (low bone mass), and these individuals are at risk for the later development of osteoporosis.

The 1.5 million bone fractures that occur to people with osteoporosis each year lead to more than a half million HOSPITALIZATIONS. In addition, about 180,000 people eventually enter NURSING HOMES as a result of osteoporotic fractures.

About 80 percent of all people with osteoporosis are women, but an estimated 2 million men in the United States also have osteoporosis. The risk of developing osteoporosis increases with aging for males and females.

For most older women the reduced production of estrogen is responsible for the development of osteoporosis. Osteoporosis may also be caused by some medications, such as anticlotting medications, anticonvulsants, chemotherapy drugs for cancer, glucocorticoids (anti-inflammatory medications that are used to treat RHEUMATOID ARTHRITIS

and other diseases), lithium (used to treat bipolar disorder, a psychiatric disease), as well as by methotrexate (a drug to treat rheumatoid arthritis), thyroxine, and other medications. Kidney disease may also cause osteoporosis.

Studies published in 2007 in the *Archives of Internal Medicine* indicated that older depressed people taking ANTIDEPRESSANTS in the selective serotonin reuptake inhibitor (SSRI) class may be at risk for decreased bone density, especially in the hip. In contrast, individuals taking tricyclic antidepressants did not show decreased bone density. The 2,722 women who were studied had an average age of 78.5 years.

According to the authors, "One potential explanation for our findings is that SSRI use may have a direct deleterious effect on bone. This theory is supported by findings of in vitro and in vivo laboratory investigations."

Symptoms and Diagnostic Path

Generally a "silent disease," most people with osteoporosis experience no symptoms until they fall and fracture a bone or when one or more vertebrae in the spine collapse. Collapsed vertebrae cause a loss of height as well as BACK PAIN and spinal malformations. Even very minor falls can fracture osteoporotic bones.

Physicians may diagnose osteoporosis in a routine physical examination, based on a physical examination; for example, a decrease in height is an indictor of osteoporosis. A bone density test may be ordered to confirm osteoporosis. The physician will ask the patient about health habits, such as SMOKING and consuming alcohol, which are both risk factors for the development of osteoporosis. If the patient also has back pain in addition to osteoporosis, the doctor may request an X-ray of the spine to check for any fractures or malformations. Laboratory tests may reveal a deficiency in vitamin D, which is another potential indicator of osteoporosis.

The most common bone density test is the dual-energy X-ray absorptiometry (DEXA) scan. This scanner can measure bone density of the entire skeleton, although generally measurements taken at the spine and hip are the most reliable means to predict the future risk of fractures as well as to diagnose osteoporosis. The DEXA scan can also tell the physician what the risk of fractures is, as well as whether bone density is normal or not.

Treatment Options and Outlook

When the underlying cause of the osteoporosis can be treated, that approach is taken; for example, if the patient is taking a medication that is causing the osteoporosis (such as glucocorticoids to treat asthma and arthritis or antiseizure drugs), the dosage may be reduced or the patient may be given a different medication. If the patient consumes alcohol or smokes, he or she is urged to abstain from these substances to delay the progression of the osteoporosis.

When the primary risk factor is something that cannot be changed, such as age or race, then the physician concentrates on treating the existing condition, recommending the patient work on factors that can be changed (such as diet and nutrition and exercise) and seeking to delay any further degeneration.

Many patients with osteoporosis have a diet that is deficient in calcium, and they should increase their consumption of low-fat dairy products high in calcium as well as their consumption of calcium-rich greens such as broccoli and calcium-fortified foods including cereal, bread, and orange juice. However, the daily calcium intake should not exceed 2,500 milligrams, because an excessive dose of calcium could lead to the development of kidney stones.

According to the National Institute of Arthritis and Musculoskeletal and Skin Diseases, individuals older than age 70 need 1,200 milligrams of calcium per day.

Patients who are deficient in vitamin D can obtain this nutrient by spending 15 minutes in the sun each day as well as by eating foods that are high in vitamin D such as fish oils and foods fortified with vitamin D, including milk and cereals. Some individuals will need to take supplemental vitamin D, although they should consult with their physician first to ensure that they do not take an excessive dose of vitamin D. According to the U.S. Surgeon General, individuals over age 70 need 600 international units (IUs) of vitamin D per day, in contrast to the 400 IUs needed by those who are ages 51 to 70.

Walking, dancing, and gardening are often recommended exercises (although the physician should be consulted first) for patients with osteoporosis, as is playing tennis.

Many patients with osteoporosis take prescribed medications to treat their osteoporosis. These drugs can reduce the risk for further bone loss. The primary drugs that are used by postmenopausal women for this purpose as of this writing are alendronate (Fosamax), raloxifene (Evista), risedronate (Actonel), and ibandronate (Boniva).

In addition, teriparatide (Forteo), an injectable drug of parathyroid hormone, is used in both postmenopausal women and in men who are at high risk for fractures from their osteoporosis. Alendronate and risedronate are also used to treat osteoporosis in men as well as in men and women who have developed osteoporosis as a result of taking glucocorticoid medications.

Calcitonin may be used to treat women who are at least five years beyond the onset of menopause. It is available as either a subdermal injection or as a daily nasal spray. Some people have an allergic reaction to the injection, whereas the nasal spray generally only causes a runny nose at worst.

Hormone therapy is another treatment option for postmenopausal women with osteoporosis, including estrogen therapy or combined estrogen and progestin. Estrogen alone is a therapy that is usually limited to women who have had a hysterectomy. If hormone therapy is used, the U.S. Food and Drug Administration (FDA) recommends that hormone therapy be given at the lowest dose and for the shortest period possible.

Risk Factors and Preventive Measures

Osteoporosis is most common in non-Hispanic white women and Asian women. Among men with osteoporosis, the risk is highest among non-Hispanic white men and Asian men. Slender women have a greater risk than women of other body sizes. Women with a family history of osteoporosis have an increased risk for the disease. Women who have had anorexia nervosa, an eating disorder in which a person starves herself in order to achieve an ideal of thinness, have an increased risk for osteoporosis.

SUBSTANCE ABUSE AND DEPENDENCE, particularly alcoholism, is another risk factor for osteoporosis, as is smoking. In addition, prolonged periods of inactivity, such as extensive bed rest, increases the risk for osteoporosis.

Other factors increase the risk of osteoporosis-related fractures, such as falls that are caused by poor balance, uncorrected or bad eyesight, and decreased muscle strength. Sedating drugs increase the risk for falls, as do some elements that are found in the environment, such as throw rugs in the house or icy sidewalks and front stairs outside. Some medical conditions also increase the risk for fractures with osteoporosis, such as chronic lung disease, hyperthyroidism, hyperparathyroidism, vitamin D deficiency, kidney disease, Cushing's disease, and chronic lung disease.

Recommended Steps to Avoid Falls Outdoors and Indoors

The NIAMS recommends that people with osteoporosis take the following steps to decrease the risk for falls:

- Wear rubber-soled shoes when outdoors.
- When sidewalks are slippery, walk on the grass.
- Use a cane or walker or even a walking stick.
- In the winter put salt or kitty litter on icy sidewalks to reduce the risk of slipping and falling.
- Wear low-heeled shoes.
- If glasses are normally worn, wear them when going to the bathroom to avoid tripping over unseen or blurred objects.
- Keep rooms free of clutter, especially on floors.

- Use plastic or carpet runners on slippery floors.
- Avoid walking around the house in socks, which may be slippery on some surfaces, such as the kitchen floor. Instead, wear nonskid shoes or slippers.
- Make sure the stairs are well lit and there are railings on both sides of the stairs.
- Put grab bars on the bathroom walls near the toilet, shower, and tub.
- Use a rubber mat in the tub or shower.
- Use a cordless phone to avoid rushing to answer the phone or keep a cell phone nearby.
- Increase the number of lights, if needed, to improve lighting.

See also ACCIDENTAL INJURIES; ARTHRITIS; DEPRESSION; GENDER DIFFERENCES; OSTEOARTHRITIS; VITAMIN AND MINERAL DEFICIENCIES/EXCESSES.

Diem, Susan J., M.D., et al. "Use of Antidepressants and Rates of Hip Bone Loss in Older Women: The Study of Osteoporotic Fractures." *Archives of Internal Medicine* 167 (June 25, 2007): 1,240–1,245.

Office of the Surgeon General. *Bone Health and Osteoporosis: A Report of the Surgeon General. Executive Summary.* Rockville, Md.: U.S. Department of Health and Human Services, 2004.

Stone, Lorraine M., and Kenneth W. Lyles. "Osteoporosis in Later Life." *Generations* 30, no. 3 (Fall 2006): 65–70.

otolaryngologist   See HEARING DISORDERS.

PACE (Programs of All-Inclusive Care for the Elderly) See MEDICARE.

painkilling medications Drugs that stop or diminish minor, moderate, and severe pain. Both over-the-counter (OTC) drugs or prescribed drugs can relieve pain, depending on its level of severity. The most commonly known OTC drugs are aspirin and acetaminophen (Tylenol). Naproxen (Aleve) is also an OTC medication, as is ibuprofen (Advil). There are also many types of prescribed painkilling medications, including oral drugs that include NARCOTICS, such as hydrocodone or oxycodone, or injected drugs such as meperidine (Demerol). Some drugs combine codeine with acetaminophen, such as Tylenol with codeine. It is important to note that some drugs are not recommended for older people, such as meperidine, because of its effect on aging bodies. (See INAPPROPRIATE PRESCRIPTIONS FOR THE ELDERLY.)

For some individuals, their pain from CANCER, chronic BACK PAIN, or other serious diseases is so severe that they are administered morphine and other injectable narcotics. In addition, some individuals with chronic severe pain rely on an implantable morphine pump that provides a steady delivery of morphine.

In some cases, individuals with CHRONIC PAIN develop a tolerance to narcotics, needing higher dosages of the drug to obtain the same level of pain relief; however, contrary to popular belief (including the belief of some physicians), a tolerance to a drug alone is not sufficient to constitute addiction. Instead, the addicted person also experiences negative consequences in his or her work and family life, such as spending much of the time thinking about, procuring, or using illegal drugs. Addiction

is often defined as the chemical and psychological craving for a drug.

Note that if the person in severe pain is receiving an adequate dosage of the drug to combat pain, his or her life usually is not fixated on drugs. (See PRESCRIPTION DRUG ABUSE/MISUSE.) However, in many cases, older people are undertreated for their pain, and when they ask the doctor for more medication or higher dosages of the medication, this behavior is sometimes mistaken for drug dependency or addiction.

See also ARTHRITIS; CHRONIC PAIN; DIABETES; DRUG ABUSE; HEALTH-CARE AGENT/PROXY; HOSPICE; PALLIATIVE CARE; SUBSTANCE ABUSE AND DEPENDENCE.

palliative care A term that refers to care that is provided to the chronically and severely ill older person that focuses primarily on relieving pain and treating distressing symptoms, such as nausea, weakness, and fatigue as well as emotional symptoms. Many people who receive palliative care, although not all of them, are terminally ill, and, consequently, they are not expected to recover. Palliative care is meant to improve the patient's quality of life and, in contrast to other forms of medicine, does not concentrate on curing the illness.

Sometimes the patient's psychological issues are overwhelming when they are severely ill. For example, according to Doctors Morrison and Meier in their article on palliative care for the *New England Journal of Medicine* in 2004, if the patient has anxiety, as indicated by restlessness, insomnia, excessive worry and agitation, the doctor may recommend counseling and may also prescribe BENZODIAZEPINES with shorter half-lives. (Benzodiazepines with long half-lives are not recommended for the elderly.) A "half-life" refers to the time that it takes for the drug to degrade and ultimately disappear from the system; those drugs with shorter half-lives leave the body faster.

If the patient has severe CONSTIPATION, the doctor determines if the patient is taking NARCOTICS (which often cause constipation) and also analyzes whether the patient may have a fecal impaction (stools that are stuck in the colon) and then treats the problem.

Palliative care also often includes emotional and spiritual support to the ill person, as needed. HOSPICE care is one form of palliative care. Note that although providers of palliative care do not provide any lifesaving measures, neither do they seek to hasten or delay the person's death. Family members are also often provided with emotional support by a facility offering palliative care.

An estimated 1,240 hospitals offered palliative care programs in 2005, and the American Board of Medical Specialties recognized palliative and hospice care as a medical subspecialty in 2006.

See also CARDIOPULMONARY RESUSCITATION; CHRONIC PAIN; DEATH; DEATH, FEAR OF; END-OF-LIFE ISSUES; HEALTH-CARE AGENT/PROXY; HEART FAILURE; LIVING WILL; TALKING TO ELDERLY PARENTS ABOUT DIFFICULT ISSUES.

Boockvar, Kenneth S., M.D., and Diane E. Meier, M.D. "Palliative Care for Frail Older Adults." *Journal of the American Medical Association* 296 (November 8, 2006): 2,245–2,253.

Kuehn, Bridget M. "Hospitals Embrace Palliative Care." *Journal of the American Medical Association* 298, no. 11 (September 19, 2007): 1,263–1,265.

Morrison, R. Sean, M.D., and Diane E. Meier, M.D. "Palliative Care." *New England Journal of Medicine* 350, no. 25 (June 17, 2004): 2,582–2,590.

Rabow, Michael W., M.D., et al. "The Comprehensive Care Team: A Controlled Trial of Outpatient Palliative Medicine Consultation." *Archives of Internal Medicine* 164 (January 12, 2004): 83–91.

Von Gunten, Charles F., M.D. "Secondary and Tertiary Palliative Care in U.S. Hospitals." *Journal of the American Medical Association* 287, no. 7 (February 20, 2002): 875–881.

pancreatic cancer According to the American Cancer Society, an estimated 18,830 men and 18,340 women were diagnosed with pancreatic cancer in 2007. The lifetime risk of developing pancreatic cancer is about 1.27 percent for both men and women. An estimated 16,840 men and 16,530 women died of pancreatic cancer in 2007. This form of cancer is the fourth leading cause of cancer death. The risk for pancreatic cancer increases with age.

Symptoms and Diagnostic Path

Jaundice (yellowing in the skin and eyes) is a classic sign of pancreatic cancer, occurring in at least 50 percent of patients. The jaundice is caused by a blocked bile duct. An earlier sign may be darkening of the urine or lighter colored stools. A buildup of bilirubin (a substance composed in the liver) can cause itching of the skin. There are other causes of jaundice, such as liver disease, HEPATITIS, and gallstones, which are all far more common disorders than pancreatic cancer.

Another symptom may be abdominal pain or back pain, which may indicate advanced pancreatic cancer. Unintended weight loss and a poor appetite are other symptoms. Another indicator is the inability to digest fat, causing the stools to be greasy and float in the toilet.

Pancreatic cancer is diagnosed by a medical examination and study of the white part of the eyes and skin to see if jaundice is present. Imaging tests, such as computerized tomography (CT) scans, may also be performed to both diagnose and stage (see how advanced) the cancer. If a biopsy is taken, CT scans can be used to insert a biopsy needle to the right area. Other tests that may help diagnose pancreatic cancer are ultrasound, magnetic resonance imaging (MRI), or positron emission tomography (PET) scans. A gastroenterologist is a physician specialist who treats pancreatic cancer and other digestive diseases.

In addition, an endoscopic retrograde cholangiopancreatography (ERCP) may be performed to insert a tube through the esophagus and stomach and into the bile duct that connects to the small intestine. This can show a blockage of the bile duct or pancreatic duct.

Treatment Options and Outlook

Treatment options for pancreatic cancer include surgery, radiation, and chemotherapy. The prognosis is often poor because pancreatic cancer is often diagnosed when it is advanced. As a result, the overall survival rate is about 4 percent. It is often "silent" in the early stages and is not clinically detectable.

Risk Factors and Preventive Measures

About 90 percent of all patients with pancreatic cancer are 55 years or older, and more than 70 percent are age 65 or older, according to the American Cancer Society. At the time of diagnosis, the average patient is 72 years old. Men are only slightly more likely to develop pancreatic cancer than women.

African Americans are more likely to develop pancreatic cancer than whites, although the reasons for this are unknown. It may be due to higher rates of smoking and diabetes in black males; smokers have a two to three times higher risk of developing pancreatic cancer than nonsmokers. Very obese people have an increased risk for pancreatic cancer, as do those who rarely exercise. People with diabetes have an increased rate of pancreatic cancer, as do people with chronic pancreatitis (a long-term inflammation of the pancreas). Some pancreatitis appears to be hereditary, and individuals with inherited pancreatitis have an elevated risk of developing pancreatic cancer (from 40 to 75 percent).

An estimated 10 percent of the cases of pancreatic cancer seem to be related to genetic mutations.

See also CANCER.

panic disorder See ANXIETY AND ANXIETY DISORDERS.

Parkinson's disease A degenerative disease of the nervous system, first described by British physician James Parkinson in 1817, which he personally referred to as the "shaking palsy."

The primary symptom of Parkinson's disease is severe tremor, as well as rigidity of the muscles and slowed movements (*bradykinesia*). In addition, people with Parkinson's disease often have impaired coordination and balance, and many have uncontrolled movements. Some people with Parkinson's will eventually develop DEMENTIA.

About 50,000 people in the United States are diagnosed with Parkinson's disease each year, according to the National Institutes of Health, and it is estimated that there are about a half million people with the disease in the United States.

Symptoms and Diagnostic Path

Early symptoms of Parkinson's disease may include a lack of facial expression (a "masked face") and the inability to move the arms and legs normally. The person may seem very stiff and slow.

As the disease worsens, the tremors and the shaking start to interfere with the individual's everyday activities. People with Parkinson's disease may have difficulty holding items steadily, such as the utensils needed to feed themselves. In addition, those with Parkinson's disease often develop a certain type of gait, which is characterized by leaning forward accompanied by small, quick steps. They often stop swinging their arms when they walk and may have trouble initiating movement. They may freeze up suddenly as they walk, temporarily unable to move further.

Many people with Parkinson's disease suffer from severe emotional changes as well as DEPRESSION. They may develop slurred speech and have difficulty making themselves understood to others. They often have a low volume of speech (hypophoria), which contributes to their difficulty with communication with others.

Some patients with Parkinson's disease develop problems with their bowels and bladder. They may have a problem with CONSTIPATION because of a general slowing down of the digestive tract.

Patients with Parkinson's may also develop chronic pain because of aching muscles and joints. Severe fatigue is another common symptom.

There are no laboratory tests to diagnose Parkinson's disease, and the disease is diagnosed based on symptoms and a neurological examination. Sometimes early signs may be dismissed as normal aging, and the disease is not diagnosed until the symptoms become pronounced.

Treatment Options and Outlook

Parkinson's disease is a degenerative disease that worsens over time, and as of this writing, there is no cure. However, medications can help, such as levodopa. However, there are many side effects with levodopa such as nausea, vomiting, and low blood pressure. The long-term use of levodopa can lead to such severe side effects as HALLUCINATIONS and even psychosis. In addition, twisting and writhing movements known as dyskinesia develop in individuals who take large doses of levodopa over time.

Anticholinergic drugs, including drugs such as trihexyphenidyl, benztropine, and ethopropazine, can help reduce the stiffness and rigidity of Parkinson's disease. Dopamine agonists, another category of medication, can mimic the action of dopamine in the brain. Medications in the category of MAO-B inhibitors cause dopamine to accumulate and reduce the symptoms of Parkinson's disease.

Catechol-O-methyltransferase (COMT) inhibitors are used to break down dopamine, and two drugs, entacapone and tolcapone, are approved in the United States.

Deep brain stimulation is a treatment option. This procedure involves electrical stimulation of specific brain tissue through implanted electrodes.

In some cases, surgery is used to treat Parkinson's disease, including the pallidotomy and thalamotomy. These surgeries destroy the parts of the brain that worsen symptoms.

Risk Factors and Preventive Measures

Women are about 50 percent more likely than men to develop Parkinson's disease, although the reason for this is unknown. Age is another risk factor, and the average age of onset of the disease is 60 years. However, some individuals have an early onset of Parkinson's disease that can occur before the age of 50 years.

There appears to be a genetic risk factor, and individuals with one or more relatives with Parkinson's disease have an increased, but still small, risk of developing the disease.

Parkinson's disease cannot be prevented, but when it is identified, it should be treated aggressively.

See also AMERICANS WITH DISABILITIES ACT; DEMENTIA; FAMILY AND MEDICAL LEAVE ACT; GENDER DIFFERENCES; HEALTH-CARE AGENT/PROXY; MANIA.

periodic limb movement disorder Similar to restless legs syndrome, periodic limb movement disorder (PLMD) causes people to jerk their legs every 20 to 40 seconds while asleep.

Symptoms and Diagnostic Path

Most people jerk slightly when first falling asleep, but periodic movement disorder occurs throughout sleep. This can cause a loss of sleep and result in fatigue.

Treatment Options and Outlook

Some medications can help improve PLMD, such as clonazepam (Klonopin), gabapentin (Neurontin), baclofen (Lioresal), or tiagabine (Gabitril), according to Dr. Anderson in his online article in eMedicine. If PLMD is caused by a medical problem that is resolved, the symptoms should also improve.

Risk Factors and Preventive Measures

The risk for PLMD increases with age. Other risk factors are the presence of sleep apnea, withdrawal from benzodiazepines or barbiturates, anemia, diabetes, and an iron deficiency. Exercise and medication, as well as warm baths, can help improve this disorder.

See also SLEEP DISORDERS.

Anderson, Wayne E., Dr. "Periodic Limb Movement Disorder." eMedicine. March 30, 2007. Available online. URL: http://www.emedicine.com/neuro/topic523.htm. Accessed February 26, 2008.

personal emergency device Special equipment that the older person can press, manipulate, or activate in some way to remotely notify others (such as emergency medical personnel) that the individual is in danger or is hurt and requires assistance. Such a device can be very helpful for older or disabled people who are at risk of physical harm from FALLS or from HEART ATTACKS or STROKES. In many cases, ASSISTED-LIVING FACILITIES provide personal emergency devices to their residents and often insist that they wear their devices at all times.

The personal emergency device is usually small, lightweight, and portable and should be kept in a place that is nearby and accessible to the older person. It may be a wearable device, such as a necklace. When activated, the personal emergency device informs a previously determined service that the individual is in trouble and the service notifies emergency services.

Anyone who is considering using a personal emergency device should find out the following information:

- How is the device used?
- Who will be contacted if the device is activated?
- What is the cost for the device?
- Is there a monthly fee or are there other fees for the service?
- If the device is accidentally set off, will there be an additional charge?

See also ACCIDENTAL INJURIES; ASSISTIVE DEVICES/ ASSISTED TECHNOLOGY.

pets   Animals that live with a family and that are often regarded with great affection, as compared to animals that are raised for food by farmers or that are used for other specific noncompanionship purposes. Some studies have shown that pet owners are healthier than non–pet owners and may have lower blood pressure. In addition, when individuals focus on caring for their pets, they often spend less time paying attention to their "aches and pains" and ultimately have an improved sense of well-being.

In one study, reported in a 1996 issue of the *Journal of Nutrition for the Elderly,* on seniors ages 60 and older, researchers found that the pet owners had lower triglyceride levels and that dog owners walked significantly more than nonowners.

People of all ages receive love from and give love to their pets. For the older person who may feel isolated and alone, pets can particularly provide companionship and meaning. The pet may also be a link to a beloved spouse or partner who has died, because they both enjoyed interacting with the pet together years ago. Some (but very few) nursing homes bring in animals, such as cats and dogs, for residents to befriend, and in a few nursing homes, pets live there permanently. If the older person

cannot bring a pet to the nursing home, experts say that it can help the older person to be allowed to talk about their grief over the loss of a pet.

It can be very difficult for older persons when their pets die or when they must give up their pets to move into a nursing home or other place where pets are not allowed. Pets provide unquestioning love and affection, and older people benefit from the tactile experience of petting their animals. Studies have shown that blood pressure actually drops when pet owners pet their animals.

Some older people will delay or refuse to have surgery because they cannot find someone to care for their pets. When older people who are not cognitively impaired say that they will not have needed surgery, or when they refuse to move to a nursing home despite their serious medical needs, family members and others should inquire if they are worried about what would happen to the pets and if that is the reason for refusing needed medical treatment.

Of older people who are concerned about their pet, Christine Adamec states in *When Your Pet Dies,* "It's also a good idea to have the person carry a card with the name of their pets and instructions on who should be called in the event the elderly person becomes ill or some emergency occurs. The possession of this card alone could give peace of mind to an elderly person and make him or her more willing to seek out needed medical attention."

For further information about the importance of pets, contact:

Delta Society, the Human-Animal Connection
289 Perimeter Road East
Renton, WA 98055
(425) 226-7357

Adamec, Christine. *When Your Pet Dies: Dealing with Your Grief and Helping Your Children Cope.* Lincoln, Neb.: iUniverse.com, 2000.
Dembicki, Diane, Ph.D., and Jennifer Anderson, Ph.D., R.D. "Pet Ownership May Be a Factor in Improved Health of the Elderly." *Journal of Nutrition for the Elderly* 15, no. 3 (1996): 15–31.

physician-assisted suicide   See ASSISTED SUICIDE.

Pick's disease Also known as frontotemporal dementia, Pick's disease is a syndrome that is associated with the shrinking of the frontal and temporal anterior lobes of the brain.

Symptoms and Diagnostic Path

This form of dementia usually presents before age 75. The syndrome generally causes either changes in behavior or difficulties with language. When the behavior is affected, the person becomes either very impulsive or very listless. There may be a marked interest in sex and the appearance of inappropriate sexual behavior as well as a decreased interest in personal hygiene. An excessive and inappropriate use of profanity may occur. Family members may be embarrassed or appalled at the seemingly inexplicable changes of behavior in their relative.

The person may also exhibit compulsive and repetitive behavior. With the form of Pick's disease that affects language, the person has difficulty understanding the speech of others as well as in speaking, although the memory remains intact.

Treatment Options and Outlook

There is no cure for Pick's disease, although behavior modification may help to control the undesirable behavior. If the person becomes aggressive or agitated, medications may also help to control these behaviors. In addition, antidepressants may also improve some of the symptoms.

The prognosis for Pick's disease is poor, and the disease generally progresses over about two to 10 years. At some point, the individual will require 24-hour supervision.

See also AGGRESSION, PHYSICAL; COGNITIVE IMPAIR-MENT; CONFUSION; DELUSIONS; DEMENTIA; END-OF-LIFE ISSUES; HALLUCINATIONS; HEALTH-CARE AGENT/PROXY; IRRITABILITY; MEMORY IMPAIRMENT.

pneumonia A very serious type of respiratory virus that may be life-threatening to elderly individuals. Pneumonia is also known as pneumococcal disease and refers to infection with *Streptococcus pneumoniae*. Louis Pasteur first isolated the pneumococcus virus in 1881 from the saliva of a patient with rabies. For various reasons, however, vac-cines against pneumonia were not developed until 1911. When the antibiotic penicillin first came into general use in the 1940s, most physicians lost interest in the pneumonia vaccine until it was realized that patients were still dying of pneumonia, despite the existence of a powerful antibiotic. As a result, efforts were relaunched to create a pneumonia vaccine, and in 1977, the first pneumonia vaccine was licensed in the United States.

It is estimated that about 175,000 hospitalizations occur each year as a result of infection with pneumonia. It is also a common complication of infection with influenza. Another complication is pneumococcal meningitis, which can cause death in up to 80 percent of infected individuals age 65 and older.

All elderly individuals should receive the pneumococcal immunization, which is a single lifetime dose rather than an annual shot; however, those who were younger than age 65 when they received the pneumonia vaccine may need a second dose when they are older than age 65, depending on their physician's recommendation.

According to the Centers for Disease Control and Prevention (CDC), compliance in obtaining the immunization among older people varies considerably from state to state in the United States. The rate of receiving the annual pneumonia vaccine ranges from a low of about 52 percent of elderly individuals in the District of Columbia to a high of about 72 percent in North Dakota. (See Table 1.) The federal goal in the United States is to have 90 percent of older people immunized against pneumonia. (It is not realistic to seek a goal of 100 percent.)

According to the National Center for Health Statistics, whether older individuals are immunized depends partly on race, and older whites in the United States are nearly twice as likely to receive a pneumonia vaccine than are Hispanics or blacks. In 2004, for example, about 61 percent of whites age 65 and older received the vaccine for pneumonia compared with 39 percent of blacks and 34 percent of Hispanics/Latinos.

Symptoms and Diagnostic Path

Most people who contract the pneumonia virus have a sudden onset of fever and chills. They may

TABLE 1. PERCENTAGE OF ADULTS AGE 65 AND OLDER WHO REPORTED EVER RECEIVING PNEUMONIA VACCINE

State/Area	2004	2005
Alabama	60.1	61.9
Alaska	57.2	61.2
Arizona	68.6	65.4
Arkansas	62.0	57.4
California	63.6	61.3
Colorado	70.1	70.2
Connecticut	67.8	69.3
Delaware	66.3	65.9
District of Columbia	51.4	51.6
Florida	64.3	62.4
Georgia	59.4	62.5
Hawaii	unknown	66.0
Idaho	60.1	61.6
Illinois	58.3	57.0
Indiana	62.1	65.3
Iowa	68.2	69.1
Kansas	62.5	66.8
Kentucky	57.7	62.9
Louisiana	67.4	71.4
Maine	65.6	64.4
Maryland	64.0	62.0
Massachusetts	65.3	64.8
Michigan	60.0	66.2
Minnesota	67.9	71.1
Mississippi	64.5	65.7
Missouri	67.1	64.8
Montana	71.6	69.9
Nebraska	65.7	68.0
Nevada	66.7	69.8
New Hampshire	66.8	69.8
New Jersey	64.3	64.0
New Mexico	64.7	64.7
New York	63.0	62.0
North Carolina	64.3	66.2
North Dakota	70.3	71.7
Ohio	61.1	61.5
Oklahoma	70.0	71.1
Oregon	69.4	71.4
Pennsylvania	63.9	67.2
Rhode Island	70.0	71.5
South Carolina	64.0	65.6
South Dakota	66.2	66.3
Tennessee	63.6	63.8
Texas	61.4	62.2
Utah	65.8	66.4
Vermont	65.7	66.7
Virginia	61.6	66.5
Washington	65.8	66.9
West Virginia	64.7	68.2
Wisconsin	70.3	65.7
Wyoming	70.7	71.2
Puerto Rico	32.7	28.3
U.S. Virgin Islands	32.8	29.1
Median, United States	64.6	65.7

Source: Adapted from Centers for Disease Control and Prevention, "Percentage of Adults Aged 65 Years and Older Who Reported Receiving Influenza Vaccine during the Preceding 12 Months and Percentage of Adults Aged 65 Years and Older Who Reported Ever Receiving Pneumococcal Vaccine, by State/Area, United States, Behavioral Risk Factor Surveillance System, 2004–2005." *Morbidity and Mortality Weekly Report* 55, no. 9 (October 6, 2006), Atlanta, Ga.: Centers for Disease Control and Prevention, p. 1,066.

also have chest pain, cough, rapid breathing, and extreme fatigue. Physicians diagnose the disease based on patient symptoms. HOSPITALIZATION may become necessary if the fever becomes high, the patient experiences any respiratory distress, or the presence of syndromes such as meningitis become apparent. The symptoms of meningitis are fever, confusion, sensitivity to light, and a stiff neck.

Treatment Options and Outlook

Once the individual is stricken with pneumonia, the symptoms (fever, coughing, muscle aches, and overall pain) must be treated until the disease runs its course. Older people who have been immunized for pneumonia but who contract the disease anyway have the best outlook and are much less likely to die. If an older person develops a high fever and/or any symptoms of meningitis, he or she needs to be hospitalized.

Risk Factors and Preventive Measures

The best prevention is to be immunized against both pneumonia and flu. Individuals in crowded conditions or in institutional living (such as NURS-ING HOMES) have a higher risk of contracting pneumonia and thus have an even more compelling reason to be immunized.

See also INFECTIONS; FLU/INFLUENZA.

Centers for Disease Control and Prevention. *Epidemiology and Prevention of Vaccine Preventable Diseases.* Tenth Ed. Washington, D.C.: National Institutes of Health, 2007, pp. 257–270.

———. "Percentage of Adults Aged 65 Years and Older Who Reported Receiving Influenza Vaccine during the Preceding 12 Months and Percentage of Adults Aged 65 Years and Older Who Reported Ever Receiving Pneumococcal Vaccine, by State/Area, United States, Behavioral Risk Factor Surveillance System, 2004–2005." *Morbidity and Mortality Weekly Report* 55, no. 9 (October 6, 2006), Atlanta, Ga.: Centers for Disease Control and Prevention.

polypharmacy The use of many medications, which is common among many older individuals because of their multiple medical needs. Polypharmacy can lead to MEDICATION INTERACTIONS, and the more medications that the individual takes, the greater the likelihood of such an interaction. For this reason, it is best for older people to obtain all their medications from the same pharmacy so that the pharmacist can watch for any possible interactions of medications. In addition, when elderly people visit their physicians, they should either bring a recent list of all their medications or (a better choice) they should bring the actual prescription bottles to show the doctor.

Many times people tell their doctor about prescribed drugs they take but they fail to mention any alternative remedies they are using. They may assume such drugs are inherently safe because they are "natural." This premise is a false one, and it is also why it is very important for older individuals to inform their physician of any supplements or herbs that they take. These remedies can sometimes cause a dangerous medication interaction. Warfarin (Coumadin), for example, is a blood-thinning drug, and when combined with vitamin E, it can cause dangerous internal bleeding and could even lead to death.

Some older people become confused by the many medications they have been prescribed, and, consequently, they may forget whether they took the drugs or not. Sometimes they may think they did not take medications and they take them again, receiving a dangerous double dosage. Weekly pill containers can help with this problem, and if the older person is unable to fill the containers, other people, such as family members or home-care workers, can assist with this task.

Some older individuals try to "help out" each other financially by sharing their prescribed medications or even giving others the drugs that they no longer need; this is an illegal act, and it is also an extremely dangerous one, because each person's health history is very different. Thus, a drug that may work well for one person could cause severe side effects and even harm to another individual.

See ADVERSE DRUG EVENT; INAPPROPRIATE PRESCRIPTIONS FOR THE ELDERLY; MEDICATION COMPLIANCE; PRESCRIPTION DRUG ABUSE/MISUSE; SUBSTANCE ABUSE AND DEPENDENCE.

post-traumatic stress disorder (PTSD) See ANXIETY AND ANXIETY DISORDERS.

poverty Very low income. Each year, the Department of Health and Human Services sets specific levels of income by family size, and individuals and families who earn below these levels are considered below the poverty level. The levels are set for each of the contiguous 48 states and the District of Columbia and also for Alaska and Hawaii. (The cost of living is considerably higher in Alaska and Hawaii than in the rest of the United States.)

For example, in 2007, a family of two living in the 48 states or the District of Columbia who had income of less than $13,690 was considered to be below the poverty level. If the family lived in Alaska, the poverty level for the same two-person family was below $17,120 and in Hawaii it was below $15,750. (See Table 1.)

In 2005, the median income for family households of all races headed by a person age 65 and older was $37,765. The median income varied by race and ethnicity; for example, households headed by older non-Hispanic Caucasians had a median income of $39,402. The median income of

TABLE 1. 2007 POVERTY LEVELS IN THE UNITED STATES

Persons in Family or Household	48 Contiguous States and D.C.	Alaska	Hawaii
1	$10,210	$12,770	$11,750
2	13,690	17,120	15,750
3	17,170	21,470	19,750
4	20,650	25,820	23,750
5	24,130	30,170	27,750
6	27,610	34,520	31,750
7	31,090	38,870	35,750
8	34,570	43,220	39,750
For each additional person add	3,480	4,350	4,000

Source: Department of Health and Human Services. *The 2007 HHS Poverty Guidelines.* Available online. URL: http//aspe.hhs.gov/poverty/07poverty.shtml. Accessed September 12, 2007.

TABLE 2. 2005 POVERTY LEVELS IN THE UNITED STATES

Persons in Family or Household	48 Contiguous States and D.C.	Alaska	Hawaii
1	$9,570	$11,950	$11,010
2	12,830	16,030	14,760
3	16,090	20,110	18,510
4	19,350	24,190	22,260
5	22,610	28,270	26,010
6	25,870	32,350	29,760
7	29,130	36,430	33,510
8	32,390	40,510	37,260
For each additional person add	3,260	4,080	3,750

Source: Department of Health and Human Services. *The 2005 HHS Poverty Guidelines.* Available online. URL: http//aspe.hhs.gov/poverty/05poverty.shtml. Accessed September 12, 2007.

Asians was higher, at $49,163. Among older African Americans, the median income was $27,270. For Hispanics, the median income was $26,681.

According to the Administration on Aging, about 3.6 million individuals in the United States age 65 and older (about 10 percent of all elderly people) lived in poverty in 2005, about the same number as in 2004. In 2005, about 7.9 percent of elderly whites were poor, as were 12.6 percent of older Asians, 19.9 percent of elderly Hispanics, and 23.2 percent of older African Americans.

In considering all states and the District of Columbia, 10.1 percent of the elderly lived below the poverty level in 2005. (See Table 2 for information on poverty levels in 2005, which were about $600 lower than in 2007.)

The percent of the elderly who live below the poverty level varies greatly from state to state; for example, according to the Administration on Aging, 17.6 percent of the elderly in the District of Columbia were below the poverty level in 2005, followed by 15.7 percent in Mississippi. The percentage living below the poverty rate was very high in Puerto Rico at 44.3 percent. The lowest levels of poverty (and, thus, the most well-off elderly individuals) lived in Utah, where the poverty level was 6.5 percent and Wisconsin (7.7 percent). See Table 3 for a state-by-state listing.

TABLE 3. PERCENTAGE OF INDIVIDUALS AGE 65 AND OLDER AT THE POVERTY LEVEL IN 2005

State/Area	Percent below Poverty Level
U.S. Total	10.1
Alabama	13.1
Alaska	9.1
Arizona	8.1
Arkansas	14.5
California	8.2
Colorado	8.6
Connecticut	7.5
Delaware	7.5
District of Columbia	17.6
Florida	10.3
Georgia	13.0
Hawaii	9.3
Idaho	8.7
Illinois	8.7
Indiana	8.0
Iowa	8.0
Kansas	7.9
Kentucky	13.5
Louisiana	15.6
Maine	11.0
Maryland	7.9
Massachusetts	10.0

(Table continues)

(Table continued)

State/Area	Percent below Poverty Level
Michigan	8.6
Minnesota	8.4
Mississippi	15.7
Missouri	9.1
Montana	9.1
Nebraska	8.7
Nevada	8.3
New Hampshire	6.9
New Jersey	8.7
New Mexico	12.5
New York	12.8
North Carolina	12.1
North Dakota	14.1
Ohio	8.4
Oklahoma	11.2
Oregon	7.9
Pennsylvania	9.0
Rhode Island	7.8
South Carolina	11.5
South Dakota	12.5
Tennessee	13.1
Texas	12.7
Utah	6.5
Vermont	10.0
Virginia	9.8
Washington	8.7
West Virginia	11.6
Wisconsin	7.7
Wyoming	8.0
Puerto Rico	44.3

Source: Administration on Aging. *A Profile of Older Americans: 2006.* Washington, D.C.: U.S. Department of Health and Human Services, 2006. Available online. URL: http://www.aoa.gov/PROF/Statistics/prifile/2006/profiles2006.asp. Accessed September 11, 2007.

In considering race, about 8 percent of elderly whites were impoverished in 2005 compared to 23 percent of older African Americans, 13 percent of Asians, and 20 percent of elderly Hispanics. More older women were impoverished (12.3 percent) than older men (7.3 percent) in 2005. Older people living alone were more likely to be living in poverty (19 percent) than older persons living with families (about 6 percent). Females living alone

are more likely to live in poverty than males living alone or than married couples. Married couples are the least likely to live in poverty, according to the U.S. Census Bureau.

See also ABUSE; ASSETS; HOMELESSNESS; MEDICAID.

Administration on Aging. *A Profile of Older Americans: 2006.* Washington, D.C.: U.S. Department of Health and Human Services, 2006. Available online. URL: http://www.aoa.gov/PROF/Statistics/profile/2006/profiles2006.asp. Accessed September 11, 2007.
Department of Health and Human Services. *The 2007 HHS Poverty Guidelines.* Available online. URL: http//aspe.hhs.gov/poverty/07poverty.shtml. Accessed September 12, 2007.
———. *The 2005 HHS Poverty Guidelines.* Available online. URL: http//aspe.hhs.gov/poverty/05poverty.shtml. Accessed September 12, 2007.

power of attorney   The designated temporary and often activity-limited legal right to act for another, as in matters of acquiring or selling property. If the person who has designated the power of attorney becomes incapacitated, the general power of attorney will end. In contrast, a DURABLE POWER OF ATTORNEY will continue even if the older person becomes mentally incompetent.

See also END-OF-LIFE ISSUES; HEALTH-CARE AGENT/PROXY; LEGAL GUARDIANSHIP; LIVING WILL; TALKING TO ELDERLY PARENTS ABOUT DIFFICULT ISSUES; WILLS.

Preferred Provider Organizations (PPOs)   See MEDICARE.

prescription drug abuse/misuse   The excessive use or misuse of prescription drugs, sometimes by individuals who are addicted to these drugs, while in other cases, the misuse is unintentional. Prescription drug abuse is sometimes a problem among elderly individuals who have become dependent on pain medications such as NARCOTICS or on sedating BENZODIAZEPINE drugs such as diazepam (Valium) or clonazepam (Klonopin).

However, intentional prescription drug abuse is a far greater problem among younger individuals than among the elderly, and only an estimated

1 percent of those age 50 and older intentionally abuse prescription drugs such as narcotics, contrasted with about 13 percent of men and 11 percent of women ages 18 to 25 who knowingly abuse drugs.

It should be noted, however, that the unintentional misuse of scheduled drugs such as narcotics and sedatives is a serious problem among the elderly. It should also be noted that, in general, older people are about three times more likely to use prescription drugs than are other age groups, and thus, the overall risk for unintentional misuse of drugs is much greater among the elderly.

Individuals who abuse their narcotic prescriptions may also abuse alcohol, and older people are more likely to abuse alcohol than drugs. This is often an extremely dangerous combination and can lead to illness and even death. Some physicians may fail to warn patients that they must not drink alcohol or take other sedating medications while taking the drug. Of course, sometimes physicians and pharmacists do warn patients about these potential risks and the patients either fail to pay attention to the warning or they forget about it.

One study of "medication misadventures" looked at trips to the emergency room as a result of the misuse of drugs. The findings were reported in a 1996 issue of the *American Journal of Health-System Pharmacy*. A medication misadventure was defined as either noncompliance with the drug regimen or inappropriate prescribing by the physician and did not include intentional substance abuse or overdoses.

The researchers found that during a course of 12 months, 1.7 percent of more than 62,000 visits to the emergency room were caused by medication misadventures. Patients with a medication misadventure were predominantly female and 33 percent were age 65 and older. The researchers noted that only about a third of all the patients with the misadventures understood the potentially adverse effects of the medication, and only 29 percent understood the risk of medication interactions.

The frequency of problems among the elderly was particularly noted, especially in terms of the adverse effects and the inappropriate dosages prescribed for this group. With the increasing size of the elderly population today compared with the time when the study was published in 1996, it is likely that the scope of medication misadventures is even greater in the 21st century.

Sometimes patients with ALZHEIMER'S DISEASE or other forms of DEMENTIA may inadvertently take the painkilling medications of other household members, which is why it is extremely important for anyone who lives with a person with dementia to lock up all medications.

In some cases, it is not the older person who misuses prescription medications, it is others; for example, in some nursing homes, psychiatric drugs have been used to excess to sedate residents who were considered disorderly and difficult. They may have exhibited agitation because of Alzheimer's disease or another form of dementia, and the staff believed it was easier if the resident was sedated or even asleep. The staff of a nursing home must take into account the needs of all residents, and one very agitated older person could be a threat to others; however, it is unlikely that the individual is always agitated and aggressive.

See also ADVERSE DRUG EVENT; ANTIDEPRESSANTS; DRUG ABUSE; INAPPROPRIATE PRESCRIPTIONS FOR THE ELDERLY; PAINKILLING MEDICATIONS; POLYPHARMACY; SUBSTANCE ABUSE AND DEPENDENCE.

Schneitman-McInture, O., et al. "Medication Misadventures Resulting in Emergency Department Visits at an HMO Medical Center." *American Journal of Health-System Pharmacy* 53, no. 12 (1996): 1,416–1,422.

prescription medication programs   Programs that offer discounted rates for individuals who purchase prescribed medications. Some large store chains offer their customers marked discounts on many common generic medications. With the onset of MEDICARE Part D, many individuals obtain their prescriptions through Medicare. However, some older individuals are not eligible for or have not applied for Medicare Part D. To avoid the high cost of many drugs, they seek prescription medication programs that offer discounted medications to those who are eligible and who are approved for the program.

See also POVERTY.

pressure sores See BEDSORES.

Privacy Rule of the Health Insurance Portability and Accountability Act of 1966 (HIPAA) See MEDICAL RECORDS.

Programs of All-Inclusive Care for the Elderly (PACE) See MEDICARE.

prostate cancer Prostate cancer is the second most fatal form of cancer among men, after lung cancer. It is also the most frequently diagnosed form of cancer in men and accounts for about one-third of all cancer diagnoses in males. A urologist is the specialist physician who treats diseases and disorders of the urinary tract and kidneys, as well as diseases of the male prostate gland, such as prostate cancer or other PROSTATE DISEASES. The urologist is also a surgeon.

About 219,000 men were diagnosed with prostate cancer in 2007 in the United States, and 27,050 men died of prostate cancer. More than 80 percent of all prostate cancers are diagnosed in men who are older than age 65.

Symptoms and Diagnostic Path

With early prostate cancer there may be no symptoms at all, which is why the digital rectal examination is an important test that the physician performs during a routine annual physical examination. Most men hate this test because it is embarrassing and uncomfortable, but they should also realize that it can be a lifesaving test. A urologist is a physician who specializes in treating prostate diseases.

If there are symptoms of prostate cancer, they may include the following:

- pain or burning during urination
- a need for frequent urination
- a weak urinary flow
- difficulty with erections
- difficulty with urination
- blood in the urine or semen
- constant pain in the lower back, pelvis, or upper thighs

If prostate cancer is suspected, the physician may perform a transrectal ultrasound of the pelvic area by inserting a small probe through the rectum. This procedure provides the doctor with a sonogram, or image, of the prostate. Further testing includes a biopsy of the prostate. The doctor may also order X-rays of the bones if he or she thinks that the cancer cells may have spread to the bones, in the case of an advanced cancer.

According to the National Cancer Institute, before treatment begins, men with prostate cancer should consider asking their doctor the following questions:

- What is the stage of the disease? Do any lymph nodes show any indication of cancer? Has the cancer spread?
- What is the grade of the tumor?
- What is the goal of treatment? What are the treatment choices? Which treatment do you recommend and why?
- What are the expected benefits of each treatment?
- What are the risks and possible side effects of each treatment that I should consider? How can side effects be managed?
- What can I do to prepare for treatment?
- Will the treatment require me to stay in a hospital? If so, for how long?
- How will treatment affect my normal activities? Will it affect my sex life? Will I have urinary problems? Will I have bowel problems?
- If I were your father, what treatment would you recommend?
- Would a clinical trial research study be the right choice for me?

Treatment Options and Outlook

The treatment of prostate cancer depends on how advanced the cancer is and whether it is confined to the prostate or not. Treatment may include surgery or prostatectomy (removal of the prostate gland) or radiation of the gland. If the cancer has spread, radiation of the pelvis may be indicated.

Hormone therapy may also be given to increase the likelihood that radiation will be successful in

TABLE 1. RISK OF MALES BEING DIAGNOSED WITH PROSTATE CANCER BY AGE

Age 45	1 in 2,500
Age 50	1 in 476
Age 55	1 in 120
Age 60	1 in 43
Age 65	1 in 21
Age 70	1 in 13
Age 75	1 in 9

Source: Centers for Disease Control and Prevention. *Prostate Cancer Screening: A Decision Guide.* Available online. URL: http://www.cec./gov/cancer/prostate/prospdf/prosguide.pdf. Accessed July 2, 2007, page 4.

killing the cancer. Because testosterone makes prostate cancer cells grow, doctors using hormone therapy utilize a long-term (also known as depot) shot of estrogen. This injection has the side effect of causing moodiness and even depression, although such effects go away when the hormones are out of the system.

Risk Factors and Preventive Measures

Individuals with fathers or brothers with prostate cancer have an increased risk for developing prostate cancer and should have a digital rectal examination annually. After about age 50, they should also have an annual test for their level of prostate specific antigen (PSA), a potential marker for prostate cancer. PSA levels that start to go up quickly and without explanation should be evaluated further.

The risk of a prostate cancer diagnosis is one in 2,500 for men who are age 45, but the risk increases to one in 476 for men who are age 50. The risk is much higher, or one in nine, for a male who is age 75. If family members have prostate cancer or the man is African American, the risks are further increased.

See also CANCER; KIDNEY DISEASE; URINARY INCONTINENCE.

prostate diseases Diseases of the male prostate gland, a walnut-sized organ (under normal conditions) that is involved in reproduction and that also directly affects urination. The most common ailments of the prostate gland that are present among older individuals are benign prostatic hypertrophy (BPH) and PROSTATE CANCER. Rarely, the prostate may become infected in the older man, a condition that is known as prostatitis.

Men with prostate diseases are treated by a urologist, a specialist physician who treats diseases and disorders of the urinary tract and kidneys, as well as diseases of the male prostate gland, such as prostate cancer or other prostate diseases. The urologist is also a surgeon.

Symptoms and Diagnostic Path

The symptoms and diagnostic path depend on the prostate disease or disorder.

Benign prostatic hypertrophy (BPH) is a noncancerous chronic condition that causes an enlargement of the prostate gland and that often leads to extreme urinary urgency. It is commonly found in older men. According to author Lisa Granville in her article in 2006 in *Generations*, there are microscopic indications of BPH in about half of all men by the age of 50 years and in 80 percent of men by the age of 80. In about 50 percent of these cases, the physician can feel the condition during a routine digital rectal examination.

Some symptoms that may be associated with BPH can become an emergency. According to Dr. Lange in *Prostate Cancer for Dummies* (which includes information on other prostate diseases), if the bladder continually fills up and feels full, and the man is unable to urinate, this is a medical emergency. Says Lange:

> That urine needs to come out, and the longer that it stays in your bladder, the more likely you're going to suffer from extreme pain, possible infection, a backing up of urine, and other serious medical consequences. Call your doctor, and if he's not available, insist that this emergency information be relayed to him immediately. If your doctor doesn't get back to you within a few hours, go to the emergency room of the nearest hospital or to a walk-in clinic so that you can be treated.

Lower urinary tract symptoms could mean BPH, but they could also be an indicator of an endocrine disorder, especially DIABETES. They could also indicate a urinary tract infection, a sexually transmitted disease, or they could result from the side effects of some medications, especially diuretics or antihistamines. A kidney disease may also be present. These diseases and disorders should be ruled out before BPH is diagnosed.

Laboratory tests such as urinalysis will rule out a urinary tract infection. If there is blood in the urine (hematuria), this may mean the man has a urinary tract infection or could mean the presence of bladder or prostate cancer. Further tests, such as a urine culture, will determine the diagnosis.

A serum creatinine test can rule out kidney disease. Other tests may measure urine flow rates or postvoid residual urine volume (how much urine is still left in the bladder after the man urinates).

Prostatitis is an infection of the prostate. Pain may be present with infection of the prostate, as may a discharge.

Many men with prostate cancer have no symptoms. However, as prostate cancer continues, symptoms may develop, such as difficulty with urination, having a hard time starting and stopping the urine flow, needing to urinate frequently, especially at night, pain or burning during urination, difficulty having an erection, blood in the semen or urine, and pain in the lower back, hips, or upper thighs. These symptoms may also be indicative of BPH, and therefore the physician needs to rule out BPH, a urinary tract infection, and other possible diagnoses.

Prostate cancer may be initially suspected with a simple rectal examination. The doctor may then order a biopsy of the tissue, which will be checked for cancer. If cancer is present, the tissue will be staged to determine how advanced it is and whether it has metastasized (spread) to other organs or to the bones.

Treatment Options and Outlook

The treatment and outcome depend on the type of disease as well as its severity.

BPH is treated with alpha-blocker medications, such as tamsulosin (Flomax), although surgery may be required if the condition worsens.

Finasteride (Proscar) is another medication that is commonly used to treat BPH as of this writing, and it is most effective in men with large prostates that are about the size of a plum. Finasteride is a hormonal drug that shrinks the prostate. A newer drug used to treat BPH is dutasteride (Avodart).

Lifestyle modifications are also important and beneficial, such as avoiding foods and drinks with caffeine, avoiding fluids within several hours of bedtime, and whenever possible, avoiding any medications that make the symptoms worse.

Prostatitis is treated with antibiotics. The individual is also advised to cut back on alcohol, caffeine, and spicy foods, all of which can aggravate prostatitis.

In the case of prostate cancer, the treatment depends on the stage of cancer as well as whether the cancer has spread beyond the prostate gland. Surgery or radiation represent two possible forms of treatment for treatable cancer. Some men may also be treated with hormone therapy and/or a combination of therapies. More information about prostate cancer is available in the entry on cancer.

Risk Factors and Preventive Measures

Increasing age is the primary risk factor for BPH. A family history of prostate cancer is a risk factor, particularly for brothers. There are no preventive measures other than regular examinations by a physician, including the digital rectal examination. Most men hate the rectal examination and may try to avoid it, but it can reveal important and even lifesaving information to the physician.

See also CANCER; FAMILY AND MEDICAL LEAVE ACT.

Granville, Lisa J. "Prostate Disease in Later Life." *Generations* 30, no. 3 (Fall 2006): 51–56.
Lange, Paul, M.D., and Christine Adamec. *Prostate Cancer for Dummies.* New York: Wiley Publishing, 2004.

proxy, health-care   See HEALTH-CARE AGENT/PROXY.

psychiatrist   See DEMENTIA; DEPRESSION.

psychotic behavior   Irrational and disturbed actions, often based on unfounded beliefs. Older individuals with ALZHEIMER'S DISEASE or other forms of DEMENTIA may exhibit psychotic behavior, such as severe CONFUSION, paranoia (believing that others are actively persecuting them), and other delusional ideas. They may also exhibit RAGE, as well as confusion.

In addition, some medications, particularly NARCOTICS such as morphine, can induce temporary visual or auditory HALLUCINATIONS and other unusual behavior in some older people. It is also true that some older adults suffer from psychotic disorders that are unrelated to aging and that had their initial onset at an earlier age (usually young adulthood), including such disorders as schizophrenia, schizoaffective disorder, or bipolar disorder. These disorders are usually treated with psychiatric medications.

According to the Substance Abuse and Mental Health Services Administration, because older individuals often metabolize their medications at a significantly slower rate than younger people, doctors should prescribe the lowest possible dose and gradually increase it if necessary when antipsychotic mediations are used. Older people who have been on antipsychotic medications for many years should be reevaluated periodically as they age, and their medication dosage readjusted if necessary.

See also AGGRESSION, PHYSICAL; COGNITIVE IMPAIRMENT; DELUSIONS; HALLUCINATIONS; IRRITABILITY; MANIA; MEMORY IMPAIRMENT.

pulmonologist   See CANCER; CHRONIC OBSTRUCTIVE PULMONARY DISEASE (COPD); LUNG CANCER.

racial and ethnic differences Older people may suffer from a broad array of diseases and disorders, and sometimes one race or ethnicity is more likely to suffer from a disease than another. For example, African Americans are more likely to suffer from HEART DISEASE, HYPERTENSION, DIABETES, OBESITY, and STROKE, while Caucasians are more likely to suffer from OSTEOPOROSIS and ALZHEIMER'S DISEASE. Note that increasing numbers of younger people are of multiple races because they are born to parents who are different races or ethnicities or their parents may be multiracial. However, this is generally not true of older individuals.

See also AFRICAN AMERICANS; ASIAN AMERICANS; CAUCASIANS; HISPANICS.

rage Extreme anger that is out of all proportion to what is occurring in the environment. Individuals with ALZHEIMER'S DISEASE and other forms of DEMENTIA may exhibit inappropriate rage and CONFUSION as part of their illness. They may imagine that others are plotting against them or that they seek to harm them in some way, when others are actually trying to help them. As a result of this paranoid thinking, they respond with rage.

It can be difficult or impossible for caregivers to provide care to the raging person. Sometimes family members feel compelled to move a family member into a nursing home because they cannot deal with the rages anymore.

See also AGGRESSION, PHYSICAL; COGNITIVE IMPAIRMENT; DELUSIONS; HALLUCINATIONS; IRRITABILITY; MANIA; MEMORY IMPAIRMENT; PSYCHOTIC BEHAVIOR.

rehabilitation Planned and often assisted recovery from an illness or accident. Many older people experience FRACTURES or other physical harm resulting from FALLS and other serious medical problems, and they may need assistance with rehabilitation after hospitalization, including receiving such services as physical therapy, occupational therapy, and speech therapy. Some patients will receive rehabilitation in facilities similar to nursing homes, although their primary goal is to return individuals back to their homes. Others suffer from STROKES and may need help in relearning basic ACTIVITIES OF DAILY LIVING, such as dressing, feeding themselves, and toileting. They may also need speech therapy and other forms of therapy.

Some NURSING HOMES provide rehabilitative services, while some hospitals concentrate solely on the rehabilitation of injured individuals.

See also ACCIDENTAL INJURIES.

respite services Services provided in order to give some time off to caregivers, especially family members, who provide assistance to individuals with ALZHEIMER'S DISEASE and other forms of DEMENTIA. Such services may include adult day care, volunteer or informal respite care (such as help from family members, friends, or church volunteers), as well as in-home respite care, such as companion services, homemaker services (providing help with meal preparation or daily chores), and personal care services (such as helping the older person get dressed, go to the bathroom, and bathe). Many caregivers report that if they could even have a few hours (let alone a few days) off, they would feel greatly relieved.

According to the Administration on Aging, family members who are considering a respite care program should ask respite care managers the following questions:

- Are families limited to a certain number of hours for the needed services?

- Can family members meet and interview the people who will be providing respite care?

- Does the program provide transportation for the older person?

- Does the program keep an active file on the senior's medical condition and other needs? Is there a written care plan?

- How are respite caregivers screened for their jobs?

- How much does respite care cost? What is included in the fee?

- How far ahead of time do family members have to call to arrange for respite services?

- How do the respite caregivers handle emergences? What instructions do they receive to prepare for unexpected situations (such as losing power during a thunderstorm or being snowed in)?

- How is the program evaluated? Are family members contacted for feedback? If so, can feedback received from other family members be reviewed?

When interviewing a respite care aide, the Administration on Aging recommends asking the following questions:

- Are you insured?

- Do you have any references? Who are they?

- Do you have any special skills that might help you with this job?

- Have you ever worked with someone with the same medical condition as my loved one?

- How would you handle the following situations? (Cite examples of challenges encountered as a family caregiver.)

- What is your background and training?

- What are your past experiences with respite care?

- When are you available? Do you have a backup or assistance if you cannot come when expected?

- Who can I talk to at your agency if I am concerned about something?

- Why are you interested in this job?

- Why did you leave your last job?

It is also important for family caregivers to realize that they need to take care of themselves and to deal with any depressive symptoms that may occur. In one study, the researchers found that family caregivers who were given information and assistance had significantly lower rates of depression than the control group members who did not receive such assistance. (See FAMILY CAREGIVERS.)

See also ADULT CHILDREN/CHILDREN OF AGING PARENTS; ADULT DAY CENTERS; BABY BOOMERS; COMPASSION FATIGUE; FAMILY AND MEDICAL LEAVE ACT; OLDER AMERICANS ACT.

restless legs syndrome (RLS) Restless legs syndrome causes an undeniable urge to move the legs while they are at rest. It is a common problem among older adults.

Symptoms and Diagnostic Path
Individuals with RLS feel like they have pins and needles in their legs or experience a crawling sensation in their legs. Symptoms are worse at night.

Treatment Options and Outlook
Moving the legs around helps temporarily. RLS may be treated with medications such as pramipexole (Mirapex), which is approved by the U.S. Food and Drug Administration (FDA) for the treatment of RLS. Another drug approved by the FDA for RLS is ropinirole (Requip).

Sometimes benzodiazepines (antianxiety drugs) such as clonazepam (Klonopin) are prescribed because of their sedating effects. Antiseizure drugs may also be prescribed by physicians, as may levodopa, a drug used with patients with Parkinson's disease. If the pain is severe, doctors may prescribe narcotics, although they are not the first choice of drug for RLS.

Risk Factors and Preventive Measures
According to the National Institute of Neurological Disorders and Stroke, the first gene linked to RLS has been discovered, and it is responsible for up to half the cases of RLS. However, there are other

risk factors. For example, low iron levels and/or anemia may worsen the symptoms of RLS, and when iron level deficiency and/or anemia is corrected, the RLS symptoms may abate, according to the National Institute of Neurological Disorders and Stroke. A deficiency in magnesium may also cause RLS. In addition, patients receiving kidney DIALYSIS may experience RLS.

Other diseases such as PARKINSON'S DISEASE and DIABETES are associated with RLS. If the nerves of the feet are damaged, as may often occur among patients with diabetes, the risk for RLS is increased. It is also important to note that up to 80 percent of those with RLS also have periodic limb movement disorder (PLMD), according to the National Institute of Neurological Disorders and Stroke.

According to the Restless Legs Syndrome Foundation, individuals with RLS should consider if they might be taking any medications that could make their RLS worse, such as some drugs for allergies, DEPRESSION, HYPERTENSION, and HEART DISEASE. They may wish to ask their doctors if they can take another medication or a reduced dosage.

Other preventive measures may be to eliminate alcohol altogether and also consider eliminating caffeine as well. According to the National Institute of Neurological Disorders and Stroke, the use of tobacco is associated with RLS, and it may trigger or aggravate the condition.

Maintaining a regular sleep pattern, including rising and going to sleep at about the same time every day, can improve the symptoms of RLS. Some individuals find that a hot bath, a leg massage, or heating pads and ice packs improve their symptoms.

See also SLEEP DISORDERS.

restraints Devices that are used to prevent individuals from most movements, and which may include beltlike devices, padding, or other items. Restraints are sometimes used with hospital patients to prevent them from pulling out life-giving tubes, such as their intravenous lines. They may also be used with psychotic patients, such as those with ALZHEIMER'S DISEASE or other forms of DEMENTIA, who resist necessary medical treatments and may be actively hallucinating and acting out against nursing home or hospital staff or residents.

In the past restraints were often used for the convenience of nursing home or hospital workers; however, restraints should only be used for the safety and protection of the restrained person.

See also AGGRESSION, PHYSICAL; AMERICANS WITH DISABILITIES ACT; COGNITIVE IMPAIRMENT; CONFUSION; DELUSIONS; HALLUCINATIONS; OMBUDSMAN.

retirement Leaving a full-time job. Many older workers are retired, although not all collect a pension, and some continue to work part-time or full-time in other jobs. The U.S. Census Bureau performed a comparison of the standard (statutory) age of retirement in 24 countries, including the United States, and found that the actual age of retirement may be higher or lower than the generally accepted standard age. For example, in the United States, the standard age of retirement is age 65. However, the actual age of retirement is 61.6 for women and 63.6 for men. (As of this writing, reduced retirement benefits may be received by eligible Americans ages 62–64.)

In Iceland, the standard retirement age is 67 for men and women, but the average age of retirement is 69.5 for men and 66.0 for women. At the other extreme, in Belgium, the standard age of retirement is 65 for men and 60 for women; however, the average male Belgian retires at age 57.6, and the average female Belgian at age 54.1 years.

Kinsella, Kevin, and Victoria A. Velkoff. *An Aging World: 2001.* Washington, D.C.: U.S. Census Bureau, 2001.

rheumatoid arthritis An autoimmune disorder affecting an estimated 2.1 million individuals in the United States, or about 1 percent of the population. About 75 percent of those with rheumatoid arthritis are women. In addition, many individuals who are the most severely affected by rheumatoid arthritis are elderly individuals.

Rheumatoid arthritis occurs when the immune system attacks the synovium, which is the thin membrane lining of the joint. It is a degenerative disease that can be severely painful, although treatments can help considerably.

Rheumatoid arthritis is often thought to be an inflammatory disease, but research reported in 2007 by David M. Lee, M.D., of Brigham and Women's Hospital in Boston and his colleagues discovered an adhesion molecule called cadherin-11 that they believe may be implicated in rheumatoid arthritis. At normal levels of cadherin-11, the cells stick together to form the lining of the synovium. If an overgrowth occurs, as may occur with rheumatoid arthritis, cadherin causes an erosion of the cartilage, which in turn causes the permanent destruction of the joint.

The researchers used mice that develop a disease similar to rheumatoid arthritis. When the mice were genetically altered so that they did not produce cadherin-11, the mice either did not develop arthritis or only developed a mild disease. The researchers also gave nongenetically altered mice that were prone to develop arthritis an agent that blocked cadherin-11. These mice also either did not develop the disease or experienced only mild symptoms. There was no damage to the cartilage. Hopefully, future studies of humans will reveal whether the same process is present in people.

Usually if one joint is affected, a similar one is also affected; for example, if one knee is affected by rheumatoid arthritis, the other knee is likely to be affected as well. Many older people suffer from rheumatoid arthritis, but younger people and even children may develop the disease. Rheumatoid arthritis is two to three times more common in women than men. A rheumatologist is a physician who specializes in treating all forms of arthritis, including the most common forms, such as OSTEOARTHRITIS and rheumatoid arthritis.

See also CHRONIC PAIN.

Symptoms and Diagnostic Path

Rheumatoid arthritis causes severe joint pain. It may also cause other symptoms, such as fevers, fatigue, and a general feeling of illness. The key symptoms of rheumatoid arthritis are

- pain and stiffness that lasts more than 30 minutes in the morning or after a long period of rest
- tender, warm, and swollen joints
- joint inflammation that often affects the wrist and finger joints

Physicians take a medical history and perform a physical examination to detect rheumatoid arthritis. There is no single laboratory test that definitively indicates the presence of rheumatoid arthritis, although the presence of rheumatoid factor, an antibody in the bloodstream, is one indicator. However, in the early stages of rheumatoid arthritis, some patients will test negative for rheumatoid factor. Others may test positive, yet never develop rheumatoid arthritis. Other laboratory tests that are frequently used are a test of the erythrocyte sedimentation rate (ESR), which is a measure of inflammation in the body. C-reactive protein may also be tested to measure disease activity in the body.

X-rays can determine the level of joint damage, although damage may not have occurred yet in the early stages of rheumatoid arthritis. Doctors may use early X-rays to monitor the progression of the disease in an individual.

Treatment Options and Outlook

People with rheumatoid arthritis should moderate between rest periods, when the disease has flared up, and periods of exercise. Exercise can help patients build up strength, improve their sleep, reduce their pain, and cause weight loss.

When the pain flares up, some patients use joint splints, particularly on the wrists and hands.

Many patients with rheumatoid arthritis need medications to treat the disease; for example, they may use anti-inflammatory medications as well as painkillers. Some examples of traditional over-the-counter (OTC) anti-inflammatory nonsteroidal drugs (NSAIDs) are ibuprofen, ketoprofen, and naproxen. There are also prescribed NSAIDs, such as celecoxib (Celebrex). NSAIDs should be used with care by patients older than age 65 and only after consulting a physician, because these drugs can upset the stomach and occasionally can reduce kidney function. NSAIDs are also sometimes associated with serious gastrointestinal problems, such as ulcers.

Corticosteroids are prescribed drugs that may be used to decrease the inflammation of rheumatoid arthritis. They may be given by mouth or by injection. Some examples of corticosteroids are methylprednisolone and prednisone. Corticosteroids may cause an upset stomach, as well as increased appetite, restlessness, and nervousness. They may also cause weight gain, may trigger or worsen diabetes or cataracts, and may also increase the risk for infection. Prolonged use of these medicines may lead to a serious loss of calcium from the bones.

Individuals with a history of tuberculosis or hypothyroidism (an underactive thyroid gland), as well as HYPERTENSION, OSTEOPOROSIS, or stomach ulcer, should inform their doctors about these conditions so that the physician can evaluate whether corticosteroids are safe for the individual.

Another category of drugs, disease-modifying antirheumatic drugs (DMARDs), are prescribed to slow the progression of rheumatoid arthritis. Some examples of DMARDs are azathioprine, cyclosporine, hydroxychloroquine, gold sodium thiomalate, leflunomide, methotrexate, and sulfasalazine. The side effects of DMARDs vary; for example, azathioprine may cause side effects such as a fever, cough, loss of appetite, nausea or vomiting, difficult urination, and lower back or side pain.

Patients who take azathioprine should have regular blood and liver function tests. Cyclosporine may cause bleeding gums, hypertension, an increase in hair growth, and trembling hands. Patients with liver or kidney disease, active infections, or hypertension should inform their doctors before taking this drug.

In addition, biologic response modifiers are prescribed drugs that may reduce inflammation and damage to the joints by blocking the proteins of the body's immune system that trigger inflammation. Examples of such drugs are etanercept (Enbrel), infliximab (Remicade), and adalimumab (Humira). Etanercept is injected subcutaneously (just under the skin) twice a week, and patients can be trained to give themselves these injections. Infliximab is given intravenously for two hours and is taken with methotrexate. Adalimumab is injected every two weeks.

Biologic response inhibitors are also known as tumor necrosis factor-alpha inhibitors because they block a protein, tumor necrosis factor-alpha, that is present in large quantities in the body when a person has an inflammatory condition such as rheumatoid arthritis. These drugs do not cure rheumatoid arthritis, but instead, when they work, they block the severity of the symptoms.

The drugs do have side effects. Etanercept may cause pain or burning in the throat or swelling, itching, and pain at the injection site. It may also cause a runny nose. Infliximab may cause cough, abdominal pain, dizziness, headache, runny nose, shortness of breath, sore throat, and vomiting. Adalimumab may cause rash, redness, swelling, itching, bruising, sinus infection, headache, and nausea. Biological response modifiers may be prescribed in combination with DMARDs, particularly methotrexate.

Another drug that is used to treat rheumatoid arthritis is anakinra (Kineret). This injected medication blocks interleukin 1, a protein that is seen in excessive levels among patients who have rheumatoid arthritis. Anakinra has side effects and may cause redness, swelling, or bruising at the injection site, as well as headache, upset stomach, diarrhea, runny nose, and stomach pain.

Sometimes surgery, particularly joint replacement of the knee or hip, is performed to relieve the severe pain of the patient with rheumatoid arthritis as well as to preserve the function of the joint. (See JOINT REPLACEMENTS.) Some individuals needing knee replacements have both knees replaced at the same time, while others choose to have a knee replacement on the more painful knee.

Other forms of surgery may be used to treat patients with rheumatoid arthritis, such as the reconstruction of damaged tendons, particularly in the hands. Another procedure, the synovectomy, may be performed, in which the inflamed synovial tissue is removed.

Risk Factors and Preventive Measures

It is not entirely known what causes rheumatoid arthritis. Some research has revealed several factors that may lead to the development of the disease, including genetic factors and environmental factors, such as a viral or bacterial infection that may trigger the disease (although the specific environmental cause is not known).

See also AMERICANS WITH DISABILITIES ACT; APPETITE, CHRONIC LACK OF; ARTHRITIS; FAMILY AND MEDICAL LEAVE ACT; GENDER DIFFERENCES; PAIN-KILLING MEDICATIONS.

Centers for Disease Control and Prevention. "Prevalence of Doctor-Diagnosed Arthritis and Arthritis-Attributable Activity Limitation—United States, 2003–2005." *Morbidity and Mortality Weekly Report* 55 (2006): 1,089–1,092.

Scott, D. L., M.D., and G. H. Kingsley. "Tumor Necrosis Inhibitors for Rheumatoid Arthritis." *New England Journal of Medicine* 355, no. 7 (August 17, 2006): 704–712.

rheumatologist   See CHRONIC PAIN; OSTEOARTHRITIS; RHEUMATOID ARTHRITIS.

safety issues   See ELDERIZING A HOME.

sandwich generation   See BABY BOOMERS.

sarcopenia   The age-related and involuntary loss of skeletal muscle mass and strength, which may affect as many as 40 percent of individuals age 80 and older. Irwin H. Rosenberg originally coined the term *sarcopenia* in his 1997 article on sarcopenia in the *Journal of Nutrition.*

Many individuals with sarcopenia have trouble with walking, climbing up stairs, getting up from a chair, or even getting in and out of bed. Sarcopenia may contribute to other serious health problems, such as heart failure or ARTHRITIS. It may also accelerate the risk for FALLS, a very serious and common problem among older adults.

Rosenberg first spoke about this issue in 1988 at a conference:

> I noted then that no decline with ages is as dramatic or potentially more significant than the decline in lean body mass. In fact, there may be no single feature of age-related decline more striking than the decline in lean body mass in affecting ambulation, mobility, energy intake, overall nutrient intake and status, independence and breathing.

According to Ronald Zacker in his 2006 article in the *Journal of the American Association of Physician Assistants,* starting in their 40s, adults lose 3 to 5 percent of muscle mass every 10 years or so, and this rate of decline accelerates further after age 50. Zacker says:

> Muscular strength is independently associated with functionality, while loss of skeletal muscle mass and strength is associated with declining

health. The loss of muscle mass and function can be both a fundamental case and a contributor to disability and disease progression.

Possible Causes of Sarcopenia

There are a variety of potential causes of skeletal muscle loss. One cause is a decrease in the ability of older muscles to regenerate when they are injured or overstressed.

Another possible cause is a decrease in hormones, such as testosterone, which is a hormone present in both men and women (albeit found at a higher level in males). Another hormone, dehydroepiandrosterone sulfate (DHEAS), is produced by the adrenal cortex and it goes into decline as people age.

DHEAS levels may decline up to 20 percent every 10 years in the elderly. According to Rachelle Bross and her colleagues in their 1999 article on sarcopenia, low DHEAS levels are linked to an increased risk for BREAST CANCER in women and a greater risk of CARDIOVASCULAR DISEASE in men. Some studies have shown that an oral administration of DHEAS has improved muscle mass in older men and women, while others have found no change. In addition, most studies have been performed on healthy older men rather than on frail older men and women. As a result, further studies are needed.

Some people also speculate that declining levels of estrogen in women may play a role in the development of sarcopenia. Growth hormone rates are decreased in older people, and this decline contributes to increasing rates of sarcopenia. However, growth hormone is generally not given to older people because it can have many negative effects, such as the development or acceleration of carpal tunnel syndrome as well as gynecomastia in men (enlarged breasts) and hyperglycemia (dangerous for those with DIABE-TES). Fluid retention is another side effect in those who have been administered growth hormone, as is malaise. More importantly, growth hormone does not appear to improve or arrest sarcopenia.

Arresting the Decline

According to Zacker, physical activity is one very good way to slow down the rate of deterioration from sarcopenia, particularly with resistance exercise, also known as strength training. Strength training involves using the muscles against resistance, such as with weights or even one's own weight. Research has shown that elderly people benefit from strength training, and that such exercise can decrease the number of falls, particularly among older women. It can also be effective at decreasing physical FRAILTY and disability among older people. Zacker says:

> Exercise is the only intervention that reliably increases muscle mass, strength, and power. The benefits of exercise, particularly ST [strength training], include a reduction in disease, better balance with fewer falls, and fewer fractures. Equally compelling, exercise is associated with increased independence and quality of life. Obtaining adequate nutrition via a healthy diet is a fundamental adjunct to physical activity in managing sarcopenia.

Testosterone replacement in men who are low in testosterone may be helpful, as may estrogen replacement in older women. Supplemental DHEAS can increase muscle strength and decrease body fat in men and women. It may also increase bone mineral density in women. However, there is insufficient research to document the possible risks and benefits of supplemental DHEAS.

In his 2004 article on interventions for sarcopenia and muscle weakness in older people published in *Age and Ageing,* Stephen E. Borst analyzed data from studies on sarcopenia and aging. He found that studies indicated that testosterone replacement in hypogonadal elderly men (men with low levels of testosterone) produced only modest increases in muscle mass and strength, at best. Since testosterone can stimulate the growth of prostate cancer cells (and older men are at high risk for prostate cancer), researchers have been hesitant to use higher dosages of testosterone to see if greater levels would produce more beneficial results in older men.

Borst found that resistance/strength training was the best intervention for the treatment of sarcopenia; however, it was also important to ensure an adequate nutritional intake, which is a problem among some elderly individuals. Borst says, "Resistance training remains the most effective intervention for increasing muscle mass and strength in older people. Elderly people have reduced food intake and increased protein requirements." Borst says that having adequate nutrition is a problem among elderly people and can prevent them from obtaining the benefits of resistance training.

See also EXERCISE; OSTEOPOROSIS.

Borst, Stephen E. "Interventions for Sarcopenia and Muscle Weakness in Older People." *Age and Ageing* 33 (2004): 548–555.

Bross, Rachelle, Marjan Javanbakht, and Shalender Bhasin. "Commentary: Anabolic Interventions for Aging-Associated Sarcopenia." *Journal of Clinical Endocrinology & Metabolism* 84, no. 10 (1999): 3,420–3,430.

Rosenberg, Irwin H. "Sarcopenia: Origins and Clinical Relevance." *Journal of Nutrition* 127 (1997): 990S–991S.

Zacker, Ronald J. "Health-Related Implications and Management of Sarcopenia." *Journal of the American Association of Physician Assistants* 19, no. 10 (October 2006): 24–29.

scams   See CRIMES AGAINST THE ELDERLY.

self-neglect   See NEGLECT/SELF-NEGLECT.

senior centers   Community organizations in the United States that offer information and opportunities for social interactions for older individuals. They also provide information on health and wellness, transportation services, educational opportunities, and chances to act as volunteers to others.

Some senior centers are defined as *multipurpose senior centers* by the Administration on Aging because they provide comprehensive information on health, education, and nutrition and opportunities for social and recreational interactions with others.

About 73 percent of all senior centers nationwide are multipurpose senior centers compared to 30 percent in the early 1980s.

There are about 10,000 senior centers in the United States, and of these about 6,100 receive federal funding under the OLDER AMERICANS ACT. Most activities that are offered at senior centers are available to seniors free of charge, or they involve low fees to cover, for example, some expenses for trips to places outside the immediate area.

shingles (herpes zoster) An outbreak in adulthood that is caused by the same virus that causes chicken pox in childhood, or the varicella-zoster virus. The chicken pox virus lies dormant in the bloodstream and, many years later, it may present as shingles, which is often a very painful disease. Vaccinations against chicken pox in children have dramatically limited the incidence of the virus in childhood; however, many adults who are senior citizens did have chicken pox in childhood.

It is not unknown why the varicella virus reactivates in adulthood, nor can it be predicted which individuals may suffer this reactivation. It appears that a weakness in the immune system may be implicated, but further studies are needed. Shingles is often very painful and affects the nerves of the body. Some patients say that even the touch of clothes on their bodies is severely painful. Shingles usually lasts from three to five weeks, although some individuals have a shorter or longer course of the disease.

An estimated 20–25 percent of people who have had chicken pox will develop shingles in later life.

Symptoms and Diagnostic Path

The first sign of shingles is often a feeling of burning or tingling on the skin, which is followed by a rash that may appear as one band on one side of the face or body. The patient may also have a general feeling of sickness, accompanied by headache, chills, and fever. The rash and the overall sick feeling are then followed by the development of painful blisters on the skin.

Treatment Options and Outlook

Patients with a rash that may stem from shingles should see their physician no later than three days after the onset of the rash to obtain the best treatment available. The doctor can make a diagnosis and begin treatment with antiviral drugs such as acyclovir (Zovirax), valacyclovir (Valtrex), or famciclovir (Famvir). Pain medications, steroids, and other medications may also be needed. If there is a great deal of inflammation, the doctor may also start a cortisone treatment, but this is determined on a case-by-case basis.

If blisters occur near or in the eye, serious eye damage and even blindness may occur. As a result, patients should see an ophthalmologist (doctor specializing in eye diseases) immediately. Rarely, PNEUMONIA, hearing problems, brain inflammation (encephalitis), and even death may occur.

In some cases, the pain from shingles accelerates and may become long lasting, as with post-herpetic neuralgia (PHN). In the case of PHN, this pain occurs in the area where the rash initially developed. This pain is said to be sharp and stabbing. The older a person is when he or she develops shingles, the more likely they are to also develop PHN. PHN may also lead to insomnia, weight loss, depression, and anxiety.

These symptoms are treated with sedatives, antidepressants (such as tricyclic antidepressants), and antianxiety medications. Anticonvulsants may also be used to treat PHN, particularly gabapentin (Neurontin) or the newer medication pregabalin (Lyrica). Topical analgesics may also be prescribed, such as lidocaine or Lidoderm, a transdermal skin patch.

Note that someone who has never had chicken pox can catch the disease from a person with shingles. As a result, people who have never had chicken pox should avoid contact with patients with shingles, even if these patients are their grandchildren (although most children are immunized against chicken pox today).

Most people who develop shingles do not suffer a recurrence, but recurrences are possible.

Risk Factors and Preventive Measures

An incidence of chicken pox in the past is a risk factor for the development of shingles in adulthood. Most people who develop shingles are older than ages 40 to 50. The risk is the highest for those older than age 70. Most children and adolescents in the United States today are vaccinated against chicken pox.

Some believe that severe stress may bring on a case of shingles.

In 2006 a vaccine to prevent shingles, Zostavax, was approved by the U.S. Food and Drug Administration (FDA) for individuals age 60 and older who have had chicken pox in the past. Researchers report that older adults who have the vaccine reduce their risk for developing shingles by 50 percent or greater. In addition, immunized adults who did develop shingles had milder cases and fewer complications.

In one unique study, supported by the National Institute on Aging (NIA) and the National Center for Complementary and Alternative Medicine (NCCAM), researchers found that performing tai chi (Chinese exercises) boosted the immune system and reduced the risk for developing shingles. In addition, when tai chi exercises were performed along with individuals receiving the varicella vaccine, the immunity was boosted by 40 percent over that produced by the vaccine alone.

Andrew Monjan, chief of the NIA's Neurobiology of Aging Branch, says that the research "demonstrated that a centuries-old behavioral intervention, Tai Chi, resulted in a level of immune response similar to that of a modern biological intervention, the varicella vaccine, and that Tai Chi boosted the positive effects of the vaccine." It is unknown why tai chi significantly improved the immune response of study subjects, but it may help to reduce stress.

See also CHRONIC PAIN; FAMILY AND MEDICAL LEAVE ACT; INFECTIONS; NARCOTICS; PAINKILLING MEDICATIONS.

sibling rivalry and conflict   When parents or other relatives are elderly and they need help, sometimes ADULT CHILDREN/CHILDREN OF AGING PARENTS will disagree among themselves on what course of action is the best one for the older person to take. Siblings may bicker and may even assume the former roles that they had as children (such as the big sister ordering her little brother around), despite the personal success (or lack thereof) that each person has long since attained in adulthood. A team approach and a united front is best, whenever possible, as adult siblings may blame each other for not helping the parent sufficiently or for exerting too much control over the parent. The parent may then not obtain the help that is needed.

It is best if the older parent's financial and legal affairs are in order before his or her death because it can be extremely difficult to determine what the parent would have wanted and to maintain family harmony in the absence of a will or other important documents. This is true even when adult siblings normally get along well.

In his book, *The Parent Care Conversation: Six Strategies for Transforming the Emotional and Financial Future of Your Aging Parents,* author Dan Taylor described a case in which two siblings sued two other siblings for taking a pottery collection from the deceased parents' home. The parents had left a will but stipulated that everything was to be divided among the four children. The end result of the law suit, which dragged on for three years and generated considerable family acrimony, was that the judge decided that the pottery collection had been unlawfully removed from state lands and that a fine of $120,000 was to be divided among all four siblings.

See also HEALTH-CARE AGENT/PROXY; TALKING TO ELDERLY PARENTS ABOUT DIFFICULT ISSUES.

Taylor, Dan. *The Parent Care Conversation: Six Strategies for Transforming the Emotional and Financial Future of Your Aging Parents.* New York: Penguin Books, 2006.

sinus headaches   These headaches are caused by enlarged and usually clogged sinuses. Often the patient has a concurrent bacterial infection that is causing the sinusitis and accompanying headache, and this infection should be treated with antibiotics. Some individuals develop chronic sinus headaches.

Symptoms and Diagnostic Path

Tearing eyes and a runny nose as well as a severe headache (often between the eyes, the forehead, or directly over the cheeks) are indicators of a sinus headache. Fever often accompanies sinus headache if the individual has sinusitis.

Treatment Options and Outlook

Antibiotics are used to treat sinusitis and will resolve the symptoms as well as the headache. Some people have chronic bouts of sinusitis, and they may need a low-maintenance dose of antibiotics.

Risk Factors and Preventive Measures

Individuals who are weather-sensitive may be at risk for sinus headaches. A drop in the barometric pressure may be associated with those who are weather-sensitive. The condition is often hereditary.

See also EXTREMELY SEVERE HEADACHES; HEADACHES.

skin cancer The National Cancer Institute estimated that, excluding basal and squamous cancer, there were 65,050 new cases of skin cancer in 2007, and an estimated 10,850 people died of skin cancer that year. If basal and squamous cancers are included, there are about a million new cases diagnosed each year. Skin cancer is generally caused by frequent overexposure to the sun. It is usually treatable.

The two most common types of skin cancer are basal cell cancer and squamous cell cancer. These types of cancer generally form on the face, head, neck, hands, and arms; however, skin cancer can form anywhere on the skin. Basal cell cancer is a slow-growing form of cancer that most commonly appears on the face. It rarely metastasizes (spreads) to the rest of the body. Squamous cell cancer may appear in areas exposed to the sun as well as other areas. It may spread to other parts of the body.

Symptoms and Diagnostic Path

A change in the skin may indicate the presence of skin cancer, such as the presence of a pale or waxy lump or a firm and red lump. Skin changes are not necessarily a sign of cancer, but they should be reported to the doctor anyway. If the doctor thinks there may be a problem, he or she may refer the patient to a dermatologist (a medical doctor who specializes in skin diseases) for further evaluation.

If the doctor believes that skin cancer may be present, he or she will perform a skin biopsy. As of this writing, there are four primary ways to biopsy the skin, including the punch biopsy, the incisional biopsy, the excisional biopsy, and the shave biopsy.

With the punch biopsy, the doctor uses a sharp hollow tool to remove a circle of tissue from the affected area. If an incisional biopsy is used, the doctor uses a scalpel to remove part of the tissue. With an excisional biopsy, the doctor removes the entire growth as well as some of the area around it with a scalpel. With a shave biopsy, the doctor uses a sharp blade to shave off the growth.

The National Cancer Institute recommends that patients ask the doctor the following questions before a biopsy is performed for skin cancer:

- Which type of biopsy do you recommend for me?
- How will the biopsy be done?
- Will I have to go to the hospital?
- How long will the biopsy take? Will I be awake? Will it hurt?
- Are there any risks? What are the chances of infection or bleeding after the biopsy?
- What will my scar look like?
- How soon will I know the results of the biopsy? Who will explain them to me?

If the biopsy shows that skin cancer is present, the doctor must stage the cancer, which means that an analysis is made of the size of the growth, how deeply it has grown beneath the outer layer of the skin, and whether it has spread to the lymph nodes or to other parts of the body. There are five stages of skin cancer, ranging from Stage 0, in which the cancer is only at the top layer of the skin, to Stage IV, when the cancer has metastasized to other areas of the body.

Treatment Options and Outlook

The treatment depends on how the cancer is staged. In some cases, the biopsy alone is the only treatment that is needed. In other cases, further surgery is required to try to remove all or as much of the cancer as possible. There are many options with surgery; for example, the doctor may use laser surgery, employing a narrow beam of light to destroy the cancer cells. Cryosurgery is another option, which uses liquid nitrogen to destroy the cancer.

The most frequently used surgery used for skin cancer is a procedure commonly known as Mohs surgery, in which the surgeon shaves away a thin layer of tissue and then immediately examines this layer under a microscope for cancer cells. This procedure is repeated until the surgeon can no longer see any cancer cells under the microscope.

Another option is topical chemotherapy when medication is placed on the skin to kill the cancer. The medication, which is a lotion or cream, is usually applied to the skin once or twice a day for several weeks. The drug may cause the skin to redden and may also cause a rash. The skin may also become hypersensitive to the sun. These effects will end when the treatment is completed.

Photodynamic therapy is another treatment choice. The doctor uses a chemical along with a laser beam to destroy the cancer. First the cream is applied for hours or days and then the laser is used.

Radiation therapy is also a choice of treatment for skin cancer. It is not normally used for this form of cancer but may be used if surgery would leave a serious scar or would be difficult to perform.

The National Cancer Institute recommends that patients ask their doctors the following questions before treatment starts:

- What is the stage of the disease?
- What are my treatment choices? Which do you recommend for me and why?
- What are the expected benefits of each kind of treatment?
- What are the risks and possible side effects of each treatment? What can we do to control my side effects?
- Will the treatment affect my appearance? If so, can a reconstructive surgeon or plastic surgeon help?
- Will treatment affect my normal activities? If so, for how long?
- How often should I have checkups?

Risk Factors and Preventive Measures

Excessive exposure to ultraviolet radiation from the sun, tanning booths, or sun lamps can cause skin cancer. Fair-skinned people who tend to burn eas-

ily have a greater risk for developing skin cancer. Those who live in sunny areas also have a greater risk for developing skin cancer, such as individuals residing in Texas and Florida. Other major risk factors for skin cancer include

- scars or burns on the skin
- radiation therapy
- exposure to arsenic
- chronic skin inflammation or skin ulcers
- diseases that cause the skin to be photosensitive, such as albinism or basal cell nevus syndrome
- drugs that suppress the immune system
- a family history of skin cancer
- a personal history of one or more cancers
- the presence of Bowen's disease, a scaly patch on the skin that can develop into squamous cell skin cancer

One of the best ways to prevent skin cancer is to avoid overexposure to the sun. Older individuals should not be seeking a dark tan, because excessive sun exposure could lead to the development of skin cancer. Individuals should stay out of the sun from mid-morning to late afternoon whenever possible. If they cannot stay out of the sun, they should wear hats and sunglasses that absorb ultraviolet radiation. Sunscreen lotion with a sun protection factor (SPF) of at least 15 is advisable.

See also CANCER.

sleep apnea/sleep-related breathing disorder
Sleep apnea causes a person to stop breathing for 10 to 60 seconds while asleep. The person awakens gasping for breath. Death can occur if the person does not awaken.

Symptoms and Diagnostic Path

Individuals with sleep apnea snore loudly and may keep others awake, such as their spouses.

According to Gooneratne et al. in their article on insomnia symptoms and sleep-related breathing disorder in elderly subjects in a 2006 issue of the *Archives of Internal Medicine*, insomnia is often found with sleep-related breathing disorder among older individuals. Thus, if older individuals complain of insomnia, they should also be evaluated for sleep-related breathing disorder.

Treatment Options and Outlook

Individuals with sleep apnea are treated with a continuous positive air pressure (CPAP) device that forces air through the airway if they stop breathing while they are sleeping. In some cases, the physician may recommend surgery to widen the airway.

Risk Factors and Preventive Measures

If sleep apnea is not identified and treated, the individual can develop HYPERTENSION or have a STROKE. If individuals are obese, weight loss can improve the sleep apnea problem.

Other recommendations from the National Heart, Lung and Blood Institute include

- avoiding alcohol and sedating medications, which make it harder for the throat to remain open during sleep
- sleeping on the side instead of the back and using special pillows, if necessary, to keep the throat open
- using nose sprays or allergy medications as directed by the physician
- avoiding smoking

In addition, some people use dental appliances that can keep their airways open during sleep.

See also SLEEP DISORDERS.

Gooneratne, Nalaka S., M.D., et al. "Consequences of Comorbid Insomnia Symptoms and Sleep-Related Breathing Disorder in Elderly Subjects." *Archives of Internal Medicine* 166 (September 18, 2006): 1,732–1,738.

sleep disorders   Difficulty getting to sleep and frequent awakenings are common sleep problems among many older individuals, as are problems with early morning awakening and excessive sleepiness during the daytime. Some abnormal sleep patterns are caused by obstructive SLEEP APNEA (also known as sleep-related breathing disorder), RESTLESS LEGS SYNDROME (RLS), and PERIODIC LIMB MOVEMENT DISORDER (PLMD). NIGHTMARES are another form of sleep disorder, although they are sometimes referred to as a parasomnia (an abnormal type of sleep pattern). Sleep disorders may be caused by stress and worry, as well as by BEREAVEMENT, DEPRESSION, or a variety of other causes, such as an individual suffering from one or more anxiety disorders. (See ANXIETY AND ANXIETY DISORDERS.)

According to Dr. Subir Vij in an article on *eMedicine* about geriatric sleep disorders, a sleep disturbance is the third most common patient complaint, after headaches and the common cold. Older women are more than twice as likely to suffer from moderate to severe insomnia as are older men, or about 35 percent of older women compared to 13 percent of older men. An estimated half of all individuals older than age 65 years who live at home and two-thirds of those older than age 65 who live in a long-term care facility have some form of sleep disturbance.

A broad array of medications can induce sleeplessness in older individuals as a side effect. Excessive consumption of food and drink items loaded with caffeine, such as coffee, tea, or cola drinks, can also cause sleeplessness. Some antidepressants are stimulating, as are decongestants, some antihypertensive drugs, bronchodilators, and corticosteroids. Sometimes the quantity of medications is a major part of the problem. According to Dr. Vij, many older people take up to nine medications per day, and as a result, one or more of these medications may cause a side effect of insomnia, nightmares, or another form of sleep disorder. For example, beta-blocker medications can cause difficulty with falling asleep, vivid dreams, and an increased number of awakenings.

Smoking causes or contributes to some sleep problems, and people who smoke are more likely than nonsmokers to have difficulty falling asleep and experience decreased sleep duration.

Other causes of sleep problems are chronic pain disorders, such as OSTEOARTHRITIS, gastroesophageal reflux disease (GERD), or PARKINSON'S DISEASE. In addition, chronic CONSTIPATION may lead to poor sleep.

Some individuals with ALZHEIMER'S DISEASE experience day/night reversal; they sleep all day and then are awake all night. This is also known as SUNDOWNING.

Others have difficulty sleeping in general because of their CHRONIC PAIN. The doctor may decrease the dosage of the medication that is causing insomnia or, in some cases, he or she may add a sedating medication to help improve the individual's sleep patterns. Sometimes a combination of problems will lead to sleep disorders, such as the combination of depression and chronic pain, or the combination of anxiety and a medication interaction.

Some elderly patients have insomnia or sleep loss because of nocturia, the need to urinate in the nighttime. Nocturia is also an aspect in FALLS and hip FRACTURES experienced by the elderly. The patient should tell the doctor about the nocturia to determine its cause and to see if any treatment is available. For example, the nocturia may be caused by undiagnosed DIABETES, by PROSTATE DISEASE (in men), or by sleep apnea or other causes. Some patients wake up in the middle of the night because of gastrointestinal problems, such as gastroesophageal reflux disease (GERD). Treatment with a proton pump inhibitor medication may resolve this problem.

The National Center of Sleep Disorders Research recommends that older individuals with sleep disorders consider taking the following actions:

- Get up in the morning and go to bed at night at the same time each day, including the weekends.
- Avoid caffeine, alcohol, and nicotine four to six hours before bedtime.
- Avoid eating large meals within two hours of bedtime.
- Use the bed for sleeping only and not for watching television, reading, knitting, or other activities.
- Do not take naps after 3 P.M.
- Avoid thinking about the problems of the day or life issues when in bed.
- Sleep in a dark and quiet room that is neither too hot nor too cold.
- Do something relaxing 30 minutes before bedtime, such as taking a warm bath.
- Do not exercise within two hours of bedtime.

- If sleep does not come in about 20 minutes, get up and do a quiet activity such as listening to quiet music.
- Individuals with snoring problems can try using nasal strips to make breathing easier.

In some cases, physicians will recommend sedating medications or sleep-specific remedies such as zolpidem (Ambien), a drug that is specifically approved for the short-term treatment of insomnia. The recommended initial dose for the elderly is 5 mg, according to *Essential Psychopharmacology: The Prescriber's Guide.* Some individuals may have an increased risk for CONFUSION or falls with taking this medication. Other prescribed sleep remedies as of this writing include zaleplon (Sonata) and estazolam (ProSom).

A nonscheduled sleep remedy named ramelteon (Rozerem) was approved in 2005. Ramelteon is in a class of medications called melatonin receptor agonists. It does not produce either drug dependence or rebound insomnia, a condition in which insomnia returns after discontinuation of a prescribed sleep remedy.

In 2007 the U.S. Food and Drug Administration requested that manufacturers of sedative-hypnotic sleep remedies provide stronger language on their product labeling, warning potential users of possible risks, such as the risk for a severe allergic reaction or of complex sleep-related behaviors. One complex sleep-related behavior is *sleep driving,* when the individual actually drives while asleep but later has no memory of it.

The medications covered by the FDA requirement included Ambien/Ambien CR, Butisol, Carbrital, Dalmane, Doral, Halcion, Lunesta, Placidyl, Prosom, Restoril, Rozerem, Seconal, and Sonata. More information on sedative hypnotic products is available at http://www.fda.gov/cdeer/drug/infopage/sedative_hypnotics/default.htm.

Analysis of Sleep Disorders

Patients with chronic and severe sleep disorders can be analyzed in a sleep laboratory, using polysomnography, or equipment that measures eye movements, heart rates, respiration, and other physiological variables. A sleep study will show the presence of sleep apnea, which is the most common disorder among obese males who snore. Another common problem is periodic limb PLMS, which causes the patient to flex the lower legs as frequently as every 20 to 40 seconds. RLS is another problem that can cause severe insomnia, and it is a disorder in which the patient's legs feel uncomfortable and the discomfort is relieved only by moving the legs about. PLMS may be treated with slow-release carbidopa/levodopa, while RLS may respond to bromocriptine.

See also SUNDOWNING.

Anderson, Wayne E., D.O. "Periodic Limb Movement Disorder." eMedicine. March 30, 2007. Available online. URL: http://www.emedicine.com/neuro/topic523.htm. Accessed February 26, 2008.

Asplund, R. "Nightmares, Sleep and Cardiac Symptoms in the Elderly." *Netherlands, the Journal of Medicine* 61, no. 7 (July 2003): 257–261.

Blay, Sergio Luis, Sergio Baxter Andreoli, and Fabio Leite Gastal. "Chronic Painful Physical Conditions, Disturbed Sleep and Psychiatric Morbidity: Results from an Elderly Survey." *Annals of Clinical Psychiatry* 19, no. 3 (2007): 169–174.

Gooneratne, Nalaka S., M.D., et al. "Consequences of Comorbid Insomnia Symptoms and Sleep-Related Breathing Disorder in Elderly Subjects." *Archives of Internal Medicine* 166 (September 18, 2006): 1,732–1,738.

Jagus, Christopher E., and Susan M. Benbow. "Sleep Disorders in the Elderly." *Advances in Psychiatric Treatment* 5 (1999): 30–38.

Neubauer, David N., M.D. "Sleep Problems in the Elderly." *American Family Physician* (May 1, 1999). Available online. URL: http://www.aafp.org/afp/990501ap/2551.html. Accessed April 8, 2008.

Stahl, Stephen M. *Essential Psychopharmacology: The Prescriber's Guide.* New York: Cambridge University Press, 2005.

Vij, Subir, M.D. "Sleep Disorder, Geriatric." eMedicine, 2005. Available online. URL: http://www.emedicine.com/Med/topic3179.htm. Accessed April 8, 2008.

Wolkove, Norman, Osama Elkholy, Marc Baltzan, and Mark Palayew. "Sleep and Aging: 2. Management of Sleep Disorders in Older People." *Canadian Medical Association Journal* 176, no. 9 (April 24, 2007): 1,449–1,454.

smoking   Use of cigarettes, cigars, or pipes (although cigarettes are the most popular product) that include tobacco. Years of smoking can cause many very serious diseases, including LUNG CANCER, ORAL CANCER, EMPHYSEMA, chronic bronchitis, and a greater risk than among nonsmokers for the development of PNEUMONIA. Smoking can exacerbate many other illnesses and disorders, such as HEART DISEASE and digestive disorders. Many older smokers began the habit in their teens, often in response to intense peer pressure, and before the dangers of smoking were widely known, and they rapidly developed an addiction to nicotine.

Most smokers age 65 and older have smoked for years and are heavy smokers. In addition, older smokers are less likely to try to stop smoking than younger smokers, although studies have shown that they are actually more likely to succeed with quitting if they do stop.

According to the Centers for Disease Control and Prevention (CDC), 10.2 percent of individuals ages 65 and older were smokers in 2006, including 12.6 percent of males ages 65 and older and 8.3 percent of females in this age group.

According to the Centers for Disease Control and Prevention (CDC), states vary considerably on the percentages of older adults who continue to smoke, from a high of 14.5 percent in Nevada to a low of 4.7 percent in Utah. The CDC goal is 12 percent, which has been successfully met by most states (47 states).

See also CANCER; EMPHYSEMA; GENDER DIFFERENCES.

Fryar, Cheryl D., et al. "Smoking and Alcohol Behaviors Reported by Adults: United States, 1999–2002." *Advance Data from Vital and Health Statistics,* no. 378 (November 29, 2006).

He, Wan, Manisha Sengupta, Victoria A. Velkoff, and Kimberly A. DeBarros. *65+ in the United States: 2005.* Washington, D.C.: U.S. Census Bureau, December 2005.

Special Needs Plan (SNP)   See MEDICARE.

stomach cancer   According to the National Cancer Institute, there were an estimated 21,260 new cases of stomach cancer in 2007, including 13,000 men and 8,260 women. An estimated 11,210 people died of stomach cancer in 2007, including 6,610 men and 4,600 women. Stomach cancer is also known as gastric cancer. The risk for this form of cancer increases with age.

Symptoms and Diagnostic Path

Often there are no symptoms in the early onset of stomach cancer. Later symptoms may include

- nausea and vomiting
- weight loss
- feeling bloated after a small meal
- stomach discomfort
- blood in the stool

Note that many other health problems can also cause these symptoms, such as an infection or an ulcer. However, it is important to see the doctor when these symptoms are present.

If stomach cancer may be present, the patient is usually referred to a gastroenterologist, a physician who specializes in treating digestive diseases. The doctor will check the abdomen for swelling and swollen lymph nodes and check the eyes for jaundice. Tests will usually be ordered, such as an upper gastrointestinal series, which are X-rays of the esophagus and stomach taken after the patient drinks a barium solution. With an endoscopy, the doctor inserts a thin lighted tube into the stomach. The patient may be sedated before this procedure. The doctor uses the endoscope to remove tissue from the stomach, which will be biopsied. A pathologist will check the tissue for cancer cells.

Patients who will be having a biopsy should ask their doctors the following questions:

- How will the biopsy be done?
- Will I need to go to the hospital?
- Will I have to do anything to prepare for it? How long will it take? Will I be awake? Will it hurt?
- Are there any risks? What are the chances of infection or bleeding after the procedure?
- How long will it take for me to recover? When can I resume my normal diet?
- How soon will I know the results? Who will explain them to me?

- If I do have cancer, who will talk to me about the next steps? When?

If cancer is present, the doctor will stage the cancer, which means he or she will determine whether the cancer has invaded nearby tissues or if it has spread elsewhere. Stomach cancer can spread to the lymph nodes, liver, pancreas, and other organs. Laboratory tests may be ordered to check for anemia and to check liver function. Other tests that may be performed include a computerized tomography (CT) scan of the organs, an endoscopic ultrasound, and a laparoscopy.

Treatment Options and Outlook

Cancer treatment for stomach cancer is either local therapy or systemic therapy. Local therapy includes surgery and radiation therapy, while chemotherapy is systemic therapy.

Questions patients should ask the doctor about treatment are

- What is the stage of the disease?
- What are my treatment choices? Which do you suggest for me and why?
- Would joining a research study be a good choice for me?
- Will I have more than one kind of treatment?
- What are the expected benefits of each kind of treatment?
- What are the risks and possible side effects of each treatment? What can we do to control my side effects? How else can I take care of myself during treatment?
- How will treatment affect my normal activities? Am I likely to have eating or other problems?
- Whom should I call if I have problems during treatment?
- How often should I have checkups?

If surgery is recommended it will be either a partial gastrectomy (partial removal of the stomach) or a total gastrectomy, when the entire stomach, nearby lymph nodes, parts of the esophagus, and small intestine and other tissues near the tumor are all removed. Patients who may have surgery should ask the following questions:

- What kind of surgery do you recommend for me?
- Will you remove lymph nodes? Will you remove other tissue? Why?
- How will I feel after surgery?
- Will I need a special diet?
- If I have pain, how will you control it?
- How long will I be in the hospital?
- Am I likely to have eating problems? Will I need a feeding tube? If so, for how long? How do I take care of it? Who can help me if I have a problem?
- Will I have any lasting side effects?

Weight loss is common after stomach surgery. Many patients may experience dumping syndrome, a condition in which food or liquids enters the small intestine very rapidly and causes nausea, bloating, cramps, and dizziness. Smaller meals may resolve this problem, as will eating fewer sweets.

If chemotherapy is the treatment, it is generally done after surgery. Radiation therapy may be given at the same time as chemotherapy. Chemotherapy affects the blood cells that fight infection and perform other important functions. As a result, chemotherapy drugs increase the risk for infections, easy bruising, and fatigue. Chemotherapy may cause poor appetite, nausea and vomiting, and hair loss. Patients for whom chemotherapy is recommended should ask the following questions:

- Why do I need this treatment?
- Which drug or drugs will I have?
- How do the drugs work?
- When will treatment start? When will it end?

Radiation therapy uses high-energy rays to destroy cancer cells. Treatments generally last five days a week for several weeks, and the treatments are given as outpatient therapy in a hospital or clinic. Radiation therapy may cause nausea and diarrhea and stomach pain. It may also cause extreme fatigue.

Patients for whom radiation therapy is recommended for their stomach cancer should ask the following questions:

- Why do I need this treatment?
- When will treatments begin? When will they end?
- How will I feel during treatment?
- How will we know if the radiation treatment is working?
- Are there any lasting effects?

Risk Factors and Preventive Measures

Most people who develop stomach cancer are age 72 and older, and men are more likely to develop stomach cancer than women. In considering racial and ethnic risk factors, stomach cancer appears more commonly among Asian, Pacific Islander, Hispanic, and African Americans than in non-Hispanic whites.

Some experts believe that a diet high in smoked, salted, or pickled foods increases the risk for stomach cancer. Eating fresh vegetables and fruits may be protective factors against the development of stomach cancer.

Other risk factors include

- the presence of *Helicobacter pylori* infection in the stomach (which increases the risk for inflammation and stomach ulcers)
- smoking
- some health problems, such as chronic gastritis or pernicious anemia
- a rare type of stomach cancer that runs in some families

See also CANCER.

stroke   A sudden and life-threatening loss of blood flow to a part of the brain that results in damage to or death of brain cells. The stroke may lead to permanent damage and disability or the patient may recover all or most of his or her abilities. A stroke is also known as a brain attack. Stroke is the third leading cause of death among all Americans.

Immediate medical attention is vitally important to the stroke patient, and the patient should be seen in the hospital, preferably by a stroke team, within 60 minutes of the onset of symptoms. Patients with symptoms of stroke should never attempt to drive themselves to the hospital nor should others drive them because precious time will be wasted and every moment counts. Instead, it is very important to call for an ambulance, usually by dialing 911 for emergency services.

Some strokes go unnoticed or ignored because they last only a few minutes and the symptoms end. These strokes are called transient ischemic attacks (TIAs) and are also known as ministrokes. They are important because an untreated stroke can be followed by a major and disabling stroke within hours. It is best if treatment occurs within the first three hours after the symptoms occur. Clot-busting drugs can be administered, but they must be given with the three-hour time frame.

Almost 75 percent of all strokes occur to individuals age 65 and older. According to the National Institute of Neurological Disorders and Stroke, the risk of suffering from a stroke increases by more than double for each decade of life after age 55. In addition, stroke represents 8 percent of all deaths among individuals age 65 and older, according to the Centers for Disease Control and Prevention (CDC).

Stroke is also a leading cause of death among the elderly. African Americans are the most likely of all races to die from a stroke. Men and women age 65 and older have about an equal risk of suffering from a stroke.

There are two primary types of strokes, including an ischemic stroke and a hemorrhagic stroke. An ischemic stroke is the most common form of stroke in which the blood supply to the brain is interrupted and there is a loss of oxygen to the brain tissue. An ischemic stroke may result from ARTEROSCLEROSIS (clogged arteries). Fatty deposits of plaque may build up on the arterial walls over time, and these deposits eventually result in an abnormal blood flow, causing the blood to clot.

A clot that stays in one place within the brain is called a cerebral thrombus, while a clot that breaks loose and moves along the bloodstream inside the brain is known as a cerebral embolism. An abnormal heart valve may also cause an ischemic stroke. Heart rhythm problems and severe alterations in blood pressure may also be responsible for a loss or diminished blood flow to the brain.

With a hemorrhagic stroke a blood vessel leading to the brain or inside the brain bursts. This rupture damages brain cells.

Some strokes are considered minor problems, while others are considered major events. However, anyone with any stroke symptoms should receive immediate medical attention. Only a physician can diagnose a stroke accurately, determine the status of the stroke, and decide how the patient should be treated.

Symptoms and Diagnostic Path

Anyone with the danger symptoms should seek medical care immediately. The danger symptoms of stroke are the sudden development of any of the following:

- sudden numbness or weakness in the face, arm, or leg, especially when it is only occurring on one side of the body
- sudden confusion or trouble in understanding speech or in speaking
- sudden problems seeing in one or both eyes
- sudden dizziness, loss of balance or coordination, or trouble walking
- sudden and severe headache with no known cause

Physicians use imaging tools to determine whether a stroke has occurred, and if so, to determine the severity of the stroke. They may use a computerized tomography (CT) scan or a magnetic resonance imaging (MRI) scan of the brain. They may also use an ultrasound to image the carotid arteries of the neck in order to check for blockages or clots. Magnetic resonance angiography (MRA) may be used to detect any blockages of the carotid arteries and vertebral arteries.

Other tests may include an echocardiogram to determine if a clot from the heart has caused the problem, as well as an electrocardiogram to identify any underlying heart disease.

Laboratory tests will be performed to determine if there is any abnormal clotting of the blood or if there are any autoimmune conditions present.

Treatment Options and Outlook

Medications are frequently used to treat stroke victims. Anticoagulants are often prescribed. The most frequently prescribed anticoagulants are warfarin (Coumadin) and heparin. Antiplatelet agents (drugs that block small blood components from sticking together) are also commonly used, including aspirin/extended-release dipyridamole (Aggrenox) and clopidogrel (Plavix). Calcium channel blockers may also be prescribed. Pain medications may be needed as well.

Intravenous feeding therapy is often instituted because the patient is admitted to the hospital and is either unable or has difficulty in self-feeding. Also the patient may have lost the swallowing reflex, thereby making it unsafe to swallow foods. Once the patient has recovered, he or she may be placed on long-term ASPIRIN THERAPY, usually taking a baby aspirin per day to prevent future strokes. Rarely, patients with severe strokes may require surgery to repair damage that has occurred.

Stroke victims may suffer long-term effects, and follow-up care with a physician (usually a neurologist) is needed. They may also need assistance with performing basic activities of daily living, such as eating, dressing, toileting, and so on. Stroke patients may need to receive care in a rehabilitative nursing home until they are well enough to receive care within the home.

Speech therapists can help stroke patients who have difficulty speaking and swallowing, while occupational therapists can provide assistance with such basic skills and ACTIVITIES OF DAILY LIVING as writing, bathing, dressing, and other key activities. Physical therapists can often help stroke patients to regain their lost abilities, such as the ability to move from one position to another or to walk. Occupational therapists can help patients with such tasks as cooking and bathing.

A stroke also often has a profound emotional impact on the patient. Many stroke patients become anxious or depressed after the stroke, traumatized by the stroke itself, and also fearful of the imminent onset of another attack. They may need to consult with a psychiatrist in collaboration with the neurologist and other physicians who are involved in providing ongoing treatment.

Some stroke victims may experience a range of complications from their stroke, including

- permanent loss of mobility in part of the body
- permanent loss of brain functions
- a reduced ability to care for himself or herself
- a decreased life span
- a reduced ability to communicate or interact with others
- muscle spasticity
- a reduced awareness of one side of his or her body

Risk Factors and Preventive Measures

The primary risk factors for the development of a stroke occur among those individuals who have

- DIABETES
- HYPERTENSION
- a history of heart disease
- a history of transient ischemic attacks (TIAs), which are ministrokes
- cigarette SMOKING; heavy smokers have the greatest risk
- OBESITY
- alcohol abuse
- past strokes
- a family history of strokes

Individuals with risk factors for stroke should be screened for hypertension and should have their blood CHOLESTEROL checked periodically. Patients with hypertension should work to reduce their blood pressure to normal levels, with a combination of medications, weight loss, exercise, and other recommendations provided by their physicians. A low-fat diet is often recommended. Patients who smoke should stop smoking immediately because smoking is linked to strokes. Regular exercise is also recommended because exercise may strengthen the heart and improve overall blood flow. Note that before starting any exercise program, individuals should check with their doctors.

See also AMERICANS WITH DISABILITIES ACT; DISABILITIES; FAMILY AND MEDICAL LEAVE ACT; HEALTH-

CARE AGENT/PROXY; HEART ATTACK; HEART FAILURE; MEMORY IMPAIRMENT.

substance abuse and dependence The excessive use of or dependence on (addiction to) alcohol or drugs. Most substance abusers who are age 65 and older either abuse or they are dependent on alcohol, followed by opiates.

According to the Substance Abuse and Mental Health Services Administration, increases from 1995 to 2005 in the admission for treatment for the abuse of opiates, cocaine, and sedatives represented the primary growth in drug treatment admissions among those age 65 and older. Most of the opiate admissions were for heroin. However, an estimated 1.4 percent of the admissions of older people in 1995 and 2.4 percent in 2005 were for treatment for the abuse of codeine, morphine, oxycodone, Dilaudid, and Demerol, which are all prescription drugs. (See PRESCRIPTION DRUG ABUSE/MISUSE.)

It is concerning that the percentage of admissions for alcohol has declined from 84.7 percent to 75.9 percent and the percentage of admissions for opiates and cocaine has increased; for example, in 1995, only 6.6 percent of elderly people were admitted for the treatment of opiate abuse. That percentage went up and down over the years but the highest percentage (10.5 percent) occurred in 2005. (See Table 1.)

Demographics of Those Entering Treatment for Substance Abuse

In general, most older people admitted for treatment for substance abuse are white males, and the largest percentage of older people who are admitted are between 65 and 69 years old (59 percent of all older people receiving substance abuse treatment).

According to the Substance Abuse and Mental Health Services Administration, 76 percent of treatment admissions were male.

However, some experts believe that substance abuse among older women may be a significantly greater problem than is realized by the general public or even by medical professionals. For example, according to a report on older women and substance abuse in the *National Women's Report* in 2006, many people are in denial that such a problem could exist. According to the authors:

A two-year survey of 400 primary care physicians found that less than 1 percent even considered a substance abuse diagnosis when typical signs of alcohol or drug abuse in older women were described to them. Instead, they were more likely to diagnose women with depression and prescribe medications that could aggravate any existing substance abuse.

These doctors may also attribute an anxiety disorder to women who are actually exhibiting signs of substance abuse. Some physicians may believe

---

TABLE 1. ADMISSION TO SUBSTANCE ABUSE TREATMENT OF INDIVIDUALS AGE 65 AND OLDER, BY PRIMARY SUBSTANCE AT ADMISSION: 1995–2005

Primary Substance	Percentage										
	1995	1996	1997	1998	1999	2000	2001	2002	2003	2004	2005
Alcohol	84.7	84.8	83.6	83.1	80.5	80.4	78.7	77.8	78.5	74.4	75.9
Opiates	6.6	6.5	7.3	7.5	7.9	8.2	9.2	9.2	9.3	8.8	10.5
Cocaine	2.1	2.0	1.9	2.3	2.6	2.9	2.6	2.9	3.2	3.9	4.4
Sedatives	0.5	0.5	0.7	0.3	0.2	0.3	0.4	0.4	0.4	0.8	1.3
Marijuana	0.9	0.9	1.0	0.9	1.2	1.2	1.0	1.2	1.4	1.3	1.0
Stimulants	0.3	0.3	0.3	0.2	0.5	0.5	0.4	0.8	0.6	0.6	0.8
Tranquilizers	0.7	0.8	0.7	0.7	0.7	0.8	1.2	0.9	0.8	0.6	0.6
Other	4.2	4.2	4.5	5.0	6.4	5.7	6.5	6.8	5.8	9.6	5.5

Source: Adapted from Substance Abuse and Mental Health Services Administration. "Adults Aged 65 or Older in Substance Abuse Treatment: 2005." *The DASIS Report,* May 31, 2007. Available online. URL: http://www.drugabusestatistics.Samhsa.gov/2k/7/olderTX/older/TXpdf, p. 2. Accessed July 6, 2007.

that signs of substance abuse are really indicators of ALZHEIMER'S DISEASE or DEMENTIA. Even if doctors do recognize the presence of a substance abuse issue, they may mistakenly believe that elderly people are just too old to receive treatment for their addiction. (See AGEISM.)

Some signs and symptoms of prescription drug abuse in older women include

- taking the drug just to get through the day
- taking the drug in escalating dosage
- using the drug with alcohol
- shopping around for new doctors and/or pharmacists to avoid suspicion
- driving while apparently impaired

According to the Substance Abuse and Mental Health Services Administration, about 64 percent of older people admitted for substance abuse treatment in 2005 were white, followed by blacks (18 percent), Hispanics (14 percent), and other races and ethnicities (4 percent).

Mental Illness and Substance Abuse

It should also be noted that a history of mental illness is often linked to substance abuse, so doctors who think that they see DEPRESSION or anxiety in a substance abuser may be right. However, many older adults with depression or other psychiatric disorders are not diagnosed with psychiatric problems, or they believe that their depressed or anxious feelings are normal for older people. (See ANXIETY AND ANXIETY DISORDERS.)

Treatment of Substance Abuse

According to the Older American Substance Abuse and Mental Health Technical Assistance Center (a division of the Substance Abuse and Mental Health Services Administration) in their 2005 report, in part because of their increasing numbers, the number of older adults who will be needing substance abuse treatment will more than double from 1.7 million in 2001 to 4.4 million by 2020.

Among those age 50 years and older, there were 184,252 admissions to treatment centers in 2005. Of these, 6,722 people (4 percent) were ages 65 to 69, and 4,622 people (3 percent) were age 70 and older. People age 50 years and older represented about 10 percent of the total 1.8 million admissions for the treatment of substance abuse in 2005.

Older people also had fewer prior admissions for treatment than individuals younger than age 65; for example, 15 percent of individuals between the ages of 50 to 54 had been admitted for treatment five or more times in the past. Among those ages 55 to 59, 12 percent had been admitted for treatment five or more times in the past. However, among older people, only 7 percent of those ages 65 and older had been admitted for treatment five or more times in the past.

Military Veterans Substance Abusers

The veteran status of the substance abusers admitted for treatment varied considerably by age; for example, among those ages 50 to 54 who were admitted for the treatment of substance abuse, only 13 percent were military veterans. However, among those ages 70 and older, 31 percent were veterans.

TABLE 2. STATES WITH THE LARGEST NUMBERS AND HIGHEST RATES OF ADMISSIONS FOR SUBSTANCE ABUSE, AGE 65 AND OLDER, BY RANK: 2005

State	Number	State	Rate per 100,000 Aged 65 or Older
New York	3,140	Colorado	166
California	908	New York	125
Colorado	773	South Dakota	111
Arizona	395	Oregon	78
Minnesota	393	Connecticut	75
Oregon	365	Maine	72
Connecticut	356	Minnesota	63
Pennsylvania	325	Vermont	61
Illinois	310	Arizona	52
Maryland	305	Montana	51
Massachusetts	283	Maryland	47
Washington	270	Nebraska	42
New Jersey	244	Washington	37
Georgia	223	Iowa	36
Ohio	210	Kentucky	25

Source: Substance Abuse and Mental Health Services Administration. "Adults Aged 65 or Older in Substance Abuse Treatment: 2005." *The DASIS Report,* May 31, 2007, page 4. Available online. URL: http://www.drugabuse statistics.Samhsa.gov/2k/7/olderTX/older/TXpdf. Accessed July 6, 2007.

In considering the state-by-state admissions to treatment facilities for substance abuse, the highest rate among 15 states reporting data was found in New York (3,140 older people per 100,000), while 210 older people per 100,000 were admitted for treatment in Ohio. (See Table 2.) The rate of admissions per 100,000 people was also considered in addition to the sheer numbers of admissions. Using the rate of admissions in 15 states, the highest rate was found in Colorado (166 per 100,000 older people), and the lowest rate was found in Kentucky, or 35 people per 100,000 older people who were treated for substance abuse. Note that although New York has the highest number of admissions, the highest rate per 100,000 was in Colorado. The reason for this is that rates take into consideration the population of the state. Thus, when state population only is considered, there was a higher rate of admissions in Colorado than in New York.

See also ADVERSE DRUG EVENT; ALCOHOLISM; DIABETES; DRUG ABUSE; GENDER DIFFERENCES; INAPPROPRIRATE PRESCRIPTIONS FOR THE ELDERLY; NARCOTICS; PAINKILLING MEDICATIONS; PRESCRIPTION DRUG ABUSE/MISUSE.

Bartels, Stephen J., Frederic C. Blow, Laurie M. Brockmann, and Aricca D. Van Citters. *Substance Abuse and Mental Health among Older Americans: The State of the Knowledge and Future Directions.* Rockville, Md.: Substance Abuse and Mental Health Services Administration, August 11, 2005.

National Women's Health Resource Center. "Older Women & Substance Abuse." *National Women's Health Report* 28, no. 6 (December 2006): 6.

Substance Abuse and Mental Health Services Administration. "Adults Aged 65 or Older in Substance Abuse Treatment: 2005." *The DASIS Report,* May 31, 2007. Available online. URL: http://www.drugabusestatistics.Samhsa.gov/2k/7/olderTX/older/TXpdf. Accessed July 6, 2007.

———. "Older Adults in Substance Abuse Treatment: 2005." *The DASIS Report,* November 8, 2007. Available online. URL: http://oas.samhsa.gov/2k7/older/older.cfm. Accessed November 9, 2007.

suicide The purposeful termination of one's own life by the individual, sometimes with the assistance or the encouragement of others. (See ASSISTED SUICIDE.) In general, older individuals are at an increased risk for committing suicide compared to younger people of all ages.

In one study on medical illness and the risk for suicide in the elderly reported in *Archives of Internal Medicine* in 2004, the researchers found that some specific illnesses were associated with an increased risk for suicide, and they also found that multiple illnesses further escalated the risk. Among these illnesses were congestive heart failure, chronic obstructive lung disease, seizure disorder, URINARY INCONTINENCE, ANXIETY AND ANXIETY DISORDERS, DEPRESSION, psychotic disorders, bipolar disorder, and moderate to severe CHRONIC PAIN.

If a person says that he or she has a plan to carry out the act of suicide, this is a red flag for family members who should not ignore such statements. The person should not be left alone. Any guns in the house should be removed, as should unsupervised access to medications. The relative should call a crisis hotline or suicide crisis center and/or should contact the elderly person's physician. If the doctor is unavailable, contact the nearest emergency room or dial 911 for emergency services.

Older people have a greater risk for suicide than younger individuals. According to the National Institute of Mental Health (NIMH), adults age 65 and older represented only 12 percent of the population in the United States in 2004, but they accounted for about 16 percent of all suicide deaths in the United States. In considering suicide rates, the national average in the general population was 10.0 suicides per 100,000 people. The rate for individuals age 65 and older was 14.3 per 100,000 people.

Non-Hispanic white men age 85 and older were the most likely to die from suicide in 2004, and they had a rate of 17.8 suicide deaths per 100,000.

The suicide attempts that are made by elderly people are more likely to be successful and to result in death, in contrast to the many failed suicide attempts that are often made by younger individuals.

The suicide risk increases among those who believe that their ability to function in society is limited (whether their belief is valid or not). The risk for depression in older people who live in the general community ranges from about one to five percent, but it increases to 13.5 percent among those who need HOME HEALTH CARE, and it is 11.5 percent among elderly patients in the hospital.

According to the Substance Abuse & Mental Health Technical Assistance Center, the following are risk factors for suicide among older Americans:

- older age
- male
- race (white)
- depression
- ubstance abuse
- use of antianxiety drugs such as diazepam (Valium)

Older White Men and Suicide/Homicide

Older men are more likely to commit suicide than older women, and they are also more likely to kill their spouses and then kill themselves than are individuals of other ages. Men represent 82 percent of all suicides among older adults. In considering racial differences and suicide, white males age 65 and older have the highest risk for suicide, according to the Centers for Disease Control and Prevention (CDC), or 33.2 deaths per 100,000 people in 2000. The next highest suicide death rate is Hispanic men (17.2 deaths per 100,000 people), at nearly half the rate for white males.

Among older women, Asian or Pacific Islander females age 65 and older had the highest rate for suicide in 2000, or 5.4 per 100,000, followed by white women at 4.3 per 100,000 women.

Depression is a key cause for suicide. Other causes are the presence of terminal diseases such as CANCER and/or severe or chronic pain.

Means of Suicide and Associated Drugs

Guns are the most commonly used means of suicide among older adults, followed by poisons. The use of some prescription drugs, such as diazepam (Valium), has also been linked with suicides among older individuals. ALCOHOLISM is also correlated with suicide among older people.

If individuals discuss their desire to commit suicide and/or they describe a plan to carry out the suicide, their physicians should be contacted immediately.

Psychotherapy and medication work well to treat depression in suicidal older adults. According to the NIMH, studies have shown that 80 percent of older adults with depression recovered with combined treatment of therapy and medication.

Homicide-Suicides

Another form of suicide is the homicide-suicide, and nearly all such cases involve a husband who murders his wife and then kills himself.

According to a paper written in 2001 by Donna Cohen of the Department of Aging and Mental Health at the Florida Mental Health Institute at the University of South Florida, about 500 combination homicide-suicides (1,000 deaths) occur each year nationwide among people who are age 55 and older. Cohen says these are not pacts made together with a partner, nor are they acts of altruism. In fact, the victim rarely knows what is planned.

In a later article in 2005 by Malphurs and Cohen for the *American Journal of Geriatric Psychiatry*, the authors noted that of 29 spousal-homicidal cases of individuals age 55 and older compared with 58 suicide victims, the homicide-suicide perpetrators were more likely to have exhibited domestic violence or they were caregivers to their wives. In contrast, the suicide victims were often receiving caregiving from their wives and had health problems. Both groups were depressed.

Family members or others who perceive that stress and conflict is present in a male caregiver to his wife, especially if he has exhibited violence in the past, should seek help to determine if the female partner is at risk.

Often the victim is murdered in her sleep. In most cases, says Cohen, the homicide-suicide occurs because the male perpetrator actively fears a threat to the relationship, such as an imminent move of one or both parties to a nursing home. Other motives are a real or imagined change in health or increased marital conflict.

Cohen says that there are clues to a risk for a homicide-suicide that others can identify and act upon. Some key clues are

- a marriage of long standing, with the husband playing a dominant role

- a male caregiver whose wife has ALZHEIMER'S DISEASE or another form of DEMENTIA
- a husband and wife who have many medical problems, one or both of whom are becoming more ill
- a move to a nursing home or assisted-living facility is under consideration and a distinct possibility
- the couple has become increasingly socially isolated from both their family and their friends

Cohen says that adult children and others should take note if the husband exhibits the following behavioral patterns:

- He says that he is feeling hopeless or helpless.
- He loses interest in former activities.
- He talks about harming his wife.

Giving away important items and crying for no reason are other indicators of a possible homicide-suicide plan. Family members should ask the individual if he has thought about suicide or homicide-suicide, and they should also offer their help so that the individual does not feel compelled to go through with the crimes.

See also ASSISTED SUICIDE; BEREAVEMENT; DEATH; FAMILY CAREGIVERS; GENDER DIFFERENCES; NARCOTICS; PAINKILLING MEDICATIONS; PRESCRIPTION DRUG ABUSE/MISUSE; SUBSTANCE ABUSE AND DEPENDENCE.

Cohen, Donna. "Homicide-Suicide in Older Persons: How You Can Help Prevent a Tragedy." Tampa, Fla.: Department of Aging and Mental Health, Florida Mental Health Institute, University of South Florida, 2001.

Juurlink, David N., M.D., et al. "Medical Illness and the Risk of Suicide in the Elderly." *Archives of Internal Medicine* 164 (June 14, 2004): 1,179–1,184.

Malphurs, Julie E., and Donna Cohen. "A State Case-Control Study of Spousal Homicide-Suicide in Older Persons." *American Journal of Geriatric Psychiatry* 13 (March 2005): 211–217.

Substance Abuse & Mental Health Technical Assistance Center. *Suicide Prevention for Older Adults.* (undated) Washington, D.C.: U.S. Department of Health and Human Services.

sundowning Refers to sleeping during the day and staying awake at night, a reversal of the common sleep patterns of most people. Sundowning is often found among individuals with ALZHEIMER'S DISEASE, and this behavior can be very difficult for caregivers to deal with, since most caregivers sleep at night and they are active in the day; hence, it is difficult for people with normal sleep patterns to monitor older people who are awake and alert all night long. However, there are some effective means to discourage sundowning behaviors, such as placing heavy draperies or shades on the windows so that the older person believes that it is evening during the day.

See also DEMENTIA; SLEEP DISORDERS.

talking to elderly parents about difficult issues

Many ADULT CHILDREN/CHILDREN OF AGING PARENTS struggle with talking to their aging parents about certain issues, and particularly with end-of-life issues (such as whether the parent wishes extreme measures to be taken if he or she becomes extremely ill or what arrangements they want for their remains after death), financial issues (such as whether the parent has a will and whether they have sufficient funds to support themselves), and health issues (such as what medications they take and what medical problem[s] they have been diagnosed with).

Some adult children may believe, for example, that if they ask a parent if he or she has made a will, the parent will think that the adult child is greedy and grasping and/or wishes that the parent was dead. In fact, some aging parents may actually have such thoughts, but in most cases, their fears can be assuaged. One way to do this is to talk about a friend or acquaintance whose parent died and how the lack of information the adult children had led to chaos and confusion for the family.

Sometimes elderly parents have not maintained adequate financial records, and they may feel embarrassed about this, or they may not even realize that there is a problem. Aging parents may have many reasons for not keeping their records current. Says Dan Taylor, author of *The Parent Care Conversation: Six Strategies for Transforming the Emotional and Financial Future of Your Aging Parents*:

> The manner in which many people go about organizing and updating their financial affairs and records often resembles that familiar vacation spot called Someday Isle. The net result for the child, who must parachute in and find everything when an emergency arises, or organize assets for distribution following the death of a parent, can sometimes be like a scavenger hunt. In order to

find the last house payment made, it may become necessary to sift through months of statements covering a host of expenses, ranging from gas bills and car payments to American Legion dues and Colonial Penn's guaranteed issue term life premiums. And typically, this must all be accomplished at a moment of maximum personal stress.

Taylor recommends that adult children who are highly organized offer to put their parents' financial affairs in order for them as a gift. If the adult child is not highly organized, he or she can hire a professional organizer to accomplish this task. Another suggestion is for the adult child to put his or her own financial affairs in order first, and then tell the parents that he or she feels so much better knowing where everything is and that everything is taken care of.

If these tactics do not work, the adult child could tell the parents that if they fail to keep their financial affairs current and accessible, when they do need help, it will be impossible for anyone to help them. No caveats should be added, but the statement should be made flatly, with no additions. It may not have an immediate effect, but in many cases, the parents may eventually provide the needed information.

In one case, an adult child told her parents that she could not obtain their personal papers if they died or were incapacitated because she had no key to their house. She made this statement simply several times and thought it had no effect, until one day her father threw a set of house keys in her direction, saying, "Here!" The adult child chose to avoid a confrontation and simply put the keys away, believing that her father had great difficulty surrendering even a part of his independence.

Another extremely difficult topic to talk about is when it is time for a parent to stop driving, because they are physically and/or mentally too incapacitated to drive anymore. Many elderly individuals have been driving since they turned 16, and they associate driving with adulthood and independence. They may fear that it will be hard or impossible to find someone to drive them places, and they may not like the idea of having to be dependent on others.

Rather than waiting for the parent to have a car accident that may injure or kill him or her or others (to build up one's resolve, imagine if a child were run over), it is best to talk to the parent about whether they have thought about letting someone else drive them where they need to go. Before this conversation occurs, the adult child should attempt to anticipate the various arguments that the parent may have, such as that they live too faraway from the bus stop to take the bus, that they need the car to go to the weekly bingo game, or simply that everything is fine and there is no problem.

The adult child should plan counterarguments such as the parent could take a taxi or get a neighbor to drive him or her and offer to pay for the gas. To the flat statement that everything is fine, the adult child could point out that the parent has already had several accidents and ask them to imagine how they would feel if they ever injured or killed a child while driving. The adult child could also ask the parent if they have discussed the driving issue with their physician.

Another difficult subject involves potential relocation. The parent may need to move to an ASSISTED-LIVING FACILITY or senior housing apartment, because their home has become too difficult to manage with increasing mental and physical incapacity. However, although this need for a move may be evident to many people, it may be far from clear to the elderly parent, who may not wish to leave a beloved home and may fear having to give up items that will not fit into an apartment or assisted-living facility.

The adult child could offer to go with the parent to view senior apartments or assisted-living facilities to see what they are like. Unless it is a pressing issue, in most cases, the adult child should not pressure the parent to relocate immediately because it may take time for the idea to become acceptable to the parent.

See also DRIVING; DURABLE POWER OF ATTORNEY; HEALTH-CARE AGENT/PROXY; LIVING WILL; MENTAL COMPETENCY; POWER OF ATTORNEY; SIBLING RIVALRY AND CONFLICT; WILLS.

Taylor, Dan. *The Parent Care Conversation: Six Strategies for Transforming the Emotional and Financial Future of Your Aging Parents.* New York: Penguin Books, 2006.

tension headaches   Despite their name, tension-type headaches are not solely caused by tension or stress in a person's life. Stress can make such headaches worse, but it does not initially cause them. According to Walker and Wadman, the tension headache is present in about half (44.5 percent) of patients age 65 and older, and most older patients have six headaches per month.

Symptoms and Diagnostic Path

The tension headache causes severe pain that occurs on both sides of the head. Often the headache is in a "hatband" distribution. This type of headache may last for hours or for much longer. It is diagnosed based on its symptoms and ruling out other causes of pain. Physicians may order a magnetic resonance imaging (MRI) scan of the head and brain to rule out a brain tumor. They may also do an X-ray or an MRI of the neck to look for a source of this kind of headache. Laboratory tests can rule out metabolic disorders and blood diseases.

Treatment Options and Outlook

Many people gain relief from tension headaches by taking over-the-counter analgesics such as acetaminophen (Tylenol) or ibuprofen. Others need prescribed drugs such as nonsteroidal anti-inflammatory drugs (NSAIDs) or muscle relaxants. Some people with tension headaches improve with triptan migraine remedies, such as sumatriptan (Imitrex). Heat or ice may also improve the condition. (Heat or ice should be wrapped in a cloth and never placed directly on the skin.)

Risk Factors and Preventive Measures

Men are more likely to suffer from tension headaches than women, but these types of headaches are relatively common in both sexes.

When possible, it is best for patients with chronic headaches to try to identify if there are any particular triggers to the tension headache (or any other type of headache). For example, stress, some foods (chocolate, caffeine, etc.), and other factors may induce a headache in some people. If particular triggers to headaches are found, those items should be avoided.

See also HEADACHES.

thyroid cancer According to the American Cancer Society, there were 33,550 new cases of thyroid cancer diagnosed in 2007, including 8,070 men and 25,480 women. An estimated 1,530 people died of thyroid cancer in 2007, including 650 men and 880 women. Adults age 60 and older are more likely to develop the most deadly form of this cancer, anaplastic thyroid cancer, than younger individuals.

The thyroid is an endocrine gland in the neck. There are four primary types of thyroid cancer: papillary thyroid cancer, follicular thyroid cancer, medullary thyroid cancer, and anaplastic thyroid cancer.

Papillary thyroid cancer, which constitutes about 80 percent of all thyroid cancers in the United States, grows slowly, and many people with this form of cancer can be cured, according to the National Cancer Institute. Follicular thyroid cancer represents about 15 percent of all thyroid cancers. If it is diagnosed in an early stage, most people can be treated successfully. Medullary thyroid cancer, which presents about 3 percent of all thyroid cancers, grows slowly and is easier to control if it is discovered and treated before spreading to other parts of the body. Anaplastic thyroid cancer, which comprises about 2 percent of all thyroid cancers, tends to grow rapidly and spread fast. It is very difficult to control.

Symptoms and Diagnostic Path

Thyroid cancer usually does not have symptoms in the early stage. As the cancer grows, symptoms may include

- a lump in the front of the neck
- voice changes and hoarseness
- swollen lymph nodes in the neck
- trouble with breathing or swallowing
- throat or neck pain that does not go away

Note that often the above symptoms are due to an infection, a benign goiter, or another health problem that is not cancer. However, if the symptoms do not disappear within several weeks, the individual should see a physician.

Thyroid cancer is diagnosed with a physical examination in which the doctor checks the thyroid for lumps (nodules) and swelling or growths in the lymph nodes nearby. An endocrinologist is a physician who specializes in treating endocrine system diseases, including thyroid cancer. The doctor may order a laboratory test for thyroid-stimulating hormone (TSH) to check for an abnormal TSH level.

An ultrasound and a thyroid scan will provide further information. A biopsy is the only way to determine if the patient has cancer. The biopsy can be performed with a fine-needle aspiration, in which the doctor removes a tiny sample of tissue with a thin needle from a thyroid nodule. An ultrasound can help the doctor see where the needle should be positioned. If the fine-needle aspiration cannot help with diagnosis, a surgeon can remove the nodule for biopsy.

Before having the biopsy for possible thyroid cancer, patients should ask the following questions:

- Will I have to go to the hospital for the biopsy?
- How long will it take?
- Will I be awake? Will it hurt?
- Are there any risks? What are the chances of infection or bleeding after the biopsy?
- How long will it take for me to recover?
- Will I have a scar on my neck?
- How soon will I know the results? Who will explain them to me?
- If I were your parent, what treatment would you recommend?
- If I do have cancer, who will talk to me about the next steps? When?

If thyroid cancer is present, the doctor must determine whether the cancer has spread and if so, to what location it has spread. In general, thyroid cancer spreads to lymph nodes, lungs, and bones. To help the doctor determine the status of the cancer (also known as staging), the patient may have one or more tests, including an ultrasound, a computerized tomography (CT) scan, a magnetic resonance imaging (MRI) scan, a chest X-ray, or a whole body scan.

Treatment Options and Outlook

The choice of treatment depends on the type of cancer, the size of the nodule, the age of the patient, and whether the thyroid cancer has spread. Surgery and/or external radiation therapy are options to remove or destroy thyroid cancer. Systemic therapies may also be used, such as thyroid hormone treatment, radioactive iodine therapy, and chemotherapy.

Before treatment for thyroid cancer begins, patients should ask the following questions:

- What type of thyroid cancer do I have? May I have a copy of the report from the pathologist?
- What is the stage of my disease? Has the cancer spread from the thyroid? If so, to where?
- What are my treatment choices? Which do you recommend for me? Why?
- Will I have more than one kind of treatment?
- What are the expected benefits of each kind of treatment?
- What are the risks and possible side effects of each treatment? What can we do to control the side effects?
- What can I do to prepare for treatment?
- Will I need to say in the hospital? If so, for how long?
- How will treatment affect my normal activities?
- What is my chance for a full recovery?
- Would a clinical trial be appropriate for me? Can you help me find one?
- How often will I need checkups?

If the patient has surgery, the surgeon may perform a total thyroidectomy through an incision in the neck. Nearby lymph nodes will also be removed. If the patient has follicular or papillary thyroid cancer, the surgeon may remove only part of the thyroid. After surgery, most people need to take thyroid hormone replacement pills, despite the form of surgery that was chosen. If the surgeon also removes the parathyroid glands, glands that are embedded in the thyroid gland, patients may need to take vitamin D pills and calcium for the rest of their lives. The calcium levels in their bodies will need to be carefully monitored.

Before the surgery patients should ask their surgeons the following questions:

- Which type of surgery do you suggest for me?
- Do I need any lymph nodes removed? Will the parathyroid glands or other tissues be removed? Why?
- What are the risks of surgery?
- How will I feel after surgery? If I have pain, how will it be controlled?
- How long will I be in the hospital?
- What will my scar look like?
- Will I have any lasting side effects?
- Will I need to take thyroid hormone pills? If so, how soon will I start taking them? Will I need to take them for the rest of my life?
- When can I get back to my normal activities?

Sometimes thyroid hormone pills are given as a treatment to block cancer, as with papillary or follicular thyroid cancer. They slow the growth of remaining thyroid cancer calls that are left in the body after surgery.

Radioactive iodine (I-131) therapy is another form of treatment for thyroid cancer and is used with patients who have papillary or follicular thyroid cancer. This therapy is given as a capsule or a liquid. It is often given as an outpatient treatment, although some people must stay in the hospital for a day or two. It is important to protect the bladder from the effects of treatment by drinking large quantities of fluids.

Patients who will be receiving radioactive iodine therapy should ask the following questions:

- Why do I need this treatment? What will it do?
- How do I prepare for this treatment? Do I need to avoid foods and medicine that have iodine in them? For how long?

- How do I protect my family members and others from the radiation? For how many days?

- Will the I-131 therapy cause side effects? What can I do about them?

- What is the chance that I will be given I-131 therapy again in the future?

Another form of radiation is external radiation therapy, which uses high-energy rays from a large machine to kill the cancer cells. Most patients receive treatment at a hospital or clinic for five days a week for several weeks. Treatments last for a few minutes. Radiation to the neck may cause the mouth to be dry and sore and may also cause hoarseness and difficulty swallowing. The skin may be red and tender. Radiation therapy often causes fatigue, particularly after several weeks.

Patients who will be receiving external radiation therapy should ask the following questions:

- Why do I need this treatment? When will the treatments begin? How often will I have them? When will they end?

- How will I feel during treatment?

- How will we know if the radiation treatment is working?

- What can I do to take care of myself during treatment?

- Can I continue my normal activities?

- Are there any lasting side effects?

Chemotherapy is the treatment that is used with anaplastic thyroid cancer, and it may also be used to relieve symptoms of medullary thyroid cancer or other forms of thyroid cancer. Chemotherapy drugs are injected into a vein, and they kill cancer cells throughout the body. Treatment may be given in a clinic, but some people are hospitalized during treatment. The most common side effects of chemotherapy are nausea and vomiting, loss of appetite, sore mouth, and hair loss.

Patients who will be receiving chemotherapy for thyroid cancer should ask the following questions:

- Why do I need this treatment? What will it do?

- Will I have side effects? What can I do about them?

- How long will I be on this treatment?

Risk Factors and Preventive Measures

Prior radiation is a risk factor for thyroid cancer. From the 1920s to the 1950s, children with acne, enlarged tonsils, and other head and neck problems were sometime treated with high dose X-rays. Doctors discovered later that some people who had received such treatment developed thyroid cancer. (Routine X-rays are generally safe, although shields may be needed to protect other parts of the body.) Radioactive fallout can produce thyroid cancer, such as with the nuclear power plant accident in Chernobyl in the Soviet Union in 1986.

A family history of medullary thyroid cancer increases the risk for the development of thyroid cancer, particularly when a change in the RET gene (officially known as the ret-proto-oncogene, according to the National Institutes of Health) occurs. Most people with the changed gene develop medullary thyroid cancer. A blood test can determine if the changed RET gene is present.

A family history of goiters (swollen thyroids) or having multiple polyps in the colon or rectum are risks for the development of papillary thyroid cancer. In addition, people who have had a goiter or benign thyroid nodules also have an increased risk for developing thyroid cancer.

Women are nearly three times more likely than men to have thyroid cancer.

Most people with thyroid cancer are older than age 45, and those with anaplastic thyroid cancer are usually older than age 60.

See also CANCER.

thyroid disease An abnormality of the thyroid, which is a butterfly-shaped gland that is located in the front of the neck. The key thyroid disorders are hyperthyroidism, which is an excess of thyroid hormone, and hypothyroidism, which is an insufficient amount of thyroid hormone. When they have thyroid disease, older people are more likely to have abnormally low levels of thyroid, although it is possible for them to have overly high levels.

Risk Factors

It is important to screen for hypothyroidism among symptomatic individuals, because the symptoms of severe hypothyroidism (lethargy, weakness, and confusion) may be confused with those of DEMENTIA. Hypothyroidism is relatively easy to treat by administering thyroid medication.

Causes of Thyroid Disease

Many thyroid diseases are autoimmune disorders, which means that the body has mistakenly attacked the thyroid gland as it would a foreign invader, either overproducing or underproducing thyroid hormone, depending on the form of the disease.

In fewer cases, thyroid disease results from reactions to some medications, such as lithium (which is usually prescribed for manic depression) or amiodarone (which may be given for some heart conditions), both of which may trigger hypothyroidism. Much more rarely, a disorder of the hypothalamus or the pituitary gland may cause hypothyroidism.

Symptoms of Hyperthyroidism

Hyperthyroidism, or excessively high levels of thyroid hormone, may be detected by a physician when a patient has some or all of the symptoms listed below. Hyperthyroidism is dangerous because it can stress the heart and the body unnecessarily.

Note: these symptoms may also indicate many other diseases, and, thus, only an experienced physician can perform the diagnosis. In most cases, an endocrinologist should treat thyroid disease.

- elevated heart rate (pulse) of more than 100 beats per minute
- enlarged thyroid
- increased requirement for insulin and worsening of blood glucose levels, if the person has diabetes
- insomnia/nightmares
- weight loss despite a greater appetite
- heavy sweating
- extreme nervousness and irritability/anxiety
- heat intolerance
- shaking hands

- decreased menstruation or no menstruation prior to menopause or surgical removal of the uterus

Symptoms of Hypothyroidism

There are basic symptoms common to many people whose thyroid levels are low. However, these symptoms may also indicate other diseases. Common symptoms of hypothyroidism are:

- chronic constipation
- puffy face, especially under the eyes
- dry and itchy skin, doughy skin
- depression/lack of energy/apathy
- sensitivity to cold temperatures
- decreased need for insulin in those who have DIABETES
- muscle cramps and aches
- more frequent bowel movements (although not diarrhea)

The most common form of hypothyroidism is Hashimoto's thyroiditis. This is an autoimmune condition in which the body mistakenly makes antibodies (proteins) against the enzyme in the thyroid. Initially, it can cause *hyper*thyroidism, but more frequently this disease will result in *hypo*thyroidism because of the ongoing damage to the thyroid gland.

Diagnosing Thyroid Disease

If doctors believe that patients may have thyroid disease based on the symptoms displayed, then they will usually order a blood test known as a TSH (thyroid-stimulating hormone) assay. This will determine whether the thyroid levels are high, low, or within the normal range. Although one might think that high TSH levels mean hyperthyroidisrn, the reverse is true. The lower the TSH outside the normal range, the more hyperthyroid a person is. The higher the TSH outside the normal range, the more hypothyroid the person is.

Treatment Options and Outlook

The treatment of thyroid disease depends on the type of disease. Treatment may be very simple, such as prescribing supplemental thyroid hormone to the hypothyroid patient and following up with periodic blood tests to ensure that the blood levels of thyroid are in the normal range. Conversely, if the person has excessive levels of thyroid, the physician may attempt to suppress the thyroid function through various means, such as with prescribing antithyroid pills or radioactive iodine. In some cases, surgery will become necessary. Generally, a subtotal thyroidectomy is performed, leaving part of the thyroid gland intact. Sometimes, a total thyroidectomy is performed.

See also THYROID CANCER.

tinnitus A constant or an intermittent ringing in the ears that affects about 50 million Americans who hear ringing, hissing, or other sounds that other people cannot hear. It is present in nearly one third of all adults older than age 70. Age-related nerve impairment is the chief cause of tinnitus among older individuals.

Other risk factors for tinnitus include

- wax in the ear canal
- stiffening of bones in the middle ear (otosclerosis)
- allergies
- hypertension or hypotension
- a tumor
- DIABETES
- thyroid abnormalities
- a head or neck injury

It is often impossible to determine the specific cause of tinnitus, and thus the condition can rarely be cured. Some strategies that may help include

- medications such as antidepressants or antianxiety drugs
- avoiding loud noises
- electrical stimulation procedures
- limiting or altogether eliminating caffeine and tobacco
- resting
- using biofeedback

- hearing aids, sleep machines, and masking devices

See also HEARING DISORDERS.

toileting It may become difficult or impossible for some older adults to get to the toilet in time because of their problems with URINARY INCONTINENCE or FECAL INCONTINENCE. These problems may be caused by a medical problem or by medications. Patients who have had STROKES may have to relearn basic ACTIVITIES OF DAILY LIVING, including toileting.

Some older people have difficulty using standard toilets and do much better with higher toilets meant for disabled individuals. These toilets can replace standard toilets in most homes or apartments. When possible, elderly individuals should be encouraged to continue to use the toilet to avoid the problem of LEARNED HELPLESSNESS.

See also BATHING AND CLEANLINESS.

transportation The means by which older people travel to essential places, such as to the supermarket, appointments with physicians, to see their friends, and so on. Individuals who live in ASSISTED-LIVING FACILITIES often have transportation provided to stores and doctors' offices as part of the services offered by the facility, but individuals who continue to live in a home or an apartment on their own usually do not receive any such assistance. Many older people drive themselves to wherever they need to go, but this functionality may become problematic as they become older and their reaction times slow considerably or illnesses make it very difficult for them to drive anymore.

Some questions to ask a transportation provider include the following, provided by the Administration on Aging. The responses to these questions will enable a caregiver to determine if the transportation is suitable for their parent or other elderly relative.

- What is the service area covered?
- How much will the service cost?
- Will insurance pay for rides provided by the service?

- Are there requirements to qualify for the services? If so, what are they?

- Is there an evaluation that must take place prior to the first ride?

- Is there a membership fee that must be paid before scheduling rides with the service?

- How far in advance must reservations be made?

- Are rides provided in the evenings, weekends, or on holidays?

- Are rides provided to social as well as medical or shopping appointments?

- Are door-through-door, door-to-door, or curb-to-curb services provided? (e.g., services to inside the house, to the door of the home, or to the curb where the home is located.)

- Are rides provided to people who use wheelchairs?

- Do riders stay in their wheelchairs, or are they transferred to a seat during the ride?

- Is there an escort or attendant in the vehicle with the driver?

- Does someone stay with my family member during appointments?

- Can a family member serve as an escort? If so, is there an extra cost associated?

- Will there be a wait when picked up from home? If so, how long?

- Will there be a wait when picked up for the return trip? If so, how long?

- Will the driver or attendant come into the office/building for the return trip?

- Will other passengers be riding? If so, what is the maximum length of time of the ride while others are being picked up/dropped off?

It may not be possible for an older person with Alzheimer's or another form of dementia to use any form of public transportation, and conse-quently, relative caregivers become the primary transportation providers. Transporting a parent or relative with Alzheimer's disease or another form of dementia can be challenging for even the most loving person. The Administration on Aging suggests the following tips to ease this task:

- Be patient and allow time to get ready and get into the car.

- Try to allow your loved one time to calm down before entering the car.

- Be prepared with relaxing music, sunglasses, photos, food, etc.

- Seat your loved one in the rear passenger side seat with a seat belt on and the child lock in the "on" position.

- Encourage your loved one to do as much as possible for himself or herself.

- Try to keep glare from the sun to a minimum.

- Give information in small bits.

- Stay calm.

- Validate your loved one's feelings whenever possible (for example, "Yes, it is really hot outside"; "Yes, there are a lot of cars on the road today").

- Give brief, step-by-step directions.

- Encourage reminiscence.

- Be aware of your own body language.

- Ask your loved one to use the bathroom before getting into the car.

- Keep a cell phone in the car in case of an emergency.

See also DRIVING; TALKING TO ELDERLY PARENTS ABOUT DIFFICULT ISSUES.

Administration on Aging. *Transportation Tips for Caregivers.* U.S. Department of Health and Human Services, November 1, 2004.

ulcers, peptic Very painful sores within the digestive system that usually appear in the stomach or elsewhere in the digestive tract, such as in the small intestine. In the recent past, it was believed and generally accepted by most doctors that most ulcers were caused by stress and that reducing stress (in addition to lowering stomach acid) would improve healing an ulcer. However, research has demonstrated that most ulcers (about two-thirds) are caused by a specific bacterium, *Helicobacter pylori*. In addition, some ulcers are induced by the frequent use of some medications, especially nonsteroidal anti-inflammatory drugs (NSAIDs), including both over-the-counter and prescribed NSAIDs. Both the bacteria and the NSAIDs weaken the stomach lining and allow acids to damage the wall of the stomach and small intestine.

Although stress does not cause ulcers, it is also true that, as with many medical conditions, stress can increase the individual's overall pain. Spicy foods, alcohol, and smoking can also worsen the pain from ulcers. Caffeine may also be a major irritant for the individual with an ulcer.

Symptoms and Diagnostic Path

Ulcers may cause a chronic burning pain in the gut, which may be severe. The pain usually feels like a dull ache, and it may come and go for a few days or weeks. It usually starts within two to three hours after eating a meal, and it may also come in the middle of the night when the stomach is empty. The pain generally disappears after eating.

Other symptoms may include

- weight loss
- lack of appetite
- pain while eating
- nausea and vomiting

If peptic ulcers are not diagnosed and treated, the symptoms can worsen. A doctor should be called immediately if any of the following symptoms are present because they may be life threatening:

- a sudden sharp pain that does not go away
- black or bloody stools
- bloody vomit or vomit that resembles coffee grounds
- profound weakness or fatigue

Doctors diagnose ulcers using an upper gastrointestinal series. A gastroenterologist is a physician who has specialized training in the treatment of digestive disorders and diseases, including ulcers. The patient drinks barium to help make the stomach and small intestine show up clearly on X-rays. Another test that can detect an ulcer is the endoscopy, in which the patient is medicated and a thin tube (the endoscope) is passed through the mouth and into the stomach and duodenum. The doctor may also remove stomach tissue to take a biopsy. In addition, the doctor may test the patient's breath to see whether *H. pylori* is present.

Treatment Options and Outlook

If an individual is diagnosed with an ulcer, he or she needs medication. Proton pump inhibitors or histamine receptor blockers are medicines to stop the stomach from making acids and give the stomach a chance to heal. Antibiotics are also given to kill the bacteria. If NSAIDs are the cause of the ulcer, the individual must stop taking them.

Risk Factors and Preventive Measures

Individuals who have had ulcers in the past are at risk for developing them again, as are people who take NSAIDs, whether they are over-the-counter or prescribed NSAIDs. In addition, people who smoke or drink are at risk for developing peptic ulcers, as are those who are age 50 and older. Individuals whose relatives have had peptic ulcers also have an increased risk for developing ulcers.

Stress does not cause ulcers, but it can worsen existing ones, as stress worsens many medical problems, such as chronic HEADACHES, BACK PAIN, and so forth.

See also ADVERSE DRUG EVENT; APPETITE, CHRONIC LACK OF; INAPPROPRIATE PRESCRIPTIONS FOR THE ELDERLY.

urinary incontinence Difficulty with retaining bladder control, often causing a loss of urine, which may be a small or a large amount. The older person may have to wear incontinence pads or even adult DIAPERS, depending on the extent of the urine loss. Individuals with urinary incontinence should seek the assistance of a urologist to diagnose the cause of the incontinence and develop a treatment plan. A urologist is a specialist physician who treats diseases and disorders of the urinary tract and kidneys, as well as diseases of the male prostate gland, such as PROSTATE CANCER or other PROSTATE DISEASES. The urologist is also a surgeon. It should not be assumed that because someone is older than age 65 that they must wear padding in the underwear or even diapers. However, an estimated one in 10 people age 65 and older have some level of urinary incontinence.

Urinary incontinence has many causes, and there may be multiple causes in one person. For example, chronic constipation can cause urinary incontinence, as can vaginal infections, urinary tract infections, and weak bladder muscles. In addition, some diseases can lead to urinary incontinence, such as PARKINSON'S DISEASE. Damage from a man's enlarged prostate can cause urinary incontinence.

Symptoms and Diagnostic Path

Dribbling of urine or outright accidents are symptoms of possible urinary incontinence. There are several different types of incontinence, including stress incontinence, urge incontinence, overflow incontinence, and functional incontinence.

With stress incontinence, urine leaks when the person laughs or coughs, exercises, lifts heavy objects, or takes action that places pressure on the bladder. This type of incontinence is more common among middle-aged women, although it may occur in women at the onset of menopause.

Urge incontinence is an embarrassing condition in which the person cannot hold the urine in time to make it to the toilet. It is most often found in individuals with DIABETES, STROKE, ALZHEIMER'S DISEASE, Parkinson's disease, or multiple sclerosis. It may also be an early sign of bladder CANCER.

Overflow incontinence is a leakage of a small amount of urine. This medical problem may occur when a man has an enlarged prostate that blocks the urethra so that much of the urine cannot be expelled. In addition, individuals with diabetes and spinal cord injury may have overflow incontinence.

Functional incontinence occurs among some older people who have difficulty getting to the toilet fast enough because arthritis or other disorders make it hard for them to move fast enough.

Treatment Options and Outlook

Medications can be prescribed to treat urinary incontinence, depending on the cause. If menopause is a factor, then vaginal estrogen cream may be helpful. Some drugs can prevent bladder spasms that contribute to urinary incontinence. If the person has stress incontinence, an implant may be injected into the area around the urethra. The doctor may also recommend exercises to help strengthen the urinary muscles, such as Kegel exercises in which the patient alternately tightens and loosens bladder muscles. In some cases, however, surgery is indicated.

See also FECAL INCONTINENCE; TOILETING.

urologist See CANCER; PROSTATE CANCER; PROSTATE DISEASES; URINARY INCONTINENCE.

vascular dementia   See BINSWANGER'S DISEASE.

veteran benefits   Benefits that are provided by the Veterans Health Administration (VHA) to veterans (individuals who have been in the military service in the United States) such as monthly payments, outpatient medical care, and hospital care. Most elderly veterans are males, but there are a very small number of female veterans. As individuals age, there will be increasing numbers of female veterans in the future.

The Veterans' Administration (VA) operates the largest integrated health-care system in the United States, with more than 1,300 care sites including clinics, hospitals, nursing homes, counseling centers, and other facilities.

Veterans may apply for benefits by completing VA Form 10-10EZ, Application for Health Benefits, which is available at benefits offices or VA health-care facilities as well as online at URL: http://www.va.gov/1010ez.htm.

The VA prioritizes veterans by their level of service-connected disabilities. Those who are evaluated at a service-connected disability of 50 percent or more, or who are determined by the VA to be unemployable due to service-connected conditions, are given this top priority. (Note that most elderly veterans will have received their rating many years ago.)

Veterans with service-connected disabilities that are rated 30 to 40 percent are in Group 2.

Those with service-connected disabilities that are rated 10 to 20 percent, as well as former prisoners of war (POWs), those who were awarded a Purple Heart medal (for being wounded in battlefield conditions), and several other categories are in Group 3.

Group 4 includes veterans receiving aid or housebound benefits or those who are classified as catastrophically disabled. Group 5 includes those who are either receiving VA pension benefits or are eligible for Medicaid, as well as non-service-connected veterans whose net worth is below established thresholds. Several other categories are also included.

Veterans who are 50 percent or more disabled from service-connected conditions, who are unemployable due to service-connected conditions, or who are receiving care for a service-connected disability have special access to care. Veterans should contact the VA for further information.

Some veterans must pay co-pays for their VA health care.

For those veterans who are blind and enrolled in the VA health-care system, they may receive the following:

- a health and benefits review
- adjustment to blindness training
- home improvements and structural alterations to their homes
- special adaptations
- low-vision aids and training
- electronic and mechanical aids for the blind
- guide costs including training costs
- talking books, tapes, and Braille literature

The VA provides nursing home care for those who need short-term care or those with a 70 percent or greater service-connected disability. The VA contracts with nursing homes for services.

Studies of Older Veterans

Some older veterans receive their health care in VHA hospitals or clinics, while others receive their care at hospitals or clinics near their homes, paid for by MEDICARE, MEDICAID, or private insurance.

A study of elderly male veterans receiving care through the Veterans Health Administration reported in 2007 in the *American Journal of Public Health* compared preventive services received through the VHA to services received in Medicare fee-for-service or Medicare health maintenance organization plans. The researchers found that the veterans receiving care through the VHA had a 10 percent greater rate of influenza vaccination, a 15 percent greater rate of vaccination for pneumonia, and a 15 percent greater use of prostate cancer screening than veterans receiving care through Medicare HMOs.

There was also reportedly less screening with Medicare fee-for-service organizations than through the VHA, and veterans who received their care through Medicare fee-for-services reported receiving less care for preventive measures than did the veterans who obtained their care through Medicare HMOs. Thus, preventive care through the VHA was superior to the other two services.

In another study of inpatient psychiatric care through the VHA that compared the race of the inpatients, published in *Psychiatric Services* in 2000, the researchers studied nearly 24,000 male veterans age 60 years and older who were admitted to acute inpatient units in 1994. They found that a significantly greater proportion of African-American veterans were diagnosed with cognitive disorders, substance use disorders, and psychotic disorders, followed by Hispanics, and last by Caucasians. However, the rate of mood disorders was markedly less among African Americans and was about half the rate found among older white patients who were admitted. The rate differential decreased with age, but African Americans age 70 and older still had much higher rates of cognitive and psychotic disorders than Hispanics or Caucasians and also had much lower rates of mood disorders.

For example, 26.9 percent of the African-American elderly veterans age 70 and older were diagnosed with psychotic disorders compared with 25.3 percent of the Hispanic veterans and 20.1 percent of the Caucasian veterans. Yet in the case of mood disorders, only 6.5 percent of the African Americans had such a diagnosis compared with

17.3 percent of Caucasians and 20.4 percent of Hispanics.

It is unknown why the rate of mood disorders was markedly lower among the elderly African-American veterans, but further studies may provide answers.

Documents Needed to Verify and Process VA Claims When a Veteran Dies

When a veteran dies, according to the VA, the following documents are needed to process claims:

- the veteran's proof of military discharge papers
- the veteran's marriage certificate for claims of a surviving spouse or children
- the veteran's death certificate if the veteran did not die in a VHA facility
- the veteran's children's birth certificates or adoption papers to determine minor children's benefits
- the veteran's birth certificate to determine parents' benefits

See also ALZHEIMER'S DISEASE; CANCER.

Department of Veterans Affairs. *Federal Benefits for Veterans and Dependents. 2007 Edition.* Washington, D.C.: Department of Veterans Affairs, 2007.

Kales, Helen C., M.D. "Race and Inpatient Psychiatric Diagnoses among Elderly Veterans." *Psychiatric Services* 51, no. 6 (June 2000): 795–800.

Keyhani, Salomeh, M.D., et al. "Use of Preventive Care by Elderly Male Veterans Receiving Care through the Veterans Health Administration, Medicare Fee-for-Service, and Medicare HMO Plans." *American Journal of Public Health* 97, no. 12 (December 2007): 2,179–2,185.

vitamin and mineral deficiencies/excesses   Either insufficient or excessive blood levels of vitamins and/or minerals, which are often common problems among many older people. In severe cases of deficiencies, the depletion of vitamins and/or minerals may lead to a DEMENTIA-like condition, as with the depletion of thiamine among individuals with long-term ALCOHOLISM who have developed WERNICKE-KORSAKOFF SYNDROME. This can manifest as a severe deficit in short-term memory function. Older individuals may also be deficient in iron or in vitamin B_{12} (also known as cobalamin), which may lead to the development of ANEMIA.

Excessive amounts of vitamins or minerals can also be harmful and are often caused by individuals taking supplements that they believe are good for them. Usually these individuals have not consulted their physicians about their supplements, believing that they are automatically "good" and safe.

Studies have shown that patients frequently fail to tell their doctors about supplements that they take. However, high levels of vitamins or minerals can be extremely harmful and even fatal, as with vitamin E supplementation in a person with a bleeding problem. (Vitamin E decreases the clotting of the blood.) It is always best to talk to a physician before adding any vitamin or mineral supplement to the diet.

The primary vitamins that are relevant to older people are vitamins A, B_6, B_{12}, D, E, and K.

Vitamin A

Vitamin A promotes bone growth, and it is also important for vision and the immune system. In addition, it promotes the healthy lining of the eyes as well as benefiting the intestinal, respiratory, and urinary tract. Vitamin A is found in animals and plants. Some animal foods that are rich in vitamin A are cooked beef liver and cooked chicken liver. Fruits and vegetables high in vitamin A include carrot juice and boiled carrots, frozen spinach, vegetable soup, and cantaloupe. Males age 19 and older need about 3,000 international units (IUs) of vitamin A per day, and females age 19 and older need about 700 IUs.

Vitamin A deficiency is rare in the United States; it is more often seen in malnourished children in other countries. However, people in the United States can have a vitamin A deficiency, particularly among heavy drinkers or those who are on a strict diet. Usually a vitamin A deficiency is also accompanied by a deficiency in zinc. Night blindness is one indicator of a vitamin A deficiency. The ancient Egyptians were aware of this, and they cured night blindness by eating liver.

Too much vitamin A (vitamin A hypervitaminosis) can occur among those taking very high dosages of vitamin A, and this excess has been linked to an increased risk for hip fractures in older women and older men. Some researchers also believe that osteoporosis may be triggered by an excessive intake of vitamin A.

Some signs of excessive amounts of vitamin A are headache, blurred vision, nausea and vomiting, and lack of muscle coordination.

Vitamin B_6

Vitamin B_6 is found in beans, fortified cereals, fish, poultry, and in some fruits and vegetables. Deficiencies of Vitamin B_6 are rare in the United States. However, they may occur in older adults or in people with alcoholism, because these individuals are at an increased risk for an insufficient intake of B_6. Symptoms of vitamin B_6 deficiency may occur when the levels have been low for an extended period, and they may include a sore tongue, skin inflammation, confusion, depression, and convulsions. A deficiency of vitamin B_6 may also cause anemia.

Excessive levels of vitamin B_6 are also dangerous because they can cause nerve damage to the arms and legs.

Vitamin B_{12}

Vitamin B_{12} deficiency is fairly common, and an estimated 20 percent of elderly people are deficient in Vitamin B_{12}. (It is also sometimes called *cobalamin,* because it contains cobalt, a metal.) The deficiency may be caused by a dietary deficiency (such as with those who are strict vegetarians and who do not use vitamin supplements) or by the malabsorption of vitamin B_{12}. In elderly patients deficient in Vitamin B_{12}, the malabsorption of vitamin B_{12} is most frequently the cause, followed by pernicious anemia.

In a study of 200 elderly patients with a proven deficiency of Vitamin B_{12}, reported in the *Canadian Medical Association Journal* in 2004, the researchers found malabsorption from food was the cause in 60 to 70 percent of the cases, and pernicious anemia (also known as Biermer's disease) was the cause in 15 to 20 percent of the cases. Other causes were dietary deficiencies, hereditary metabolic diseases, and so forth.

Vitamin B_{12} helps to maintain healthy red blood cells and nerve cells. Foods high in vitamin B_{12}

include fish, poultry, meat, eggs, and milk. A deficiency of vitamin B_{12} may occur in vegetarians, although most cases of deficiency occur among people with an underlying gastrointestinal disorder that inhibits vitamin B_{12} absorption.

An initial symptom of a vitamin B_{12} deficiency is reduced cognitive function, which is later followed by anemia and DEMENTIA. Individuals with a vitamin B_{12} deficiency may also have numbness and tingling in the hands or feet, a poor memory, difficulty in maintaining their balance, CONSTIPATION, a loss of appetite, and weight loss.

According to the Office of Dietary Supplements, as many as 30 percent of adults age 50 years and older may have atrophic gastritis, which is an excessive growth of intestinal bacteria that makes the body unable to absorb the vitamin B_{12} in food. They can, however, absorb synthetic vitamin B_{12} that is added to their foods or as a dietary supplement.

Some drugs interfere with the absorption of vitamin B_{12}, such as proton pump inhibitors, which are used to treat both peptic ulcers and gastroesphageal reflux disease (GERD). Histamine 2 inhibitors are also used to treat peptic ulcer disease and can interfere with the absorption of vitamin B_{12}. Metformin (Glucophage) is a drug that is given to treat DIABETES, and it may interfere with the metabolism of calcium and indirectly reduce the absorption of vitamin B_{12}.

Experts say that there is little risk of vitamin B_{12} toxicity (as long as the kidneys function adequately), although the individual's physician should monitor all supplements.

Vitamin D Deficiency

Some older people are deficient in vitamin D, which is associated with muscle weakness and may be the cause of FALLS in the elderly. Vitamin D deficiency is common among many older people, and some housebound elderly people are severely deficient according to a 2005 article in the *British Medical Journal.*

The author points out that sometimes people are still deficient in vitamin D despite taking supplements, but this may mean that their supplement strength is too low. (Individuals should consult with their physicians before taking any over-the-counter supplements to ensure that the supplement will not be harmful to them.)

Author Geoff Venning in the *British Medical Journal* writes:

> Vitamin D deficiency among elderly people is much more common than previously recognized. It constitutes a serious public health problem for residents of old people's homes, and long stay wards [elderly individuals staying for long periods in geriatric units in European hospitals] and housebound people in the community. The consequences include muscle weakness, body sway, and a tendency to falls and fractures, as well as osteomalacia [softening of the bones, also known as rickets in children].

Vitamin D is found in food, and it can also be made by the body through exposure to the sun's ultraviolet light. Vitamin D maintains a normal blood level of both calcium and phosphorus and, as a result, promotes the maintenance of strong bones. Milk is fortified with vitamin D, and one cup of milk per day supplies about 25 percent of the vitamin D needs for those between ages 51 and 70 and about 15 percent of the needs of adults age 71 and older. Some cereals are fortified with vitamin D. Cod liver oil, salmon, mackerel, tuna, and sardines are high in vitamin D.

A vitamin D deficiency may be caused by a dietary inadequacy, increased excretion (loss), or impaired absorption and utilization. Individuals with lactose intolerance may also develop a vitamin D deficiency, as well as those who are strict vegetarians. A vitamin D deficiency in adults can lead to osteomalacia, which causes weak bones and muscle weakness. The individual may have bone pain but may also have symptoms that are so minor as to be unnoticed.

As individuals age, their ability to synthesize vitamin D declines. Some experts say that as many as 40 percent of adults with hip fractures are deficient in vitamin D. Individuals with limited sun exposure are also at risk for a vitamin D deficiency. People with darkly pigmented skin, such as African Americans, have a higher risk of developing a vitamin D deficiency than paler individuals.

A deficiency of vitamin D increases the risk for the development of OSTEOPOROSIS. Vitamin D may also be protective against cancer, and lower levels of vitamin D may increase the risk for CANCER, particularly colorectal cancer.

There are also risks with taking excessive intakes of vitamin D, and vitamin D toxicity can lead to constipation, nausea and vomiting, weight loss, poor appetite, and weakness. It may also escalate the blood levels of calcium to a higher level, causing confusion.

Vitamin E

Vitamin E is found in leafy green vegetables, vegetable oils, nuts, and fortified cereals. Other foods high in vitamin E are wheat germ oil, almonds, sunflower seed kernels, peanut butter, and spinach. A vitamin E deficiency is rare, although it may accompany a zinc deficiency. Some people cannot absorb fat, and they require a vitamin E supplement, such as those with Crohn's disease, an inflammatory bowel disease.

Vitamin E is an ANTIOXIDANT and is believed to help protect against the development of cancer. Vitamin E supplementation may also help protect against CATARACTS, although further research is needed. However, individuals should check with their doctors, because vitamin E supplements can increase the risk of bleeding and should not be taken with anticlotting drugs such as coumadin (Warfarin).

Vitamin K

Some studies have indicated that a suboptimal level of Vitamin K correlates with an increased risk for FRACTURES, which are a major problem for many older people. In a meta-analysis of studies on this issue, published in 2006 in the *Archives of Internal Medicine*, the researchers assessed whether oral vitamin K (phytonadione and menaquinone) supplements could apparently reduce bone loss and also prevent fractures. They found evidence that supplementation with vitamin K did reduce bone loss, and there was also evidence of fewer fractures among Japanese patients.

The study authors said that routine supplementation with vitamin K is not indicated until further research is performed; however, patients at risk for fracture should be advised to eat a diet rich in vitamin K, which is primarily obtained from leafy green vegetables and some vegetable oils.

The primary minerals that are relevant to older people are calcium, iron, and magnesium. In most cases, older individuals can obtain sufficient amounts of these needed minerals from their diets. However, some people need supplements. As with vitamins, it is essential to inform the physician ahead of time about any minerals that the individual plans to take as supplements, to ensure that they will be safe.

Calcium

Calcium is used by the body to build up the bones. Most of the calcium in the body (99 percent) is stored in the bones and teeth, and the remainder is found in the blood and muscles. Calcium is a necessary element for muscle and blood vessel contraction, as well as for the secretion of hormones and enzymes. Bone is constantly being broken down and deposited, although in some older people, bone breakdown may exceed bone buildup, particularly among older women with osteoporosis.

Both males and females age 51 years and older need about 1,200 mg of calcium per day. Calcium is found in milk, cheese, and yogurt. Individuals with lactose intolerance (those who cannot consume dairy products because they cannot digest lactose) need to consume alternative calcium sources, such as broccoli or kale.

A calcium deficiency (hypocalcemia) may occur when a person has kidney failure, the surgical removal of the stomach, or the use of diuretic medications. Hypocalcemia causes numbness and tingling in the fingers and muscle cramps. If severe, hypocalcemia can cause mental confusion, abnormal heart rhythms, and even death. Rarely, hypocalcemia is caused when the parathyroid glands embedded in the thyroid gland are damaged or destroyed. Individuals with hypocalcemia must take calcium supplements.

Most people who take calcium supplements take either calcium carbonate or calcium citrate. Calcium carbonate is inexpensive. (Calcium lactate is also available, but generally only by mail order.) Calcium supplements can cause bloating and constipation.

It is also possible to have excessively high levels of calcium, which leads to hypercalcemia (excessive calcium in the bloodstream). Hypercalcemia can harm the kidneys and decrease the absorption of other minerals; however, hypercalcemia is rare. Hypercalcemia may be caused by excessive use of calcium supplements, but is it more likely to occur from a malignant tumor in the advanced stages. It may also be caused by disease of the parathyroid glands.

Iron

Iron is a mineral that regulates cell growth, and an iron deficiency causes fatigue and decreased immunity. However, excessive iron levels can lead to iron toxicity and may even cause the individual's death.

There are two primary types of iron, including heme and nonheme iron. Heme iron comes from hemoglobin or the protein in red blood cells. Heme iron is found in such food products as red meats, fish, and poultry, as well as seafood. In contrast, nonheme iron is found in plants such as lentils, beans, molasses, spinach, and raisins. Most dietary iron is nonheme. Men and women older than age 51 need about 8 mg of iron per day, less than young adults need.

According to the World Health Organization, iron deficiency is the number-one nutritional deficiency in the world. Iron deficiency anemia is a common problem worldwide and also occurs in the United States. However, most older people are not iron-deficient unless they are being treated with kidney DIALYSIS or they have problems with gastrointestinal malabsorption and cannot absorb iron normally.

People with ARTHRITIS or cancer may develop anemia, but this form of anemia is usually different from iron deficiency anemia, and, thus, iron supplements will not improve the condition. Older people should never take iron supplements without first discussing it with their physician because of the unintentional risk of iron overload, which can lead to organ damage and death.

Magnesium

About half of the magnesium in the human body is found in the bones, and the rest is inside body tissues and organs. Magnesium helps to maintain normal nerve and muscle function and keep the blood strong. It also is involved in blood sugar levels. Spinach has a high magnesium content, as do beans and peas. The average male age 31 and older needs about 420 mg of magnesium per day, and the average female age 31 and older needs 320 mg of magnesium.

Magnesium deficiencies are not common in the United States, but gastrointestinal disorder may limit the ability to absorb magnesium. Excessive diarrhea and vomiting can also cause magnesium levels to drop.

Some signs of magnesium deficiency are nausea and vomiting, fatigue, weakness, and a loss of appetite. As the magnesium deficiency becomes worse, the person may experience muscle contractions and cramps, and numbness and tingling. Even worse symptoms are abnormal heart rhythms, personality changes, and coronary spasms. A severe magnesium deficiency can cause low levels of blood calcium. It is also associated with low levels of blood potassium.

People who take some diuretics (also known as "water pills" because they decrease the fluid level in the body) may develop a magnesium deficiency. Individuals with poorly controlled diabetes may need magnesium supplements, as may patients with alcoholism. Older adults have a higher risk for a magnesium deficiency than younger adults, often because they are more likely to take medications that interact with magnesium.

Very low levels of magnesium are treated with intravenously replaced magnesium. It is also possible to consume excessive levels of magnesium, as when individuals take numerous antacids that contain magnesium.

See also ADVERSE DRUG EVENT; APPETITE, CHRONIC LACK OF; NUTRITION; OBESITY.

Andres, Emmanuel, et al. "Vitamin B12 (Cobalamin) Deficiency in Elderly Patients." *Canadian Medical Association Journal* 171, no. 3 (August 3, 2004): 251–259.

Cockayne, Sarach, et al. "Vitamin K and the Prevention of Fractures: Systematic Review and Meta-analysis of Randomized Controlled Trials." *Archives of Internal Medicine* 166 (June 26, 2006): 1,256–1,261.

Vennig, Geoff. "Recent Developments in Vitamin D Deficiency and Muscle Weakness Among Elderly People." *British Medical Journal* 3, no. 30 (2005): 524–526.

wandering Generally refers to an older person walking away from the home or apartment and then forgetting how to find the way back home and continuing to walk about. Wandering is a common problem among many patients with ALZHEIMER'S DISEASE or other forms of DEMENTIA; individuals who may wish to walk about yet they quickly become disoriented and unable to find their way home.

Wandering may also occur to individuals with dementia who drive their vehicles and lose their way. Some individuals with dementia have driven far from home, out of their state, and even to other states without realizing that they are lost. Some older individuals have died from heat stroke or dehydration as a result of becoming lost and unable to obtain timely assistance from others.

See also AGGRESSION, PHYSICAL; COGNITIVE IMPAIRMENT; CONFUSION; DELUSIONS; HALLUCINATIONS; IRRITABILITY; MANIA; MEMORY IMPAIRMENT; RAGE.

water A common everyday substance that is absolutely essential to the lives of older individuals. Yet contaminated water can be harmful, and older individuals and their caregivers need to be aware of the potential risks associated with water.

According to the Environmental Protection Agency (EPA) in their fact sheet on water, most drinking water is safe, but there are some potential problems to watch out for. For example, drinking water that is not clean may contain disease-causing microbes that older adults are particularly susceptible to, such as *E. coli,* salmonella, and shigella, as well as parasites such as cryptosporidium and giardia.

Sometimes drinking water may contain other substances, such as arsenic. Arsenic is very dangerous over the long term and can cause CANCER, increase DIABETES rates, and worsen cardiovascular problems. Arsenic may occur naturally as part of the local geology or may occur as a result of arsenic-containing chemicals used locally. The EPA has a standard for public drinking water, but the standard does not apply to private wells or systems serving 25 or fewer people. Water can be tested for arsenic.

The EPA recommends taking the following actions to avoid water-related problems:

- Learn where your water comes from. If it comes from a public system, it must meet EPA standards. If it comes from a well, it is not subject to EPA standards and should be tested annually to make sure that it is safe.

- Follow public notices on drinking water. They may be distributed by the media, including newspapers, radio, and television, or by mail to notify the public if there is a waterborne disease emergency. Follow the advice of your water supplier. Boiling water for one minute will kill most microorganisms but will not help with chemical contamination.

- Contact your water supplier to see if you should test for lead. Do not boil your water to get rid of lead because it will only make the problem worse by increasing the concentration of any existing lead as the water evaporates. If the plumbing system could contain lead, use cold water only for drinking and cooking. Run the cold water until it become as cold as possible, especially if the water has not been used for several hours. Contact the National Lead Information Center at (800) 424-LEAD for more information.

- Test for radon. Radon gas is the second leading cause of lung cancer in the United States, and nearly one in 15 homes have high levels of radon. It is odorless and invisible. Radon test kits can be purchased through the mail or in hardware stores, or qualified professionals can perform the test.

Water Infiltration Hazards at Home, Especially after Floods

After floods in the home, excessive moisture or water may accumulate, causing mold growth. In addition, contact with water pollutants may occur if there is a sewage backflow in the home, which is especially common after severe rain that led to flooding. The following actions should be taken:

- Inspect the older person's home for water leaks in the bathroom, laundry, and around the windows and doors. Ask for help checking the roof gutters and eaves.

- Eliminate water and you will eliminate mold. To prevent mold from starting, make sure the older person gets help with fixing plumbing leaks and other water problems immediately. If mold is already present, scrub if off with detergent and water and dry it completely. Some cleaning products treat mold growth.

- If there is a flood, sewage and other materials can enter the home. Even if the water is clean, standing water and wet items offer a breeding ground for microorganisms. Make sure the older person gets help with eliminating standing water, drying out the home, and removing wet materials. Clean and disinfect the damaged area. Furniture, rugs, and curtains may need to be replaced if sewage entered the home.

Environmental Protection Agency. *Fact Sheet: Water Works: Information for Older Adults and Family Caregivers.* December 2005.

Wernicke-Korsakoff syndrome A disorder that is usually caused by long-term ALCOHOLISM and that ultimately leads to a severe deficiency of thiamine (vitamin B$_1$). Wernicke's encephalopathy is the first of the two stages of this syndrome, and it is then followed by Korsakoff psychosis. Wernicke-Korsakoff syndrome is also known as alcoholic encephalopathy or Wernicke's disease.

Symptoms and Diagnostic Path

This syndrome causes CONFUSION, memory gaps, lack of coordination, weakness, and the tendency to make up information (confabulate) when the person cannot remember what actually happened. Other symptoms that may occur with Wernicke-Korsakoff syndrome are vision changes (including double vision and eyelid drooping), an inability to form new memories, and HALLUCINATIONS.

During the physical examination, the physician may note that the individual's muscle reflexes are abnormal or decreased. The gait and coordination of the person are often abnormal. Some muscles may be weak or even atrophied. The individual may have HYPOTENSION (low blood pressure), and the body temperature may also be low. The individual may appear to be malnourished.

Other causes of thiamine deficiency should be ruled out before Wernicke-Korsakoff syndrome is diagnosed, including long-term kidney DIALYSIS, congestive heart failure that is treated with long-term diuretics, thyrotoxicosis (extremely high thyroid hormone levels), and acquired immune deficiency syndrome (AIDS).

Treatment Options and Outlook

Hospitalization is often required for the initial treatment because the person's symptoms are usually so severe. The goal of hospitalization is to gain control over these symptoms. The patient is treated with thiamine that is administered orally, by injection, or intravenously. The thiamine may help to improve the poor muscle coordination and confusion or delirium; however, it will usually not improve any loss of memory or intelligence that is associated with Wernicke-Korsakoff syndrome.

The individual with this syndrome must be totally abstinent from alcohol to prevent any further loss of physical or brain functioning.

Risk Factors and Preventive Measures

Individuals who have been heavy drinkers for years and who have poor diets are at risk for this syndrome. The only preventive measure is to avoid heavy drinking.

See also ALCOHOL; HEALTH-CARE AGENT/PROXY; MEMORY IMPAIRMENT; SUBSTANCE ABUSE; VITAMIN AND MINERAL DEFICIENCIES/EXCESSES.

wills Legal documents that stipulate to whom an individual wishes to leave his or her money and real and personal property upon his or her death. If the person does not have a will (also referred to as dying intestate), the state or county will determine who will receive the deceased individual's assets.

See also DURABLE POWER OF ATTORNEY; END-OF-LIFE ISSUES; HEALTH-CARE AGENT/PROXY; LIVING TRUST; LIVING WILL; POWER OF ATTORNEY; TALKING TO ELDERLY PARENTS ABOUT DIFFICULT ISSUES.

APPENDIXES

APPENDIX I
IMPORTANT ORGANIZATIONS

AAA Foundation for Traffic Safety
607 Fourteenth Street NW
Suite 201
Washington, DC 20005
(202) 638-5944
http://www.seniordrivers.org

AARP
601 E Street NW
Washington, DC 20049
(888) 687-2277
http://www.aarp.org

Administration on Aging
U.S. Health and Human Services
200 Independence Avenue SW
Washington, DC 20201
(202) 619-0724
http://www.aoa.gov

Ageless Design
3197 Trout Place Road
Cumming, GA 30041
(800) 752-3238
http://www.agelessdesign.com

Agency for Healthcare Research & Quality
Office of Communications & Knowledge Transfer
540 Gaither Road
Suite 2000
Rockville, MD 20850
(800) 358-9295
http://www.ahrqu.gov

Aging with Dignity
P.O. Box 1661
Tallahassee, FL 32302-1661
(888) 5WISHES (594-7437)
http://www.agingwithdignity.org

AIDSinfo
P.O. Box 6303
Rockville, MD 20849
(800) 448-0440
http://www.aidsinfo.nih.gov

Alliance for Retired Americans
815 16th Street NW
Fourth Floor
Washington, DC 20006
(202) 637-5399
http://www.retiredamericans.org

Alcoholics Anonymous
Grand Central Station
New York, NY 10163
(212) 870-3400
http://www.aa.org

Alliance for Aging Research
2021 K Street NW
Suite 305
Washington, DC 20006
(202) 293-2856
http://www.agingresearch.org

Alzheimer's Association
225 North Michigan Avenue, Floor 17
Chicago, IL 60601
(800) 272-3900
http://www.alz.org

Alzheimer's Disease Cooperative Study
University of California, San Diego
La Jolla, CA 92093-5880
(858) 622-5880
http://adcs.ecsd.edu

Alzheimer's Disease Education & Referral (ADEAR) Center
P.O. Box 8250
Silver Spring, MD 20907-8250
(800) 438-4380
http://www.alzheimersnia.nih.gov

Alzheimer's Drug Discovery Foundation
1414 Avenue of the Americas
Suite 1502
New York, NY 10019
(212) 935-2402
http://www.alzdiscovery.org

Alzheimer's Foundation of America
322 8th Avenue, 6th Floor
New York, NY 10001
(866) 232-8484
http://www.alzfdn.org

American Academy of Dermatology
P.O. Box 4014
Schaumburg, IL 60618-4014
(886) 503-7546
http://www.aad.org

American Academy of Family Physicians
11400 Tomahawk Creek Parkway
Leawood, KS 66211
(800) 274-2237
http://www.aafp.org

American Academy of Hospice and Palliative Medicine
4700 West Lake Avenue
Glenview, IL 60025
(847) 375-4712
http://www.aahpm.org

American Academy of Neurology
1080 Montreal Avenue
St. Paul, MN 55116
(800) 879-1960
http://www.aan.com

American Academy of Ophthalmology
P.O. Box 7424
San Francisco, CA 94120-7424
(415) 561-8500
http://www.aao.org

American Academy of Orthopaedic Surgeons
6300 North River Road
Rosemont, IL 60018
(847) 823-7186
http://www.aaos.org

American Academy of Pain Medicine
4700 West Lake Avenue
Glenview, IL 60025
(847) 375-4731
http://www.painmed.org

American Academy of Physical Medicine and Rehabilitation
330 North Wabash Avenue
Suite 2500
Chicago, IL 60611-7617
(312) 464-9700
http://www.aapmr.org

American Academy of Sleep Medicine
One Westbrook Corporate Center
Suite 920
Westchester, IL 60154
(708) 492-0930
http://www.aasmnet.org

American Association for Geriatric Psychiatry
7910 Woodmont Avenue
Suite 1050
Bethesda, MD 20814-3004
(301) 654-7850
http://www.aagpgpa.org

American Association for the Study of Liver Diseases
1729 King Street
Suite 200
Alexandria, VA 22314
(703) 299-9766
http://www.aasid.org

American Association of Cardiovascular and Pulmonary Rehabilitation
401 North Michigan Avenue
Suite 2200
Chicago, IL 60611
(312) 321-5146
http://www.aacvpr.org

American Association of Clinical Urologists
1111 North Plaza Drive
Suite 550
Schaumburg, IL 60201
(847) 517-1050
http://www.aacuweb.org

American Association of Critical Care Nurses
101 Columbia
Aliso Viejo, CA 92656
(800) 899-2226
http://www.aacn.org

American Association of Homes and Services for the Aging (AAHSA)
2519 Connecticut Avenue NW
Washington, DC 20008
(202) 783-2242
http://www.aahsa.org

American Association of Kidney Patients
3505 East Frontage Road
Suite 315
Tampa, FL 33607
(800) 749-AAKP
http://www.aakp.org

American Association of Neurological Surgeons
5550 Meadowbrook Drive
Rolling Meadows, IL 60008
(847) 378-0500
http://www.ans.org

American Association of Suicidology
5221 Wisconsin Avenue NW
Washington, DC 20015
(202) 237-2280
http://www.suicidology.org

American Bar Association Commission on the Law and Aging
740 15th Street NW
Washington, DC 20005-1019
(202) 662-1000
http://www.abanet.org/aging

American Brain Tumor Association
272 River Road
Des Plaines, IL 60018
(847) 827-9910
http://www.abta.org

American Cancer Society
1599 Clifton Road NE
Atlanta, GA 30329-4251
(404) 320-3333
http://www.cancer.org

American Chiropractic Association
1701 Clarendon Boulevard
Arlington, VA 22209
(703) 276-8800
http://www.amerchiro.org

American Chronic Pain Association
P.O. Box 850
Rocklin, CA 95677
(800) 533-3231
http://www.theacpa.org

American College of Cardiology
9111 Old Georgetown Road
Bethesda, MD 20814
(301) 897-2694
http://www.acc.org

American College of Emergency Physicians
1125 Executive Circle
Irving, TX 75038
(972) 550-0911
http://www.acep.org

American College of Gastroenterology
P.O. Box 342260
Bethesda, MD 20827
(301) 263-9000
http://www.acg.gi.org

American College of Health Care Administrators
300 North Lee Street
Alexandria, VA 22314
(703) 739-7900
http://www.achca.org

American College of Nutrition
300 South Duncan Avenue
Suite 225
Clearwater, FL 33755
(727) 446-6086
http://www.cert-nutrition.org

American College of Obstetricians and Gynecologists (ACOG)
409 Twelfth Street SW
P.O. Box 96920
Washington, DC 20090-6920
(202) 638-5577
http://www.acog.org

American College of Physicians
190 North Independence Mall West
Philadelphia, PA 19106-1572
(800) 523-1546, extension 2600
http://www.acponline.org

American College of Rheumatology
Association of Rheumatology Health Professionals
1800 Century Place
Suite 250
Atlanta, GA 30345
(404) 633-3777
http://www.rheumatology.org

American College of Sports Medicine
P.O. Box 1440
Indianapolis, IN 46206
(317) 637-9200
http://www.acsm.org

American College of Surgeons
633 North Saint Clair Street
Chicago, IL 60611
(312) 202-5000
http://www.facs.org

American Congress of Rehabilitation Medicine
6801 Lake Plaza Drive
Suite B-205
Indianapolis, IN 46220
(317) 915-2250
http://www.acrm.org

American Council of the Blind
1155 15th Street NW
Suite 1004
Washington, DC 20005
(202) 467-5081
http://www.acb.org

American Council on Alcoholism
1000 East Indian School Road
Phoenix, AZ 85014

(800) 527-5344
http://www.aca-usa.org

American Council on Consumer Interests
415 South Duff
Suite C
Ames, IA 50010
(515) 956-4666
http://www.consumerinterests.org

American Council on Science and Health
1995 Broadway
Second Floor
New York, NY 10023
(212) 362-7044
http://www.acsh.org

American Counseling Association
5999 Stevenson Avenue
Alexandria, VA 22304
(800) 347-6647
http://www.counseling.org

American Dental Association
211 East Chicago Avenue
Chicago, IL 60611
(312) 440-2500
http://www.ada.org

American Diabetes Association
National Call Center
1701 North Beauregard Street
Alexandria, VA 22311
(800) 342-2383
http://www.diabetes.org

American Dietetic Association
120 South Riverside Plaza
Suite 2000
Chicago, IL 60606-6995
(800) 877-1600
http://www.eatright.org

American Federation for Aging Research (AFAR)
1414 Sixth Avenue, 18th Floor
New York, NY 10019-2514
(212) 752-2327
http://www.afar.org

American Foundation for the Blind
11 Penn Plaza, Suite 300
New York, NY 10001

(212) 502-7600
http://www.afb.org

American Foundation for Suicide Prevention
120 Wall Street, 22nd Floor
New York, NY 10005
(888) 333-AFSP
http://www.afsp.org

American Gastroenterological Association
4930 Del Ray Avenue
Bethesda, MD 20814
(301) 654-2055
http://www.gastro.org

American Geriatrics Society
The Empire State Building
350 Fifth Avenue
Suite 801
New York, NY 10118
(212) 308-1414
http://www.americangeriatrics.org

American Headache Society
19 Mantua Road
Mt. Royal, NJ 08061
(856) 423-0043
http://www.ahsnet.org

American Health Assistance Foundation
22512 Gateway Center Drive
Clarksburg, MD 20871
(800) 437-2423
http://www.ahaf.org

American Health Care Association (AHCA)
1201 L Street NW
Washington, DC 20005
(202) 842-4444
http://www.ahca.org

American Heart Association (AHA)
7272 Greenville Avenue
Dallas, TX 75231
(800) 242-8721
http://www.americanheart.org

American Horticultural Therapy Association
3570 East Twelfth Avenue
Suite 206
Denver, CO 80206
(800) 634-1630
http://www.ahta.org

American Hospice Foundation
2120 L Street NW
Suite 200
Washington, DC 20037
(202) 223-0204
http://americanhospice.org

American Hospital Association
One North Franklin
Chicago, IL 60606-3421
(312) 422-3000
http://www.aha.org

American Insomnia Association
One Westbrook Corporate Center
Suite 920
Westchester, IL 60154
(708) 492-0930
http://www.americaninsomniaassociation.org

American Institute for Cancer Research
1759 R Street NW
Washington, DC 20009
(800) 843-8114
http://www.aicr.org

American Liver Foundation
75 Maiden Lane
Suite 603
New York, NY 10038
(800) 465-4837
http://www.liverfoundation.org

American Lung Association
61 Broadway, 6th Floor
New York, NY 10006
(212) 315-8700
http://www.lungusa.org

American Medical Association
515 N. State Street
Chicago, IL 60610
(800) 621-8335
http://www.ama-assn.org

American Medical Directors Association
10480 Little Patuxent Parkway
Suite 760
Columbia, MD 21044
(800) 876-2632
http://www.amda.org

American Menopause Foundation
350 Fifth Avenue
Suite 2822
New York, NY 10118
(212) 714-2398
http://www.americanmenopause.org

American Mental Health Counselors Association
801 N. Fairfax Street, Suite 304
Alexandria, VA 22314
(800) 326-2642
http://www.amhca.org

American Music Therapy Association
8455 Colesville Road
Suite 1000
Silver Spring, MD 20910
(301) 589-3300
http://www.musictherapy.org

American Nurses Association
8515 Georgia Avenue
Suite 400
Silver Spring, MD 20910
(800) 274-4262
http://www.nursingworld.org

American Occupational Therapy Association, Inc.
4720 Montgomery Lane
P.O. Box 31220
Bethesda, MD 20824-1220
(301) 652-2682
http://www.aota.org

American Optometric Association
1505 Prince Street, Suite 300
Alexandria, VA 22314
(800) 365-2219
http://www.aoa.org

American Orthopaedic Foot and Ankle Society
6300 North River Road
Suite 510
Rosemont, IL 60018
(800) 235-4855
http://www.aofas.org

American Osteopathic Association
142 East Ontario Street
Chicago, IL 60611

(800) 621-1773
http://www.osteopathic.org

American Pain Society
4700 W. Lake Ave.
Glenview, IL 60025
(847) 375-4715
http://www.ampainsoc.org

American Parkinson Disease Association
135 Parkinson Avenue
Staten Island, NY 10305
(800) 223-2732
http://www.apdaparkinson.org

American Pharmaceutical Association
2215 Constitution Avenue NW
Washington, DC 20037
(800) 237-2742
http://www.aphanet.org

American Physical Therapy Association
1111 North Fairfax Street
Alexandria, VA 22314-1488
(800) 999-2782
http://www.apta.org

American Podiatric Medical Association, Inc.
9312 Old Georgetown Road
Bethesda, MD 20814-1621
(301) 581-9221
http://www.apma.org

American Psychiatric Association
1000 Wilson Boulevard
Suite 1825
Arlington, VA 22209-3901
(703) 907-7300
http://www.psych.org/

American Psychological Association
750 First Street NE
Washington, DC 20002-4242
(800) 374-2721
http://www.apa.org

American Public Health Association
800 Eye Street NW
Washington, DC 20001
(202) 777-2478
http://www.apha.org/meetings

American Red Cross
2025 E Street NW
Washington, DC 20006
(800) 435-7669
http://www.redcross.org

American Self-Help Group Clearinghouse
1002 East Hanover Avenue
Suite 202
Cedar Knolls, NJ 07927
(973) 326-8853
http://www.mentalhelp.net/selfhelp

American Seniors Housing Association
5100 Wisconsin Avenue NW
Suite 307
Washington, DC 20016
(202) 237-0900
http://www.seniorshousing.org

American Sleep Apnea Association
1424 K Street NW
Suite 302
Washington, DC 20005
(202) 293-3650
http://www.sleepapnea.org

American Social Health Association
P.O. Box 13827
Research Triangle Park, NC 27709
(800) 227-8922
http://www.ashastd.org

American Society for Bone and Mineral Research
2025 M Street NW
Suite 800
Washington, DC 20036-3309
(202) 367-1161
http://www.asbmr.org

American Society of Bariatric Physicians
2921 South Parker Road
Suite 625
Aurora, CO 80014
(303) 770-2526
http://www.asbp.org

American Society of Cataract and Refractive Surgery
4000 Legato Road
Suite 700

Fairfax, VA 22033
(703) 591-2220
http://www.ascrs.org

American Society of Neurorehabilitation
5841 Cedar Lake Road
Suite 204
Minneapolis, MN 55416
(952) 646-2022
http://www.asnr.com

American Society on Aging
833 Market Street
Suite 511
San Francisco, CA 94103
(415) 974-9604

American Speech-Language-Hearing Association
10801 Rockville Pike
Rockville, MD 20852
(800) 638-8255
http://www.asha.org

American Stroke Association
National Center
7272 Greenville Avenue
Dallas, TX 75231
(888) 478-7653
http://www.strokeassociation.org

American Thyroid Association
6066 Leesburg Pike
Suite 550
Falls Church, VA 22041
(703) 998-8890
http://www.thyroid.org

American Tinnitus Association
ATA National Headquarters
P.O. Box 5
Portland, OR 97207-0005
(800) 634-8978
http://www.ata.org

American Urological Association Foundation, Inc.
1000 Corporate Boulevard
Suite 410
Linthicum, MD 21090
(410) 689-3700
http://www.urologyhealth.org

Americans for Better Care of the Dying
1700 Diagonal Road
Suite 635
Alexandria, VA 22314
(703) 647-8505
http://www.abcd-caring.org

America's Health Insurance Plans
601 Pennsylvania Ave WN
South Building
Suite 500
Washington, DC 20004
(202) 778-3200
http://www.hiaa.org

Anxiety Disorders Association of America
8730 Georgia Avenue
Suite 600
Silver Spring, MD 20910
(240) 485-1001
http://wwww.adaa.org

Aplastic Anemia and MDS International Foundation, Inc.
P.O. Box 613
Annapolis, MD 21404-0613
(410) 867-0242
http://www.aamds.org

ARCH National Respite Network and Resource Center
800 Eastowne Drive
Suite 105
Chapel Hill, NC 27514
(919) 490-5577
http://www.archrespite.org

Arthritis Foundation
P.O. Box 7669
Atlanta, GA 30357
(800) 568-4045
http://www.arthritis.org

Assisted Living Federation of America
1650 King Street
Suite 602
Alexandria, VA 22314
(703) 894-1805
http://www.ala.org

Associated Professional Sleep Societies
One Westbrook Corporate Center
Suite 920
Westchester, IL 60154
(708) 492-0930
http://www.apss.org

Association for Death Education and Counseling
638 Prospect Avenue
Hartford, CT 06105-4298
(203) 232-4825

Association for Frontotemporal Dementias (AFTD)
100 North 17th Street
Suite 600
Philadelphia, PA 19103
(267) 514-7221
http://www.FTD-Picks.org

Association for Gerontology in Higher Education
1030 Fifteenth Street NW
Suite 240
Washington, DC 20005
(202) 289-9806
http://www.aghe.org

Association of American Physicians and Surgeons
1601 North Tucson Boulevard
Suite 9
Tucson, AZ 85716
(800) 635-1196
http://www.aapsonline.org

Association of State and Territorial Health Officials
1275 K Street NW
Suite 800
Washington, DC 20005
(202) 371-9090
http://www.astho.org

Asthma and Allergy Foundation of America
1233 Twelfth Street NW
Washington, DC 20036
(800) 727-8642
http://www.aafa.org

Bacghmann-Strauss Dystonia & Parkinson Foundation
Mt. Sinai Medical Center

One Gustave L. Levy Place
P.O. Box 1490
New York, NY 10029
(212) 241-5614
http://www.dystonia-parkisons.org

Better Hearing Institute
515 King Street
Alexandria, VA 22314
(800) 327-9355
http://www.betterhearing.org

Better Sleep Council
501 Wythe Street
Alexandria, VA 22314
(703) 683-8371
http://www.bettersleep.org

Beverly Foundation
566 El Dorado Street
Suite 100
Pasadena, CA 91101
(626) 792-2292
http://www.beverlyfoundation.org

B'nai B'rith
2020 K Street NW, 7th Floor
Washington, DC 20006
(202) 857-6600
http://www.bnaibrith.org

**Brookdale Center on Aging (BCOA) of
    Hunter College**
425 East 25th Street
13th Floor North
New York, NY 10010
(212) 451-2780
http://www.brookdale.org

CancerCare
275 7th Avenue
Floor 22
New York, NY 10001
(800) 813-4673
http://www.cancercare.org

Catholic Charities USA
1731 King Street
Alexandria, VA 22314
(703) 549-1390
http://www.catholiccharitiesusa.org

Census Bureau
4700 Silver Hill Road
Washington, DC 20233
http://www.census.gov

Center for Social Gerontology
2307 Shelby Avenue
Ann Arbor, MI 4810
(734) 665-1126
http://www.tcsg.org

Center for the Study of Aging
International Association of Physical Activity,
    Aging and Sports
706 Madison Avenue
Albany, NY 12208
(518) 465-6927
http://www.centerforthestudyofaging-albany.org

**Center for Substance Abuse Treatment
    (CSAT)**
Substance Abuse and Mental Health Services
    Administration
1 Choke Cherry Road
Room 2-1075
Rockville, MD 20857
(240) 276-2700

Centers for Disease Control and Prevention
1600 Clifton Road
Atlanta, GA 30333
(800) 311-3435
http://www.cdc.org

**Centers for Medicare and Medicaid Services
    (CMS)**
7500 Security Boulevard
Baltimore, MD 21244
(800) 633-4227
http://www.medicare.gov

Children of Aging Parents (CAPS)
P.O. Box 167
Richboro, PA 18954
(800) 227-7294
http://www.caps4caregivers.org

CJD Aware!
2527 South Carrollton Ave.
New Orleans, LA 70118-3013
(504) 861-4627
http://www.cjdaware.com

Clearinghouse on Abuse and Neglect of the Elderly (CANE)
University of Delaware
Newark, DE 19716
(302) 831-3525
http://www.elderabusecenter.org/clearinghouse/index.html

College of American Pathologists
325 Waukegan Road
Northfield, IL 60093
(800) 323-4040
http://www.cap.org

Community Nutrition Institute
419 West Broad Street, #204
Falls Church, VA 22046
(703) 532-0030
http://www.communitynutrition.org

Community Transportation Association of America
1341 G Street NW, 10th Floor
Washington, DC 20005
(202) 628-1480
http://www.ctaa.org

Consumer Action
717 Market Street
Suite 310
San Francisco, CA 94103
(415) 777-9635
http://www.consumer-action.org

Consumer Consortium on Assisted Living
2342 Oak Street
Falls Church, VA 22046
(703) 533-8121
http://www.ccal.org

Consumer Federation of America
1424 Sixteenth Street NW
Suite 604
Washington, DC 20036
(202) 387-6121
http://www.consumerfed.org

Continuing Care Accreditation Commission
1730 Rhode Island Avenue NW
Suite 209
Washington, DC 20036

(202) 587-5001
http://www.carf.org

Cooper Institute and Brown University Center for Behavioral and Preventive Medicine Human Kinetics
P.O. Box 5076
Champaign, IL 61825
(800) 747-4457
http://www.activeliving.info

Corporation for National Service
1201 New York Avenue NW
Washington, DC 20525
(800) 424-8867
http://www.seniorcorps.org

Council of Better Business Bureaus
4200 Wilson Boulevard
Suite 800
Arlington, VA 22203
(703) 525-8277
http://www.bbb.org

Council of Citizens with Low Vision International
5707 Brockton Drive
Suite 302
Indianapolis, IN 46220
(800) 733-2258

Cremation Association of North America
401 North Michigan Avenue
Chicago, IL 60611
(312) 245-1077
http://www.cremationassociation.org

Creutzfeldt-Jakob Disease (CJD) Foundation Inc.
P.O. Box 5312
Akron, OH 44334
(800) 659-1991
http://www.cjdfoundation.org

The Dana Alliance for Brain Initiatives
745 Fifth Avenue
Suite 900
New York, NY 10151
(212) 223-4040
http://www.dana.org

Delta Society
975 124th Avenue NE

Suite 101
Bellevue, WA 98055
(425) 226-7357
http://www.deltasociety.org

Department of Housing and Urban Development
451 Seventh Street SW
Washington, DC 20410
(202) 708-1112
http://www.hud.gov

Department of Justice
950 Pennsylvania Avenue NW
Washington, DC 20530
(202) 514-2000
http://www.usjoj.gov

Department of Veterans Affairs (VA)
Veterans Benefits Administration
Veterans Health Administration
810 Vermont Avenue NW
Washington, DC 20420
(800) 827-1000
http://www.va.gov

Depression and Bipolar Support Alliance
730 North Franklin Street
Suite 501
Chicago, IL 60610
(800) 826-3632
http://www.dbsalliance.org

Depression and Related Affective Disorders Association
8201 Greensboro Drive
Suite 300
McLean, VA 22102
(703) 610-9026
http://www.drada.org

Digestive Disease National Coalition
507 Capitol Court NE
Suite 200
Washington, DC 20002
(202) 544-7497
http://www.ddnc.org

Disabled American Veterans
P.O. Box 14301
Cincinnati, OH 45250

(202) 554-3501
http://www.dav.org

Elder Craftsmen
610 Lexington Avenue
New York, NY 10022
(212) 319-8128
http://www.eldercraftsmen.org

Elder Care Initiative in Consumer Law
National Consumer Law Center, Inc.
Boston, MA 02110
(617) 542-8010
http://www.consumerlaw.org

Elderweb
1305 Chadwick Drive
Normal, IL 61761
(309) 451-3319
http://www.elderweb.com

Emergency Nurses Association
815 Lee Street
Des Plaines, IL 60016
(800) 900-9659
http://www.ena.org

Endocrine Society
8401 Connecticut Avenue
Suite 900
Chevy Chase, MD 20815
(301) 482-1384
http://www.endo-society.org

Epilepsy Foundation
4531 Garden City Drive
Landover, MD 20785
(800) 332-1000
http://www.epilepsyfoundation.org

Family Caregiver Alliance
180 Montgomery Street
Suite 1100
San Francisco, CA 94104
(800) 445-8106
http://www.caregiver.org

Federal Citizen Information Center
P.O. Box 100
Pueblo, CO 81002
(800) FED-INFO
http://www.pueblo.gsa.gov

Fifty-Plus Lifelong Fitness
2843 East Bayshore Road
Suite 202
Palo Alto, CA 94303
(650) 843-1750
http://www.500plus.org

Florida Geriatrics Society
2563 Capital Medical Boulevard
Tallahassee, FL 32308
(850) 531-8349
http://www.fgsonline.org

Food Allergy and Anaphylaxis Network
11781 Lee Highway
Suite 160
Fairfax, VA 22033
(800) 929-4040
http://www.foodallergy.org

Food and Drug Administration (FDA)
5600 Fishers Lane
Rockville, MD 20857
(888) 463-6332
http://www.fda.gov

Foundation for Biomedical Research
818 Connecticut Avenue NW
Suite 900
Washington, DC 20006
(202) 457-0654
http://www.fbresearch.org

Funeral Consumers Alliance
33 Patchen Road
South Burlington, VT 05403
(800) 765-0107
http://www.funerals.org

Generations Online
108 Ralston House
Philadelphia, PA 19104
(215) 222-6400
http://www.genearationsonline.com

Gerontological Society of America
1220 L Street NW
Suite 901
Washington, DC 20005-1503
(202) 842-1275
http://www.geron.org

Glaucoma Research Foundation
251 Post Street
Suite 600
San Francisco, CA 94108
(800) 826-6693
http://www.glaucoma.org

Gray Panthers
1612 K Street NW
Suite 300
Washington, DC 20006
(800) 280-5362
http://www.graypanthers.org

HealthierUS.Gov
U.S. Department of Health and Human Services
Office of Public Health and Science
Office of Disease Prevention and Health
    Promotion
200 Independence Avenue SW
Hubert H. Humphrey Building
Room 738G
Washington, DC 20201
(202) 401-6295
http://www.healthierus.gov

Heart Rhythm Society
1400 K Street NW
Suite 500
Washington, DC 20005
(202) 464-3400
http://www.hrsonline.org

Hepatitis B Foundation
3805 Old Easton Road
Doylestown, PA 18902
(215) 489-4900
http://www.hepb.org

Hepatitis Foundation International
504 Blick Drive
Silver Spring, MD 20904
(800) 891-0707
http://www.hepfi.org

Hospice Association of America
228 Seventh Street SE
Washington, DC 20003
(202) 546-4759
http://www.hospice-america.org

Hospice Foundation of America
2001 S Street NW
Suite 300
Washington, DC 20009
(800) 854-3402
http://www.hospicefoundation.org

Huntington's Disease Society of America
505 Eighth Avenue
Suite 902
New York, NY 10018
(800) 345-4372
http://www.hdsa.org

Indian Health Service
The Reyes Building
Rockville, MD 20852-1627
(301) 443-3593
http://www.ihs.gov

Institute for Cancer Prevention
1 Dana Road
Valhalla, NY 10595
(914) 592-2600
http://www.ahf.org

Institute for Health and Aging
University of California, San Francisco
3333 California Street
Suite 340
San Francisco, CA 94143
(415) 502-5207
http://www.ucsf.edu/champs

International Association Hospice and Palliative Care
5535 Memorial Drive
Suite F, PMB 509
Houston, TX 77007
(936) 321-9846
http://www.hospicecare.com

International Essential Tremor Foundation
P.O. Box 14005
Lenexa, KS 66285-4005
(888) 387-3667
http://www.essentialtremor.org

International Foundation for Functional Gastrointestinal Disorders
P.O. Box 170864
Milwaukee, WI 53217

(888) 964-2001
http://www.iffgd.org

International Foundation for Research & Education on Depression (iFRED)
7040 Bembe Beach Road
Suite 100
Annapolis, MD 21403
(410) 268-0044
http://www.ifred.org

International Hearing Society
16880 Middlebelt Road
Suite 4
Livonia, MI 48154
(800) 521-5247
http://www.ihsinfo.org

International Network for the Prevention of Elder Abuse
University of Massachusetts Memorial Health Care
119 Belmont
Worcester, MA 01605
(508) 793-6166

Intestinal Diseases Foundation, Inc.
The Landmarks Building
Suite 525
One Station Square
Pittsburgh, PA 15219
(412) 261-5888

John Douglas French Alzheimer's Foundation
11620 Wilshire Boulevard
Suite 270
Los Angeles, CA 90025
(800) 477-2243
http://www.jdfaf.org

Laurent Clerc National Deaf Education Center
Gallaudet University
800 Florida Avenue NE
Washington, DC 20002
(202) 651-5000
http://www.clerccenter.gallaudet.edu

Legal Services for the Elderly
140 West 42nd Street, 17th Floor
New York, NY 10036

(212) 391-0120
http://www.lawhelp.org

Leukemia and Lymphoma Society, Inc.
1311 Mamaroneck Avenue
White Plains, NY 10605
(800) 955-4572
http://www.lls.org

Lewy Body Dementia Association
P.O. Box 451429
Atlanta, GA 31145-9429
(404) 935-6444
http://www.lewybodydementia.org

Lighthouse National Center for Vision and Aging
The Sol & Lillian Goldman Building
111 East 59th Street
New York, NY 10022
(800) 829-0500
http://www.lighthouse.org

Low-Income Home Energy Assistance Program (LIHEAP) Clearinghouse National Center for Appropriate Technology
3040 Continental Drive
Butte, MT 59702
(406) 494-8662
http://liheap.ncat.org

Lupus Foundation of America
2000 L Street NW
Suite 710
Washington, DC 20036
(800) 558-0121
http://www.lupus.org

Meals on Wheels Association of America
203 South Union Street
Alexandria, VA 22314
(703) 548-5558
http://www.mowaa.org

MedicAlert Foundation
2323 Colorado Avenue
Turlock, CA 95382
(888) 633-4298
http://www.medicalert.org

Medicare Rights Center
520 Eighth Ave.

North Wing, 3rd Floor
New York, NY 10018
(212) 869-3850
http://www.medicarerights.org/

Mental Health America
2000 North Beauregard Street, 6th Floor
Alexandria, VA 22311
(800) 969-6642
http://www.mentalhealthamerica.net

Michael J. Fox Foundation for Parkinson's Research
Grand Central Station
P.O. Box 4777
New York, NY 10163
(212) 509-0995
http://www.michaeljfox.org

Mood and Anxiety Disorder Programs (MAP)
National Institute of Mental Health
9000 Rockville Pike
Bethesda, MD 20892
(866) 627-6464
http://intramural.nimh.nih.gov/mood

Narcolepsy Network, Inc.
P.O. Box 294
Pleasantville, NY 10570
(888) 292-6522
http://www.narcolepsynetwork.org

National Academy of Elder Law Attorneys, Inc.
1604 North Country Club Road
Tucson, AZ 85716
(520) 881-4005
http://www.naela.org

National Adult Day Services Association
2519 Connecticut Avenue NW
Washington, DC 20008
(800) 558-5301
http://www.nadsa.org

National Alliance for Caregiving
4720 Montgomery Lane, 5th Floor
Bethesda, MD 20814
http://www.caregiving.org

National Alliance for Hispanic Health
1501 Sixteenth Street NW
Washington, DC 20036

(202) 387-5000
http://www.hispanichealth.org

National Alliance for the Mentally Ill (NAMI)
Colonial Place Three
Arlington, VA 22201
(800) 950-6264
http://www.nami.org

National Arthritis and Musculoskeletal and Skin Disease Information Clearinghouse
1 AMS Circle
Bethesda, MD 20892-3675
(301) 495-4484
http://www.niams.nih.gov/default.asp

National Asian Pacific Center on Aging
1511 Third Avenue
Suite 914
Seattle, WA 98101
(206) 624-1221
http://www.napca.org

National Association for Continence
P.O. Box 1019
Charleston, SC 29402
(843) 377-0900
http://www.nafc.org

National Association for Health & Fitness
c/o Be Active New York State
65 Niagara Square, Room 607
Buffalo, NY 14202
(716) 583-0521
http://www.physicalfitness.org

National Association for Hispanic Elderly
234 East Colorado Boulevard
Suite 300
Pasadena, CA 91101
(626) 564-1988
http://anppm.org

National Association for Home Care
228 Seventh Street SE
Washington, DC 20003
(202) 547-7424
http://www.nahc.org

National Association for Practical Nurse Education and Services
P.O. Box 25647
Alexandria, VA 22313

(703) 933-1002
http://www.napnes.org

National Association for Visually Handicapped
22 West 21st Street, Sixth Floor
New York, NY 10010
(212) 889-3141
http://www.navh.org

National Association of Activity Professionals
P.O. Box 5530
Sevierville, TN 37864
(865) 429-0717
http://www.thenaap.com

National Association of Area Agencies on Aging
1730 Rhode Island Avenue NW
Suite 1200
Washington, DC 20026
(202) 872-0888
http://www.n4a.org

National Association of Community Health Centers
7200 Wisconsin Avenue
Suite 210
Bethesda, MD 20814
(301) 347-0400
http://www.nachc.com

National Association of Nutrition and Aging Service Programs
1612 K Street NW
Suite 400
Washington, DC 20006
(202) 682-6899
http://www.nanasp.org

National Association of Professional Geriatric Care Managers
1604 North Country Club Road
Tucson, AZ 86716
(520) 881-8008
http://www.caremanger.org

National Association of Social Workers
750 First Street NE
Suite 700
Washington, DC 20002

(800) 638-8799
http://www.naswdc.org

National Association of State Units on Aging
1201 Fifteenth Street NW
Suite 350
Washington, DC 20005
(202) 898-2578
http://www.nasua.org

National Association of the Deaf
8630 Fenton Street
Suite 820
Silver Spring, MD 20910
(301) 587-1788
http://www.nad.org

National Association on HIV Over Fifty
23 Miner Street
Boston, MA 02215
(617) 233-7107
http://www.hivoverfifty.org

National Bar Association
1225 Eleventh Street NW
Washington, DC 20001
(202) 842-3900
http://www.nationalbar.org

National Cancer Institute
6116 Executive Boulevard
Bethesda, MD 20892
(800) 422-6237
http://www.nci.nih.gov

National Caucus and Center on Black Aged, Inc.
1220 L Street NW
Suite 800
Washington, DC 20005
(202) 637-8400
http://www.ncba-aged.org

National Center for Assisted Living
1201 L Street NW
Washington, DC 20005
(202) 824-4444
http://www.ncal.org

National Center for Complementary and Alternative Medicine
NCCAM Clearinghouse
P.O. Box 7923
Gaithersburg, MD 20898-7923
(301) 519-3153 or (888) 644-6226
http://www.nccam.nih.gov

National Center for Health Statistics
Presidential Building, Room 1064
6525 Belcrest Road
Hyattsville, MD 20782
(301) 458-4636
http://cdc.gov/nchs

National Center on Elder Abuse
1201 Fifteenth Street NW
Suite 350
Washington, DC 20005
(202) 898-2586
http://www.elderabusecenter.org

National Center on Minority Health and Health Disparities
National Institutes of Health
6707 Democracy Boulevard
Suite 800, MSC 5465
Bethesda, MD 20892
(301) 402-1366
http://www.ncmhd.nih.gov

National Center on Poverty Law, Inc.
50 East Washington Street
Suite 500
Chicago, IL 60602
(312) 263-3830
http://www.povertylaw.org

National Citizens' Coalition for Nursing Home Reform
1828 L Street NW
Suite 801
Washington, DC 20036
(202) 332-2276
http://www.nccnhr.org

National Coalition for Adult Immunization
National Foundation for Infectious Diseases
4733 Bethesda Avenue
Suite 750
Bethesda, MD 20814
(301) 656-0003
http://www.nfid.org

National Coalition for Cancer Survivorship
1010 Wayne Avenue

Suite 770
Silver Spring, MD 20910
(888) 650-9127
http://www.canceradvocacy.org

National Committee to Preserve Social Security and Medicare
10 G Street NE
Suite 600
Washington, DC 20004
(800) 966-1935
http://www.ncpssm.org

National Consumer Law Center
77 Summer Street, Tenth Floor
Boston, MA 02111
(617) 542-8010
http://www.consumerlaw.org

National Consumers League
1701 K Street NW
Suite 1200
Washington, DC 20006
(202) 835-3323
http://www.nclnet.org

National Council Against Health Fraud
119 Foster Street
Peabody, MA 01960
(978) 532-9393
http://www.ncahf.org

National Council on Aging
1901 L Street NW
Fourth floor
Washington, DC 20036
(202) 479-1200
http://www.ncoa.org

National Council on Alcoholism and Drug Dependence
22 Cortlandt Street
Suite 801
New York, NY 10007
(800) 622-2255
http://www.ncadd.org

National Council on Patient Information and Education
Medication Use Safety Training (MUST) for Seniors
4915 Saint Elmo Avenue
Suite 505

Bethesda, MD 20814
(301) 656-8565
http://www.mustforseniors.org

National Diabetes Information Clearinghouse
National Institute of Diabetes and Digestive and Kidney Diseases (NIDDK)
1 Information Way
Bethesda, MD 20892-3560
(800) 860-8747
http://www.diabetes.niddk.nih.gov

National Digestive Disease Information Clearinghouse
2 Information Way
Bethesda, MD 20892-3570
(800) 891-5389
http://www.digestive.niddk.nih.gov

National Domestic Violence Hotline
P.O. Box 161810
Austin, TX 78716
(800) 799-7233
http://www.ndvh.org

National Drug and Treatment Referral Routing Service
National Clearinghouse for Alcohol and Drug Information
P.O. Box 2345
Rockville, MD 20847
(800) 729-6686
http://www.health.org

National Eye Health Education Program
National Eye Institute Information Center
2020 Vision Place
Bethesda, MD 20892
(301) 496-5248
http://www.nei.nih.gov/nehep

National Family Caregivers Association
10400 Connecticut Avenue
Suite 500
Kensington, MD 20895
(800) 896-3650
http://www.nfcacares.org

National Foundation for Infectious Diseases
4733 Bethesda Avenue
Suite 750
Bethesda, MD 20814

(301) 656-0003
http://www.nfid.org

**National Foundation for the Treatment
of Pain**
P.O. Box 70045
Houston, TX 77270
(713) 862-9332
http://www.paincare.org

National Gerontological Nursing Association
7250 Parkway Drive, #510
Hanover, MD 21076-1377
(301) 949-8377
http://www.ngna.org

**National Heart, Lung, and Blood Health
Information Center**
P.O. Box 30105
Bethesda, MD 20824-0105
(800) 575-9355
http://www.nhlbi.nih.gov

**National Highway Traffic Safety
Administration**
400 Seventh Street SW
Washington, DC 20590
(888) 327-4236
http://www.nhtsa.dot.gov

National Hispanic Council on Aging
734 15th Street NW
Suite 1050
Washington, DC 20005
(202) 429-0787
http://www.nhcoa.org

National Hospice Foundation
1700 Diagonal Road
Suite 625
Alexandria, VA 22314
(703) 837-1500
http://www.nhpco.org

National Human Genome Research Institute
National Institutes of Health
Bethesda, MD 20892
(301) 402-0911
http://www.nhgrinih.gov

National Indian Council on Aging
10501 Montgomery Boulevard NE

Suite 210
Albuquerque, NM 87111
(505) 292-2001
http://www.nicoa.org

**National Information and Referral Support
Center**
1225 I Street
Suite 725
Washington, DC 20005
(202) 898-2578
http://www.nasua.org

**National Institute of Allergy and Infectious
Diseases**
Building 31, Room 7A50
31 Center Drive, MSC 2520
Bethesda, MD 20892
(301) 496-5717
http://www.niad.nih.gov

**National Institute of Arthritis and
Musculoskeletal and Skin Diseases
(NIAMS)**
1 AMS Circle
Bethesda, MD 20892-3675
(877) 226-4267
http://www.niams.nih.gov

**National Institute of Dental and Craniofacial
Research**
National Institutes of Health
Bethesda, MD 20892
(301) 496-4261
http://www.nidcr.nih.gov

**National Institute of General Medical
Sciences**
45 Center Drive, MSC 6200
Bethesda, MD 20892
(301) 496-7301
http://www.nigms.nih.gov

**National Institute of Health Osteoporosis
and Related Bone Diseases National
Resource Center**
2 AMS Circle
Bethesda, MD 20892-3676
(800) 624-2663
http://www.niams.nih.gov/bone

National Institute of Mental Health
6001 Executive Boulevard
Room 8184, MSC 9663
Bethesda, MD 20892
(301) 443-4513
http://www.nimh.nih.gov

National Institute of Neurological Disorders and Stroke
NIH Neurological Institute
Bethesda, MD 20824
(800) 352-9424
http://www.ninds.nih.gov

National Institute of Nursing Research
Office of Science Policy and Public Liaison
Bethesda, MD 20892
(301) 496-0207
http://www.nih.gov/ninr

National Institute on Aging (NIA)
Information Center
P.O. Box 8057
Gaithersburg, MD 20898-8057
(800) 222-2225
http://www.nia.nih.gov

National Institute on Alcohol Abuse and Alcoholism
5635 Fishers Lane, MWS 9304
Bethesda, MD 20892
(301) 443-3860
http://www.niaaa.nih.gov

National Institute on Deafness and Other Communications Disorders
31 Center Drive, MSC 2320
Bethesda, MD 20892
(800) 241-1044
http://www.nidcd.nih.gov

National Institute on Drug Abuse
National Institutes of Health
Bethesda, MD 20892-9561
(800) 729-6686
http://www.nida.nih.gov

National Kidney Foundation
30 East 33rd Street
New York, NY 10016
(800) 622-9010
http://www.kidney.org

National Kidney and Urological Diseases Information Clearinghouse
National Institute of Diabetes and Digestive and Kidney Diseases
Bethesda, MD 20892
(800) 891-5390
http://www.kidney.niddk.nih.gov

National Legal Support for Elderly People with Mental Disabilities Project
Judge David L. Bazelon Center for Mental Health Law
Washington, DC 20005-5002
(202) 467-5730
http://www.bazelon.org

National Library of Medicine
National Institutes of Health
8600 Rockville Pike
Bethesda, MD 20894
(888) 346-3656
http://www.nlm.nih.gov

National Library Service for the Blind and Physically Handicapped
Library of Congress
Washington, DC 20111
(800) 657-7323
http://www.lcweb.loc.gov/nls

National Long-Term Care Ombudsman Resource Center
ORC Office
1828 L Street NW
Suite 801
Washington, DC 20036
(202) 332-2275
http://www.ltcombudsman.org

National Medical Association
1012 Tenth Street NE
Washington, DC 20001
(202) 347-1895
http://www.nmanet.org

National Mental Health Association
2000 North Beauregard Street, Sixth Floor
Alexandria, VA 22311
(800) 969-6642
http://www.nmha.org

National Mental Health Consumers' Self-Help Clearinghouse
1211 Chestnut Street
Suite 1207
Philadelphia, PA 19107
(215) 751-1810

National Multiple Sclerosis Society
733 Third Avenue, Sixth Floor
New York, NY 10017
(800) 344-4867
http://www.nmss.org

National Organization for Rare Disorders
55 Kenosia Avenue
P.O. Box 1968
Danbury, CT 06813
(800) 999-6673
http://www.rarediseases.org

National Organization for Victim Assistance
510 King Street
Suite 424
Alexandria, VA 23314
(703) 535-6682
http://www.try-nova.org

National Osteoporosis Foundation
1232 22nd Street NW
Washington, DC 20037-1292
(202) 223-2226
http://www.nof.org

National Parkinson Foundation, Inc.
1501 NW 9th Avenue
Bob Hope Road
Miami, FL 33136
(800) 327-4545
http://www.parkinson.org

National Policy & Resource Center on Nutrition & Aging
Florida International University
OE 200
Miami, FL 33199
(305) 348-1517
http://nutritionandaging.fiu.edu/index.asp

National Policy and Resource Center on Women and Aging
The Heller School for Social Policy and Management

Waltham, MA 02454-9110
(800) 929-1995
http://www.brandeis.edu/heller/national

National Psoriasis Foundation
6600 SW 92nd Avenue
Suite 300
Portland, OR 97223
(800) 723-9166
http://www.psoriasis.org

National Rehabilitation Information Center (NARIC)
4200 Forbes Boulevard
Suite 202
Lanham, MD 20706
(800) 346-2742
http://www.naric.com

National Resource Center: Diversity and Long-Term Care
Schneidger Institute for Health Policy
The Heller School for Social Policy & Management
Waltham, MA 02454
(781) 736-3900
http://www.sihp.brandeis.edu

National Resource Center on Native American Aging
P.O. Box 9037
Grand Forks, ND 58202-9037
(701) 777-3848
http://www.med.und.nodak.edu/depts/rural/nrcnaa

National Respite Network and Resource Center
800 Eastowne Drive
Suite 105
Chapel Hill, NC 27514
(919) 490-5577, ext. 222
http://www.archrespite.org

National Resource Center on Supportive Housing & Home Modifications
3715 McClintock Avenue
Los Angeles, CA 90089
(213) 740-1364
http://www.homemods.org

National Rural Health Association
521 East 63rd Street

Kansas City, MO 64111
(816) 756-3140
http://www.nrharural.org

National Self-Help Clearinghouse
365 Fifth Avenue
Suite 3300
New York, NY 10016
(212) 817-1822
http://www.selfhelpweb.org

National Senior Citizens Law Center
1101 Fourteenth Street NW
Suite 400
Washington, DC 20005
(202) 289-6976
http://www.nsclc.org

National Senior Games Association
P.O. Box 82059
Baton Rouge, LA 70884
(225) 766-6800
http://www.nationalseniorgames.org

National Sleep Foundation
1522 K Street NW
Suite 500
Washington, DC 20005
(202) 347-3471
http://www.sleepfoundation.org

National STD and AIDS Hotlines
American Social Health Association
P.O. Box 13827
Research Triangle Park, NC 27709
(800) 342-2437
http://www.ashastd.org

National Stroke Association
9707 East Easter Lane
Englewood, CO 80112
(800) 787-6537
http://www.stroke.org

National Urban League
120 Wall Street, Eighth Floor
New York, NY 10005
(212) 558-5300
http://www.nul.org

National Women's Health Network
8550 Arlington Boulevard

Suite 300
Washington, DC 20004
(202) 347-1140
http://www.nwhn.org

North American Association for the Study of Obesity
8630 Fenton Street
Suite 918
Silver Spring, MD 20910
(301) 563-6526
http://www.naaso.org

North American Menopause Society
P.O. Box 94527
Cleveland, OH 44101
(440) 442-7550
http://www.menopause.org

National ElderHealth Area Resource Center
American Indian & Alaska Native Programs
University of Colorado Health Science Center
Department of Psychiatry
Nighthorse Campbell Native Health Building
P.O. Box 6508
Aurora, CO 80045
(303) 724-1414
http://www.uchsc.edu/ai/nehcrc/nehcrc_index.htm

OASIS Institute
7710 Carondelet Avenue
St. Louis, MO 63105
(314) 862-2933
http://www.oasisnet.org

Office of Dietary Supplements
National Institutes of Health
Bethesda, MD 20892
(301) 435-2920
http://dietary-supplements.info.nih.gov

Office of Medical Applications of Research (OMAR)
National Institutes of Health
Building 31, Room 1B03
31 Center Drive, MSC 2082
Bethesda, MD 20892
(301) 496-5641
http://odp.od.nih.gov/omar

Office of Research on Women's Health
900 Rockville Pike, Building 1, Room 201
Bethesda, MD 20892
(301) 402-1770
http://orwh.od.nih.gov

Office on Smoking and Health
Centers for Disease Control and Prevention
Atlanta, GA 30341
(800) 232-4636
http://www.cdc.gov/tobacco

Older Women's League
3300 North Fairfax Drive
Suite 218
Arlington, VA 22201
(800) 825-3695
http://www.owl-national.org

Oley Foundation for Home Parenteral (IV) and Enteral (Tube-fed) Nutrition
214 Hun Memorial, A-28
Albany Medical Center
Albany, NY 12208
(800) 776-6539
http://www.oley.org

Opticians Association of America
441 Carlisle Drive
Herndon, VA 20170
(703) 437-8780
http://www.oaa.org

Organization of Chinese Americans
1001 Connecticut Avenue NW
Suite 601
Washington, DC 20036
(202) 223-5500
http://www.ocanatl.org

Paget Foundation for Paget's Disease of Bone and Related Disorders
120 Wall Street
Suite 1602
New York, NY 10005
(212) 509-5335
http://www.paget.org

Parkinson Alliance
P.O. Box 308
Kingston, NH 08528

(609) 688-0870
http://www.parkinsonalliance.org

Parkinson's Action Network (PAN)
1025 Vermont Avenue NW
Suite 1120
Washington, DC 20005
(800) 850-4726
http://www.parksonsaction.org

Parkinson's Disease Foundation
1359 Broadway
Suite 1509
New York, NY 10018
(800) 457-6676
http://www.pdf.org

Parkinson's Institute
1170 Morse Avenue
Sunnyvale, CA 94089
(800) 786-2958
http://www.thepi.org

Parkinson's Resource Organization
74090 El Paseo
Suite 102
Palm Desert, CA 92260
(760) 773-5628
http://www.parkinsonsresource.org

Partners in Care Foundation
732 Mott Street
Suite 150
San Fernando, CA 91340
(818) 837-3775
http://www.picf.org/contact

President's Council on Physical Fitness and Sports
200 Independence Avenue
Department W, Room 738 H
Washington, DC 20201
(202) 690-9000
http://www.fitness.gov

Prevent Blindness America
211 West Wacker Drive
Suite 1700
Chicago, IL 60606
(800) 331-2020
http://www.preventblindness.org

Pulmonary Fibrosis Foundation
1332 North Halsted Street
Suite 201
Chicago, IL 60622
(312) 587-9272
http://www.pulmonaryfibrosis.org

Rebuilding Together
1536 Sixteenth Street NW
Washington, DC 20036
(800) 473-4229
http://www.rebuildingtogether.org

Restless Legs Syndrome Foundation
1610 Fourteenth Street NW
Suite 300
Rochester, MN 55901
(507) 287-6465
http://www.rls.org

Robert Wood Johnson Foundation
P.O. Box 2316
Princeton, NJ 08543
(888) 631-9989
http://www.rwjf.org

Self-Help for Hard of Hearing People, Inc.
7910 Woodmont Avenue
Suite 1200
Bethesda, MD 20814
(301) 657-2248
http://www.shhh.org

Self-Reliance Foundation
1126 Sixteenth Street NW
Suite 350
Washington, DC 20036
(202) 360-4131
http://www.selfreliancefoundation.org

Senior Action in a Gay Environment
305 Seventh Avenue, 16th Floor
New York, NY 10001
(212) 741-2247
http://www.sageusa.org

Senior Service America
8403 Colesville Road
Suite 1200
Silver Spring, MD 20910
(301) 578-8900
http://www.seniorserviceamerica.org

Setting Priorities for Retirement Years (SPRY) Foundation
10 G Street NE
Suite 600
Washington, DC 20002
(202) 216-8466
http://www.spry.og

Silver Sneakers Fitness Program
9280 South Kyrene Road
Suite 134
Tempe, AZ 85284
(888) 423-4632
http://www.silversneakers.com

Simon Foundation for Continence
P.O. Box 815
Wilmette, IL 60091
(800) 237-4666
http://www.simonfoundation.org

Skin Cancer Foundation
245 Fifth Avenue
Suite 1403
New York, NY 10016
(800) 754-6490
http://www.skincancer.org

Social Security Administration
Office of Public Inquiries
6401 Security Boulevard
Baltimore, MD 21235
(800) 772-1213
http://www.socialsecurity.gov

Society for Neuroscience
1121 Fourteenth Street
Suite 1010
Washington, DC 20005
(202) 962-4000
http://www.sfn.org

Southern Medical Association
35 Lakeshore Drive
Birmingham, AL 35209
(800) 423-4992
http://www.sma.org

Substance Abuse and Mental Health Services Administration
1 Choke Cherry Road
Rockville, MD 20850

(800) 729-6686
http://www.samhsa.gov

Transplant Recipient International Organization (TRIO)
1000 Sixteenth Street NW
Suite 602
Washington, DC 20036
(202) 293-0980
http://www.trioweb.org

United Network for Organ Sharing
P.O. Box 2484
Richmond, VA 23218
(888) 894-6361
http://www.nos.org

United States Consumer Product Safety Commission
4330 East West Highway
Bethesda, MD 20814
(800) 638-2772
http://www.cpsc.gov

United States Department of Agriculture Food and Nutrition Information Center
10301 Baltimore Avenue, Room 304
Beltsville, MD 20705
(301) 504-5719
http://www.nal.usda.gov/fnic

United States Department of Housing and Urban Development (HUD)
451 Seventh Street SW
Washington, DC 20410
(202) 708-1112
http://www.hud.gov

United States Living Will Registry
523 Westfield Avenue, P.O. Box 2789
Westfield, NJ 07091-2789
(800) 548-9455
http://www.uslivingwillregistry.com

United States Postal Inspection Service
Criminal Investigations Service Center (Mail Fraud)
222 South Riverside Plaza

Suite 1250
Chicago, IL 60606
http://www.usps.com/postalinspectors/fraud

United Way of America
701 North Fairfax Street
Alexandria, VA 22314
(800) 892-2757
http://www.unitedway.org

Visiting Nurse Association of America
99 Summer Street
Suite 1700
Boston, MA 02110
(888) 866-8773
http://www.vnaa.org

Washington Health Promotion Research Center
Project Enhance Senior Services
2208 Second Avenue
Suite 100
Seattle, WA 98121
(206) 727-6219
http://www.projectenhance.org

Weight-Control Information Network (WIN)
National Institute of Diabetes and Digestive and Kidney Diseases
1 WIN Way
Bethesda, MD 20892
(877) 946-4627
http://www.niddk.nih.gov/health/nutrit/win.htm

Well Spouse Foundation
63 West Main Street
Suite H
Freehold, NJ 07228
(800) 838-0879
http://www.wellspouse.org

World Health Organization
Avenue Appia 20
1211 Geneva 27
Switzerland
(+41 22) 791-2111
http://www.who.int

APPENDIX II
STATE AGING AGENCIES IN THE UNITED STATES AND ITS TERRITORIES

Each state has its own aging office, which provides information, assistance, and referrals on issues of elder care to older individuals, family members, and others.

ALABAMA

Alabama Department of Senior Services
P.O. Box 301851
770 Washington Avenue, Suite 470
Montgomery, AL 36130-1851
(334) 242-5743 or (800) 243-5463
Fax: (334) 242-5594
http://www.adss.state.al.us

ALASKA

Alaska Commission on Aging
Department of Health and Social Services
150 Third Street, No. 103
P.O. Box 110693
Juneau, AK 99811-0693
(907) 465-4879
Fax: (907) 465-4716
http://www.hss.state.ak.us/acoa

ARIZONA

Arizona Aging and Adult Administration
Department of Economic Security
1789 W. Jefferson, No. 950A
Phoenix, AZ 85007
(602) 542-4446
Fax: (602) 542-6575
http://www.de.state.az.us/aaa

ARKANSAS

Arkansas Division of Aging and Adult Services
Department of Human Services

P.O. Box 1437
700 Main Street, 5th Floor, S530
Little Rock, AR 72203-1437
(501) 682-2441
Fax: (501) 682-8155
http://www.arkansas.gov/dhhs/aging/index.html

CALIFORNIA

California Department of Aging
1300 National Drive, #200
Sacramento, CA 95834
(916) 419-7500
Fax: (916) 928-2268
http://www.aging.ca.gov

COLORADO

Colorado Division of Aging and Adult Services
Department of Human Services
1575 Sherman Street
Ground Floor
Denver, CO 80203-1714
(303) 866-2636
Fax: (303) 866-2696
http://www.cdhs.state.co.us/aas

CONNECTICUT

Connecticut Bureau of Aging Community & Social Work Services
Department of Social Services
25 Sigourney Street
Hartford, CT 06106
(860) 424-5277
Fax: (860) 424-5301
http://www.ct.gov/dss/site/default.asp

DELAWARE

Delaware Division of Services for Aging and Adults with Physical Disabilities
Department of Health and Social Services
1901 North DuPont Highway
New Castle, DE 19720
(302) 255-9390
Fax: (302) 255-4445
http://www.dhss.delaware.gov/dhss/dsaapd/index.html

DISTRICT OF COLUMBIA

District of Columbia Office on Aging
One Judiciary Square
441 4th Street NW, Ninth Floor
Washington, DC 20001
(202) 724-5622
Fax: (202) 724-4979
http://www.dcoa.dc.gov

FLORIDA

Florida Department of Elder Affairs
4040 Esplanade Way
Suite 315
Tallahassee, FL 32399
(850) 414-2000
Fax: (850) 414-2004
http://elderaffairs.state.fl.us

GEORGIA

Georgia Division for Aging Services
2 Peachtree Street NW, 9th Floor
Atlanta, GA 30303
(404) 657-5258
Fax: (404) 657-5285
http://www.aging.dhr.georgia.gov

GUAM

Guam Division of Senior Citizens
Department of Public Health and Social Services
Government of Guam
123 Chalan Kareta Route 10
Mangilao, Guam 96923
011 (671) 475-0263
Fax: 011 (671) 734-5910
http://dphss.guam.gov/about/senior_citizens.htm

HAWAII

Hawaii Executive Office on Aging
No. 1 Capitol District
250 South Hotel Street, Suite 406
Honolulu, HI 96813-2831
(808) 586-0100
Fax: (808) 586-0185
http://www4.hawaii.gov/eoa/index.html

IDAHO

Idaho Commission on Aging
3380 Americana Terrace, No. 120
P.O. Box 83720
Boise, ID 83720-0007
(208) 334-3833
Fax: (208) 334-3033
http://www.idahoaging.com/abouticoa/index.htm

ILLINOIS

Illinois Department on Aging
421 East Capitol Avenue
Springfield, IL 62701
(217) 785-2870
Fax: (217) 785-4477
http://www.state.il.us/aging

INDIANA

Indiana Division on Aging
Division of Disability, Aging and Rehabilitative Services
Family and Services Administration
402 W. Washington Street
P.O. Box 7083
Indianapolis, IN 46207-7083
(317) 232-7123
Fax: (317) 232-7867
http://www.in.gov/fssa/da/index.htm

IOWA

Iowa Department of Elder Affairs
Jessie Parker Building
510 East 12th Street, Suite 2
Des Moines, IA 50319-9025
(515) 725-3301
Fax: (515) 725-3300
http://www.state.ia.us/elderaffairs

KANSAS

Kansas Department on Aging
New England Building
503 South Kansas Avenue
Topeka, KS 66603-3404
(785) 296-5222
Fax: (785) 296-0256
http://www.agingkansas.org

KENTUCKY

Kentucky Division of Aging Services
Cabinet for Health Services
275 East Main Street, 5C-D
Frankfort, KY 40621
(502) 564-6930
Fax: (502) 564-4595
http://chfs.ky.gov/agencies/os/dail/Programs.htm

LOUISIANA

Governor's Office of Elderly Affairs
P.O. Box 80374
412 N. 4th Street
Baton Rouge, LA 70802
(225) 342-7100
Fax: (225) 342-7133
http://goea.louisiana.gov

MAINE

Maine Office of Elder Services
Department of Human Services
442 Civic Center Drive
11 State House Station
Augusta, ME 04333-0011
(207) 287-9200
Fax: (207) 287-9229
http://maine.gov/dhhs/beas

MARIANA ISLANDS

CNMI Office on Aging
Commonwealth of the Northern Mariana Islands
P.O. Box 502178
Saipan, MP 96950-2178
(670) 233-1320 or (670) 233-1321
Fax: (670) 233-1327
http://www.dcca.gov.mp/index.cfm?pageID=86

MARYLAND

Maryland Department of Aging
301 West Preston Street, Suite 1007
Baltimore, MD 21201
(410) 767-1100
Fax: (410) 333-7943
http://www.mdoa.state.md.us

MASSACHUSETTS

Massachusetts Executive Office of Elder Affairs
One Ashburton Place
Boston, MA 02108
(617) 222-7451
Fax: (617) 727-6944
http://www.mass.gov/?pageID=eldershomepage&
    L=1&L0=Home&sid=Eelders

MICHIGAN

Michigan Office of Services to the Aging
P.O. Box 30676
7109 West Saginaw, First Floor
Lansing, MI 48909-8176
(517) 373-8230
Fax: (517) 373-4092
http://www.michigan.gov/miseniors

MINNESOTA

Minnesota Board on Aging
Aging and Adult Services Division
P.O. Box 64976
St. Paul, MN 55164-0976
(651) 431-2500 or (800) 882-6262
Fax: (651) 431-7453
http://www.mnaging.org

MISSISSIPPI

Mississippi Council on Aging
Division of Aging and Adult Services
750 N. State Street
Jackson, MS 39202
(601) 359-4925
Fax: (601) 359-4370
http://www.mdhs.state.ms.us/aas.html

MISSOURI

Missouri Division of Senior & Disability Services
Department of Health & Senior Services
P.O. Box 570

Jefferson City, MO 65102-0570
(573) 526-3626
Fax: (573) 751-8687
http://www.dhss.mo.gov

MONTANA

Montana Office on Aging
Senior and Long Term Care Division
Department of Public Health and Human
    Services
111 Sanders Street
P.O. Box 4210
Helena, MT 59604
(406) 444-7788
Fax: (406) 444-7743
http://www.dphhs.mt.gov/sltc

NEBRASKA

Nebraska Health and Human Services—State Unit on Aging
Department of Health & Human Services
P.O. Box 95044
301 Centennial Mall, South
Lincoln, NE 68509
(402) 471-2307
Fax: (402) 471-4619
http://www.hhs.state.ne.us/ags/agsindex.htm

NEVADA

Nevada Division for Aging Services
Department of Human Resources
3416 Goni Road, Building D-132
Carson City, NV 89706
(775) 687-4210
Fax: (775) 687-4264
http://aging.state.nv.us

NEW HAMPSHIRE

New Hampshire Bureau of Elderly and Adult Services
Brown Buildin, 129 Pleasant Street
Concord, NH 03301-3857
(603) 271-4394
Fax: (603) 271-4643
http://www.dhhs.state.nh.us/DHHS/BEAS/default.htm

NEW JERSEY

New Jersey Division of Aging & Community Services
Department of Health & Senior Services
240 W. State Street (FedEx zip 08608-1002)
P.O. Box 807
Trenton, NJ 08625-0807
(609) 292-4027
Fax: (609) 943-3343
http://www.state.nj.us/health/senior/index.shtml

NEW MEXICO

New Mexico Aging & LTC Services Department
2550 Cerrillos Road
Santa Fe, NM 87505
(505) 476-4799 (main)
(505) 476-4738 (direct)
Fax: (505) 827-7649
http://www.nmaging.state.nm.us

NEW YORK

New York State Office for the Aging
Two Empire State Plaza
Albany, NY 12223-1251
(518) 474-7012
Fax: (518) 474-1398
http://aging.state.ny.us

NORTH CAROLINA

North Carolina Division of Aging & Adult Services
Department of Health and Human Services
2101 Mail Service Center
Raleigh, NC 27699-2101
(919) 733-3983
Fax: (919) 733-0443
http://www.dhhs.state.nc.us/aging

NORTH DAKOTA

North Dakota Aging Services Division
Department of Human Services
600 East Boulevard Avenue
Department 325
Bismarck, ND 58505-0250
(701) 328-4601
Fax: (701) 328-2359
http://www.nd.gov/dhs

OHIO

Ohio Department of Aging
50 West Broad Street, 9th Floor
Columbus, OH 43215-5928
(614) 466-7246
Fax: (614) 995-1049
http://www.goldenbuckeye.com

OKLAHOMA

Aging Services Division
OK Department of Human Services
P.O. Box 25352
2401 N.W. 23rd Street
Suite 40
Oklahoma City, OK 73107
(405) 521-2281
Fax: (405) 521-2086
http://www.okdhs.org

OREGON

Oregon Seniors and People with Disabilities
Department of Human Services
500 Summer Street NE, E02
Salem, OR 97301-1073
(503) 945-5811
Fax: (503) 373-7823
http://www.oregon.gov/DHS/spwpd/index.shtml

PENNSYLVANIA

Pennsylvania Department of Aging
555 Walnut Street, 5th Floor
Harrisburg, PA 17101-1919
(717) 783-1550
Fax: (717) 772-3382
http://www.aging.state.pa.us

PUERTO RICO

Puerto Rico Governor's Office for Elderly Affairs
P.O. Box 191179
San Juan, PR 00919-1179
(787) 721-5710
Fax: (787) 721-6510
http://www.aoa.gov/smp/media/MLamoso.ppt

RHODE ISLAND

Rhode Island Department of Elderly Affairs
John O. Pastore Center

Benjamin Rush Building, No. 55
35 Howard Avenue
Cranston, RI 02920
(401) 462-0500
Fax: (401) 462-0503
http://www.dea.state.ri.us

(AMERICAN) SAMOA

Territorial Administration on Aging
American Samoa Government
Pago Pago, American Samoa 96799
011 (684) 633-1251 or 633-1252
Fax: 011 (684) 633-2533
http://americansamoa.gov/departments/agencies/
taoa.htm

SOUTH CAROLINA

South Carolina Lieutenant Governor's Office on Aging
Bureau of Senior Services
1301 Gervais Street
Suite 200
Columbia, SC 29201
(803) 734-9900
Fax: (803) 734-9886
http://www.aging.sc.gov

SOUTH DAKOTA

South Dakota Office of Adult Services & Aging
Department of Social Services
700 Governors Drive
Pierre, SD 57501
(605) 773-3656
Fax: (605) 773-6834
http://dss.sd.gov/elderlyservices

TENNESSEE

Tennessee Commission on Aging and Disability
Andrew Jackson Building
500 Deaderick Street, No. 825
Nashville, TN 37243-0860
(615) 741-2056
Fax: (615) 741-3309
http://www.state.tn.us/comaging

TEXAS

Texas Department of Aging and Disability Services
701 West 51st Street
MCW616
Austin, TX 78751
(512) 438-4293
http://www.dads.state.tx.us

U.S. VIRGIN ISLANDS

Virgin Islands Senior Citizen Affairs Administration
Department of Human Services
19 Estate Diamond Fredericksted
St. Croix, VI 00840
(340) 692-5950
Fax: (340) 692-2062

UTAH

Utah Division of Aging & Adult Services
Department of Human Services
120 North 200 West, Room 325
Salt Lake City, UT 84103
(801) 538-3910
Fax: (801) 538-4395
http://www.hsdaas.utah.gov

VERMONT

Vermont Department of Disabilities, Aging and Independent Living
103 South Main Street, Osgood #1
Waterbury, VT 05671-2301
(802) 241-2400
Fax: (802) 241-2325
http://dail.vermont.gov

VIRGINIA

Virginia Department for the Aging
1610 Forest Avenue, Suite 100
Richmond, VA 23229
(804) 662-9333
Fax: (804) 662-9354
http://www.vda.virginia.gov

WASHINGTON

Washington Aging and Disability Services
Department of Social & Health Services
Mail Stop 45050
14th and Jefferson, Office Bldg. 2
Olympia, WA 98504-5010
(360) 902-7797
Fax: (360) 902-7848
http://www.aasa.dshs.wa.gov

WEST VIRGINIA

West Virginia Bureau of Senior Services
1900 Kanawha Boulevard, East
3003 Town Center Mall
Charleston, WV 25305-0160
(304) 558-3317
Fax: (304) 558-5609
http://www.wvseniorservices.gov

WISCONSIN

Wisconsin Bureau of Aging and Disability Resources
Department of Health and Family Services
One West Wilson Street, Room 450
P.O. Box 7851
Madison, WI 53707-7851
(608) 266-2536
Fax: (608) 267-3203
http://dhfs.wisconsin.gov/aging

WYOMING

Wyoming Aging Division
Department of Health
6101 Yellow Stone Road, Room 259B
Cheyenne, WY 82002
(307) 777-7986 or (800) 442-2766
Fax: (307) 777-5340
http://wdhfs.state.wy.us/aging/index.html

APPENDIX III
STATE OMBUDSMEN REGULATING LONG-TERM CARE FACILITIES SUCH AS NURSING HOMES

State ombudsmen are specific individuals whose mission is to assist older people and their families with disputes with long-term care facilities, particularly those disputes involving nursing homes. Each state has its own ombudsman office, although the department under which the office operates varies from state to state.

ALABAMA

Alabama Department of Senior Services
State Long-Term Ombudsman
100 North Union Street
RSA Union Building
Suite 770
Montgomery, AL 36130
(334) 242-5770
http://www.ageline.net

ALASKA

Office of the State Long-Term Care Ombudsman
Alaska Mental Health Trust Authority
3745 Community Park Loop
Suite 200
Anchorage, AK 99508
(907) 334-4480
http://www.akoltco.org

ARIZONA

State Long-Term Care Ombudsman
Arizona Aging & Adult Administration
1789 West Jefferson, #950A
Phoenix, AZ 85007
(602) 542-6454
http://www.de.state.az.us/aaa/programs/ombudsman/default.asp

ARKANSAS

State Long-Term Care Ombudsman
Arkansas Division of Aging & Adult Services
P.O. Box 1437
Little Rock, AR 72203
(501) 682-8952
http://www.arombudsman.com/pay.html

CALIFORNIA

State Long-Term Care Ombudsman
California Department of Aging
1300 National Drive
Suite 200
Sacramento, CA 95834
(916) 419-7510
http://www.aging.ca.gov/html/programs/ombudsman.html

COLORADO

State Long-Term Care Ombudsman
The Legal Center
455 Sherman Street
Suite 130
Denver, CO 80203
(800) 288-1376, extension 217
http://www.thelegalcenter.org/services_older.html

CONNECTICUT

State Long-Term Care Ombudsman
Office of the State Long-Term Care Ombudsman
Connecticut Department of Social Services
25 Sigourney Street, 12th Floor
Hartford, CT 06106
(860) 424-5239
http://www.ltcop.state.ct.us

DELAWARE

State Long-Term Care Ombudsman
Division of Services for Aging & Adults
1901 North Dupont Highway
Main Administration Building Annex
New Castle, DE 19720
(302) 255-9390
http://www.dhss.delaware.gov/dsaapd

DISTRICT OF COLUMBIA

State Long-Term Care Ombudsman
Legal Counsel for the Elderly
601 E Street NW
Suite A4-315
Washington, DC 20049
(202) 434-2140

FLORIDA

State Long-Term Care Ombudsman
Department of Elder Affairs
Florida State Long-Term Care Ombudsman
    Council
4040 Esplanade Way
Tallahassee, FL 32399
(888) 831-0404
http://www.myflorida.com/ombudsman

GEORGIA

State Long-Term Care Ombudsman
Office of the State LTCO
2 Peachtree Street NW, Ninth Floor
Atlanta, GA 30303
(888) 454-5826
http://www.georgiaombudsman.org

GUAM

State Long-Term Care Ombudsman
Division of Senior Citizens, Guam DPHSS
P.O. Box 2816
Hagatna, GU 96932
(671) 735-7832, extension 5

HAWAII

State Long-Term Care Ombudsman
Executive Office on Aging
250 South Hotel Street, Suite 406
Honolulu, HI 96813
(808) 586-0100

IDAHO

State Long-Term Care Ombudsman
Idaho Commission on Aging
P.O. Box 83720
3380 American Terrace, Suite 120
Boise, ID 83720
(208) 334-3833
http://www.idahoaging.com/programs/ps_
    ombuds.htm

ILLINOIS

State Long-Term Care Ombudsman
Illinois Department on Aging
421 East Capitol Avenue, Suite 100
Springfield, IL 62701-1789
(217) 785-3143
http://www.state.il.us/aging

INDIANA

State Long-Term Care Ombudsman
Indiana Division Disabilities/Rehabilitative
    Services
402 West Washington Street, Room W-454
P.O. Box 7083, MS21
Indianapolis, IN 46207
(800) 622-4484

IOWA

State Long-Term Care Ombudsman
Iowa Department of Elder Affairs
510 East 12th Street
Jessie M. Parker Building, Suite 2
Des Moines, IA 50319
(515) 725-3327

KANSAS

State Long-Term Care Ombudsman
Office of the State Long-Term Care Ombudsman
900 SW Jackson Street, Suite 1041
Topeka, KS 66612
(877) 662-8362
http://da.state.ks.us/care

KENTUCKY

State Long-Term Care Ombudsman
Office of the Ombudsman
Cabinet for Health & Family Services
275 East Main Street, Suite 1E-B

Frankfort, KY 40621
(502) 564-5497

LOUISIANA

State Long-Term Care Ombudsman
Office of Elderly Affairs
412 North 4th Street, Third Floor
P.O. Box 61
Baton Rouge, LA 70821
(866) 632-0922

MAINE

State Long-Term Care Ombudsman
Maine Long-Term Care Ombudsman Program
1 Weston Court
P.O. Box 128
Augusta, ME 04332
(207) 621-1079
http://www.maineombudsman.org

MARYLAND

State Long-Term Care Ombudsman
Maryland Department of Aging
301 West Preston Street
Room 1007
Baltimore, MD 21201
(410) 767-1100
http://www.mdoa.state.ms.us/ombudsman.html

MASSACHUSETTS

State Long-Term Care Ombudsman
Massachusetts Executive Office of Elder Affairs
1 Ashburton Place, 5th Floor
Boston, MA 02108-1518
(617) 727-7750

MICHIGAN

State Long-Term Care Ombudsman
Michigan Office of Services to the Aging
7109 West Saginaw
P.O. Box 30676
Lansing, MI 48909
(517) 335-0148
http://www.miseniors.net

MINNESOTA

State Long-Term Care Ombudsman
Office of Ombudsman for Older Minnesotans
P.O. Box 64971

St. Paul, MN 55164-0971
(651) 431-2552
http://www.mnaging.org/admin/ooom.htm

MISSISSIPPI

State Long-Term Care Ombudsman
Mississippi Department of Human Services
Division of Aging
750 North State Street
Jackson, MS 39202
(601) 359-4927
http://www.mdhs.state.ms.us

MISSOURI

State Long-Term Care Ombudsman
Department of Health & Senior Services
P.O. Box 570
Jefferson City, MO 65102
(800) 309-3282
http://www.dhss.mo.gov/Ombudsman

MONTANA

State Long-Term Care Ombudsman
Montana Department of Health & Human Services
P.O. Box 4210
111 North Sanders
Helena, MT 59604-4210
(406) 444-7785

NEBRASKA

State Long-Term Care Ombudsman
Division of Aging Services
P.O. Box 95044
Lincoln, NE 68509-5044
(402) 471-2307

NEVADA

State Long-Term Care Ombudsman
Nevada Division for Aging Services
3416 Goni Road
Building D, Number 132
Carson City, NV 89706
(775) 687-4210, extension 254

NEW HAMPSHIRE

State Long-Term Care Ombudsman
New Hampshire Office of the Long-Term Care
    Ombudsman
129 Pleasant Street

Concord, NH 03301-3857
(603) 271-4704

NEW JERSEY
State Long-Term Care Ombudsman
Office of Ombudsman for Institutional Elderly
P.O. Box 807
Trenton, NJ 08625-0807
(609) 943-4026
http://www.state.nj.us/health/senior/sa_ombd.
   htm

NEW MEXICO
State Long-Term Care Ombudsman
New Mexico Aging and Long-Term Care Services
   Department
2550 Cerrillos Road
Santa Fe, NM 87505
(505) 476-4790

NEW YORK
State Long-Term Care Ombudsman
New York State Office for the Aging
2 Empire State Plaza
Agency Building 2
Albany, NY 12223
(518) 474-7329
http://www.ombudsman.state.ny.us

NORTH CAROLINA
State Long-Term Care Ombudsman
North Carolina Division of Aging and Adult
   Services
2101 Mall Service Center
Raleigh, NC 27699-2101
(919) 733-8395, extension 227
http://www.dhhs.stae.nc.us/aging/ombud.htm

NORTH DAKOTA
State Long-Term Care Ombudsman
Aging Services Division
Health and Human Services Office Center
Dorothea Dix Hospital Campus—Taylor Hall
693 Palmer Drive
Raleigh, NC 27699
(919) 733-3983
http://www.dhhs.state.nc.us/aging/ombud.htm

OHIO
State Long-Term Care Ombudsman
Ohio Department of Aging
50 West Broad Street, Ninth Floor
Columbus, OH 43215-3363
(614) 644-7922
http://www.goldenbuckeye.com

OKLAHOMA
State Long-Term Care Ombudsman
Long-Term Care Ombudsman Program
DHS Aging Services Division
2401 NW 23rd Street, Suite 40
Oklahoma City, OK 73107

OREGON
State Long-Term Care Ombudsman
Oregon Office of the Long-Term Care
   Ombudsman
3855 Wolverine NE, Suite 6
Salem, OR 97305-1251
(503) 378-6533
http://www.oregon.gov/LTCO

PENNSYLVANIA
State Long-Term Care Ombudsman
Pennsylvania Department of Aging
555 Walnut Street, Fifth Floor
P.O. Box 1089
Harrisburg, PA 17101
http://www.aging.state.pa.us/aging/site/default.asp

PUERTO RICO
State Long-Term Care Ombudsman
Puerto Rico Governor's Office of Elder Affairs
P.O. Box 191179
San Juan, PR 00919-1179
(787) 725-1515

RHODE ISLAND
State Long-Term Care Ombudsman
Alliance for Better Long-Term Care
422 Post Road
Suite 204
Warwick, RI 02888
(401) 785-3340

SOUTH CAROLINA

State Long-Term Care Ombudsman

Governor's Office on Aging
1301 Gervais Street, Suite 200
Columbia, SC 29201
(803) 734-988
http://www.aging.sc.gov

SOUTH DAKOTA

State Long-Term Care Ombudsman

Department of Social Services
South Dakota Office of Adult Services and Aging
700 Governors Drive
Pierre, SC 57501-2291
(605) 773-3656
http://dss.sd.gov

TENNESSEE

State Long-Term Care Ombudsman

Tennessee Commission on Aging and Disability
Andrew Jackson Building
500 Deaderick Street
Suite 825
Nashville, TN 37243
(615) 741-2056

TEXAS

State Long-Term Care Ombudsman

Center for Consumer and External Affairs
P.O. Box 149030
Mail Code 250
Austin, TX 8714
(512) 438-4356
http://www.dads.state.tx.us/news_info/ombuds-
  man/index.html

UTAH

State Long-Term Care Ombudsman

Department of Human Services
Utah Division of Aging and Adult Services
120 North 200 West
Room 325
Salt Lake City, UT 84103
(801) 538-3924

VERMONT

State Long-Term Care Ombudsman

Vermont Legal Aid, Inc.
264 North Winooski Avenue

P.O. Box 1367
Burlington, VT 05402
(802) 863-5620
http://www.dad.state.vt.us/ltcinfo/ombudsman.
  html

VIRGINIA

State Long-Term Care Ombudsman

Virginia Association of Area Agencies on Aging
24 East Cary Street
Suite 100
Richmond VA 23219
(804) 565-1600
http://www.vaaa.org

WASHINGTON

State Long-Term Care Ombudsman

State Long-Term Care Ombudsman Program
  Multi-Service Center
1200 South 336th Street
P.O. Box 23699
Federal Way, WA 98093
(800) 422-1384
http://www.ltcsop.org

WEST VIRGINIA

State Long-Term Care Ombudsman

West Virginia Bureau of Senior Services
1900 Kanawha Boulevard East
Building 10
Charleston, WV 25305-0160
(304) 558-3317
http://www.state.wv.us/seniorservices

WISCONSIN

State Long-Term Care Ombudsman

Wisconsin Board on Aging and Long-Term Care
1402 Pankratz Street
Madison, WI 53704-4001
(800) 815-0015
http://longtermcare.state.wi.us

WYOMING

State Long-Term Care Ombudsman

Wyoming Senior Citizens, Inc.
865 Gilchrist,
P.O. Box 94
Wheatland, WY 82201
(307) 322-5553

APPENDIX IV

STATE HELPLINE AND HOTLINE CONTACTS TO REPORT ELDER ABUSE OR NEGLECT WITHIN THE STATE

If abuse or neglect of an elderly person is suspected, this abuse should be reported to the appropriate agency for investigation in order to protect the person from further abuse or neglect. The chart in this appendix offers telephone numbers to call on behalf of individuals who may be suffering from abuse in their homes or in nursing homes where they reside.

Note: Many states have toll-free numbers beginning with 800, 866, or 877.

State	Reporting Elder Abuse in the Home or Community	Reporting Elder Abuse in a Nursing Home or Long-Term Care Facility
Alabama	(800) 458-7214	(800) 458-7214
Alaska	(800) 478-9996	(800) 730-6393
Arizona	(877) 767-2385	(877) 767-2385
Arkansas	(800) 332-4443	(800) 582-4887
California	(888) 436-3600	(800) 231-4024
Colorado	(800) 773-1366	(800) 773-1366 or (800) 886-7689, ext. 2800
Connecticut	(888) 385-4225 or (860) 424-5241	(860) 424-5241
Delaware	(800) 223-9074	(800) 223-9074
District of Columbia	(202) 541-3950	(202) 434-2140
Florida	(800) 962-2873	(800) 962-2873
Georgia	(888) 774-0152	(800) 878-6442
Guam	(671) 475-0268	(671) 475-0268
Hawaii	(808) 832-5115 (Oahu)	(808) 832-5115 (Oahu)
	(808) 243-5151 (Maui, Molokai, and Lanai)	(808) 832-5151 (Maui, Molokai, and Lanai)
	(808) 241-3432 (Kauai)	(808) 241-3432 (Kauai)
	(808) 933-8820 (East Hawaii)	(808) 933-8820 (East Hawaii)
	(808) 327-6280 (West Hawaii)	(808) 327-6280 (West Hawaii)
Idaho	(877) 471-2777	(877) 471-2777
Illinois	(866) 800-1409	(800) 252-4343
Indiana	(800) 992-6978	(800) 992-6978
Iowa	(800) 362-2178	(877) 686-0027
Kansas	(800) 922-5330	(800) 842-0078
Kentucky	(800) 752-6200	(800) 752-6200

(continues)

(Continued)

State	Reporting Elder Abuse in the Home or Community	Reporting Elder Abuse in a Nursing Home or Long-Term Care Facility
Louisiana	(800) 259-4990	(800) 259-4990
Maine	(800) 624-8404	(800) 383-2441
Maryland	(800) 917-7383	(800) 917-7383
Massachusetts	(800) 922-2275	(800) 462-5540
Michigan	(800) 996-6228	(800) 882-6006
Minnesota	(800) 333-2433	(800) 333-2433
Mississippi	(800) 222-8000	(800) 227-7308
Missouri	(800) 392-0210	(800) 392-0210
Montana	(800) 551-3191	(800) 551-3191
Nebraska	(800) 652-1999	(800) 652-1999
Nevada	(800) 992-5757	(800) 992-5757
New Hampshire	(800) 351-1888	(800) 442-5640
New Jersey	(800) 792-8820	(800) 792-8820
New Mexico	(800) 797-3260	(800) 797-3260
New York	(800) 342-3009	(888) 201-4563
North Carolina	(800) 662-7030	(800) 662-7030
North Dakota	(800) 451-8693	(800) 451-8693
Ohio	(866) 635-3748	(800) 342-0533
Oklahoma	(800) 522-3511	(800) 522-3511
Oregon	(800) 232-3020	(800) 522-2602
Pennsylvania	(800) 490-8505	(800) 254-5164
Puerto Rico	(787) 721-5710	not available
Rhode Island	(401) 462-0550	(401) 785-3340
South Carolina	(803) 898-7318	(800) 868-9095
South Dakota	(605) 773-3656	(605) 773-3656
Tennessee	(888) 277-8366	(888) 277-8366
Texas	(800) 252-5400	(800) 458-9858
Utah	(800) 371-7897	(800) 371-7897
Vermont	(800) 564-1612	(800) 564-1612
Virginia	(888) 832-3858	(888) 832-3858
Washington	(866) 363-4276	(800) 562-6078
West Virginia	(800) 353-6513	(800) 352-6513
Wisconsin	(608) 266-2536	(800) 815-0015
Wyoming	(800) 457-3659	(800) 457-3659

APPENDIX V
STATE HEALTH DEPARTMENTS

Although they have different names, each state has its own health department, which is responsible for many different functions and assists people of all ages. However, sometimes seniors receive extra help; for example, in Wisconsin, the state offers SeniorCare, a prescription drug assistance program for Wisconsin residents who are 65 years old and older. The Nevada State Health Division publishes complaints about adult day-care facilities. Other states have other programs and information on or for elderly individuals. Check the state's Web site for the most recent information on programs and benefits for elderly residents.

ALABAMA

Alabama Department of Public Health
P.O. Box 303017
Montgomery, AL 36130-3017
(334) 206-5300
http://www.adph.org

ALASKA

Health and Social Services
350 Main Street, Room 404
P.O. Box 110601
Juneau, AK 99811-0601
(907) 465-3030
http://health.hss.state.ak.us

ARIZONA

Arizona Department of Health Services
150 North 18th Avenue
Phoenix, AZ 85007
(602) 542-1000
http://www.azdhs.gov

ARKANSAS

Department of Health
4815 West Markham
Little Rock, AR 72205
(501) 661-2000
http://www.healthyarkansas.com/health.html

CALIFORNIA

California Office of Clinical Preventive Medicine
P.O. Box 997413
Sacramento, CA 95899-7413
(916) 440-7616
http://www.dhcs.ca/gov/services/pages/OCPM.aspx

COLORADO

Colorado Department of Public Health and Environment
4300 Cherry Creek Drive South
Denver, CO 80246-1530
(303) 692-2000
http://www.cdphe.state.co.us

CONNECTICUT

Department of Public Health
410 Capitol Avenue
Hartford, CT 06134
(860) 509-8000
http://www.ct.gov/dph/site/default.asp

DELAWARE

Department of Health and Human Services
841 Silver Lake Boulevard
Dover, DE 19904
(302) 674-7300
http://dhss.delaware.gov/dhss/main/aging.htm

DISTRICT OF COLUMBIA

Department of Health
825 North Capitol Street NE
Washington, DC 20002
(202) 671-5000
http://doh.dc.gov/doh/site/default.asp

FLORIDA

Department of Health
4052 Bald Cypress Way
Tallahassee, FL 32399
(850) 245-4147
http://www.doh.state.fl.us

GEORGIA

Division of Public Health
Two Peachtree Street NW
Atlanta, GA 30303-3186
(404) 657-2700
http://health.state.ga.us

HAWAII

Hawaii State Department of Health
1250 Punchbowl Street
Honolulu, HI 96813
(808) 586-4400
http://hawaii.gov/health

IDAHO

Idaho Department of Health and Welfare
450 West State Street
Fifth Floor
Boise, ID 83720
(800) 926-2588
http://healthandwelfare.idaho.gov

ILLINOIS

Illinois Department of Public Health
535 W. Jefferson Street
Springfield, IL 62761
(217) 782-4977
http://www.idph.state.il.us

INDIANA

Indiana State Department of Health
2 N. Meridian Street
Indianapolis, IN 46204
(317) 233-1325

http://www.in.gov/isdh

IOWA

Iowa Department of Public Health
321 E. 12th Street
Des Moines, IA 50319
(515) 281-7689
http://idph.state.ia.us

KANSAS

Kansas Department of Health and Environment
Curtis State Office Building
1000 SW Jackson
Topeka, KS 66612
(785) 296-1500
http://www.kdheks.gov

KENTUCKY

Cabinet for Health and Family Services
Office of the Secretary
275 East Main Street
Frankfort, KY 40621
(800) 372-2973
http://chfs.ky.gov

LOUISIANA

Louisiana Department of Health & Hospitals
628 N. 4th Street
P.O. Box 629
Baton Rouge, LA 70802
(225) 342-9500
http://www.dhh.louisiana.gov

MAINE

Department of Health and Human Services
286 Water Street
State House Station 11
Augusta, ME 04333-0011
(800) 606-0215
http://www.maine.gov/dhhs/elderly.shtml#abuse

MARYLAND

Maryland Department of Health & Mental Hygiene
201 West Preston Street
Baltimore, MD 21201
(410) 767-6860

http://www.dhmh.state.md.us/health

MASSACHUSETTS

Department of Public Health
250 Washington Street
Boston, MA 02108-4619
(617) 624-6000
http://www.mass.gov/dph

MICHIGAN

Michigan Department of Community Health
Capitol View Building
201 Townsend Street
Lansing, MI 48913
(517) 373-3740
http://www.michigan.gov/mdch

MINNESOTA

Minnesota Department of Health
P.O. Box 64975
St. Paul, MN 55164-0975
(651) 201-5000
http://www.health.state.mn.us

MISSISSIPPI

Mississippi State Department of Health
570 East Woodrow Wilson Drive
Jackson, MS 39216
(601) 576-7400
http://www.msdh.state.ms.us

MISSOURI

Missouri Department of Health & Senior Services
P.O. Box 570
Jefferson City, MO 65102
(573) 751-6400
http://www.dhss.mo.gov

MONTANA

Montana Department of Public Health & Human Services
111 North Sanders Street (SRS Building)
Helena, MT 59601
(406) 444-0936
http://www.dphhs.mt.gov

NEBRASKA

Nebraska Department of Health & Human Services
301 Centennial Mall South
Lincoln, NE 68509
(402) 471-3121
http://www.hhs.state.ne.us

NEVADA

Department of Health & Human Services
4126 Technology Way, Room 100
Carson City, NV 89706-2009
(775) 684-4000
http://dhhs.nv.gov

NEW HAMPSHIRE

New Hampshire Department of Health and Human Services
29 Hazen Drive
Concord, NH 03301
(603) 271-5557
http://www.dhhs.state.nh.us/DHHS/DHHS_SITE/default.htm

NEW JERSEY

Department of Health and Senior Services
P.O. Box 360
Trenton, NJ 08625-0360
(609) 292-7837
http://www.state.nj.us/health

NEW MEXICO

New Mexico Department of Health
1190 South Saint Francis Drive
Santa Fe, NM 87502
(505) 827-2613
http://www.health.state.nm.us

NEW YORK

New York State Department of Health
Corning Tower
Empire State Plaza
Albany, NY 12237
(866) 881-2809 (weekends and emergency only)
http://www.health.state.ny.us

NORTH CAROLINA

Division of Public Health
1931 Mail Service Center

Raleigh, NC 27699-1931
(919) 707-5000
http://www.ncpublichealth.com

NORTH DAKOTA

North Dakota Department of Health
600 East Boulevard Avenue
Bismarck, ND 58505-0200
(701) 328-2372
http://www.health.state.nd.us

OHIO

Ohio Department of Health
246 North High Street
Columbus, OH 43215
(614) 644-7858
http://www.odh.ohio.gov

OKLAHOMA

Oklahoma State Department of Health
1000 Northeast Tenth Street
Oklahoma City, OK 73117
(405) 271-5600
http://www.health.state.ok.us

OREGON

Public Health Division
800 NE Oregon Street
Portland, OR 97232
(971) 673-1222
http://oregon.gov/DHS/ph/index.shtml

PENNSYLVANIA

Pennsylvania Department of Health
Health and Welfare Building
7th & Forster Streets
Harrisburg, PA 17120
(877) 724-3258
http://www.dsf.health.state.pa.us/health/site/
default.asp

RHODE ISLAND

Rhode Island Department of Health
3 Capitol Hill
Providence, RI 02908
(401) 222-2231
http://www.health.state.ri.us

SOUTH CAROLINA

South Carolina Department of Health and Environmental Control
2600 Bull Street
Columbia, SC 29201
(803) 898-3432
www.scdhec.gov

SOUTH DAKOTA

Department of Health
600 East Capitol Avenue
Pierre, SD 57501
(605) 773-3361
http://doh.sd.gov

TENNESSEE

Bureau of Health Services
Cordell Hull Building
425 5th Avenue North
Nashville, TN 37243
(615) 741-7305
http://health.state.tn.us

TEXAS

Department of State Health Services
P.O. Box 149347
Austin, TX 78714-9347
(512) 458-7111
http://www.dshs.state.tx.us/contact.shtm

UTAH

Utah Department of Health
Cannon Health Building
288 North 1460 West
Salt Lake City, UT
(801) 538-6111
http://health.utah.gov

VERMONT

Vermont Department of Health
108 Cherry Street
Burlington, VT 05402
(802) 863-7200
http://healthvermont.gov

VIRGINIA

Virginia Department of Health
109 Governor Street
Richmond, VA 23218-2448

(877) 482-3468
http://www.vdh.state.va.us

WASHINGTON

Washington State Department of Health
P.O. Box 47890
Olympia, WA 98504-7890
(360) 236-4030
http://www.doh.wa.gov

WEST VIRGINIA

**West Virginia Department of Health &
  Human Resources**
State Capitol Complex
Building 3, Room 206
Charleston, WV 25305

(304) 558-0684
http://www.wvdhhr.org/contact.cfm

WISCONSIN

Department of Health and Family Services
1 W. Wilson Street
Madison, WI 53703
(608) 266-1865
http://www.dhfs.state.wi.us

WYOMING

Wyoming Department of Health
401 Hathaway Building
Cheyenne, WY 82002
(307) 777-7656
http://wdh.state.wy.us

APPENDIX VI

NUMBER AND PERCENTAGE OF ADULTS AGE 65 AND OLDER BY SELECTED HEALTH STATUS, CONDITION, OR IMPAIRMENT, AND OTHER CHARACTERISTICS, AVERAGE ANNUAL, 2000–2003

This table provides important comparative information by percentage on age, gender, race, poverty status, health insurance coverage, and marital status in relation to many common chronic health conditions and impairments in older people in the United States, such as hypertension, diabetes, and heart disease, as well as hearing impairment, vision impairment, and the loss of all natural teeth.

Four age categories are considered, including all individuals ages 65 and older in the United States, as well as subgroups of ages 65 to 74, 75 to 84, and 85 and older.

	HEALTH STATUS, CONDITION, OR IMPAIRMENT							
Selected Characteristic	Population (in thousands)	Fair or Poor Health	Hyper-tension	Heart Disease	Diabetes	Hearing Impairment	Vision Impairment	Lost All Natural Teeth
65 and over								
Sex:								
Men	14,147	26.4	46.7	36.3	18.1	47.5	16.0	26.2
Women	19,072	25.7	52.6	27.2	14.2	31.9	18.5	28.6
Race and Hispanic origin								
White, not Hispanic	27,529	23.5	48.5	32.4	14.4	41.0	17.0	26.7
Black, not Hispanic	2,685	41.1	66.9	25.8	24.2	24.4	20.5	35.4
Asian, not Hispanic	649	25.7	53.5	24.6	14.6	34.0	15.2	24.3
Hispanic	2,015	39.6	46.9	21.5	23.5	24.5	19.1	28.7
Poverty status								
Poor	2,479	42.5	56.2	32.7	20.4	36.8	24.7	44.6
Near poor	6,083	33.8	55.2	33.5	18.4	40.6	22.4	38.2
Not poor	12,791	19.7	48.6	31.2	14.8	40.0	15.7	20.9
Health insurance coverage								
Private	21,095	22.0	49.6	32.1	15.0	39.6	16.0	24.1
Medicare/other public only	1,989	55.4	63.1	38.7	26.7	38.3	29.3	46.6
Medicare only	7,953	27.8	48.6	31.2	14.8	40.0	15.7	20.9

Selected Characteristic	Population (in thousands)	Fair or Poor Health	Hyper-tension	Heart Disease	Diabetes	Hearing Impairment	Vision Impairment	Lost All Natural Teeth
Marital status								
Currently married	18,456	24.4	47.6	31.6	16.1	38.7	15.0	22.6
Formerly married	13,160	28.4	53.2	31.1	15.7	38.8	21.1	34.8
Never married	1,177	24.8	53.4	27.3	13.7	34.4	17.1	26.9
Ages 65–74								
Sex:								
Men	8,116	23.5	46.7	31.7	19.4	40.9	12.9	23.7
Women	9,760	22.5	48.9	22.5	15.1	23.5	14.6	24.1
Race and Hispanic origin:								
White, not Hispanic	14,440	20.1	46.0	27.8	15.2	33.9	13.2	23.5
Black, not Hispanic	1,578	37.0	65.5	23.3	26.5	18.9	17.0	29.3
Asian, not Hispanic	378	19.8	51.6	19.0	14.7	24.0	12.9	15.5
Hispanic	1,287	37.1	45.6	19.1	24.2	18.7	16.1	23.4
Poverty status:								
Poor	1,284	41.7	55.2	29.0	21.6	29.9	21.1	41.4
Near poor	2,897	33.9	54.9	30.6	21.3	33.3	19.3	35.5
Not poor	7,594	16.9	46.4	26.9	15.3	33.4	12.8	18.4
Health insurance coverage:								
Private (with and without Medicare)	11,326	18.6	47.1	27.4	16.1	32.5	12.3	20.8
Medicare/other public only	1,036	53.3	60.7	36.6	27.4	31.9	26.2	43.1
Medicare only	4,190	25.4	47.3	23.6	15.9	28.4	13.5	25.9
Marital status:								
Currently married	11,595	21.6	46.2	27.3	16.7	33.3	12.6	20.9
Formerly married	5,368	25.5	50.8	26.0	17.7	27.7	16.6	30.5
Never married	629	23.7	53.8	21.7	17.6	29.6	14.2	24.6
Ages 75–84								
Sex:								
Men	4,905	29.0	48.1	42.9	17.4	54.9	17.9	27.6
Women	7,170	28.2	56.6	30.6	14.2	36.4	20.0	30.9
Race and Hispanic origin:								
White, not Hispanic	10,294	26.2	51.7	36.7	14.4	45.8	18.7	28.2
Black, not Hispanic	869	46.5	71.0	30.1	21.9	29.8	24.1	39.5
Asian, not Hispanic	205	30.3	58.6	33.4	14.6	39.8	15.3	36.2
Hispanic	593	42.3	49.3	25.8	23.5	32.7	21.4	35.4
Poverty status:								
Poor	892	43.0	57.1	36.6	21.2	40.5	25.5	47.3
Near poor	2,500	33.8	56.7	35.5	16.5	43.6	23.1	39.1
Not poor	4,308	22.2	52.1	36.6	14.6	47.5	18.1	22.9
Health insurance coverage:								
Private (with and without Medicare)	7,796	24.9	52.6	36.7	14.8	45.0	18.0	26.3
Medicare/other public only	724	59.0	66.9	41.2	26.7	39.9	28.8	47.6
Medicare only	2,828	29.3	51.5	31.3	14.9	40.8	19.1	33.0

(Table continues)

(Table continued)

Selected Characteristic	Population (in thousands)	Fair or Poor Health	Hyper-tension	Heart Disease	Diabetes	Hearing Impairment	Vision Impairment	Lost All Natural Teeth
Marital status:								
Currently married	6,030	28.2	50.6	38.4	15.9	46.9	18.0	24.5
Formerly married	5,508	29.1	55.8	33.4	15.4	41.2	20.8	35.4
Never married	414	27.2	55.5	26.3	10.1	36.7	17.0	27.5
Age 85 and older								
Sex:								
Men	1,126	35.9	40.3	40.3	11.8	63.0	29.3	37.4
Women	2,142	32.4	56.0	37.5	10.6	55.4	30.8	41.7
Race and Hispanic origin:								
White, not Hispanic	2,795	31.0	49.6	40.4	10.1	59.9	29.7	37.9
Black, not Hispanic	238	48.5	61.3	26.6	16.9	41.3	31.0	60.4
Asian, not Hispanic	66	45.6	49.3	29.3	13.6	73.0	27.4	37.4
Hispanic	135	52.6	48.4	25.7	16.8	44.0	37.6	49.8
Poverty status:								
Poor	303	44.2	57.7	37.0	13.0	55.5	37.2	50.3
Near poor	686	33.8	51.0	38.6	13.1	60.6	32.5	46.5
Not poor	890	31.4	49.9	41.6	11.3	60.1	28.0	32.0
Health insurance coverage:								
Private (with and without Medicare)	1,972	29.8	52.3	41.5	9.9	59.0	29.2	34.9
Medicare/other public only	229	54.1	62.3	40.8	23.7	62.5	45.0	58.8
Medicare only	935	34.1	45.1	32.0	9.8	54.9	28.5	45.9
Marital status:								
Currently married	831	35.8	45.8	42.3	10.1	55.8	25.8	31.8
Formerly married	2,284	33.3	52.4	37.6	11.4	59.3	32.0	43.6
Never married	134	22.6	44.9	27.0	6.3	50.6	30.9	36.0

Source: Adapted from Schoenborn, Charlotte A., Jackline L. Vickerie, and Eva Powell-Griner. "Health Characteristics of Adults 55 Years of Age and Over: United States, 2000–2003." *Advance Data from Vital and Health Statistics,* Number 370. Hyattsville, MD: National Center for Health Statistics, 2006, pp. 14–17.

APPENDIX VII
COUNTRIES WITH MORE THAN 2 MILLION PEOPLE AGE 65 AND OLDER: 2000 AND 2030

Many countries worldwide anticipate a major surge in the numbers of their population age 65 and older by 2030, including China, India, and the United States, among other countries listed in the table below.

(Numbers in Thousands)									
	Rank		65 and Older			Rank		65 and Older	
Country	2000	2030	2000	2030	Country	2000	2030	2000	2030
China	1	1	87,538	239,480	Poland	16	24	4,736	8,292
India	2	2	46,545	127,429	Bangladesh	17	14	4,304	13,211
United States	3	3	35,061	71,453	Vietnam	18	16	4,300	11,960
Japan	4	5	21,671	33,527	Thailand	19	15	3,968	12,045
Russia	5	7	18,354	27,768	Canada	20	22	3,964	8,972
Germany	6	8	13,515	21,840	Turkey	21	17	3,931	10,876
Italy	7	10	10,394	15,084	Argentina	22	27	3,841	6,902
Indonesia	8	4	10,046	34,058	Nigeria	23	25	3,456	8,241
France	9	11	9,499	14,978	Korea, South	24	18	3,301	10,638
United Kingdom	10	13	9,284	14,463	Iran	25	26	3,031	7,963
Brazil	11	6	9,267	29,186	Romania	26	34	2,990	4,081
Ukraine	12	23	6,847	8,312	Philippines	27	20	2,956	9,652
Spain	13	19	6,820	9,874	Egypt	28	21	2,824	9,584
Pakistan	14	12	5,829	14,683	Australia	29	30	2,382	4,953
Mexico	15	9	4,946	15,582	Netherlands	30	33	2,165	4,159

Source: Adapted from He, Wan, Manisha Sengupta, Victoria A. Velkoff, and Kimberly A. DeBarros. *65+ in the United States: 2005.* Washington, D.C.: U.S. Census Bureau, December 2005, p. 30.

APPENDIX VIII

COUNTRIES WITH MORE THAN 1 MILLION PEOPLE AGE 80 AND OLDER: 2000 AND 2030

As seen in the chart below, other countries in Asia and Europe have a rapidly growing population of individuals age 80 and older. China had the largest very elderly population in 2000, followed by the United States. In 2030, however, China will have the largest very elderly population, followed by India and then the United States.

(Numbers in thousands)		
	80 and older	
Country	2000	2030
China	12,041	44,463
United States	9,252	19,517
India	6,107	19,974
Japan	4,761	13,379
Germany	3,008	6,369
Russia	2,919	5,511
United Kingdom	2,381	4,263
Italy	2,316	4,838
France	2,218	4,684
Spain	1,524	2,979
Brazil	1,412	5,680
Ukraine	1,096	1,783
Indonesia	1,006	5,326

Source: Adapted from He, Wan, Manisha Sengupta, Victoria A. Velkoff, and Kimberly A. DeBarros. *65+ in the United States: 2005.* Washington, D.C.: U.S. Census Bureau, December 2005, p. 31.

APPENDIX IX

RATE OF SELECTED CHRONIC HEALTH CONDITIONS CAUSING LIMITATION OF ACTIVITY AMONG OLDER ADULTS, BY AGE AND RATE PER 1,000 POPULATION: UNITED STATES, 2003–2004

As seen in the chart, the risk for chronic health conditions among the elderly, such as senility (also known as dementia), lung disease, diabetes, vision problems, hearing problems, heart disease, and arthritis all increase with age.

Type of Chronic Health Condition	Age 65–74	Age 75–84	Age 85 and older
Senility/dementia	7.1	31.6	97.8
Lung disease	32.9	41.2	39.7
Diabetes	42.6	49.1	47.2
Vision	19.0	38.7	82.8
Hearing	9.9	24.1	66.7
Heart or other circulatory	100.9	156.7	223.7
Arthritis or other musculoskeletal	127.1	181.1	268.3

Source: Adapted from National Center for Health Statistics. *Health, United States, 2006, with Chartbook on Trends in the Health of Americans.* Hyattsville, MD: National Institutes of Health, 2006, p. 105.

APPENDIX X

LIFE EXPECTANCY AT BIRTH AND AT AGE 65 FOR SELECTED COUNTRIES, 2000

As can be seen in the table below, life expectancies between countries varied considerably in 2000. The country with the highest male life expectancy at birth was Sweden (77.6 years); the country with the highest male life expectancy at age 65 was Singapore, with an expected life expectancy of 17.6 additional years. The United States had a male life expectancy at birth of 74.1 years and at age 65 of 15.6 additional years.

Among females, the country with the highest life expectancy at birth was Japan, with a life expectancy of 84.1 years. At age 65, Japan also had the highest life expectancy of 22.0 additional years, or a life expectancy of age 87. In the United States, the female life expectancy at birth was 79.5 years. The female life expectancy in the United States at age 65 was 19.2 additional years, or to age 84.2.

	Male			Female	
Country	At Age 0	At Age 65	Country	At Age 0	At Age 65
Sweden	77.6	16.7	Japan	84.1	22.0
Japan	77.3	17.2	Singapore	83.2	21.8
Singapore	77.1	17.6	Canada	83.0	21.8
Austria	76.9	17.2	Australia	82.7	21.0
Hong Kong	76.9	17.3	France	82.7	21.1
Switzerland	76.9	16.9	Switzerland	82.7	20.8
Israel	76.6	17.0	Spain	82.6	20.5
Italy	76.4	16.7	Hong Kong	82.4	20.9
Canada	76.0	16.9	Sweden	82.3	20.2
Norway	76.0	16.1	Italy	82.1	20.2
Greece	75.9	16.3	Norway	81.4	19.7
Spain	75.8	16.6	Austria	81.2	19.6
Netherlands	75.6	15.4	Finland	81.2	19.3
United Kingdom	75.5	15.6	Germany	81.2	19.5
Austria	75.4	16.2	Belgium	81.0	19.7
Kuwait	75.3	15.9	Greece	80.9	19.0
Germany	75.2	15.8	New Zealand	80.9	20.3
France	75.1	16.6	Puerto Rico	80.9	20.8
Jordan	74.9	16.1	Netherlands	80.8	19.3
New Zealand	74.9	16.2	Israel	80.7	19.5
Belgium	74.5	15.4	United Kingdom	80.3	18.9

	Male			Female	
Country	At Age 0	At Age 65	Country	At Age 0	At Age 65
Denmark	74.4	15.2	Jordan	79.9	19.0
Cuba	74.1	16.1	Portugal	79.5	18.3
United States	74.1	16.3	United States	79.5	19.2
Finland	74.0	15.3	Ireland	79.4	18.0
Ireland	73.9	14.4	Taiwan	79.3	18.7
Taiwan	73.6	16.4	Chile	79.2	18.7
Costa Rica	73.3	15.7	Denmark	79.1	18.2
Jamaica	73.3	15.3	Slovenia	79.0	18.6

Source: Adapted from He, Wan, Manisha Sengupta, Victoria A. Velkoff, and Kimberly A. DeBarros. *65+ in the United States: 2005.* Washington, D.C.: U.S. Census Bureau, December 2005, p. 40.

APPENDIX XI

NATIONAL REPORT CARD ON HEALTHY AGING: HOW HEALTHY ARE OLDER ADULTS IN THE UNITED STATES?

The table below shows federal health targets for older individuals nationwide and whether they were met, exceeded, or not met. For example, the national goal was for 12 percent of older individuals to be smokers, but the actual rate was 9.3 percent, which was a lower and better rate. In contrast, 20.2 percent of older people were obese in comparison to the target rate of 15 percent, so that goal was not met.

Indicator	Data for Persons Age 65 and Older	Data Year	Healthy People 2010 Target	Grade Met/ Not met
Oral health: Complete tooth loss (percentage)	21.3	2004	20	Not met
No leisure time activity in past month (percentage)	31.9	2004	20	Not met
Obesity (percentage)	20.2	2004	15	Not met
Current smoking (percentage)	9.3	2004	12	Met
Flu vaccine in past year (percentage)	68.1	2004	90	Not met
Ever had pneumonia vaccine (percentage)	64.7	2004	90	Not met
Mammogram within past two years (percentage)	75.1	2004	70	Met
Colorectal cancer screening (percentage)	63.1	2004	50	Met
Cholesterol checked within past five years (percentage)	90.4	2003	80	Met
Hip fracture hospitalizations (per 100,000 persons)	558 men 1,113 women	2004	474 men 416 women	Not met

Source: Centers for Disease Control and Prevention. *The State of Aging and Health in America 2007.* Bethesda, MD: National Institutes of Health, 2007, p. 9.

APPENDIX XII
NATIONAL ORGANIZATIONS FOR OLDER CANADIANS

The numbers of older people in Canada are rapidly rising, and there are many national organizations available to meet their needs. Some of these organizations are listed below.

Advocacy Centre for the Elderly
2 Carlton Street
Suite 701
Toronto, ON M5B 1J3
(416) 598-2656
http://advocacycentreelderly.org

Alzheimer Flame of Hope
Suite 222 5929L Jeanne D'Arc Boulevard
Ottawa, ON K1C 7K2
(866) 277-7704
http://www.alzheimerinfo.ca

Canada Safety Council
1020 Thomas Spratt Place
Ottawa, ON K1G 5L5
(613) 739-1535

Canadian Association of Retired People (CARP)
National Head Office
Suite 1304
27 Queen Street E.
Toronto, ON M5C 2M6
(416) 363-8748
http://www.carp.ca

Canadian Association on Gerontology
222 College Street
Suite 106
Toronto, ON M5T 3J1
(416) 978-7977
http://www.cagacg.ca

Canadian Geriatrics Society
232–329 March Road
Box 11
Kanata, ON K2K 2E1
(613) 592-7111
http://www.canadiangeriatrics.com/index.html

Canadian National Institute for the Blind
1929 Bayview Avenue
Toronto, ON M4G 3E
(800) 563-2642
http://www.chib.ca

Canadian Psychiatric Association
141 Laurier Avenue West
Suite 701
Ottawa, ON K1P 5J3
(613) 234-2815
http://www.cpa-apc.org

Dietitians of Canada
480 University Avenue
Suite 604
Toronto, ON M5G 1V2
(416) 596-0857
http://www.dietitians.ca

Division of Aging and Seniors
Public Health Agency of Canada
Address Locator (A.L.) 1908A1
Ottawa, ON K1A 1B4
(613) 952-7606
http://www.phac-aspc.gc.ca

Gerontology Research Centre
2800-515 West Hastings Street
Vancouver, BC V6B 5K3
(778) 782-5062
http://www.sfu.ca/grc

Health Canada
Headquarters
Address Locator (A.L.) 0900C2
Ottawa, ON K1A 0K9
(613) 957-2991
http://www.hc-sc.gc.ca

Heart and Stroke Foundation of Canada
222 Queen Street
Suite 1402
Ottawa, ON K1P 5V9
(613) 569-4361
http://ww2.heartandstroke.ca

Help the Aged Canada
1300 Carling Avenue, Unit 205
Ottawa, ON K1Z 7L2
http://www.helptheaged.ca

Institute for Life Course and Aging
University of Toronto
222 College Street Suite 106
Toronto, ON M5T 3J1
(416) 978-0377
http://www.aging.utoronto.ca

Public Health Agency of Canada
130 Colonnade Road
A.L. 6501H
Ottawa, ON K1A 0K9
http://www.phac-aspc.gc.ca

Senior Years
479 5th Avenue East
Owen Sound, ON N4K 2R4
(519) 371-6766
http://www.senioryears.com

Society of Rural Physicians of Canada
P.O. Box 893
Shawville, QC J0X 2Y0

PROVINCIAL AND TERRITORIAL DEPARTMENTS AND MINISTRIES OF HEALTH

ALBERTA

Alberta Health and Wellness
10025 Jasper Avenue
Edmonton, AB T5J 1S6

(780) 427-7164
http://www.health.gov.ab.ca

BRITISH COLUMBIA

Ministry of Health
1515 Blanshard Street
Victoria, BC V8W 3C8
(205) 952-3456
http://www.gov.bc.ca/healthservices

MANITOBA

Manitoba Health Department
(204) 945-3744
http://www.gov.mb.ca/health

NEW BRUNSWICK

Department of Health and Wellness
P.O. Box 5100
Fredericton, NB E3B 5G8
(506) 453-4800
http://www.gnb.ca

NEWFOUNDLAND AND LABRADOR

Health and Community Services
Coordinator of Inquiries and Health Planning
Confederation Building
P.O. Box 8700
St. Johns, NL A1B 4J6
(709) 729-4984
http://www.health.gov.nl.ca/health

NORTHWEST TERRITORIES

Department of Health and Social Services
P.O. Box 1320
Yellowknife, NT X1A 2L9
(867) 920-6173
http://www.hlthss.gov.nt.ca

NOVA SCOTIA

Nova Scotia Department of Health
1690 Hollis Street
P.O. Box 388
Halifax, NS B3J 2R8
(902) 424-5818
http://www.gov.ns.ca/health

NUNAVUT

Department of Health and Social Services
P.O. Box 1000

Iqaluit, NU X0A 0H0
(867) 975-5700
http://www.gov.nu.ca/hsssite/hssmain.shtml

ONTARIO

Ministry of Health and Long-term Care
McDonald Block
Suite M1-57
900 Bay Street
Toronto, ON M7A 1R3
(416) 314-5518
http://www.health.gov.on.ca

PRINCE EDWARD ISLAND

Health and Social Services
Jones Building—Second Floor
11 Kent Street
P.O. Box 2000
Charlottetown, PE C1A 7N8
(902) 368-4900
http://www.gov.pe.ca/hss

QUEBEC

Ministère de la Sante et des Service Sociaux
Édifice Catherine-de-Longpre
1075 Sainte-Foy Road
Québec, QC G1S 2M1
(418) 266-8900
http://www.msss.gouv.qc.ca

SASKATCHEWAN

Saskatchewan Health
3475 Albert Street
Regina, SK S4S 6X6
(306) 787-3013
http://www.health.gov.sk.ca

YUKON

Department of Health and Social Services
P.O. Box 2703
Whitehorse, YT Y1A 2C6
(867) 667-3673
http://www.hss.gov.yk.ca

APPENDIX XIII
STATE CONSUMER PROTECTION OFFICES IN THE UNITED STATES

State consumer protection offices can conduct investigations, mediate complaints, provide information, and perform other functions. Criminals and fraudsters sometimes target elderly individuals, and they (or others on behalf of the elderly person) should contact consumer protection agencies to determine what actions they may take in such cases. It is best to call the consumer protection office to request a complaint form and to make sure they handle the type of complaint that the older person has.

ALABAMA
Consumer Affairs Section
Office of the Attorney General
11 South Union Street
Montgomery, AL 35130
(334) 242-7335
http://www.ago.state.al.us

ALASKA
Consumer Protection Unit
Office of the Attorney General
1031 West Fourth Avenue
Suite 200
Anchorage, AK 99501
(907) 269-5100
http://www.law.state.ak.us

ARIZONA
Consumer Protection and Advocacy Section
Office of the Attorney General
1275 West Washington Street
Phoenix, AZ 85007
(602) 542-3702
http://www.asag.gov

ARKANSAS
Consumer Protection Division
Office of the Attorney General
323 Center Street
Suite 200
Little Rock, AR 72201

CALIFORNIA
Director, California Department of Consumer Affairs
400 R Street
Suite 2000-1080
Sacramento, CA 95814
(916) 445-1254
http://www.dca.ca.gov

COLORADO
Consumer Protection Division
Colorado Attorney General's Office
1525 Sherman Street, Fifth Floor
Denver, CO 80203
(303) 866-5079

CONNECTICUT
Department of Consumer Protection
165 Capitol Avenue
Hartford, CT 06106
(860) 713-6050
http://www.ct.gov/dcp/site/default.asp

DELAWARE
Fraud and Consumer Protection Division
Office of the Attorney General
Carvel State Office Building
820 North French Street, Fifth Floor
Wilmington, DE 19801

(302) 577-8600
http://www.state.de.us/attgen

DISTRICT OF COLUMBIA

Consumer & Trade Protection Section
Office of the Attorney General
441 Fourth Street NW
Suite 450N
Washington, DC 20001
(202) 442-9828

FLORIDA

Economic Crimes Division
Office of the Attorney General
PL-01 The Capitol
Tallahassee, FL 32399
(850) 414-3600

GEORGIA

Governor's Office of Consumer Affairs
2 Martin Luther King, Jr. Drive
Suite 356
Atlanta, GA 30334
(404) 656-3790
http://consumer.georgia.gov

HAWAII

Office of Consumer Protection
Department of Commerce and Consumer Affairs
235 South Beretania Street, Room 801
Honolulu, HI 96813
(808) 586-2636

IDAHO

Consumer Protection Unit
Idaho Attorney General's Office
650 West State Street
Boise, ID 83720
(208) 334-2424
http://www.state.id.us/ag

ILLINOIS

Governor's Office of Citizen's Assistance
222 South College, Room 106
Springfield, IL 62706
(217) 782-0244

INDIANA

Consumer Protection Division
Office of the Attorney General
Indiana Government Center South
4402 West Washington Street, Fifth Floor
Indianapolis, IN 46204
(317) 232-6201
http://www.in.gov/attorneygeneral

IOWA

Consumer Protection Division
Office of the Attorney General
1305 East Walnut Street, Second Floor
Des Moines, IA 50319
(515) 281-5926
http://www.IowaAttorneyGeneral.org

KANSAS

Consumer Protection and Antitrust Division
Office of the Attorney General
120 SW Tenth, Second Floor
Topeka, KS 66612
(785) 296-3751
http://www.ink.org/public/ksag

KENTUCKY

Consumer Protection Division
Office of the Attorney General
1024 Capital Center Drive
Frankfort, KY 40601
(502) 696-5389

LOUISIANA

Consumer Protection Section
Office of the Attorney General
P.O. Box 94005
Baton Rouge, LA 70804
(800) 351-4889
http://www.ag.state.la.us

MAINE

Consumer Protection Division
Office of the Attorney General
6 State House Station
Augusta, ME 04333
(207) 626-8800
http://www.maine.gov

MARYLAND

Consumer Protection Division
Office of the Attorney General
200 Saint Paul Place, 16th Floor

Baltimore, MD 21202
(410) 576-6550
http://www.oag.state.md.us/consumer

MASSACHUSETTS

Executive Office of Consumer Affairs and Business Regulation
10 Park Plaza, Room 5170
Boston, MA 02116
(617) 973-8700
http://www.mass/gov/Consumer

MICHIGAN

Consumer Protection Division
Office of Attorney General
P.O. Box 30213
Lansing, MI 48909
(517) 373-1140

MINNESOTA

Consumer Services Division
Attorney General's Office
1400 NCL Tower
445 Minnesota Street
St. Paul, MN 55101
(612) 296-3353
http://www.ag.state.mn.us/consumer

MISSISSIPPI

Consumer Protection Division
Attorney General's Office
P.O. Box 22497
Jackson, MS 39225
(601) 359-4230
http://www.ago.state.ms.usa

MISSOURI

Consumer Protection and Trade Offense Division
P.O. Box 899
1530 Rax Court
Jefferson City, MO 65102
(573) 751-6887
http://www.ago.stae.mo.us

MONTANA

Consumer Protection Office
Department of Administration
1219 Eighth Avenue

P.O. Box 200151
Helena, MT 59620
(406) 444-4500
http://www.state.mt.us/doa/consumerprotection

NEBRASKA

Office of the Attorney General
Department of Justice
2115 State Capitol
P.O. Box 98920
Lincoln, NE 68509
(402) 471-2682
http://www.nol.org/home/ago

NEVADA

Consumer Affairs Division
1850 East Sahara Avenue
Suite 101
Las Vegas, NV 89104
(702) 486-7355
http://www.fyiconsumer.org

NEW HAMPSHIRE

Consumer Protection and Antitrust Bureau
Attorney General's Office
33 Capitol Street
Concord, NH 03301
(603) 271-3641
http://www.doj.nh.gov/consumer/index.html

NEW JERSEY

Division of Consumer Affairs
Department of Law and Public Safety
124 Halsey Street
P.O. Box 45025
Newark, NJ 07102
(973) 504-6200
http://www.state.nj.us/lps/ca/home.htm

NEW MEXICO

Consumer Protection Division
P.O. Drawer 1508
407 Galisteo Street
Santa Fe, NM 87504
(505) 827-6060
http://www.ago.state.nm.us

NEW YORK

Bureau of Consumer Frauds and Protection
Office of the Attorney General
State Capitol
Albany, NY 12224
(518) 474-5481
http://www.oag.state.ny.us

NORTH CAROLINA

Consumer Protection Division
Office of the Attorney General
9001 Mail Service Center
Raleigh, NC 27699
(919) 716-6400
http://www.ncdoj.com

NORTH DAKOTA

Consumer Protection and Antitrust Division
Office of the Attorney General
4205 State Street
P.O. Box 1054
Bismarck, ND 58502
(701) 328-3404
http://www.ag.state.nd.us

OHIO

Ohio Consumers' Counsel
10 West Broad Street, 18th Floor
Columbus, OH 43215
(614) 466-8574
http://www.pickoca.org

OKLAHOMA

Consumer Protection Unit
Oklahoma Attorney General
4545 North Lincoln Avenue
Suite 260
Oklahoma City, OK 73105
(405) 521-2029
http://www.oag.tate.ok.us

OREGON

Financial Fraud/Consumer Protection Section
Department of Justice
1162 Court Street NE
Salem, OR 97310
(503) 947-4333
http://www.doj.state.or.us

PENNSYLVANIA

Bureau of Consumer Protection
Office of Attorney General
14th Floor, Strawberry Square
Harrisburg, PA 17120
(717) 787-9707
http://www.attorneygeneral.gov

RHODE ISLAND

Consumer Protection Unit
Department of Attorney General
150 South Main Street
Providence, RI 02903
(401) 274-4400
http://www.riag.state.ri.us

SOUTH CAROLINA

South Carolina Department of Consumer Affairs
3600 Forest Drive
Suite 300
P.O. Box 5757
Columbia, SC 29250
(803) 734-4200
http://www.scconsumer.gov

SOUTH DAKOTA

Consumer Affairs
Office of the Attorney General
State Capitol Building
500 East Capitol
Pierre, SD 57501
(605) 773-4400
http://www.state.sd.us/atg

TENNESSEE

Consumer Advocate and Protection Division
Office of the Attorney General
P.O. Box 20207
Nashville, TN 37202
(615) 741-1671
http://www.tn.gov/attorneygeneral/cpro/cpro.htm

TEXAS

(The state has regional offices. Only the Dallas office is listed here.)

Dallas Regional Office
Office of the Attorney General

1600 Pacific Avenue
Suite 1700
Dallas, TX 75201
(214) 969-5310

UTAH

Division of Consumer Protection
Department of Commerce
160 East 300 South
Box 146704
Salt Lake City, UT 84114
(801) 530-6601
http://www.consumerprotection.utah.gov

VERMONT

Consumer Assistance Program
Office of the Attorney General
104 Morrill Hall
University of Vermont
Burlington, VT 05405
(802) 656-3183
http://www.atg.state.vt.us

VIRGINIA

Office of Consumer Affairs
Department of Agriculture and Consumer Services
P.O. Box 1163
Richmond, VA 23218
(804) 786-2042
http://www.vdacs.state.va.us

WASHINGTON

Office of the Attorney General
1125 Washington Street SE
Olympia, WA 98504
(800) 551-4636
http://www.atg.wa.gov

WEST VIRGINIA

Consumer Protection Division
Office of the Attorney General
812 Quarrier Street, Sixth Floor
P.O. Box 1789
Charleston, WV 25326
(304) 558-8986
http://www.wvago.gov

WISCONSIN

Department of Agriculture, Trade and Consumer Protection
2811 Agriculture Drive
P.O. Box 8911
Madison, WI 53708
(608) 224-4949
http://www.datcp.state.wi.us

WYOMING

Consumer Protection Unit
Office of the Attorney General
123 State Capitol Building
Cheyenne, WY 82002
(307) 777-7874
http://attorneygeneral.state.wy.us/consumer.htm

APPENDIX XIV
RELAXATION EXERCISES TO RELIEVE PAIN AND STRESS

Relaxation exercises can provide relief from pain and stress, whether the pain is from cancer, arthritis, frequent headaches, or other chronic medical problems. They can also be very helpful for an older person as well as for a caregiver to an older person. These instructions are adapted from a National Cancer Institute pamphlet on coping with cancer, but they are applicable to anyone with major stress.

Ask your doctor or nurse if the following relaxation exercises can help you. Before trying the full exercise below, first practice steps 1 through 5, so you can get used to deep breathing and muscle relaxation. You may find that your mind wanders. When you notice yourself thinking of something else, gently direct your attention back to your deepening relaxation. Be sure to maintain your deep breathing. If any of these steps make you feel uncomfortable, feel free to leave it out.

EXERCISE 1

1. Find a quiet place where you can rest undisturbed for 20 minutes. Let others know you need this time for yourself.

2. Make sure the setting is relaxing. For example, dim the lights if you like and find a comfortable chair or couch.

3. Get into a comfortable position where you can relax your muscles. Close your eyes and clear your mind of distractions.

4. Breathe deeply, at a slow and relaxing pace. People usually breathe shallowly, high in their chests. Concentrate on breathing deeply and slowly, raising your belly rather than just your chest with each breath.

---

5. Next go through each of your major muscle groups, tensing (squeezing) them for 10 seconds and then relaxing. If tensing any particular muscle group is painful, skip the tensing step and just concentrate on relaxing. Focus completely on releasing all the tension from your muscles and notice the differences you feel when they are relaxed. Focus on the pleasant feeling of relaxation.

TENSE, HOLD, AND RELAX ALL THE PARTS OF YOUR BODY

Right and left arm—make a fist and bring it up to your shoulder, tightening your arm.

Lips, eyes, and forehead—scowl, raise your eyebrows, pucker your lips, and then grin.

Jaws and neck—thrust your lower jaw out, and then relax. Then tilt your chin down toward your chest.

Shoulders—shrug your shoulders up toward your ears.

Chest—push out your chest.

Stomach—suck in your stomach.

Lower back—stretch your lower back so that it forms a gentle arch, with your stomach pushed outward. Make sure to do this gently, as these muscles are often tight.

Buttocks—squeeze your buttocks together.

Thighs—press your thighs together.

Calves—point your toes up, toward your knees.

Feet—point your toes down, like a ballet dancer.

Review these parts of your body again and release any tension that remains. Be sure to maintain your deep breathing.

Now that you are relaxed, image a calming scene. Choose a spot that is particularly pleasant to you. It may be a favorite comfortable room, a sandy beach, a chair in front of a fireplace, or any other relaxing place.

Spend a few more minutes enjoying the feeling of comfort and relaxation.

When you are ready, start gently moving your hands and feet and bringing yourself back to reality. Open your eyes and spend a few minutes becoming more alert. Notice how you feel now that you have completed the relaxation exercise, and try to carry these feelings with you into the rest of your day.

CONCENTRATE ON THESE DETAILS IN YOUR IMAGINATION

What can you see around you?

What do you smell?

What are the sounds that you hear? For example, if you are [imagining yourself] on the beach, how does the sand feel on your feet, how do the waves sound, and how does the air smell?

Can you taste anything?

Continue to breathe deeply as you imagine yourself relaxing in your safe, comfortable place.

EXERCISE 2

Sit comfortably. Loosen any tight clothes. Close your eyes. Clear your mind and relax your muscles using steps 4 and 5 described in Exercise 1 above.

Focus your mind on your right arm. Repeat to yourself, "My right arm feels heavy and warm." Stick with it until your arm *does* feel heavy and warm.

Repeat with the rest of your muscles until you are fully relaxed.

Some people find it helpful at this point to focus on thoughts that enhance their relaxation. For example: My arms and legs are very comfortable. I can just sink into this chair and focus only on the relaxation.

Source: National Cancer Institute. *Facing Forward: Life After Cancer Treatment.* Bethesda, Md.: National Institutes of Health, September 2006, pp. 60–61.

APPENDIX XV
FAMILY CAREGIVER WEB SITES

ALABAMA
http://www.adss.state.al.us/AlaCare/index.htm

ALASKA
http://health.hss.state.ak.us/dsds/hcb.htm

ARIZONA
https://www.azdes.gov/aaa/programs/care/default.asp

ARKANSAS
http://www.arkansascaregivers.com/

CALIFORNIA
http://www.aging.ca.gov/html/programs/I_and_A.html

COLORADO
http://www.cdhs.state.co.us/aas/agingservicesunit_caregiver.htm

CONNECTICUT
http://www.ct.gov/agingservices/cwp/view.asp?a=2513&q=313064

DELAWARE
http://www.dhss.delaware.gov/dhss/dsaapd/care.html

DISTRICT OF COLUMBIA
http://dcoa.dc.gov/dcoa/site/default.asp?dcoaNav=|31409|

FLORIDA
http://elderaffairs.state.fl.us/english/caregiver.html

HAWAII
http://www2.state.hi.us/eoa/programs/caregiver/index.html

IDAHO
http://www.idahoaging.com/programs/ps_caregiver.htm

ILLINOIS
http://www.state.il.us/aging/1caregivers/caregivers-main.htm

INDIANA
http://www.iaaaa.org/resources/caregiver.asp

IOWA
http://www.iowafamilycaregiver.org

KANSAS
http://www.agingkansas.org/kdoa/programs/progdescriptions.htm#Caregiver

KENTUCKY
http://chfs.ky.gov/agencies/os/dail/familycaregiver.htm

LOUISIANA
http://ltp-76b.portal.louisiana.gov/elderlyaffairs/caregiver_support.html

MAINE
http://www.maine.gov/dhs/beas/caregivers.htm

MARYLAND
http://www.mdoa.state.md.us/caregivers.htm

MASSACHUSETTS
http://www.mass.gov/?pageID=elderstopic&L=2&L0=Home&L1=Caregiver+Support&sid=Eelders

343

MICHIGAN

http://www.miseniors.net/We+Assist/Caregivers2.htm

MINNESOTA

http://www.mnaging.org/advocate/caregiver.htm

MISSISSIPPI

http://www.mdhs.state.ms.us/aas_mfcsp.htm

MISSOURI

http://www.dhss.mo.gov/AAA/index.html

MONTANA

http://www.dphhs.mt.gov/sltc/

NEBRASKA

http://www.answers4families.org/eldercare/eldercare.home.html

NEVADA

http://www.nveldercare.org/index.php?page=home

NEW HAMPSHIRE

http://www.dhhs.state.nh.us/DHHS/BEAS/family-caregivers-adult.htm

NEW JERSEY

http://www.state.nj.us/caregivernj

NEW MEXICO

http://www.nmaging.state.nm.us/talk.html

NEW YORK

http://aging.state.ny.us/caring/index.htm

NORTH CAROLINA

http://www.fullcirclecare.org/needhelp/welcome.htm

NORTH DAKOTA

http://www.nd.gov/humanservices/services/adultsaging/caregiver.html

OHIO

http://goldenbuckeye.com/infocenter/publications/profile_caregiver.html

OKLAHOMA

http://www.okdhs.org/programsandservices/aging/ci/

OREGON

http://www.oregon.gov/DHS/spwpd/caregiving/home.shtml

PENNSYLVANIA

http://caregiverpa.psu.edu

RHODE ISLAND

http://adrc.ohhs.ri.gov/caregivers/index.php

SOUTH CAROLINA

http://www.dhhs.state.sc.us/dhhsnew/NR/exeres/ED990B6B-CA67-4B83-9600 -DD1832A180DA.asp

SOUTH DAKOTA

http://dss.sd.gov/elderlyservices/services/caregiver.asp

TENNESSEE

http://www.state.tn.us/comaging/caregiving.html

TEXAS

http://www.dads.state.tx.us/services/agingtexaswell/caregiving/index.html

UTAH

http://www.hsdaas.utah.gov/caregiver_support.htm

VERMONT

http://www.dad.state.vt.us/ConsumerPages/InformationAssistance.htm

VIRGINIA

http://www.vda.virginia.gov/index.asp

WASHINGTON

http://www.aasa.dshs.wa.gov/caregiving

WEST VIRGINIA

http://www.state.wv.us/seniorservices/wvboss_article2.cfm?atl=D089BE89-9617-11D5-92160020781CA477&fs=1

WISCONSIN

http://www.dhfs.state.wi.us/Aging/caregiver.htm

WYOMING

http://wdhfs.state.wy.us/aging/services/nfcp.htm

BIBLIOGRAPHY

AARP and the National Center for Complementary and Alternative Medicine. *Complementary and Alternative Medicine: What People 50 and Older Are Using and Discussing with Their Physicians.* Washington, D.C.: AARP, 2007. Available online. URL: http://assets.aarp.org/rgcenter/health/cam_2007.pdf. Downloaded on January 18, 2007.

Adamec, Chris. *The Unofficial Guide to Elder Care.* New York: Macmillan, 1999.

Adamec, Christine. "When Parents of Parents Remarry." *Single Parent* 27, no. 9 (October 1984): 20–21.

Administration on Aging. *Fact Sheet: The Long-Term Ombudsman Program.* Washington, D.C.: U.S. Department of Health and Human Services, 2006.

———. *Adult Day Services: How Can They Help You?* Washington, D.C.: U.S. Department of Health and Human Services, November 4, 2004.

———. *Snapshot: Statistical Profile of Black Older Americans Aged 65+.* Washington, D.C.: U.S. Department of Health and Human Services, February 2006.

———. *Snapshot: A Statistical Profile of Hispanic Older Americans Aged 65+.* Washington, D.C.: U.S. Department of Health and Human Services, September 10, 2007.

———. *A Profile of Older Americans: 2006.* Washington, D.C.: U.S. Department of Health and Human Services, 2006. Available online. URL: http://www.aoa.gov/PROF/Statistics/prifile/2006/profiles2006.asp. Downloaded September 11, 2007.

———. *Caring for Someone in the Last Years of Life.* Washington, D.C.: U.S. Department of Health and Human Services, November 1, 2004.

———. *Transportation Tips for Caregivers.* Washington, D.C.: U.S. Department of Health and Human Services, November 1, 2004.

American Bar Association. *The American Bar Association Legal Guide for Americans over 50.* New York: Random House Reference, 2006.

American Cancer Society. *Cancer Facts & Figures 2007.* Atlanta, Ga.: American Cancer Society, 2007.

American Hospital Association. *When I'm 64: How Boomers Will Change Health Care.* Chicago: American Hospital Association, 2007.

Andres, Emmanuel, et al. "Vitamin B12 (Cobalamin) Deficiency in Elderly Patients." *Canadian Medical Association Journal* 171, no. 3 (August 3, 2004): 251–259.

Asplund, R. "Nightmares, Sleep and Cardiac Symptoms in the Elderly." *Netherlands, the Journal of Medicine* 61, no. 7 (July 2003): 257–261.

Aung, Koko, et al. "Vitamin D Deficiency Associated with Self-Neglect in the Elderly." *Journal of Elder Abuse & Neglect* 18, no. 4 (2006): 63–78.

Bartels, Stephen J., Frederic C. Blow, Laurie M. Brockmann, and Aricca D. Van Citters. *Substance Abuse and Mental Health among Older Americans: The State of the Knowledge and Future Directions.* Rockville, Md.: Substance Abuse and Mental Heal Services Administration. August 11, 2005.

Belle, Steven H., et al. "Enhancing the Quality of Life of Dementia Caregivers from Different Ethnic or Racial Groups: A Randomized Controlled Trial." *Annals of Internal Medicine* 145, no. 10 (2006): 727–738.

Bethel, M. Angelyn, et al. "Longitudinal Incidence and Prevalence of Adverse Outcomes of Diabetes Mellitus in Elderly Patients." *Archives of Internal Medicine* 167 (May 14, 2007): 921–927.

Bitondo Dyer, Carmel, et al. "Self-Neglect among the Elderly: A Model Based on More Than 500 Patients Seen by a Geriatric Medicine Team." *American Journal of Public Health* 97, no. 9 (September 2007): 1,671–1,676.

Bitondo Dyer, Carmel, M.D.; Sabrina Pickens; and Jason Burnet. "Vulnerable Elders: When It Is No Longer Safe to Live Alone." *Journal of the American Medical Association* 298, no. 12 (September 26, 2007): 1,448–1,449.

Blay, Sergio Luis, Sergio Baxter Andreoli, and Fabio Leite Gastal. "Chronic Painful Physical Conditions, Disturbed Sleep and Psychiatric Morbidity: Results from an Elderly Survey." *Annals of Clinical Psychiatry* 19, no. 3 (2007): 169–174.

Blow, Frederick C., and Kristen Lawton Barry, "Use and Misuse of Alcohol Among Older Women." *Alcohol Research & Health* 26, no. 4 (2002): 308–315.

Bonnie, Richard J., and Robert B. Wallace, eds. *Elder Mistreatment: Abuse, Neglect, and Exploitation in an Aging America.* Washington, D.C.: National Academies Press, 2003.

Boockvar, Kenneth S., M.D.; and Diane E. Meier, M.D. "Palliative Care for Frail Older Adults: 'There Are Things I Can't Do Anymore That I Wish I Could . . .'" *Journal of the American Medical Association* 296, no. 18 (November 8, 2006): 2,245–2,253.

Borst, Stephen E. "Interventions for Sarcopenia and Muscle Weakness in Older People." *Age and Ageing* 33 (2004): 548–555.

Brogden, Mike and Preeti Nijhar. *Crime, Abuse and the Elderly.* Portland, Oreg.: Willan Publishing, 2000.

Bross, Rachelle, Marjan Javanbakht, and Shalender Bhasin. "Commentary: Anabolic Interventions for Aging-Associated Sarcopenia." *Journal of Clinical Endocrinology & Metabolism* 84, no. 10 (1999): 3,420–3,430.

Buijsse, Brian, Edith J. M. Feskens, Frans J. Kok, and Daan Kromhout. "Cocoa Intake, Blood Pressure, and Cardiovascular Mortality: The Zutphen Elderly Study." *Archives of Internal Medicine* 166 (February 27, 2006): 411–417.

Burkhardt, Jon E., et al. "Mobility and Independence: Changes and Challenges for Older Drivers: Executive Summary." Administration on Aging (July 1998).

Butler, Robert N., et al. "Anti-Aging Medicine: Efficacy and Safety of Hormones and Antioxidants." *Geriatrics* 55, no. 7 (2000): 48.

Cassell, Dana K.; Robert C. Salinas, M.D.; and Peter A. S. Winn, M.D. *The Encyclopedia of Death and Dying.* New York: Facts On File, Inc., 2005.

Centers for Disease Control and Prevention. *Epidemiology and Prevention of Vaccine Preventable Diseases.* 10th ed. Washington, D.C.: National Institutes of Health, 2007.

Centers for Disease Control and Prevention. "Percentage of Adults Aged 65 and Older Who Reported Receiving Influenza Vaccine During the Preceding 12 Months and Percentage of Adults Aged 65 Year and Older Who Reported Ever Receiving Pneumococcal Vaccine, by State/Area, United States, Behavioral Risk Factor Surveillance System, 2004–2005." *Morbidity and Mortality Weekly Report* 55, no. 9 (October 6, 2006) 1,065–1,068.

———. *Prostate Cancer Screening: A Decision Guide.* Available online. URL: http://www.cec./gov/cancer/prostate/prospdf/prosguide.pdf. Downloaded July 2, 2007.

———. "Fatalities and Injuries from Falls among Older Adults—United States, 1993–2003 and 2001–2005." *Morbidity and Mortality Weekly Report* 55, no. 45 (November 17, 2006): 1,221–1,224.

———. "Prevalence of Doctor-Diagnosed Arthritis and Arthritis-Attributable Activity Limitation-United States, 2003–2005." *Morbidity and Mortality Weekly Report* 55 (2006). 1,089–1,092.

Centers for Medicare and Medicaid Services. "Medicare and You: 2007." Washington, D.C.: Department of Health and Human Services, 2007.

Cesari, Matteo, et al. "Sarcopenia, Obesity, and Inflammation—Results from the Trial of Angiotension Converting Enzyme Inhibition and Novel Cardiovascular Risk Factors Study." *American Journal of Clinical Nutrition* 82 (2005): 428–434.

Cockayne, Sarach, et al. "Vitamin K and the Prevention of Fractures: Systematic Review and Meta-analysis of Randomized Controlled Trials." *Archives of Internal Medicine* 166 (June 26, 2006): 1,256–1,261.

Cohen, Donna, "Homicide-Suicide in Older Persons: How You Can Help Prevent a Tragedy." Tampa, Fla.: Department of Aging and Mental Health, Florida Mental Health Institute, University of South Florida, 2001.

Commission on Law and Aging. *Consumer's Tool Kit for Health Care Advance Planning.* 2nd ed. Washington, D.C.: American Bar Association, 2005.

Cremation Association of North America. *Final 2005 Statistics and Projections to the Year 2025, 2006 Preliminary Data.* Chicago, Ill.: Cremation Association of North America, September 4, 2007. Available online. URL: http://www.cremationsassociation.org/docs/CANA-Final06Prelim.pdf. Downloaded September 7, 2007.

Curtis, Lesley H., et al. "Inappropriate Prescribing for Elderly Americans in a Large Outpatient Population." *Archives of Internal Medicine* 164 (August 9/23, 2004): 1,621–1,625.

DeFrances, Carol J., and Michelle N. Podgornik. "2004 National Hospital Discharge Survey." *Advance Data from Vital and Health Statistics* no. 371 (May 4, 2006): 1–19.

Department of Health and Human Services. *The 2007 HHS Poverty Guidelines.* Available online. URL: http//aspe.hhs.gov/poverty/07poverty.shtml. Downloaded September 12, 2007.

Department of Justice. "Nondiscrimination on the Basis of Disability by Public Accommodations and in Commercial Facilities: Excerpt from 28 CFR Parts 36: ADA Standards for Accessible Design." Washington, D.C.: Code of Federal Regulations. Available online. URL: http://www.usdoj.gov/crt/ada/stdspdf.htm. Downloaded November 23, 2007.

Department of Labor, Employment Standards Administration, Wage and Hour Division. "29 DFR Part 825, Family and Medical Leave Act Regulations: A Report on the Department of Labor's Request for Information; Proposed Rule." *Federal Register,* June 28, 2007.

Department of Veterans Affairs. *Federal Benefits for Veterans and Dependents. 2007 Edition.* Washington, D.C.: Department of Veterans Affairs, 2007.

Dharmarajan, T.S., M.D., and Edward P. Norkus. "Approaches to Vitamin B12 Deficiency: Early Treatment May Prevent Devastating Complications." *Postgraduate Medicine* 110, no. 1 (July 2001): 99–105.

Diem, Susan J. M.D., et al. "Use of Antidepressants and Rates of Hip Bone Loss in Older Women: The Study of Osteoporotic Fractures." *Archives of Internal Medicine* 167, no. 12 (June 25, 2007): 1,240–1,245.

Division of Aging and Seniors, Health Canada. *Canada's Aging Population.* Ottawa, Ont.: Minister of Public Works and Government Services Canada, 2002.

Division of Aging and Seniors, Public Health Agency of Canada. *Report on Seniors' Falls in Canada.* Ottawa, Ont.: Minister of Public Works and Government Services, Canada, 2005.

Dodal, Saritha, and William L. Lyons. "Chronic Pain in Later Life." *Generations* 30, no. 3 (Fall 2006): 77–82.

Dyer, Carmel Bitondo, Marie-Therese Connolly, and Patricia McFeeley. "The Clinical and Medical Forensics of Elder Abuse and Neglect." In *Elder Mistreatment: Abuse, Neglect, and Exploitation in an Aging America.* Washington, D.C.: National Academies Press, 2003, pp. 339–381.

Environmental Protection Agency. *Fact Sheet: Environmental Hazards Weigh Heavy on the Heart: Information for Older Americans and Their Caregivers.* Washington, D.C.: EPA. September 2005.

———. *Fact Sheet: Diabetes and Environmental Hazards: Information for Older Adults and Their Caregivers.* Washington, D.C.: EPA, August 2007.

———. *Fact Sheet: Age Healthier, Breathe Easier: Information for Older Adults and their Caregivers.* Washington, D.C.: EPA, June 2007.

———. *Fact Sheet: "It's Too Darn Hot"—Planning for Excessive Heat Events: Information for Older Adults and Family Caregivers.* Washington, D.C.: EPA, October 2007.

———. *Fact Sheet: Water Works: Information for Older Adults and Family Caregivers.* Washigton, D.C.: EPA, December 2005.

Federal Emergency Management Agency. *Fire Risks for the Blind or Visually Impaired.* Washington, D.C.: Department of Homeland Security, December 1999.

Feinberg, Steven D., M.D. "Prescribing Analgesics: How to Improve Function and Avoid Toxicity When Treating Chronic Pain." *Geriatrics* 55, no. 12 (2000): 44–62.

Food and Drug Administration. *Eating Well as We Age.* Rockville, Md.: Department of Health and Human Services. (Undated.) Available online. URL: http://www.fda.gov/opacom/lowlit/eatage.pdf. Downloaded November 2, 2007.

Fryar, Cheryl D., et al. "Smoking and Alcohol Behaviors Reported by Adults: United States, 1999–2002." *Advance Data from Vital and Health Statistics* no. 378 (November 29, 2006).

General Accounting Office. *Assisted Living: Examples of State Efforts to Improve Consumer Protections.* Washington, D.C.: GAO, April 2004.

Gist, Yvonne J., and Lisa I. Hertzel. *We the People: Aging in the United States.* Washington, D.C.: U.S. Census Bureau, December 2004.

Gooneratne, Nalaka S., M.D., et al. "Consequences of Comorbid Insomnia Symptoms and Sleep-Related Breathing Disorder in Elderly Subjects." *Archives of Internal Medicine* 166 (September 18, 2006): 1,732–1,738.

Gorbien, Martin J., M.D., and Amy R. Eisenstein. "Elder Abuse and Neglect: An Overview." *Clinics in Geriatric Medicine* 21 (2005): 279–292.

Gorospe, Emmanuel, and Jatin K. Dave. "The Risk of Dementia with Increased Body Mass Index." *Age and Ageing* 36 (2007): 23–29.

Gostin, Lawrence O., J.D., LL.D. "Physician-Assisted Suicide: A Legitimate Medical Practice?" *Journal of the American Medical Association* 295, no. 16 (April 26, 2006): 1,941–1,943.

Granville, Lisa J. "Prostate Disease in Later Life." *Generations* 30, no. 3 (Fall 2006): 51–56.

Gwinnell, Esther, M.D., and Christine Adamec. *The Encyclopedia of Addictions and Addictive Behaviors.* New York: Facts On File, 2005.

———. *The Encyclopedia of Drug Abuse.* New York: Facts On File, 2008.

He, Wan. *The Older Foreign-Born Population in the United States: 2000.* Washington, D.C.: Aging Studies Branch, International Programs Center, Population Division, U.S. Census Bureau. September 2002.

He, Wan, Manisha Sengupta, Victoria A. Velkoff, and Kimberly A. DeBarros. *65+ in the United States: 2005.* Washington, D.C.: U.S. Census Bureau, December 2005.

Hedrick, Susan, et al. "Characteristics of Resident and Providers in the Assisted Living Pilot Program." *The Gerontologist* 47, no. 3 (2007): 365–377.

International Longevity Center. *Ageism in America.* New York: International Longevity Center, 2006.

Istre, Gregory R., M.D., et al. "Deaths and Injuries from House Fires." *New England Journal of Medicine* 344, no. 24 (June 25, 2001): 1,911–1,916.

Jano, Elda, and Rajender R. Aparasu. "Healthcare Outcomes Associated with Beers' Criteria: A Systematic Review." *The Annals of Pharmacotherapy* 41 (March 2007): 438–448.

Jassal, Sarbjit Vanita, M.D., et al. "Changes in Survival among Elderly Patients Initiating Dialysis from 1990 to 1999." *Canadian Medical Association Journal* 177, no. 9 (October 23, 2007): 1,033–1,038.

Johnson, Richard W., Desmond Tooney, and Joshua M. Wiener. *Meeting the Long-Term Care Needs of the Baby Boomers: How Changing Families Will Affect Paid Helpers and Institutions.* Washington, D.C.: The Urban Institute, 2007.

Juurlink, David N., M.D., et al. "Medical Illness and the Risk of Suicide in the Elderly." *Archives of Internal Medicine* 164 (June 14, 2004): 1,179–1,184.

Kahn, Ada, and Ronald Doctor. *The Encyclopedia of Phobias, Fears and Anxieties.* 3rd ed. New York: Facts On File, 2008.

Kales, Helen C., M.D. "Race and Inpatient Psychiatric Diagnoses among Elderly Veterans." *Psychiatric Services* 51, no. 6 (June 2000): 795–800.

Kandel, Joseph, M.D., and David B. Sudderth, M.D. *Back Pain—What Works! A Complete Guide to Back Problems.* Prima Publishing, 1996.

Kandel, Joseph, M.D., and David Sudderth, M.D. *The Headache Cure.* New York: McGraw-Hill, 2005.

Kearl, Michael C. "Cremation: Desecration, Purification, or Convenience?" *Generations* 27, no. 11 (Summer 2004): 15–20.

Kennedy, Gary. *Geriatric Mental Health Care: A Treatment Guide for Health Professionals.* New York: Guilford Press, 2000.

Keyhani, Salomeh, M.D., et al. "Use of Preventive Care by Elderly Male Veterans Receiving Care through the Veterans Health Administration, Medicare Fee-for-Service, and Medicare HMO Plans." *American Journal of Public Health* 97, no. 12 (December 2007): 2,179–2,185.

Kuehn, Bridget M. "Hospitals Embrace Palliative Care." *Journal of the American Medical Association* 298, no. 11 (September 19, 2007): 1,263–1,265.

Kurella, Manjula, et al. "Octogenarians and Nonagenarians Starting Dialysis in the United States." *Annals of Internal Medicine* 146 (2007): 177–183.

Lang, Ariel J., and Murray B. Stein, M.D. "Anxiety Disorders: How to Recognize and Treat the Medical Symptoms of Emotional Illness." *Geriatrics* 56, no. 5 (2001): 24–34.

Lange, Paul H., M.D., and Christine Adamec. *Prostate Cancer for Dummies.* New York: Wiley, 2003.

Lau, Denys T., et al. "Hospitalization and Death Associated with Potentially Inappropriate Prescriptions Among Elderly Nursing Home Residents." *Archives of Internal Medicine* 165 (January 10, 2005): 68–74.

Leipzig, Rosanne M., M.D. "Prescribing Keys to Maximizing Benefit While Avoiding Adverse Drug Effects." *Geriatrics* 56, no. 2 (2001): 30–34.

Matkin Dolan, Chantal, et al. "Associations between Body Composition, Anthropometry, and Mortality in Women Aged 65 and Older," *American Journal of Public Health* 97, no. 5 (2007): 913–918.

Mellor, M. Joanna, and Patricia Brownell, eds. *Elder Abuse and Mistreatment: Policy, Practice, and Research.* New York: The Haworth Press, 2006.

Michaelsson, Karl, et al. "Genetic Liability to Fractures in the Elderly." *Archives of Internal Medicine* 165 (September 12, 2005): 1,825–1,830.

Miraldi, Cinzia, M.D., et al. "Diabetes Mellitus, Glycemic Control, and Incident Depressive Symptoms among 70–79-Year-Old Persons: The Health, Aging, and Body Composition Study." *Archives of Internal Medicine* 167 (June 11, 2007): 1,137–1,144.

Mora Henry, Stella, R.N., with Ann Convery. *The Elder Care Handbook: Difficult Choices, Compassionate Solutions.* New York: Collins, 2006.

Moran, S. A., C. J. Caspersen, G. D. Thomas, D. R. Brown, and The Diabetes and Aging Work Group (DAWG). *Reference Guide of Physical Activity Programs for Older Adults: A Resource for Planning Interventions.* Atlanta, Ga.: National Center for Chronic Disease Prevention and Health Promotion, Centers for Disease Control and Prevention, 2007.

Morrison, R. Sean, M.D., and Diane E. Meier, M.D. "Palliative Care." *New England Journal of Medicine* 350, no. 25 (June 17, 2004): 2,582–2,590.

Mouton, Charles P., M.D., et al. "Common Infections in Older Adults." *American Family Physician* 63 (2001): 257–268.

National Cancer Institute. *Facing Forward: Life after Cancer Treatment.* Bethesda, Md.: National Institutes of Health, September 2006.

———. *What You Need to Know About Breast Cancer.* Bethesda, Md.: National Institutes of Health, May 2005.

———. *What You Need to Know About Kidney Cancer.* Bethesda, Md.: National Institutes of Health, April 2003.

———. *What You Need to Know About Oral Cancer.* Bethesda, Md.: National Institutes of Health, June 2003.

———. *What You Need to Know About Kidney Cancer.* Bethesda, Md.: National Institutes of Health, April 2003.

———. *What You Need to Know About Liver Cancer.* Bethesda, Md.: National Institutes of Health, 2002.

———. *What You Need to Know About Stomach Cancer.* Bethesda, Md.: National Institutes of Health, August 2005.

———. *What You Need to Know About Thyroid Cancer.* Bethesda, Md.: National Institutes of Health, August 2007.

National Center for Health Statistics. *Health, United States, 2006 with Chartbook on Trends in the Health of Americans.* Hyattsville, Md.: National Institutes of Health, 2006.

———. "Hospice Discharges and Their Length of Service." *Vital and Health Statistics Series* 13, no. 154 (August 2003).

National Heart, Lung, and Blood Institute. *Aim for a Healthy Weight.* Bethesda, Md.: National Institutes of Health, August 2005.

———. *Clinical Guidelines on the Identification, Evaluation, and Treatment of Overweight and Obesity in Adults: The Evidence Report.* Bethesda, Md.: National Institutes of Health, September 1998.

———. *High Blood Cholesterol: What You Need to Know.* Washington, D.C.: National Institutes of Health, June 2005.

———. *Aim for a Healthy Weight.* Washington, D.C.: National Institutes of Health, 2005.

———. *The Practical Guide: Identification, Evaluation, and Treatment of Overweight and Obesity in Adults.* Bethesda, Md.: National Institutes of Health, October 2000.

National Institute of Arthritis and Musculoskeletal and Skin Diseases. *Joint Replacement Surgery and You: Information for Multicultural Communities.* Washington, D.C.: National Institutes of Health, 2005.

National Institute of Mental Health. *When Unwanted Thoughts Take Over: Obsessive-Compulsive Disorder.* National Institutes of Health: Bethesda, Maryland, 2006.

National Institute on Aging. *Caregiver Guide: Tips for Caregivers of People with Alzheimer's Disease.* Hyattsville, Md.: National Institutes of Health. n.d. Available online. URL: http://www.nia.nih.gov/Alzheimers/Publications/caregiverguide.htm. Downloaded July 10, 2007.

———. *Exercise: A Guide from the National Institute on Aging.* Washington, D.C.: U.S. Department of Health and Human Services, September 2006.

———. *So Far Away: Twenty Questions for Long-Distance Caregivers.* National Institutes of Health. Available online. URL: http://www.nia.nih.gov/HealthInformation/Publications/LongDistanceCaregiving/. Downloaded October 14, 2007.

National Institute on Alcohol Abuse and Alcoholism. *Harmful Interactions: Mixing Alcohol with Medicines.* NIH Publication No. 03-5329. Washington, D.C.: National Institutes of Health, 2007.

National Women's Health Resource Center. "Older Women & Substance Abuse." *National Women's Health Report* 28, no. 6 (December 2006): 6.

Office of Community Planning and Development. *The Annual Homeless Assessment Report to Congress.* Washington, D.C.: U.S. Department of Housing and Urban Development, February 2007.

Office of Dietary Supplements. "Vitamin B_{12}," Dietary Supplement Fact Sheet, 2006. Available online. URL: http://ods.od.nih.gov/factsheets/VitaminB12_pf.asp. Downloaded August 22, 2007.

Office of the Surgeon General. *Bone Health and Osteoporosis: A Report of the Surgeon General. Executive Summary* Rockville, Md.: U.S. Department of Health and Human Services, 2004.

Older American Substance Abuse and Mental Health Services Administration. "Adults Aged 65 or Older in Substance Abuse Treatment: 2005." *The DASIS Report,* May 31, 2007. Available online. URL: http://www.drugabusestatistics.Samhsa.gov/2k/7/iolderTX/older/TXpdf. Downloaded July 6, 2007.

———. *Depression and Anxiety Prevention for Older Adults.* Washington, D.C.: U.S. Department of Health and Human Services, n.d.

———. *Suicide Prevention for Older Adults.* Washington, D.C.: U.S. Department of Health and Human Services, n.d.

Palmore, Erdman. "The Ageism Survey: First Findings." *The Gerontologist* 41, no. 5 (2001): 572–575.

Petit, William A., Jr., and Christine Adamec. *The Encyclopedia of Diabetes.* New York: Facts On File, 2002.

Pietrzak, Robert H., et al. "Gambling Level and Psychiatric and Medical Disorders in Older Adults: Results from the National Epidemiologic Survey on Alcohol and Related Conditions." *American Journal of Geriatric Psychiatry* 15, no. 4 (2007): 301–313.

Pompei, Peter. "Diabetes Mellitus in Later Life." *Generations* 30, no. 3 (Fall 2006): 39–44.

Rabow, Michael W., M.D., et al. "The Comprehensive Care Team: A Controlled Trial of Outpatient Palliative Medicine Consultation." *Archives of Internal Medicine* 164 (January 12, 2004): 83–91.

Rhoades, J. A. *Overweight and Obese Elderly and Near Elderly in the United States, 2002: Estimates for the Noninstitutionalized Population Age 55 and Older.* Rockville, Md.: Agency for Healthcare Research and Quality. Available online. URL: http://www.meps.ahrq.gov/papers/st68/stat68.pdf. Downloaded October 25, 2007.

Ries, L., et al. *SEER Cancer Statistics Review 1975–2004.* Bethesda, Md.: National Cancer Institute. Available online. URL: http://seer.cancer.gov/csr/1975_2004/. Downloaded July 29, 2007.

Rochon, Paula A., et al. "Variation in Nursing Home Antipsychotic Prescribing Rates." *Archives of Internal Medicine* 167 (April 9, 2007): 676–683.

Rott, Keith T., M.D., and Carlos A. Agudelo, M.D. "Gout." *Journal of the American Medical Association* 289, no. 21 (June 4, 2003): 2,857–2,860.

Schneitman-McInture, O., et al. "Medication Misadventures Resulting in Emergency Department Visits at an HMO Medical Center." *American Journal of Health-System Pharmacy* 53, no. 12 (1996): 1,416–1,422.

Schoenborn, Charlotte A., Jackline L. Vickerie, and Eva Powell-Griner. "Health Characteristics of Adults 55 Years of Age and Over: United States, 2000–2003." *Advance Data from Vital and Health Statistics,* Number 370. Hyattsville, Md.: National Center for Health Statistics, 2006.

Schwab, Reiko. "Acts of Remembrance, Cherished Possessions, and Living Memorials." *Generations* 27, no. 11 (Summer 2004): 26–30.

Scott, D. L., M.D., and G. H. Kingsley. "Tumor Necrosis Inhibitors for Rheumatoid Arthritis." *New England Journal of Medicine* 355, no. 7 (August 17, 2006): 704–712.

Singer, Peter A., M.D., et al. "Reconceptualizing Advance Care Planning from the Patient's Perspective." *Archives of Internal Medicine* 158 (April 27, 1998): 879–884.

Soldo, B. J., et al. *Cross-Cohort Differences in Health on the Verge of Retirement.* Cambridge, Mass.: National Bureau of Economic Research, 2007.

Soumerai, Stephen B., et al. "Cost-Related Medication Nonadherence among Elderly and Disabled Beneficiaries: A National Survey 1 Year Before the Medicare Drug Benefit." *Archives of Internal Medicine* 166 (September 25, 2006): 1,829–1,835.

Stahl, Stephen M. *Essential Psychopharmacology: The Prescriber's Guide.* New York: Cambridge University Press, 2005.

Stone, Lorraine M., and Kenneth W. Lyles. "Osteoporosis in Later Life." *Generations* 30, no. 3 (Fall 2006): 65–70.

Straus, Peter J., and Nancy M. Lederman. *The Complete Retirement Survival Guide.* 2nd ed. New York: Checkmark Books, 2003.

Substance Abuse and Mental Health Services Administration. "Adults Aged 65 or Older in Substance Abuse Treatment: 2005." May 31, 2007. Available online. URL: http//oas.samhsa.gov/2k7/olderTX/olderTX.htm. Downloaded October 12, 2007.

———. "Older Adults in Substance Abuse Treatment: 2005." *The DASIS Report.* November 8, 2007. Available online. URL: http://oas.samhsa.gov/2k7/older/older. cfm. Downloaded November 9, 2007.

———. *Results from the 2006 National Survey on Drug Use and Health: National Findings.* Rockville, Md.: Office of Applied Studies.

Supiano, Mark A. "Hypertension in Later Life." *Generations* 30, no. 3 (Fall 2006): 11–16.

Teaster, Pamela B., et al. *The 2004 Survey of State Adult Protective Services: Abuse of Vulnerable Adults 18 Years of Age and Older.* Washington, D.C.: National Center on Elder Abuse, March 2007.

Thomas, Sabu, and Michael W. Rich. "Heart Failure in Older People." *Generations* 30, no. 4 (Fall 2006): 25–32.

Tjepkema, Michael. *Measured Obesity: Adult Obesity in Canada: Measured Height and Weight.* Ottawa, Canada: Analytical Studies and Reports.

Tomita, Mackiko R., William C. Mann, Linda F. Fraas, and Kathleen M. Stanton. "Predictors of the Use of Assistive Devices That Address Physical Impairments Among Community-Based Frail Elders." *Journal of Applied Gerontology* 23, no. 2 (June 2004): 141–155.

Vaccarino, Viola, Lisa F. Berkamn, and Harlan M. Krumholz. "Long-term Outcome of Myocardial Infarction in Women and Men: A Population Perspective." *American Journal of Epidemiology* 152, no. 10 (2000): 965–973.

Valiyava, Elmira, et al. "Lifestyle-Related Risk Factors and Risk of Future Nursing Home Admission." *Archives of Internal Medicine* 166 (May 8, 2006): 985–990.

Vennig, Geoff. "Recent Developments in Vitamin D Deficiency and Muscle Weakness among Elderly People." *British Medical Journal* 3, no. 30 (2005): 524–526.

Villarel, Dennis T., M.D., et al. "Effect of Weight Loss and Exercise on Frailty in Obese Older Adults." *Archives of Internal Medicine* 166 (April 24, 2006): 860–866.

Von Gunten, Charles F., M.D. "Secondary and Tertiary Palliative Care in U.S. Hospitals." *Journal of the American Medical Association* 287, no. 7 (February 20, 2002): 875–881.

Walker, R. A. and M. C. Wadman. "Headache in the Elderly." *Clinics in Geriatric Medicine* 23, no. 2 (May 2007): 291–305.

Weight-Control Information Network. *Healthy Eating & Physical Activity across Your Lifespan: Young at Heart.* Bethesda, Md.: National Institute of Diabetes and Digestive and Kidney Diseases, January 2007.

Weiss, Guenter, M.D., and Lawrence T. Goodnough, M.D. "Anemia of Chronic Disease." *New England Journal of Medicine* 352, no. 10 (March 10, 2005): 1,011–1,023.

Wijk, Helle, and Agneta Grimby. "Needs of Elderly Patients in Palliative Care." *American Journal of Hospice & Palliative Medicine* 25, no. 2 (2008): 106–111.

Wolkove, Norman, Osama Elkholy, Marc Baltzan, and Mark Palayew. "Sleep and Aging: 2. Management of Sleep Disorders in Older People." *Canadian Medical Association Journal* 176, no. 9 (April 24, 2007): 1,449–1,454.

Zacker, Ronald J. "Health-Related Implications and Management of Sarcopenia." *Journal of the American Association of Physician Assistants* 19, no. 10 (October 2006): 24–29.

INDEX